Mycotoxins
and Other Fungal Related
Food Problems

Mycotoxins and Other Fungal Related Food Problems

Joseph V. Rodricks, EDITOR

Food and Drug Administration

A symposium sponsored by the
Division of Agricultural and
Food Chemistry at the 168th
Meeting of the American Chemical
Society, Atlantic City, N.J.,
Sept. 11–13, 1974.

ADVANCES IN CHEMISTRY SERIES 149

AMERICAN CHEMICAL SOCIETY

WASHINGTON, D. C.   1976

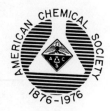

QD
1
.A355
no. 149

Library of Congress CIP Data

Mycotoxins and other fungal related food problems.
(Advances in chemistry series; 149. ISSN 0065-2393)

Includes bibliographical references and index.

1. Mycotoxins—Congresses. 2. Food-Microbiology—
Congresses.
I. Rodricks, Joseph V., 1938-   . II. American Chemi-
cal Society. Division of Agricultural and Food Chemistry.
III. Series: Advances in chemistry series; 149.

QD1.A355   no. 149   (QP632.M9)   540'8s
(615.9'52'92)   76-4547
ISBN 0-8412-0222-2   ADCSAJ 149 1-409   (1976)

Advances in Chemistry Series

Robert F. Gould, *Editor*

FOREWORD

ADVANCES IN CHEMISTRY SERIES was founded in 1949 by the American Chemical Society as an outlet for symposia and collections of data in special areas of topical interest that could not be accommodated in the Society's journals. It provides a medium for symposia that would otherwise be fragmented, their papers distributed among several journals or not published at all. Papers are refereed critically according to ACS editorial standards and receive the careful attention and processing characteristic of ACS publications. Papers published in ADVANCES IN CHEMISTRY SERIES are original contributions not published elsewhere in whole or major part and include reports of research as well as reviews since symposia may embrace both types of presentation.

CONTENTS

PREFACE

After the discovery of the aflatoxins in the early 1960s, research on fungal toxins and their roles in human and animal diseases intensified greatly and also became more systematized. Before the discovery of the aflatoxins, a number of fungal toxins had been shown to be etiologic agents in some important, though relatively sporadic, outbreaks of food-borne diseases of humans and animals. Most of these diseases are more appropriately designated as acute poisonings. But the discovery of the aflatoxins added an important new dimension to the problem of fungal toxins as food and feed contaminants, since these compounds have been shown to be probable causative agents in an important disease in humans (liver cancer) which can be induced by long-term and relatively low-level ingestion of the toxins. The concern has been compounded by further discoveries that levels of aflatoxins of probable health significance to humans have been found in a number of important foods and that many of these foods are stocks which, outwardly at least, are of high enough quality to be consumed directly by humans.

Some have described the mycotoxin research phase which began in the 1960s as "quantitative" in that the major objectives became not only the identification of which mold or mycotoxin was a contaminant of what food or feed (in the earlier phase this "qualitative" aspect of the research usually followed the outbreak of an episode of acute poisoning, usually in farm animals, sometimes in humans), but also a determination of how much of the mycotoxin was present and what dietary level would represent an animal or human health risk—acute or chronic. Thus, development and validation of analytical methods and confirmatory tests, and the deployment of such methods and tests on a massive scale became a major goal, and a number of scientific societies, federal agencies and research institutions took up the task of monitoring the development of methods and their use in data collection. Quantitative toxicity studies in experimental animals also began to appear with greater frequency. The natural products chemist began to tap the field as a source of fascinating new structural work.

Concurrently, for both practical and more purely academic reasons, other types of research on mycotoxins were activated by the continuing need to deal with aflatoxin contamination of food. Much of this research has expanded to other mycotoxins, particularly those of the genera *Asper-*

gillus, Penicillium, and *Fusarium.* Research activities on mycotoxins are of necessity interdisciplinary in nature. While no single research project can be all-encompassing, there is an overall need to coordinate the work of agricultural experts, plant pathologists, plant geneticists, mycologists, organic chemists, analytical chemists, biochemists, toxicologists, medical experts, epidemiologists, nutritionists, veterinarians, food processing experts, and statisticians (these last to ensure the development of adequate plans for sampling agriculural commodities for mycotoxin contamination and also to assess the results of toxicity tests). In addition to these research activities, there must be action on the part of policy makers to ensure that, wherever potential health problems are shown to exist, actions will be taken to minimize the risks. These policy makers have to address a number of issues which transcend the scientific questions. For instance, control of the mycotoxin problem probably depends to a great extent on the resources available to a nation for the proper harvesting, drying, transportation, and storage of agricultural commodities. Legal questions must be considered. The decision to destroy food which contains a material known to produce chronic disease in man—when the alternative is famine or starvation—is another question which transcends scientific discourse but which also must be deliberated.

It is within the context of these general considerations that the present symposium was organized by the Division of Agricultural and Food Chemistry of the American Chemical Society. It was not the goal of the symposium to deal with the myoctoxin problem in a broad way, but rather to focus closely on the chemical aspects of the subject. And while, in the main, the contributors held to this concept, most could not avoid touching upon some of the other scientific disciplines attached to mycotoxin research. It is the nature of the subject. Moreover, even with the emphasis on chemistry, there is a wide range of approaches, reflecting the interests of the authors themselves: some deal heavily with biosynthesis, others with structural characteristics of mycotoxins; some focus on analytical methods, and still others attempt to balance all chemical aspects of the problem. Because of this, the book provides, I hope, a good picture of the range of chemical research activities which support the current multidisciplinary attack on the mycotoxin problem.

The organization of the book is straightforward. It begins with C. W. Hesseltine's discussion of how mycotoxins enter the food chain, and proceeds to Leonard Stoloff's review of what is now known about their occurrence in food. There is then a series of papers dealing with specific mycotoxins or groups of mycotoxins. Aflatoxin chemistry is dealt with only tangentially: this subject has been adequately covered in many symposia, reviews, and books. However, R. C. Shank does provide an excellent summary of what is now known about the role of this "king" of mycotoxins in human disease.

Finally, there are papers dealing with compounds which are not classified as mycotoxins but which can be present in food as a result of mold invasion. First there are the compounds which are primarily known for their toxic effects in plants; these are the fungal-produced phytopathogenic toxins discussed by H. H. Luke and R. H. Biggs. Specific fungal genera which are known to produce phytopathogenic compounds are the subjects of the succeeding two papers. As a subject for speculation: can these compounds enter the food chain and are any of them toxic to animals? J. Kuć provides a fascinating look at a subject which will surely emerge as a major area of scientific work in the future: the alteration of the biochemical characteristics of plants as a result of mold invasion or other forms of physiological stress. The book ends with discussions of two specific examples of the phenomenon reviewed by J. Kuć.

Systematic research on mycotoxins and other mold related food problems is still in its infancy. This is not to denigrate the work of the many dedicated investigators, particularly veterinarians and agriculturalists, who have recognized and been at work on these problems for many years. Rather, it emphasizes that only within the past ten years has this problem begun to attract the attention it deserves from the total scientific community interested in the problems of food safety and, more generally, of human and animal health. It is hoped that this book makes a contribution to this growing science.

Food and Drug Administration
Washington, D.C.
December 1974

JOSEPH V. RODRICKS

Conditions Leading to Mycotoxin Contamination of Foods and Feeds

CLIFFORD W. HESSELTINE

Northern Regional Research Laboratory, Agricultural Research Service, U.S. Department of Agriculture, Peoria, Ill. 61604

Toxigenic mold invasion is affected during plant growth, at harvest, and after harvest. Invasion by fungi is affected by the amount of spore inoculum in the field, stresses on the plant, invertebrate infections, damage by other fungi, plant resistance, mechanical damage, mineral nutrition of the plant, and temperature. During harvest, grain is exposed to mechanical damage and mold inoculum. After harvest, mold growth depends on moisture level of the grain, temperature and humidity, rapidity of drying, aeration, the microbiological ecosystem, insects, mixing of grain, chaff and dirt, chemical treatment, internal infection, accidental rewetting of the grain by condensation or leakage, and the development of hot spots.

The key to preventing toxigenic fungi from developing in foods and feeds is to understand how they enter and develop in plant material. The alternative to preventing them from developing is to destroy or to remove the mycotoxin from the food or feed. However this approach is fraught with a number of problems: (a) any chemical or physical treatment that removes mycotoxins adds to the cost of a product already damaged from mold growth; besides the initial processing cost, additional material may be lost from separating the mycotoxin-infected parts mechanically or chemically (solvent extraction). For example, scabby wheat is cleaned by removing the chaffy kernels. (b) Most processes that remove mycotoxins are not 100% efficient. (c) When chemical processes are used, extensive testing is required to establish that a second biologically active compound with a different mode of action has not been formed. (d) Processes that remove mycotoxins may reduce the food value of the final product.

I prefer the first, and perhaps less popular, approach of preventing mold from developing in crops. However, this approach requires a thorough understanding of the conditions under which each of the mycotoxin molds grows—*i.e.*, information from one species of fungi cannot be transferred to another species. *Penicillium duponti* has an optimum growth at 45°C and does not grow at room temperature, the optimum growth temperature for *P. citrinum*. Our basic information about fungal growth is surprisingly meager and incomplete. For example, early in our work on aflatoxin in cereals, we searched the literature for the kind of sugars that *Aspergillus flavus* utilized: we found only a short and incomplete statement on the subject (*1*).

In this brief review of conditions leading to mycotoxin formation in foods and feeds, I usually use only one reference for each factor to conserve space; however, I enumerate all factors affecting mycotoxin formation without describing the optimum conditions for maximum production of mycotoxins by any particular mold species; I follow the outline of Jarvis (*2*) who divided the environmental conditions into chemical, physical, and biological.

Table I. Fungi Which Produce Mycotoxins Classified by Habitat

Fungi Growing in the Living Plant

Claviceps purpurea	*Aspergillus flavus*
Sclerotinia sclerotiorum	*Rhizoctonia leguminicola*
Fusarium graminearum	*Helminthosporium*
(*Gibberella zeae*)	*biseptatum*

Fungi Growing in Decaying Plant Material

Pithomyces chartarum	*Fusarium graminearum*
Stachybotrys atra	*Chaetomium globosum*
Periconia minutissima	*Dendrodochium toxicum*
Fusarium sporotrichoides	*Myrothecium verrucaria*
Cladosporium sp.	*Trichothecium roseum*
Alternaria longipes	*Trichoderma viride*

Fungi Growing on Stored Plant Material

Aspergillus flavus	*Penicillium islandicum*	*Chaetomium*
A. parasiticus	*P. citrinum*	*globosum*
A. versicolor	*P. rubrum*	*Fusarium*
A. ochraceus	*P. citreoviride*	*graminearum*
A. clavatus	*P. cyclopium*	*F. tricinctum*
A. fumigatus	*P. viridicatum*	*F. nivale*
A. rubrum	*P. urticae*	*F. moniliforme*
A. chevalieri	*P. verruculosum*	
	P. puberulum	
	P. expansum	
	P. rugulosum	
	P. palitans	
	P. roqueforti	

Another approach is to study the different conditions which influence mold growth in the field and during the harvest and storage. For example, factors affecting mold invasion of the developing corn kernel include the amount of spore inocula, stress factors on the growing plant, insect and mite populations, damage from other fungi, varietal susceptibility or resistance, mechanical damage from farming, storm damage, bird damage, mineral nutrition of the plant, and temperature. During harvest, the grain is exposed to mechanical injury and extensive spore inoculation. After harvest, mold growth and mycotoxin production can be affected by the moisture level, temperature, aeration, microbiological ecosystem, storage insects, blending of corn, amount of chaff and dirt, chemical treatment, amount of internal infection, rewetting from condensation and leakage, amount of damage, chemical composition of the substrate, and heating. Mycotoxin production is also a variable factor. Numerous fungi produce mycotoxins in the living plant, on decaying plant material, and in stored material (Table I). Table II contains the physical, chemical, and biological factors that influence mold growth and mycotoxin formation.

Table II.   Factors Affecting Mycotoxin Formation

	In Field	*At Harvest*	*In Storage*
Physical			
Moisture	+	+	+
rapidity of drying	−	+	+
rewetting	−	+	+
relative humidity	+	+	+
Temperature	+	+	+
Mechanical damage	+	+	+
Blending of grain	−	+	+
Hot spots	−	−	+
Time	+	+	+
Chemical			
CO_2	−	−	+
O_2	−	−	+
Nature of substrate	+	−	+
Mineral nutrition	+	−	+
Chemical treatment	−	−	+
Biological			
Plant stress	+	−	+
Invertebrate vectors	+	−	+
Fungus infection	+	−	+
Plant varietal differences	+	−	+
Fungal strain differences	+	−	+
Spore load	+	+	+
Microbiological ecosystem	+	−	+

Physical Factors

Moisture. If other factors are equal, the saprophytic fungi that grow in the field require a higher moisture level than those found in storage. Jarvis (2) states that decay fungi require a higher moisture content in the substrate (22–25% wet weight) than storage fungi, which can grow on stored substrates (13–18%). Two aspects of the effect of moisture on fungi must be considered: the moisture required for spore germination, and moisture required for growth. There is some suggestion that an optimal moisture level exists for aflatoxin formation in solid substrates. Sussman (3) cites a number of references to fungi, such as *Fusarium* and *Myrothecium,* whose spores will not germinate without an exogenous source of energy even though moisture levels are adequate and spores contain an energy source. On the other hand, spores of some fungi, such as the rust fungi and *Helminthosporium,* germinate in distilled water. Ayerst (4) studied the effect of moisture on the growth of a number of fungi. His data on the mycotoxin-producing fungi are shown in Table III.

Table III.   Approximate Temperature and Moisture Limits and Optima for Growth of Several Mycotoxin-Producing Fungi[a]

Species	Optima		Limits	
	°C	aw[b]	°C	aw
Aspergillus chevalieri	33	0.93	10–42	0.71
Aspergillus flavus	33	0.98	12–43	0.78
Aspergillus fumigatus	40	0.97	12–53	0.82
Penicillium cyclopium	23	0.98	<5–32	0.82
Penicillium martensii	23	0.98	<5–32	0.79
Penicillium islandicum	31	0.97	10–38	0.83
Stachybotrys atra	23	0.98	7–37	0.94

[a] Data from Ref. 4.
[b] aw = Ratio of the vapor pressure of the water in the substrate to that of pure water at the same temperature and pressure.

When several isolates of the same species were examined, they behaved similarly in their physical limits and optima of growth. When growth was most rapid, spore germination was most rapid. The range of minimal moisture levels required by different fungi varies greatly. At the lower levels are species of Aspergilli which grow slowly at 13–14% moisture levels. Ashworth *et al.* (5) studied the moisture required for growth and aflatoxin production in peanuts as compared with the growth of the *Aspergillus glaucus* group and *A. niger* (Figure 1). Under moisture effects, the following three aspects are noted.

RAPIDITY OF DRYING. If other conditions affecting mold growth are equal, the time required to dry a commodity is a critical aspect in preventing mycotoxin formation. Since mycotoxins are secondary metabo-

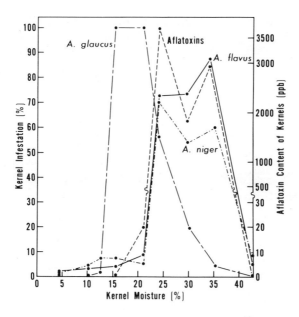

Figure 1.   Influence of kernel moisture on development of Aspergillus flavus, A. glaucus *group,* A. niger, *and aflatoxin. Data from Ref. 5.*

lites, typically they are not formed until the mold has grown through the log phase. For example, aflatoxin is not formed until at least 48 hr after spore germination (6a). This delay means that corn, with a moisture level optimal for the growth of A. *flavus,* will not be dangerous even when heavily inoculated if the corn can be dried to below 13% within 48 hr. This time element can be considered in developing better digging and drying for peanuts at harvest. In digging peanuts, drying below the level for growth of A. *flavus* can be rapidly accomplished if the fruits can be placed at the top of the rows of dug plants in the sun.

REWETTING. Often mycotoxins develop when dried and stored products are remoistened by leaks in the bins, floods, or condensation. Sometimes plant material is placed in waterproof plastic bags which are sealed at a high temperature and high humidity and stored. Later if the bags are exposed to low temperatures, moisture forms next to the plastic, and caking from fungal growth results. Dew forming on plant material in the field will allow spore germination and consequent mold invasion of the substrate.

RELATIVE HUMIDITY. This aspect will be discussed below under the heading of carbon dioxide (Table V). Hesseltine (6b) and Semeniuk (7) have reviewed moisture as an environmental factor.

Temperature. Temperature effects on the growth of microorganisms have broad literature coverage; thus this discussion focuses on the production of mycotoxins and types of mycotoxins produced. Sorenson *et al.* (8) studied the effect of temperature on aflatoxin formation in rice and showed that aflatoxin could be produced at about 11°C to slightly above 36°C (Figure 2). Under these conditions aflatoxin G_1 formation does

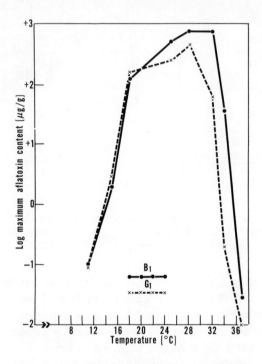

Figure 2.   Effect of incubation temperature on formation of aflatoxins B_1 and G_1 (8)

not exactly parallel aflatoxin B_1 formation. This fungus will grow at 6°–8° to 44°–45°C; however at temperatures above 37°C, no aflatoxin is formed. Note that under actual field conditions, daily temperature and moisture levels may vary considerably. They may only inhibit fungal growth and not kill the fungi. Our experience has been that infected corn can be dried and held for several months without any reduction in the viability of typical storage molds. Once this corn is remoistened, growth rapidly resumes.

Literature (9) on zearalenone suggests that *Gibberella zeae* infestation in the field on ears of corn may not produce toxin. However in the following spring, when the temperature is above freezing and when moisture increases, the fungus may produce large quantities of mycotoxin on corn in the bin or in the field. Sherwood and Peberdy (*10*) found that incubation at 12°C after a period of growth at 25°C increased zearalenone production in barley, oats, and wheat. They suggest this enhanced yield at 12°C may be associated with a reduction in growth and subsequent switching of carbon metabolism to other biosynthetic pathways. Unfortunately, their experiments were limited to the two temperatures.

Mechanical Injury. Griffin (*11*), who studied the germination of conidia of *A. flavus* on peanuts, showed that only trace germination occurred in the geocarposphere, the portion of soil influenced by the developing pod. However, if the peanut pods were injured mechanically, a high rate (63.4%) of germination occurred. Germination of conidia of *A. flavus* in pure culture nearly completely depends on an exogenous carbon source.

At the Northern Laboratory, Lillehoj *et al.* (*12*) investigated inoculated or physically damaged ears of corn in the field. Four hybrids, two normal and two *opaque-2* endosperm hybrids, were grown in four different locations. Three weeks after silking, test ears were either inoculated with *A. flavus* spores or physically damaged. Undamaged and uninoculated ears were controls. They were harvested at 15, 30, 45, and 70 days after treatment. The aflatoxin positives in the inoculated ears were different from area to area: Illinois, 22%; Missouri, 67%; Texas, 87%; and Georgia, 91%. Most of the infection and toxin formation occurred within 30 days after inoculation. Sixty of the 512 damaged, uninoculated ears contained aflatoxin; only 21 of the 512 control ears contained aflatoxin. Eighty percent of the aflatoxin-positives associated with physically damaged but uninoculated ears were observed at one location, an area known to have a high *A. flavus* spore load.

Blending (Commingling) of Grain. A common practice in grain handling is to blend grain from two or more sources to improve its condition. Corn with high moisture is mixed with dry grain to make its moisture level too low for storage mold to develop. Grain may be blended to reduce the moisture level to meet a U.S. Grade standard. Sometimes lower quality grain is blended with higher grade grain to give an intermediate grade or to maintain the higher grade. Thus U.S. Grade No. 1 corn is blended with U.S. Grade No. 3 to make Grade No. 2, a grade of corn commonly used in foods. Certainly the blending of unmolded moist corn with extremely good dry corn is desirable since the final dry product will keep well and have good quality. However, if improperly blended, the good corn will also deteriorate if the moisture level is above that required for mold growth. Storability of grains depends not only on the average moisture levels in a bin but also on the moisture concentrations in individual seeds. Commingling of grain to reach an average safe moisture level results in a heterogenous blend of seed in which some kernels contain sufficient moisture for mold growth. Also high-moisture grain such as corn infected with fungi when blended may continue to develop during moisture equilibration or drying and therefore become a source of inoculation for an entire bin.

To study the problem of blending of high-moisture corn with dry corn, the Northern Regional Research Laboratory has blended white and yellow corn with high (26–27.9%) and low (9.8%) moisture levels and different loads of spores of A. flavus (13). Their purpose was to acquire data on the spread of A. flavus infection and aflatoxin production in high and low moisture fractions of corn blends with average moisture levels believed to be safe for storage.

By using white and yellow corn, individual kernels from any blend could be separated to determine infection and aflatoxin content. Samples were removed for analysis at 2, 6, 9, 16, 30, and 58 day intervals after incubation at 25°C. Most of the equilibration of the mixture of high-moisture and dry corn occurred in the first 2 to 4 days. This study demonstrated that A. flavus will infect and subsequently form aflatoxin in dry fractions of corn blends which have a mean moisture level of 14% or less. This is especially significant because previous reports indicated that moisture levels of 16 or 17% were necessary for A. flavus to grow. It appears, however, that distinctly lower levels of moisture will support A. flavus growth at least when high-moisture corn and dry kernels are blended. Table IV shows some typical results.

Hot Spots. Hot spots are discussed separately from moisture because a small area of only a few kernels which are moist can start mold growth. As a result the molds generate more moisture from the substrate and consequently a large area becomes molded. Moisture is generated from the dry substrate and not from an external source. During the past year we found two different bins of corn in which hot spots developed spontaneously, and in both cases aflatoxin was present. We could not find detailed studies on the development of naturally occurring hot spots. The first bin involved 1500 bushels of high moisture yellow corn that had been treated experimentally with an organic acid preservative. We have data on the initial mold and bacterial counts, moisture level, chemical treatment, monthly microbiological counts, and heating which will be published by R. J. Bothast from the Northern Laboratory.

The second bin, near Peoria contained both zearalenone and aflatoxin (14). This bin, discovered in June 1973 contained 1972 yellow shelled corn harvested in January 1973. The harvest was late because of extremely wet weather which caused much Fusarium mold to develop. At harvest, the corn had been dried to below 15% and placed in a rectangular wooden bin with space between the bottom of the bin and the soil which allowed ventilation on all sides of the bin. The roof and walls were rainproof except on the east side where a window had been removed to allow the elevator to put corn into the bin. Since the window was opened during the winter, rain and snow had blown onto the center of the shelled corn. The first corn sample, taken from the center of the corn at the surface, contained 1600 ppb aflatoxin B_1 and 150 ppb B_2. The bin was 6.5×7 ft; the shelled corn was 7 in. deep at the front and 20 in. deep at the back. The aflatoxin levels found from probe sampling of the bin in August 1973 are shown in Figure 3.

Yeast extract agar in petri plates was exposed inside and around the outside of the building before any of the corn was disturbed to detect *A. flavus* spores. *A. flavus* spores were detected above the corn and at the door of the bin. None were detected outside the building.

Table IV.   Blending of High Moisture and Dry Corn Uninoculated and Inoculated with *Aspergillus flavus*[a]

		Days After Blending					
	Blend	*2*	*6*	*9*	*16*	*30*	*58*
		Uninoculated					
White d[b]	*Aspergillus flavus*[d]	0	1	1	2	0	20
	Aflatoxin[e]	0	0	0	0	0	0
Yellow hm[c]	*Aspergillus flavus*	0	2	0	0	0	6
	Aflatoxin	0	0	0	0	0	0
		Inoculated					
White d	*Aspergillus flavus*	24	66	74	70	52	58
	Aflatoxin	0	5	10	10	10	10
Yellow hm	*Aspergillus flavus*	60	94	92	80	86	78
	Aflatoxin	0	5	5	10	10	50
		Uninoculated					
White hm	*Aspergillus flavus*	0	0	0	0	0	0
	Aflatoxin	0	0	0	0	0	0
Yellow d	*Aspergillus flavus*	4	2	0	0	2	4
	Aflatoxin	0	0	0	0	0	0
		Inoculated					
White hm	*Aspergillus flavus*	58	70	68	68	64	80
	Aflatoxin	5	5	5	10	10	100
Yellow d	*Aspergillus flavus*	72	64	86	82	54	98
	Aflatoxin	5	10	100	500	500	500

[a] Data from Ref. *13*.
[b] d = Dry corn (9.8% moisture).
[c] hm = High-moisture corn (26.6–27.9% moisture).
[d] Internal infection of corn kernels expressed as percent.
[e] Aflatoxin expressed in μg/g. There was an initial infection of 1% *A. flavus* in the yellow corn but none in the white. Bushel lots of blended corn were prepared by blending (a) 14 lb high moisture white + 42 lb dry yellow (mean moisture = 14%) and (b) 13 lb high moisture yellow + 43 lb dry white (mean moisture = 14%).

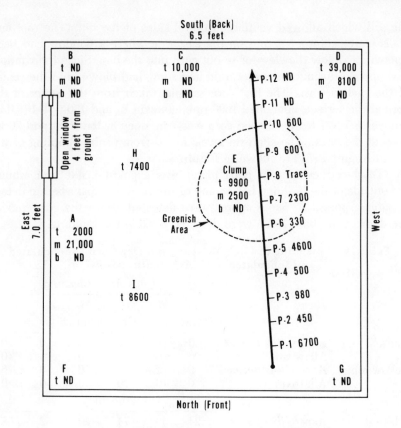

*Figure 3.   Aflatoxin levels found from probe samples of a hot spot
in a bin of corn (14)*

In addition to the individual corn samples, clumps of corn kernels
showing sporulation of *A. flavus* were carefully removed, and the adjacent
kernels were individually assayed for total aflatoxins. Aflatoxin levels
increased between July 12 and August 27. Not all of the kernels bound
together by *A. flavus* mycelium contained aflatoxin even though the surface was covered with growth. For example, in a clump of 13 kernels,
5 kernels assayed from 980 to 11,000 ppb, and 8 showed nothing. Of the
140 kernels assayed for both aflatoxin and zearalenone, 16 had aflatoxin
(260–38,000 ppb) and 12 had zearalenone (9000–1,700,000 ppb). No
kernel contained both mycotoxins. Zearalenone, unlike aflatoxin, was not
localized in the bin, but was distributed throughout the bin at 1100–
92,000 ppb.

Time. Time becomes a factor when we consider the fungus in relation to the substrate. Several aspects of time might be mentioned:
(a) Grain can be safely stored for a short time at high moisture levels.

Christensen and Kaufmann (*15*) show that grain, if carefully controlled, can be held more safely for a few weeks at higher moisture and temperature levels than grain stored for months or years at lower levels. (b) Mold grows slowly at temperatures near their minimum—*i.e.*, it takes additional time for toxin to form. (c) The age of fungal spores is important because older spores require a longer period to germinate and consequently to develop mycelium and to form toxin. (d) Over long periods of grain storage under conditions that inhibit mold growth, viable microbial inoculum will gradually decrease because of the death of spores. (e) Even in optimum conditions, some time is required for germination, growth of mycelium, penetration of the substrate, and toxin production. (f) Penetration of the kernel will take longer if it is intact rather than cracked or broken. (g) If there is extensive competition from other fungi, growth and invasion of the substrate will be reduced. (h) If the substrate is not ideal, the quantity of mycelium is reduced although the nature of the substrate will not necessarily reduce the speed of fungus invasion.

Chemical Factors

Carbon Dioxide. The effect of CO_2 on the prevention of aflatoxin formation in peanuts was studied by Sanders *et al.* (*16*) at Auburn University. Peanuts were sprayed with spores of *A. flavus* of a known aflatoxin-producing strain. When temperature was kept constant and only CO_2 and the relative humidity were varied, the levels of aflatoxin were greatly reduced at high CO_2 values and low relative humidities. At 60% CO_2, no visible growth or sporulation occurred at 86% relative humidity but both fungal phases were abundant in air at this humidity. They concluded that 20 or 40% CO_2 in combination with a reduced temperature (17°C) or reduced relative humidity or both prevented aflatoxin formation in peanuts. In Table V the effect of an atmosphere of 60% CO_2 is compared with the normal content of CO_2 in the air. Generally results were similar at 40% CO_2.

The inhibitory effect of CO_2 on molds is used in farm storage in India where cereal grains are stored below ground in a godown which is then sealed with a mixture of mud and cow manure. Undoubtedly CO_2 accumulates, and spoilage from molds and insects is prevented. In the U.S., a similar practice involves storing wet shelled corn in large concrete trenches. At harvest the wet corn is packed down with caterpillar treaded tractors and then sealed with weighted plastic covers. Corn is fed from the trench at one end so that the exposed corn is used daily. Under these conditions only yeasts and bacteria develop; mold growth is inhibited.

Table V.   Effect of Various Gas Mixtures and Relative Humidities
(Kernel Moisture) on Free Fatty Acids and Aflatoxin in Peanuts
Inoculated with *Aspergillus flavus* and Stored 14 Days at 25°C[a]

Gas Concentration, %			Relative Humidity, %	Free Fatty Acid, %	Total Aflatoxin
CO_2	O_2	N_2			
0.003	21	79	99	69.2	206.3
0.003	21	79	92	58.5	185.2
0.003	21	79	86	44.1	72.1
60	20	20	99	8.1	0.2
60	20	20	92	3.3	+
60	20	20	86	0.6	0
Untreated control				0.5	0

[a] Data from Ref. *16*.

Oxygen. All mycotoxin-producing fungi are strongly aerobic (*7*).
Below a minimum oxygen level, molds fail to sporulate, their spores fail
to germinate, and mycelium fails to develop. However, the lack of O_2
does not mean that mycelia or spores are killed. The lack of oxygen and
high CO_2 levels undoubtedly account for the success under the storage
conditions described. Control of oxygen as well as moisture is certainly
essential to producing large quantities of mycotoxins by agitated solid
state fermentation (*17*).

Nature of Substrate. Since this paper deals with the practical aspects of conditions that affect mycotoxin-producing molds, I refer to
papers dealing with cereals and oilseeds as substrates for toxin formation
(*18*). We inoculated a number of toxigenic strains of A. *flavus* and
A. *parasiticus* on autoclaved cereals and oilseeds to determine differences
in their ability to support toxin formation. The results with A. *parasiticus*
(Table VI) show that soybeans were a poor substrate under the best
toxin-producing conditions (solid state fermentation at 28°C with harvest
at six days). On the other hand, two of the three strains gave compara-

Table VI.   Production of Total Aflatoxins (μg/g) by Strains of
Aspergillus parasiticus on Agricultural Commodities[a, b]

	NRRL 3000	NRRL 2999	NRRL 3145
Peanuts	107	104	8.5
Soybeans	19	2.8	0.06
Corn	53	47	5.5
Wheat	72	19	7.1
Rice	107	185	10.6
Sorghum	72	88	57

[a] Data from Ref. *18*.
[b] Autoclaved prior to inoculation.

tively high yields of aflatoxin on rice, with peanuts a close second. A further study should be made to discover if all soybean varieties show as much resistance to aflatoxin formation. Incidentally, growth and sporulation of *A. flavus* and *A. parasiticus* were excellent on the steam sterilized soybeans, indicating that low toxin production was not caused by lack of growth.

Mineral Nutrition. It is well-established that fungi, like other living things, require a number of trace elements such as iron and zinc for growth. One would expect that these and other trace elements would be required for mycotoxin production. Whether or not these elements are in suboptimal levels in various grains is not known. However several studies have investigated the optimal levels in artificial culture media. Steele *et al.* (19) investigated the production of ochratoxin A in a synthetic medium in shake flasks. The optimal conditions for producing ochratoxin A by *A. ochraceus* NRRL 3174 were 0.055–2.2 mg/l. zinc, 0.004–0.04 mg/l. copper, and 1.2–24 mg/l. iron. Concentrations of zinc and copper above these levels reduced ochratoxin yields but did not alter the use of either sucrose or glutamate. The omission of any of these elements resulted in poor growth and no ochratoxin formation.

Prior Chemical Treatment. Treatment of grain by various chemicals, especially those used to control insects in stored products, may in some instances affect the amount of mycotoxin produced if the grain is moistened sufficiently for growth of toxigenic molds.

Vandegraft *et al.* (20) studied this problem in detail with compounds used commercially for treating grain. Wheat was treated at commercially used levels with phosphine and with carbon tetrachloride–carbon disulfide (80:20 wt %). After treatment the wheat was aerated and stored. Cracked wheat was moistened to 25%, and individual batches were inoculated with pure cultures of *A. flavus, A. parasiticus*, and ochratoxin-producing strains of *A. ochraceus* and *Penicillium viridicatum*. After six days incubation at 28°C on a gump shaker, the two mycotoxins were assayed (Table VII).

Mycotoxins often increased appreciably. For example, with carbon tetrachloride–carbon disulfide treatment, the amount of ochratoxin increased more than three times with the *P. viridicatum* strain. All *A. flavus* strains produced more aflatoxin in both treatments. However, with other fungi such as *A. parasiticus* NRRL 2999, the toxin formation decreased after phosphine treatment.

Biological Factors

Plant Stress. Previous investigations prove that plants under stress are highly susceptible to infection by some fungi. Wheat scab caused by

Table VII.   Effect of Phosphine and Carbon Tetrachloride–Carbon
Disulfide Treatment of Wheat on Aflatoxin and
Ochratoxin Production $(\mu g/g)^{a,\,b}$

	Aflatoxin B_1					Ochratoxin	
	Aspergillus flavus			Aspergillus parasiticus		Aspergillus ochraceus	Penicillium viridicatum
Wheat[c]	NRRL 3251	NRRL 3357	NRRL 3517	NRRL 2999	NRRL 3145	NRRL 3174	NRRL 3712
Control	2850	190	390	1030	150	2890	1740
Phosphine	3380	260	430	910	120	3380	1680
Control	2910	230	550	510	90	3060	510
Carbon tetrachloride–carbon disulfide	3050	490	680	680	100	3160	1820

[a] Data from Ref. 20.
[b] Geometric means of duplicate flasks.
[c] Wheat was sterilized with heat.

Gibberella zeae results when blossoming wheat plants are subjected to cool, humid weather. Pettit *et al.* (21) studied the influence of irrigation *vs.* lack of water on aflatoxin formation in peanuts before digging. Two areas were selected for study: one in north central Texas at Stephenville and one in south central Texas at Yoakum. At both locations Spanish peanuts were planted in adjacent plots, one irrigated and one nonirrigated. Peanuts were harvested at three different times. From each plot 100 kernels were surface-sterilized and both the degree of infection of *A. flavus* and the amount of aflatoxin were determined.

The data for 1967 and 1969 are summarized in Table VIII from the

Table VIII.   Infection and Aflatoxin Formation in

		Yoakum				
	Dry Land			Irrigated		
Days After Planting	120	130	140	120	130	140
			1967			
Frequency of infection by *A. flavus*, %	10	14	36	1	4	0
Levels of aflatoxin in ppb	30	400	—	0	0	0
			1969			
Frequency of infection by *A. flavus*, %	33	37	16	48	16	0
Levels of aflatoxin in ppb	80	0	2240	0	0	0

[a] Data from Ref. 21.

tables given in this paper. Obviously in the two years shown, infection was higher in dry land plots where the plants were under drought stress than in nonstressed plants in the adjacent plots at both locations. Yield of peanuts in the dry-land plot at Yoakum was only 375 lb/acre; the irrigated plot averaged 2853 lb/acre. Sixty-six percent of the kernels in the dry land were sound *vs.* 71% in the irrigated plot. This difference indicates that the amount of damage to the peanuts in the soil could not account for the amount of infection observed. In 1968 a similar study was made, but since rainfall was adequate, the differences were not pronounced. The authors concluded that when the kernel moisture averages are above 30% or below 10%, *A. flavus* activity is restricted.

Insect Vectors. Ragunathan *et al.* (*22*) studied the association of storage fungi with the rice weevil. When eggs, grubs, pupae, and adults were surface-sterilized and plated on three media, only the eggs were free of fungi. *Aspergillus ochraceus, A. flavus,* and a number of other fungi were found in the grubs, pupae, and adults. Data on adults only are given in Table IX. In weevils from sorghum, the most common species was *A. restrictus,* but in weevils from wheat and rice, *A. flavus* predominated. The incidence of infected weevils was 25–100% in sorghum, 32–100% in wheat, and 20–94% in rice. These authors state that the saprophytic fungi, which include some mycotoxin producers, are mechanically carried in the alimentary canal of the insect along with the food. Also, the weevils collected in the field at the time of corn harvest carried *A. flavus.*

Fungus Infection. As early as 1807, Prevost recognized that the infection of one fungus makes a plant more susceptible to invasion by a second (*23*). According to Fischer and Holton, wheat plants infected with the smut, *Tilletia caries,* are very susceptible to attack by root rot

Peanuts Grown in Texas Dry Land and Irrigated Soils[a]

	Stephenville				
Dry Land			Irrigated		
120	130	140	120	130	140
		1967			
8	8	0	0	0	0
0	68	27	0	0	0
		1969			
0	1	0	0	0	0
0	Trace	0	0	Trace	0

Table IX. Internal Fungi of *Sitophilus oryzae* (Rice Weevil) Adults
Breeding in Wheat, Sorghum, and Rice[a,b]

	Wheat	Sorghum	Rice
Range in fungal infection, %	32–100	25–100	20–94
Average fungal infection, %	67	66	55
Predominant fungus	Aspergillus flavus	Aspergillus restrictus	Aspergillus flavus

[a] Data from Ref. 22.
[b] Based on 10 commercial samples.

organisms such as *Fusarium*. This observation has been made many times. For instance, in plots of wheat inoculated with *Tilletia* 40% of the plants became infected with *Fusarium* as contrasted to control plots (nonsmut-infected plants) which had only 12% infection. Presumably this condition of one fungus infection making the plant more susceptible to infection by a second mycotoxin fungus is a condition worth investigating.

Ashworth and Langley (24) studied the relationship of pod damage to kernel damage by molds in Spanish peanuts. They concluded that pod lesions caused by *Rhizoctonia solani,* a root rot pathogen, are important preharvest points of entry to peanut kernels for other fungi such as *Aspergillus niger* and the aflatoxin producing fungus *A. flavus*. Of course the converse is also true—one infection may prevent the growth of a second fungus.

Doupnik (25) reported on more than 100 samples of seed corn infected by *Helminthosporium maydis* from the 1970–1971 harvests in Georgia. In each sample 25 seeds were examined for aflatoxin. Of the blight-damaged kernels 47.2% were infected with *A. flavus,* and only 9.6% of the nonblight-damaged had *A. flavus*. This type of correlation also applies to infection by *Fusarium, Penicillium* species, and other Aspergilli. When the blighted samples were analyzed for aflatoxin, 25% contained aflatoxin, and only 5% of the nonblighted samples were contaminated. Furthermore the levels were higher (728 μg/kg aflatoxin) in the blighted samples than in the nonblighted samples (19 μg/kg).

Plant Varietal Differences. The development of plant varieties that resist infective fungi is a proved success in disease control. The introduction of wheat strains resistant to wheat rust is a classic example. This approach for controlling mycotoxins, especially aflatoxin, should be investigated in the breeding of corn and peanut varieties. Because peanuts were the first crop found to contain aflatoxin, more work on their resistance to *A. flavus* infection has been done than for other crops. Mixon and Rogers (26) studied the susceptibility of new peanut accessions to seed infection by *A. flavus*. They took 1406 varieties or lines of peanuts, moistened 50 g of seed, inoculated the peanuts in petri dishes with a spore suspension of one or two high producing aflatoxin strains, and let the peanuts stand at about 30% moisture for seven days at 25°C and 98% relative humidity. During screening, two varieties of Valencia-type peanuts, P.I. 33,7394 and P.I. 33,7409, showed resistance to infection. During the test period, no infection occurred with P.I. 33,7394 and only 10% with P.I. 33,7409. This incidence is contrasted to other varieties in which 100% infection occurred. Of the 1406 lines listed, 3.3% had 10% or less infection while 240 selections had 91–100% infection (Figure 4). Mixon and Rogers' paper shows the distribution of resistance of 1406 peanut lines to *A. flavus* infection. Unfortunately, both of these varieties are low-yielding and are commercially unsuitable. In a 1973 report on the two resistant varieties, Taber *et al.* (27) state that the hila is small and closed. If the hila are longer and more open the line is susceptible to *A. flavus* entry. When the seedcoat is removed, both susceptible and resistant lines readily support *A. flavus* growth.

Fungal Strain Differences. Within a single species various strains will produce different amounts of secondary metabolites. *Penicillium chrysogenum* strains contain a range of yields of penicillin. The same is true of mycotoxins which are also secondary metabolites. For example, *A. flavus* strains show strains, such as NRRL 1957, that produce no aflatoxin whereas other strains consistently give high titers of toxin. Strain differences in yields of aflatoxin are shown in the tables appearing in our paper on a study of the variation of *A. flavus* and related species from various parts of the world (28).

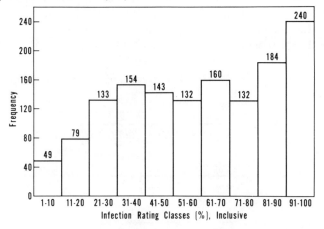

Figure 4. Frequency distribution of selections and varieties of peanuts in infection rating classes following inoculation and incubation with Aspergillus flavus *strain NRRL A-13,794. Eight lines not included had zero infection. Data from Ref. 26.*

An informative and well-documented investigation was reported by Schroeder and Boller (29) who, with their associates, collected A. *flavus* isolates from peanuts, cottonseed, rice, and sorghum. Their isolates were tested individually for their ability to produce aflatoxins under the same conditions. The summary of this study, based on 349 isolates, appears in Table X. It is obvious that a sufficient number of strains was studied

Table X.   Percent of Aflatoxin-Producing Isolates of the *Aspergillus flavus* Group Isolated from Four Field Crops (1969–1970)[a]

Source	Isolates Tested, No.	Isolates Producing Aflatoxin, %	Maximum Yield of Aflatoxin B_1, μg/Flask
Peanut	100	98	3300
Cottonseed	59	81	3200
Rice	127	20	1100
Sorghum	63	24	3300

[a] Data from Ref. 29.

from each commodity to be statistically significant and that there was a marked difference in the ability of various strains to produce aflatoxin. Since aflatoxin occurs in some corn samples, similar data should be obtained from corn and should determine if isolates from one area differ from those of other areas in their ability to form toxins.

Spore Load. Spore load refers to the amount of inoculum present to infect the substrate. If the spores are airborne, their quantity and type can be readily determined in a given amount of air. However, if the inoculum is in a substrate, such as in the corn kernel or in the soil (where it is important to know something about the inoculum) surrounding the peanut pods, the inoculum is more difficult to measure. A good discussion

Table XI.   Production of Aflatoxin and Ochratoxin

	Aspergillus flavus			
Wheat	NRRL 3251	NRRL 3353	NRRL 3357	NRRL 3517
	Aflatoxin B_1			
Sterilized	2850[c]	0.8	190	390
Unsterilized	620	1.9	100	90
	Aflatoxin G_1			
Sterilized	ND[d]	0.6	ND	ND
Unsterilized	ND	0.8	ND	ND

[a] Data from Ref. 20.
[b] Fermentation conditions: 150 g/Fernbach, 28°C, six days, Gump shaker, 200 rpm; except NRRL 3712, 20°C, 12 days.

of the non-airborne inoculum problem can be found in Ref. *30*. If many infective units of inoculum exist, more extensive infection occurs in the host or stored grain because of the additional growth sites. Other factors affecting infectivity include the longevity of the inoculum (its life span and viability) and the type of environment (supportive or inhibitive), but in nature spores usually do not find an ideal environment.

From a practical standpoint knowledge of the source of inoculum is important in preventing the development of mycotoxin-producing fungi. *A. flavus* spores may be carried by invertebrate vectors directly from the place they are produced to a new substrate. Evidence (*22*) indicates that corn in the field may be infected in this fashion. *Fusarium* species cause ear rot of corn; their conidia are airborne onto the silks of corn (*31*), and insects are attracted by the honey dew produced by the ergot fungus. The germ tubes of the fungus grow down the silks, enter the tip of the ear, and eventually infect the whole ear. As noted earlier, the blending of grain can bring infected kernels in contact with noninfected grain. Undoubtedly some infection results from viable spores that remain in bins after the removal of grain. Also, inoculum of storage fungi may develop from molds growing in pockets in conveyor pipes and elevators and may infect other grain.

Interaction of Microorganisms. Much mycotoxin research is based on pure culture studies of mold strains; sufficient information is not available on the interaction of other microorganisms, especially fungi, on the ability of molds to produce mycotoxins. Vandegraft *et al.* (*20*) investigated the effect of insecticide treatments of wheat on aflatoxin and ochratoxin formation by Aspergilli and Penicillia; some of their control experiments were conducted on nonsterile wheat containing the normal bacterial and mold flora. Cracked or lightly abraded wheat was inoculated with

on Sterilized and Nonsterilized Wheat (γ/g)^{a,b}

Aspergillus parasiticus		*Aspergillus ochraceus*	*Penicillium viridicatum*
NRRL 2999	*NRRL 3145*	*NRRL 3174*	*NRRL 3712*
Aflatoxin B$_1$		Ochratoxin A	
1030	150	2890	1740
220	30	1720	1030
Aflatoxin G$_1$		Ochratoxin B	
540	230	80	540
120	40	30	230

^{c} Geometric means of duplicate flasks.
^{d} ND = not detected.

four strains of *A. flavus:* two strains of *A. parasiticus* and one strain each
of *A. ochraceus* and *P. viridicatum* (Table XI). Generally, little toxin
was produced in flasks in which the inoculated fungi had to compete
with the normal flora, as in sterile wheat where the appropriate mold had
no competition. The only exception was the very low aflatoxin-producing
strain *A. flavus* NRRL 3353. Usually, the reduction in mycotoxin yield
was less than half of that yielded in the sterilized wheat.

Probably the best papers on the effect of microorganisms on infection
of grain and production of aflatoxin by *A. flavus* are by Boller and
Schroeder (*32, 33*). They studied the influence of two Aspergilli, *A.
chevalieri* and *A. candidus,* on production of aflatoxin in rice by *A. parasiticus.* Conidia of either *A. chevalieri* or *A. candidus* were mixed with
A. parasiticus spores on rice at 11.2% moisture. One hundred grams of
inoculated rice was placed in wire baskets that were suspended in wide-
mouthed jars containing water or a saturated aqueous solution of KCl to
maintain relative humidities of 100 and 85%. These jars were incubated
at 25°, 30°, and 35°C. At the end of the experiment, the degree of
infection was determined by surface sterilization, plating the kernels on
a malt salt agar, and determining the mold growing from each kernel.
In most instances, infection of the kernels by *A. parasiticus* was reduced,
especially at 35°C. For example at 35°C, 100% relative humidity, and
after 42 days when only *A. parasiticus* was inoculated, 95% of the kernels
were infected, but when *A. chevalieri* and *A. parasiticus* were both used
for inoculum, only 84% of the kernels of rice became infected with
A. parasiticus.

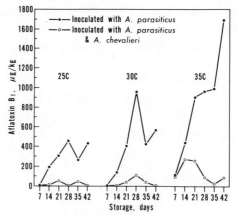

*Figure 5.   The effect of simultaneous in-
oculation with* Aspergillus parasiticus *and*
A. chevalieri *on the production and accumulation of aflatoxin B$_1$ in rice stored
at 100% relative humidity. Data from
Ref. 32.*

Another portion of each sample was assayed for aflatoxin (*see* Figure 5). Only small quantities of aflatoxin were produced at 85% relative humidity. Boller and Schroeder suggest that *A. chevalieri* may partially replace *A. flavus* in the jointly infected kernels or may metabolize aflatoxin. A second explanation is that *A. chevalieri* may compete more actively for a nutrient essential for the production of aflatoxin. When *A. candidus* was used with *A. parasiticus* to inoculate rice with the same number of conidia, *A. candidus* became the dominant mold after seven days at 23°–25°C with relative humidities of 85, 90, and 100%. Only small or negligible amounts of aflatoxin were detected.

Conclusion

The factors influencing the growth and toxin formation in fungi do not act singly but in multiples. The amount of inoculum, temperature, substrate moisture, physical condition of the substrate, and growth of other microorganisms all interact. Within hours these conditions may be greatly altered with certain factors having more influence than others. One is dealing with a dynamic ecological state.

Certainly this paper does not include all the conditions influencing mycotoxin formation. For example, pH has not been covered since most toxigenic fungi can invade and grow over a range of pH's. Also temperature factors should include fungi that grow slowly on stored foods even at freezing or below freezing temperatures. In any attempt to control the development of mycotoxins, the ways of regulating the various factors listed must be considered, and the range of limitations must be known.

Literature Cited

1. Hesseltine, C. W., Sorenson, W. G., Smith, Mabel, *Mycologia* (1970) **62**, 123.
2. Jarvis, B., *J. Appl. Bacteriol.* (1971) **34**, 199.
3. Sussman, A. S., in "The Fungi," Vol. II, Chap. 23, pp. 733–764, 1966.
4. Ayerst, G., *J. Stored Prod. Res.* (1969) **5**, 127.
5. Ashworth, L. J., Jr., Schroeder, H. W., Langley, B. C., *Science* (1965) **148**, 1228.
6a. Hayes, A. W., Davis, N. D., Diener, U. L., *Appl. Microbiol.* (1966) **14**, 1019.
6b. Hesseltine, C. W., *Mycopathol. Mycol. Appl.* (1969) **39**, 371.
7. Semeniuk, G., in "Storage of Cereal Grains and Their Products," J. A. Anderson and A. W. Alcock, Eds., pp. 77–151, Amer. Ass. Cereal Chem. Monograph Series, Vol. II, 1954.
8. Sorenson, W. G., Hesseltine, C. W., Shotwell, Odette L., *Mycopathol. Mycol. Appl.* (1967) **33**, 49.
9. Christensen, C. M., Nelson, G. H., Mirocha, C. J., *Appl. Microbiol.* (1965) **13**, 653.
10. Sherwood, R. F., Peberdy, J. F., *J. Stored Prod. Res.* (1972) **8**, 71.
11. Griffin, G. J., *Phytopathology* (1972) **62**, 1387.

12. Lillehoj, E. B., Kwolek, W. F., Vandegraft, E. E., Zuber, M. S., Calvert, O. L., Widstrom, N., Littrell, R. H., Futrell, M. C., Bockholt, A. J., *Crop Sci.*, in press.
13. Lillehoj, E. B., Fennell, D. I., Hesseltine, C. W., *J. Stored Prod. Res.*, in press.
14. Shotwell, O. L., Goulden, M. L., Bothast, R. J., Hesseltine, C. W., *Cereal Chem.*, in press.
15. Christensen, C. M., Kaufmann, H. H., in "Master Manual on Molds and Mycotoxins," pp. 22a–29a, Farm Technology/Agri-Fieldman, 1972.
16. Sanders, T. H., Davis, N. D., Diener, U. L., *J. Amer. Oil Chem. Soc.* (1968) **45**, 683.
17. Hesseltine, C. W., *Biotechnol. Bioeng.* (1972) **14**, 517.
18. Hesseltine, C. W., Shotwell, O. L., Ellis, J. J., Stubblefield, R. D., *Bacteriol. Rev.* (1966) **30**, 795.
19. Steele, J. A., Davis, N. D., Diener, U. L., *Appl. Microbiol.* (1973) **25**, 847.
20. Vandegraft, E. E., Shotwell, O. L., Smith, M. L., Hesseltine, C. W., *Cereal Chem.* (1973) **50**, 264.
21. Pettit, R. E., Taber, R. A., Schroeder, H. W., Harrison, A. L., *Appl. Microbiol.* (1971) **22**, 629.
22. Ragunathan, A. N., Srinath, D., Majumder, S. K., *J. Food Sci. Technol.* (1974) **11**, 19.
23. Fischer, G. W., Holton, C. S., in "Biology and Control of the Smut Fungi," Chap. 4, pp. 111–143, Ronald Press, New York, 1957.
24. Ashworth, L. J., Jr., Langley, B. C., *Plant Dis. Rep.* (1964) **48**, 875.
25. Doupnik, B., Jr., *Phytopathology* (1972) **62**, 1367.
26. Mixon, A. C., Rogers, K. M., *Agron. J.* (1973) **65**, 560.
27. Taber, R. A., Pettit, R. E., Benedict, C. R., Dieckert, J. W., Ketring, D. L., *J. Amer. Peanut Res. Educ. Ass.* (1973) **5**, 206.
28. Hesseltine, C. W., Shotwell, O. L., Smith, M. L., Ellis, J. J., Vandegraft, E., Shannon, G., in *Proc. U.S.–Jap. Conf. Toxic Micro-Organisms, Honolulu, Hawaii, Oct. 7–10, 1968*, M. Herzberg, Ed., pp. 202–210 (1970).
29. Schroeder, H. W., Boller, R. A., "The Aflatoxin Problem in the Southwest in 1969–70," presented at the *Joint Meetg. U.S.–Jap. Toxic Micro-Organisms Panel, 6th, Tokyo, Japan,* October 1971.
30. Dimond, A. E., Horsfall, J. G., in "Ecology of Soil-Borne Plant Pathogens: Prelude to Biological Control," K. F. Baker and W. C. Snyder, Eds., pp. 404–419, University of California, Los Angeles, 1965.
31. Dickson, J. G., "Diseases of Field Crops," pp. 91, 175, McGraw-Hill, New York, 1956.
32. Boller, R. A., Schroeder, H. W., *Phytopathology* (1973) **63**, 1507.
33. *Ibid.* (1974) **64**, 121.

RECEIVED November 8, 1974.

Occurrence of Mycotoxins in Foods and Feeds

LEONARD STOLOFF

Division of Food Technology, Food and Drug Administration, Washington, D. C. 20204

The year 1960 divides the descriptive phase of mycotoxin investigations from the analytical one. The descriptive episodes are related in this review to current knowledge of specific toxins. The analytical information covers commodities susceptible to aflatoxin contamination (oil-seeds, tree nuts, grains, dried fruits, legumes) and mycotoxins other than aflatoxins (ochratoxin, zearalenone, citrinin, penicillic acid, patulin, sterigmatocystin) for which analytical methods have been devised and applied in surveys. Incidence and level data are given in each case.

The current concern about the possible occurrence of toxins in moldy foods and feeds is a far cry from the conclusion of an eminent professor of bacteriology (1) published in 1932 that "there is very little evidence that moldy food causes illness."

Mold-Related Human Incidents

In fact when this statement was published, the role of a saprophytic fungus (*Claviceps purpurea*) in the formation of the poisonous ergot grains on rye had been established; the first conjecture to this effect was made in 1711 (2). Reviews of cause and effect relationships between human consumption of moldy food and illness (3, 4) cite numerous cases during the period 1826-1888 of poisoning from the consumption of moldy bread, an 1843 incident caused by moldy army rations in Paris, an 1878 poisoning attributed to moldy pudding, and numerous deaths between 1906 and 1909 from eating moldy corn meal. Scabby grain has a long history of causing illness in those areas such as Eastern Europe, China, and Japan where some form of grain is a dietary staple (5, 6, 7). Scab refers to that type of kernel blight caused by species of *Fusarium*.

More recently, considerable effort was expended in Russia to investigate recurring endemic instances of a syndrome described as alimentary toxic aleukia (ATA) (4) traced to the consumption of foods made from cereals which had overwintered in fields under snow. The etiology of the disease was established in 1948 as being related to invasion of the grain by *Fusarium sporotrichiella* (*F. trincinctum,* Synder and Hansen). The disease was not transmissible, and a rabbit skin test for toxicity was devised and used to divert toxic grain to alcoholic fermentation (the toxin does not distill). This is the second instance of a correlation between a specific mold and a specific syndrome. From the symptoms and the molds involved, investigators in the United States (8) and in Japan (7) conjectured, based on current knowledge, that the toxins belong to the trichthecene group of mold metabolites. This conjecture has been substantiated by direct testing of an extract from a culture of one of the Russian mold isolates (9).

Reports of illness in Japan from eating moldy rice were apparently rare until imports of rice from other countries increased during and after World War II (10). A yellow discoloration of kernels was associated with some toxic lots. Toxin-producing molds isolated from lots of yellow rice were *Penicillium citreo-viride, P. islandicum, P. citrinum,* and *P. rugulosum.* Toxins produced by these molds in laboratory culture have been isolated and characterized (11) and their effects on animals described, but no description of the human symptoms from eating moldy rice is available for comparison.

Mold-Related Animal Incidents

Moldy feed has received considerably more attention than has moldy food, probably because of the greater frequency of animal exposure and the dramatic manifestations of the massive challenge that animals usually receive. The early literature has been thoroughly reviewed (3, 4, 12, 13). Special note is taken here only of those situations where a specific mold has been incriminated in a number of similar incidents. If a source is not specifically cited, reference to one of the cited reviews is implied.

Hemorrhagic sweet clover disease is atypical of other mycotoxicoses encountered in that a specific precursor, coumarin, rather than a specific mold, is required in the substrate plant to make the toxin. The disease is mentioned here because it is the first instance since the long forgotten isolation of the ergot alkaloids that a specific toxin was identified. The compound is dicoumarol. This hemorrhagic disease affected cattle in the North Central States and Canada during the 1920's when sweet clover was introduced as a forage crop.

Stachybotryotoxicosis was originally described as a usually fatal disease of horses and less frequently of sheep and goats. Typical case histories during the 1930's indicated that the problem was widespread in Eastern Europe. Russian investigators identified the causative organism as *Stachybotrys alternans* (*S. atra*, Bisby). They also demonstrated that the typical symptoms could be produced by feeding grain invaded by *F. sporotrichiella* (*see* preceding discussion of ATA). These observations are not surprising in the light of current knowledge that both organisms produce related toxic compounds of the trichothecene group (*8, 14*).

Scabby grain has been associated with both animal and human problems. Scabby grain fed to swine is often rejected, but if eaten, causes vomiting (*15, 16*). The same effect was obtained with corn intentionally molded by *Fusarium graminearum* (*F. roseum*, Snyder and Hansen, perfect form *Gibberella zeae*) while growing. These observations are reminiscent of recent experiences of farmers in the north central United States with *Gibberella*-infected corn (*17*). The pieces of information fit with what we know today. A number of trichothecenes, toxins produced by many *Fusaria*, are demonstrated emetics (*4, 18, 19, 20, 21*) at a relatively low dosage. At higher levels the symptoms are those of stachybotryotoxicosis or of ATA, referred to earlier.

A disease in swine and cattle, caused by eating moldy corn, was reported as endemic in Florida, Alabama, and Georgia. It was also related to feed-associated hepatitis of dogs (*22*). Increased research attention in the 1950's implicated *Aspergillus flavus* and *Penicilium rubrum* as the causative molds. The symptoms of the field and experimentally developed moldy corn diseases, as described in the 1950 literature, are remarkably similar to the symptoms of acute aflatoxicosis developed experimentally in swine with pure aflatoxins (*23*).

Moldy feed toxicosis, also called hemorrhagic syndrome, of poultry has been a consistent problem in the United States; it exhibits extreme variability in clinical signs, course, mortality, and gross and histopathological manifestation between birds and between flocks (*12*). Among the fungi that have been isolated from suspected feed are several now known to produce specific toxins—*viz. Aspergillus clavatus, A flavus, A. fumigatus, Penicillium citrinum, P. purpurogenum,* and *P. rubrum.* Feed on which each of these molds had been cultured produced the typical syndrome.

Facial eczema, a major photosenitization disease of ruminants (*12*), was first reported from New Zealand in 1897 and was thought peculiar to that area. A similar disease has since been reported in the southeastern United States. In 1958 the cause of the New Zealand problem was traced to the growth of *Pithomyces chartarum* on dead pasture grass and later to the elaboration by that mold of any of a series of liver toxins (sporidesmins) characterized as epipolythiodioxopiperazines (*24*). The organism associated with the problem in the United States is *Perconia minutissima*,

also saprophytic on dead herbage, but the study has not been carried
beyond that point.

Era of Mycotoxins

An incident in 1960 marks a change in the general attitude to mycotoxins and an awareness of the scope of the problem. It was not the loss
of 100,000 turkey poults (25) in this English incident, nor the severe losses
of ducklings in Kenya from a similar, less-publicized, concomitant incident (26) that led to the change. These were but the initial incidents in
a series of events that established the general toxicity of peanut meals to
poultry and livestock, the relation of the toxicity to a group of fluorescent
compounds that could be extracted from toxic meals, and the ability of a
fungus, Aspergillus flavus, isolated from a toxic meal to produce the same
compounds (26). This would still have been only a veterinary problem,
if the toxic meal had not been shown capable of producing cancer of the
liver (27, 28), stimulating a study of the isolated compounds now called
aflatoxins. This study established the extreme oncogenicity of the compounds to the rat. Coincidental studies in France (29) further established the role of F. flavus as a producer of compounds hepatocarcinogenic
to the rat. These observations appeared at the same time that the World
Health Organization (FAO/UNICEF) was considering peanut meal as a
protein supplement in foods for undernourished children (30). While
that organization was pondering the question of protein starvation vs.
cancer, a report (31) of an apparently unrelated study from Auburn
University dispelled the "it can't happen here" attitude in the U.S. The
Auburn report related U.S.-produced peanut meal in laboratory animal
feed to the occurrence of liver cancer in rats. The similarity to the English
observations (27, 28), noted in the paper describing the study, was also
observed by those in government and industry concerned with the safety
of the food supply and the production of peanuts and peanut products.
The result was a spate of activity that produced isolated compounds to
work with and simple, sensitive, analytical methodology for research,
survey, and control. It is this development that characterizes the difference
between the old and new mycotoxin investigations. The new concern was
for the possibility of cancer or organ damage from chronic ingestion of
initially subclinical amounts of mold toxins. The extent of exposure to a
toxin whose effects might be evident only years after ingestion and the
safety of the food supply could be determined only by direct analysis for
the toxic compound. We entered a new era, an era of analytical determination of the incidence and level of mycotoxins in susceptible foods and a
search for specific chemical entities produced by molds that might in some
way be linked to idiopathic disease.

Incidence, as used in this paper, refers to the number of samples with detectable mycotoxin, usually as a percent of the number of samples examined and sometimes as a ratio. The level will be expressed as an average of all samples with detectable mycotoxin and as a range of the levels found. The lower figure in the range will usually be the lower limit of detection for the method used.

Of the biologically active mold metabolites that have come to our attention, significant occurrence in food or feed has been established for aflatoxins, citrinin, ochratoxin A, patulin, penicillic acid, trichothecenes, and zearalenone. Adequately sensitive analytical methods have been developed and validated for aflatoxins (32), ochratoxin A (33), and patulin (34), and unvalidated but useful methods for citrinin (35), penicillic acid (36) and zearalenone (37) are being used. There has been some concern about sterigmatocystin because of its demonstrated carcinogenicity (38) and structural relation to aflatoxins (39). A method for sterigmatocystin has been validated (40) and used in FDA surveys of suspect foods and feeds, but no occurrence has been detected, nor was sterigmatocystin found in any of 173 samples of various foods susceptible to mold attack in a study of liver cancer epidemiology in the Inhambane region of Mozambique (41), although aflatoxin was detected in 5% of the samples. Sterigmatocystin has been identified in a badly molded sample of wheat (42) and in moldy green coffee (43).

The deduced presence of trichothecenes in grains has been noted, but its detection as a natural contaminant has been recorded for only one sample of severely molded corn (44). Adequately sensitive analytical methods have not yet been developed for trichothecenes.

Aflatoxins

Aflatoxin contamination appears to be a problem with commodities such as nuts and grains which are preserved by reduction of water activity, and is more likely to occur at high prevailing temperatures. The producing molds, *Aspergillus flavus* and *A. parasiticus,* compete best with other microflora when the water activity is marginal for preservation ($a_w = 0.84$–0.86) and when the temperature is relatively high ($25°$–$45°C$) (45). Inadequate drying at harvest and poor storage practices were originally thought to be the major reason for contamination and probably are in many instances, but evidence is accumulating that significant contamination can occur prior to harvest. In some instances there is a demonstrable insect vector; in others no cause for the mold invasion is immediately apparent.

Those commodities consumed in the United States in which some aflatoxin contamination of market place samples has been found are

Table I. Farmers' Stock Peanuts Rejected for Visible *Aspergillus flavus* by Year and by Area, as Percent of Total Crop

Area	Year					
	1968	1969	1970	1971	1972	1973
Southeast	6.3	1.4	3.4	2.6	13.5	2.6
Southwest	1.2	2.4	1.4	2.5	1.9	0.8
Virginia-Carolina	0.5	0.07	0.4	0.3	0.2	0.1
All Areas	3.7	1.4	2.1	2.1	8.1	1.6

peanuts, Brazil and pistachio nuts, almonds, walnuts, pecans, filberts, cottonseed, copra, corn, grain sorghum, rice, and figs.

Peanuts. The peanut is the most thoroughly studied of the commodities susceptible to aflatoxin contamination, for a number of unassociated reasons. It was the original problem source; it is a major food crop; and marketing in the United States is under the control of the Department of Agriculture (USDA). For this last reason and also because the responsible units of government (FDA, USDA) and industry (National Peanut Council) had agreed to a system of certification for shelled peanuts when the problem was first recognized, there is comprehensive year-to-

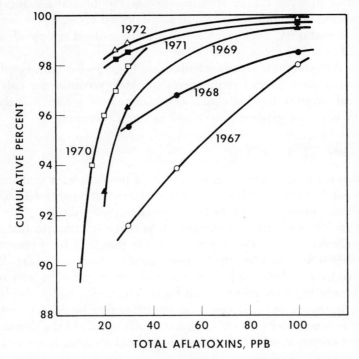

Figure 1. Cumulative percent of lots with aflatoxin levels below the given values for each crop year—1967 to 1972, southwest, all varieties

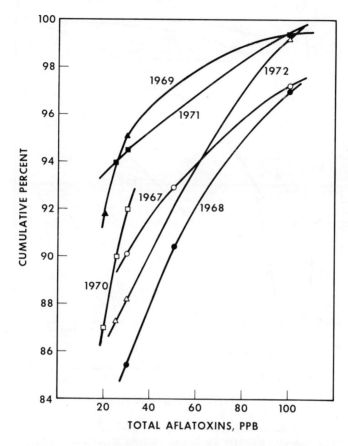

Figure 2.   Cumulative percent of lots with aflatoxin levels below the given values for each crop year—1967 to 1972, southeast, all varieties

year data for practically the entire crop as farmers' stock (Table I) or as shelled nuts (Figures 1–4). These data show considerable year-to-year and area-to-area differences in the incidence and levels encountered. The relatively small portion of the crop consumed as roasted in-shell peanuts has been free of aflatoxins because of the variety, region, and quality involved in their production. Because only shelled nuts with aflatoxins below a specified guidline are used for edible products and because the normal sorting and roasting processes substantially reduce the aflatoxin level, consumer peanut products in the United States should be relatively free of aflatoxins. Routine FDA monitoring has verified this assumption. A more comprehensive FDA survey, carried out in the spring of 1973 (46), has provided data in general agreement with that from the FDA monitoring and with independent survey data from Canada on aflatoxin

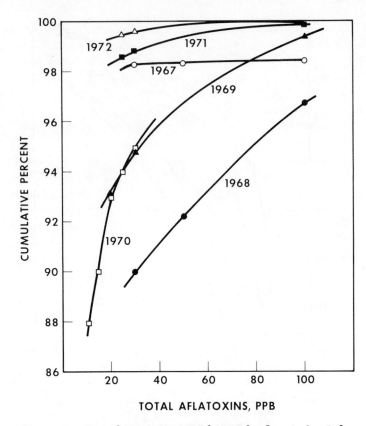

Figure 3. Cumulative percent of lots with aflatoxin levels below the given values for each crop year—1967 to 1972, Virginia and Carolinas, all varieties

in peanut butter (Table II). Some samples of finished products with levels that exceed the raw material certification guideline can be attributed to the great variance inherent in sampling and analyzing peanuts for aflatoxin contamination (47). These figures are in marked contrast to the contamination of peanuts in Thailand (48) where 49% of the market samples tested contained aflatoxin with an average B_1 level of 1530 $\mu g/kg$, or to peanut butter in the Philippines (49, 50) where 97% of the samples contained aflatoxins with an average B_1 level of 213 $\mu g/kg$, or to peanuts in Uganda where 17% of the samples tested had an average aflatoxin B_1 level of 363 $\mu g/kg$ (51).

Brazil Nuts. The presence of aflatoxins in some samples of Brazil nuts offered for entry was first observed in 1965 by the Vancouver Regional Laboratory of the Canadian Food and Drug Directorate following a general program of investigation of all nuts for aflatoxins. The U.S. FDA was alerted and, after confirming the observation, instituted a 100%

sampling of Brazil nut imports in 1967. As a result, 27% of the lots
offered for entry were detained for reconditioning or return. Subsequently
a voluntary control agreement was worked out between the importers and
the USDA with the assistance and concurrence of the FDA. When the
agreement was implemented in 1968, 32% of the lots were detained.
Through the influence of importers in educating their sources of supply,
the detention rate has declined so that in the past three years only 1%
of the lots offered for entry has been detained.

Pistachio Nuts. Pistachio nuts now imported into the United States
are produced in Turkey and Iran. Most pistachio nuts enter through the
port of New York. On the initiative of personnel of the FDA New York
District Office, an examination of pistachio nuts for aflatoxins was conducted as part of the general survey for commodities susceptible to
aflatoxin contamination. Since positive findings of violative levels of
aflatoxins were encountered, the coverage of pistachio nuts was increased
until in early 1972 more than 80% of the lots offered for entry were

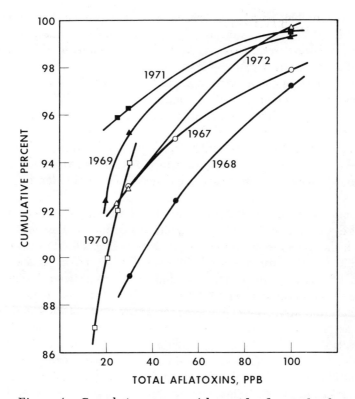

*Figure 4.   Cumulative percent of lots with aflatoxin levels
below the given values for each crop year—1967–1972, all
areas, all varieties*

Table II. Consumer Peanut Products—Cumulative Percent of Samples Examined in Various Aflatoxin Contamination Categories

	United States, Shelled Products		Canada, Peanut Butter
	Surveillance FY[a] 1973	Survey Spring 1973	Surveillance FY 1973
No. Samples Examined	98	361	428
Range, Total Aflatoxins, $\mu g/kg$	Cumulative % of Samples		
20–50	5	3	2
15–19	7	4	4
10–14	9	6	5
5– 9	12	8	11
trace – 4	16	15	25
	% of Samples		
None Detectable	84	85	75

[a] FY = fiscal year.

detained. The bottleneck was broken when the pistachio nut importers organized a voluntary certification agreement similar to the one worked out with the Brazil nut importers. At the same time a team of U.S. government aflatoxin experts visited Turkey and Iran at their request to determine how aflatoxin contamination might be prevented and to instruct key technical personnel in analytical control methods. Following the visit, detentions of pistachio nuts for aflatoxin contamination dropped to virtually zero and have remained that way for Turkish shipments; however in the first half of 1974, 13% of 246 lots shipped from Iran were detained. This reversion was attributed in part to lax control at the point of shipment and in part to an increased incidence of contamination on the tree (52).

Almonds, Walnuts, Pecans, Filberts. These nuts were examined as part of the general FDA survey of aflatoxin-susceptible commodities. Almost all the almonds, walnuts, pecans, and in-shell filberts consumed in the United States are produced domestically. A major portion of the shelled filberts consumed in the United States come from Turkey. No aflatoxin was detected in any of the domestic filberts sampled over two crop years, but approximately 8% of the 142 samples of imported filberts tested were positive for aflatoxins (total aflatoxins averaged 33 $\mu g/kg$ nut meats; range, 2–100 $\mu g/kg$). Aflatoxins have been found in market samples of domestic almonds, pecans, and walnuts (Table III) at an incidence of about 6% of the samples and an average total aflatoxin level of 23 $\mu g/kg$ nut meats. When alerted to the problem, the responsible industries investigated the cause and instituted procedures to prevent contaminated nuts from reaching the market place. The major aflatoxin con-

tamination of almonds was traced to damage by navel orange worms (53).
Sorting of the shelled almonds for specific types of damage was effective
in segregating those nuts containing aflatoxins. The major contamination
of walnuts was traced to those varieties prone to sunburn (54), and as
with almonds, sorting oriented to the specific damage effectively removed
contaminated kernels. Aflatoxin contamination of pecan kernels does not
correlate with any type of damage that can be observed; aflatoxin contamination has been found in pecan lots with no visible kernel damage. Research is in progress to determine the cause and subsequent method for
control.

Cottonseed. In the same year that turkey X disease decimated the
newly hatched birds in the English flocks, an epizootic of hepatoma
occurred in trout hatcheries in the United States. The cause was traced
to the cottonseed meal component of the trout ration and eventually to
aflatoxin in the meal (55). Even before the association was firmly established, surveys of cottonseed and cottonseed meal for incidence of aflatoxins had been started. The first surveys (56) covered three crop years
and involved samples of cottonseed and cottonseed meal collected on a
weekly basis during the crushing season from plants selected as a representative cross-section of process and production (57). The survey data
for the three-year period (Table IV) showed an 8% incidence of detectable aflatoxin (>3 μg/kg, aflatoxin B_1) in cottonseed and a 19% incidence in meal derived from that seed, with average aflatoxin B_1 levels of
143 and 99 μg/kg. There was a marked year-to-year variation in incidence and level of contamination. The higher incidence of aflatoxin in
the meal compared with the cottonseed is probably an artifact of the
difficulty in obtaining a representative sample of seed. The higher average
level in the seed compared to the meal indicates a preferential partition
of aflatoxin into the oil.

The survey results also showed a markedly higher incidence and level
of aflatoxin contamination in samples from the southern valleys of California and the lower altitude areas of Arizona compared with samples
from the remainder of the cotton belt (58). Later surveys (59, 60) confirmed the contamination problem in these areas. The surveys were aided

Table III. Almonds, Pecans, Walnuts—Incidence and Level of
Aflatoxin Contamination in Domestic Production
Sampled Fiscal Years 1970–1974

			Detectable Aflatoxins, Total	
	No.	%	μg/kg Nut Meats	
Nut	of Samples	of Samples	Average	Range
Almond	345	8	20	2– 94
Pecan	406	6.5	26	2–172
Walnut	205	3.5	27	2– 70

Table IV.   Cottonseed and Cottonseed Meal—Incidence and Level of
Aflatoxin Contamination in Three Successive Crop Years

Detectable Aflatoxin B_1

Crop Year	No. of Samples	% of Samples	Average	Highest Range ($\mu g/kg$)
		Cottonseed		
1964–5	928	6.5	220	>1500
1965–6	1319	8.2	44	151– 500
1966–7	943	8.8	228	500–1500
		Cottonseed Meal		
1964–5	964	21.1	136	500–1500
1965–6	1293	21.5	33	151– 500
1966–7	961	12.8	150	500–1500

by the observation of a field boll rot caused by *Aspergillus flavus*, its association with bright greenish-yellow (BGY) fluorescing spots on the fiber and seed (*61*), and the association of the BGY fluorescence with the presence of aflatoxins (*62, 63, 64*). The BGY fluorescence, which was later related to the action of peroxidase in the invaded tissue on kojic acid produced in copious quantity by *Aspergillus flavus* (*65*), became a valuable screening tool. The mechanical damage caused by the pink boll worm has been identified as one route of entry to the boll for *A. flavus* (*66*). Prolonged high temperature and high humidity caused by irrigation practices also contribute to *A. flavus* invasion (*67, 68*). Intensive local sampling in one of the high risk areas has shown 100% incidence of aflatoxin contamination of lots of seed going into storage with the mean total aflatoxins level of incoming seed up to 2600 $\mu g/kg$ (*69*).

Aflatoxin contamination of cottonseed is not confined to the United States although the worldwide problem appears to be less serious than in the U.S. Southwest. A Danish survey (*70*) of imported cottonseed products from eight major exporting countries (not including the United States) found aflatoxins in 1/3 of the 120 samples tested (total aflatoxins average 30 $\mu g/kg$; range, 5–120 $\mu g/kg$). The incidence by country ranged from 21 to 100% of the samples tested.

A report (*71*) of a survey in India, a country not included in the Danish survey, confirmed the correlation between aflatoxin and BGY fluorescence in cottonseed. Aflatoxin was found in 54% of 388 samples examined; 12% of the samples had aflatoxin B_1 levels greater than 500 $\mu g/kg$. There was a strong relation between the area humidity and the level and incidence of aflatoxin contamination.

Copra. Crude coconut oil has replaced copra imports to the United States since FDA surveillance activity found aflatoxin in 88% of 72 samples of copra and copra meal tested (total aflatoxins average 46 μg/ kg; range, trace–200 μg/kg). A study of Finnish copra imports (72) provided much the same picture. Aflatoxins were found in 63% of the 16 samples tested (average 37 μg/kg; range 10–100 μg/kg). No cause for the contamination has been established although inadequate drying and improper handling in transport are suspected.

Seed Oil. Peanuts, cottonseed, and copra are major sources of edible oils. A considerable portion of the aflatoxin in the seed is found in the expressed or extracted oil. Such oils, if used in the crude state, can contribute to human aflatoxin exposure (73, 74). Normal refining of edible oils effectively removes aflatoxins (73, 75).

Corn. In the pre-1960 period, moldy corn was frequently implicated in animal toxicosis; *Aspergillus flavus* was a common toxic corn isolate, and the symptoms of moldy corn toxicosis are much like those described for aflatoxicosis. Corn is the only grain normally harvested at a moisture level that can support mold growth. The requirements of mechanical harvesting have further increased that level, putting greater demands on the drying operations normally overburdened at harvest time. The possibility of aflatoxin contamination of corn was a natural conjecture particularly when a relation to epizootics of toxic hepatitis had been demonstrated (23). To determine the possibility and incidence, the Agricultural Research Service (ARS) of USDA undertook surveys of corn from crop years 1964, 1965, and 1967 (76, 77). The surveys covered 1594 samples of all grades and from all growing areas. Aflatoxin was detected in 2.5% of the samples (total aflatoxins average 9 μg/kg; range 3–37 μg/kg), most of them in the Sample Grade category. A subsequent survey (78) of 293 samples of corn destined for export during the 1968–1969 period found 2.7% of the samples with detectable aflatoxins (total aflatoxins average 18 μg/kg; range 2–31 μg/kg), a picture similar to that developed in the previous wider survey except that the contamination of the export corn involved all grades almost equally. Concentrating on corn from the southeastern states, even though that area accounts for only about 6% of total U.S. production, the next USDA survey (79) brought the problem of aflatoxin in corn into better focus. Aflatoxin was found in 35% of 60 samples of corn marketed in the 1969–1970 period (total aflatoxins average 66 μg/kg; range 6–348 μg/kg). A high incidence of contamination was found in all grade categories.

Further survey was facilitated by the observation that a BGY fluorescence, analogous to that seen in cottonseed, was associated with aflatoxin contaminated kernels (80). The USDA's Agricultural Marketing Service (AMS) used this simple observation in conjunction with a semiquantitative screening method for aflatoxin assay (81) at 15 selected stations to examine 2866 samples of 1973 crop corn submitted for grade de-

termination (82). The assay method has a sensitivity limit for total aflatoxins of about 5 μg/kg; it was used with a 15 μg/kg reference standard
to determine detectable aflatoxins greater or less than the reference
standard in all samples of corn in which some BGY fluorescence had been
observed. Aflatoxin was detected in 8.2% of the samples examined; 2.5%
of the samples had total aflatoxin levels greater than 15 μg/kg. The incidence varied from station to station; the highest was in corn received at
Mobile, Chicago, Norfolk, Omaha, Peoria, and Sacramento, in that order.
The average incidence of detectable aflatoxins from these stations was
15.6% of the 1128 samples examined; 5.6% of the samples from these six
stations had levels greater than 15 μg/kg. Because of the small sample size
(2 lb), these figures probably underestimate the real incidence.

The appearance of BGY fluorescence in corn has a high correlation
with the presence of aflatoxins (82, 83, 84), but the observation should
accompany the knowledge that the formation of the fluorescent compound
depends on a peroxidase in the viable kernel. Since current evidence indicates that aflatoxin contamination of corn is primarily a field and farm
problem (85, 86, 87, 88), most contamination can probably be picked up
by this method.

Aflatoxin in corn seems to be a worldwide problem. Limited surveys show a 40% incidence of aflatoxin in corn samples taken in Uganda
(aflatoxin B_1 average 133 μg/kg) (51), a 35% incidence in Thailand
(aflatoxin B_1 average 400 μg/kg) (48), and a 97% incidence in the Philippine island of Cebu (aflatoxin B_1 average 213 μg/kg) (49, 50). In some
areas conventional methods for using corn result in destruction or diver-
sion of the aflatoxin. Alkali processing of corn destroys much of the aflatoxin (89). Both wet milling and dry milling of corn concentrate the
aflatoxins in those fractions used for feed or oil recovery (90, 91).

Wheat, Grain, Sorghum, Oats, Rice. Other cereal grains included
in USDA–ARS surveys for aflatoxins are wheat, grain sorghum, and oats
(92, 93). Samples were obtained from USDA–AMS grader stations representing all grades and growing areas. No aflatoxins were detected in any
of the 1379 samples of wheat, 533 samples of grain sorghum, or 304 samples of oats. FDA surveillance activity found no aflatoxins in 106 samples
of wheat, but aflatoxin was detected in two of 66 samples of grain
sorghum (13 and 50 μg/kg) and in one of 157 samples of rice at 5 μg/kg.
Grain sorghum was susceptible to aflatoxin contamination in Uganda
where 23% of 69 samples examined had an average aflatoxin B_1 level of
152 μg/kg (51). Rice in the markets in Uganda, Thailand, and the
Philippines was remarkably clean (48, 49, 50, 51); aflatoxin was found
in only eight of 447 samples at an average under 10 μg/kg, but cooked rice
kept under primitive conditions proved to be a major source of human
exposure to aflatoxins (94). The small grains in general do not appear to

be an important source of aflatoxin exposure unless abused in storage or after preparation.

Legumes. Legumes in the United States appear to be relatively free of aflatoxin contamination. A USDA–ARS survey of 866 soybean samples (76) found two samples contaminated at total aflatoxins levels of 10 and 11 μg/kg. An FDA survey of 117 samples of dried beans (blackeye, black turtle, garbanzo, great northern, lima, navy, pink, pinto, and red) found no detectable aflatoxins in any sample. A study of the susceptibility of soybeans to invasion by *Aspergillus flavus* (95) indicated the presence of an *A. flavus* growth inhibitor. However in Uganda 23% of 64 bean samples assayed had an average aflatoxin B_1 level of 500 μg/kg (51), and in Thailand 3% of 322 samples had an average aflatoxin B_1 level of 106 μg/kg (48). The factors creating these differences in observation have not been determined.

Peppers. Published reports of a high incidence of *Aspergillus flavus* isolates from various types of peppers provided the impetus for a Canadian Health Protection Branch survey of black, white, and capsicum peppers (96). No aflatoxins were found in 24 samples of black or white pepper. Of the *Capsicum* based peppers, 14 of 33 samples of cayenne pepper and all six Indian chili powder samples contained aflatoxins at levels from *ca.* 2 to 8 μg/kg. Another 30 samples of *Capsicum* pepper (paprika, chili powder, Singapore chili powder) had no detectable aflatoxins.

Dried Fruits, Wine. Some fruits such as dates, figs, and raisins are preserved by drying, and unpublished mold profiles of the dried commodities listed *Aspergillus flavus* among the commonly encountered species. A limited FDA survey found no aflatoxins in 108 samples of raisins and 62 samples of dates, but aflatoxins were found in six of 165 samples of figs (total aflatoxins average 13 μg/kg; range, 2–29 μg/kg). The consideration of *Aspergillus flavus* as an invader of grapes also led to the examination of wines. In one study of 33 German wines from the South Baden vineyard country (97), aflatoxin was found in two samples at levels less than 1 μg/l. In another study (98) of 17 German Rhine country wines from the years when grape rot was a problem, no aflatoxins were detected; nor were aflatoxins detected in 13 samples of various wines imported into the United States (99) using a method sensitive to 0.3 μg/l.

Dairy Products. Aflatoxin M_1, a mammalian hydroxylation product of aflatoxin B_1, is found in the milk of lactating animals exposed to aflatoxin B_1 in their feed. An FDA survey (100) of milk products (cottage cheese dry curd, nonfat dry mnlk, evaporated milk) produced in the United States in the first three months of 1973 found M_1 in samples taken from areas where aflatoxin contamination of feed ingredients had been suspected. In one milk shed area, aflatoxin M_1 was detected in all of 16 samples taken. A lesser incidence was found in two other areas. Aflatoxin M_1 was found in 8% of the 320 samples assayed from 0.05 to 0.5 $\mu g/l$ (all calculations were based on the original milk for easy intercomparison). The first report of aflatoxin M_1 in market milk was in 1968 from South Africa (101) where detectable aflatoxin was found in five of 21 samples of fluid milk from retail outlets at a trace (<0.02 to 0.2 $\mu g/l$). A German study of commercially dried milk products (102) found aflatoxin M_1 in 5% of 166 samples at 0.07–0.2 $\mu g/l$ (recalculated to fluid milk basis). Two years later a survey of dried milk products in Germany by another team of investigators (103) found aflatoxin M_1 in 62% of 120 samples picked up at monthly intervals over a period of 1½ years. The levels (fluid milk basis) ranged from 0.02 to 0.4 $\mu g/l$ with a distinct seasonal trend to a higher incidence when the cows would normally be on stored feed. These data are supported further by an FDA examination of 35 samples of various cheeses imported from Europe. Aflatoxin M_1 was found in two of eight samples from Germany, two of four samples from Switzerland, and one of 11 samples from France. Levels ranged from 0.1 to 0.6 $\mu g/kg$ cheese. No aflatoxin was found in the 12 samples from Italy and Greece. From conversion data (104, 105, 106, 107, 108), it may be estimated that aflatoxin M_1 in the milk at 0.1 $\mu g/l$ came from aflatoxin B_1 in the feed at about 25 $\mu g/kg$ dry feed weight.

Other Mycotoxins

Although it appears that most of the mycotoxin survey work has been confined to aflatoxins, the search has included other mycotoxins for which analytical methodology of some sort was available and for which some reason existed to suspect a potential for harm. Each disturbing incidence of a mycotoxin in a food commodity has triggered a toxicological effort to determine the real potential for harm from chronic ingestion.

Zearalenone. The occurrence of zearalenone is related to the invasion of grain by various species of *Fusarium* (109, 110, 111) such as *F. tricinctum* and *F. moniliforne* but particularly by *F. roseum* var. *graminearium* (=*Gibberella zeae*) called Gibb in farm vernacular. These organisms invade developing corn at the silking stage in periods of heavy rainfall and proliferate on mature grains that have not dried because of wet weather at harvest or on grains that are stored wet (17, 112, 113). In stored corn the *Fusaria* occupy the water activity niche between the *Penicillia* and bacteria (114). Field observation of a pink discoloration of kernels signals the presence of *F. roseum* in corn; scab is associated with *F. roseum* in small grains. Since low temperature is needed to initiate and maintain the production of zearalenone (*115*) from mold, the presence of mold is insufficient evidence for the presence of the metabolite.

In the USDA surveys of corn from the 1967 crop (*77*) and of corn for export during 1968–1969 (*78*), zearalenone was found in six of the 576 samples at an average level of 625 μg/kg (range 450–800 μg/kg). In some years conditions are conducive to *Fusarium* ear rot in epidemic proportions (*17*). One such year was 1972. In the spring of the following year, the FDA collected samples of corn at terminal elevators servicing areas where there had been some evidence of *F. roseum* damage (*116*). Zearalenone was found in 17% of the 223 samples assayed, at an average level of 0.9 mg/kg (range 0.1–5.0 mg/kg) with no relation to grade or intended use including food use. Within the area surveyed there was a geographical concentration of the contamination inside a 150 mile radius of the southern tip of Lake Michigan. Zearalenone contamination of feed grains is not confined to the United States; instances of feed contamination have been reported from Finland (*117*), Denmark (*118*), France (*119*), and England (*120*).

The concentration of zearalenone within the corn kernel is distributed, as expected, in the same fashion as aflatoxin (*121*). On dry milling of contaminated corn, the highest concentrations of zearalenone were in the high fat fractions usually used for oil and feed. An FDA follow-up to a finding of zearalenone-contaminated corn (120 μg/kg) used for production of starch found zearalenone at 15 μg/kg in the starch.

Ochratoxin. Although ochratoxins A and B and the ethyl ester of ochratoxin A (ochratoxin C) have been isolated from laboratory cultures, only ochratoxin A has been detected in most cases of natural occurrence. The toxins were originally isolated from strains of *Aspergillus ochraceus* found to be toxin producers, as part of a screening program for toxigenic molds (*122, 123*). *Penicillium viridicatum* has also been identified as a producer of ochratoxin (*124, 125*) and has been associated with the natural occurrence of ochratoxin A in most situations where an association could be made. Both species are widely distributed and frequently encountered on grains, legumes, and other commodities usually protected by a reduction of water activity. A water activity that favors the growth of *P. viridicatum* on wheat and barley (*126*) is *ca.* 0.90, a level far higher than that recommended for safe storage of grains and a higher rung in the water activity ladder than that favorable for the growth of *A. flavus* (0.84–0.86).

The first detection of ochratoxin A as a natural contaminant was in a USDA–ARS survey of corn for aflatoxins, ochratoxins, and zearalenone (*77, 127*). Ochratoxin was found at 130 μg/kg in one Sample Grade sample of 283 samples of various grades of corn received from commercial markets in 1967. Three more samples with ochratoxin (83, 119, and 166 μg/kg) were encountered in a later survey of 293 samples of corn intended for export (78). In a three-year USDA–ARS survey for aflatoxin and ochratoxin in wheat (291 hard red winter, 286 hard red spring, 271 soft red winter) from graders' samples (93), ochratoxin was found in two samples of hard red winter wheat at 25 and 35 μg/kg and in seven samples of hard red spring wheat at 20–114 μg/kg. All contaminated samples were in the poorer grades. *Penicillium viridicatum* was the associated mold. Because of reports from Denmark (128) of ochratoxin in barley associated with porcine nephropathy, the FDA undertook a survey of domestic barley using samples submitted to USDA–AMS for grading. Ochratoxin was found in 14% of 159 samples with no relation to grade. Half the detections were trace amounts (<10 μg/kg); the average level of ochratoxin in the measurable detections was 18 μg/kg (range 10–29 μg/kg). Because ochratoxin had been detected in 22% of 37 samples of malt barley, a follow-up survey was made of malt barley and beer picked up at 138 U.S. breweries. No ochratoxin was detected in either barley or beer. Experimental Danish beers made from ochratoxin A contaminated barley retained approximately 4% of the original ochratoxin (129). At this rate of ochratoxin loss, barleys with sufficient ochratoxin A to result in detectable ochratoxin in the beer made from them would be rejected for malting because of inadequate germination.

A Danish survey of barley and oats (125) provided a much different picture. Ochratoxin was found in 58% of 33 samples of feed grains, mostly barley, taken in districts experiencing a high incidence of swine nephropathy; the average level was 3 mg/kg (range 0.03–28 mg/kg). Ochratoxin B in addition to ochratoxin A was detected in two of the barley samples (130). Ochratoxin was also found in 6% of 50 samples of barley selected as high quality grain at 9, 44, and 189 μg/kg. Subsequent to these findings, a farm was located at which the grain being fed to pigs was contaminated with ochratoxin. Residues of ochratoxin were found at slaughter in the kidneys of 18 of 19 pigs examined (131). No explanation has been offered for the high incidence of ochratoxin contamination of Danish barley.

In a Canadian survey of moldy feedstuffs (42) ochratoxin was found in 18 of 29 samples of heated grain (wheat, oats, and rye) at 0.03–27 mg/kg and in three of four samples of dried white beans at 0.02, 0.03, and 1.9 mg/kg. *Penicillium viridicatum* was consistently found to be the mold related to the presence of ochratoxin, as was also the case in the Danish studies. In an FDA survey of dried beans for aflatoxins and mold population, all samples with a high incidence of *A. ochraceus* were analyzed for ochratoxins; none were detected. The evidence points to *P. viridicatum* as the usual case of ochratoxin contamination.

Ochratoxin has also been found in green coffee beans (132), initially in four of five samples of heavily molded beans at <20–400 μg/kg. The study continued with an examination of samples from 267 bags of beans originating in six countries. Samples were taken after obviously spoiled beans had been removed. Ochratoxin was found in 19 samples at an average of 47 μg/kg (range 20–360 μg/kg). Another 68 samples were analyzed. Half of the samples had been flown in from the country of origin to remove the factor of ocean transport; the other half were laboratory samples of clean green coffee. Ochratoxin was found in two samples at about 20 μg/kg and in one sample at 80 μg/kg. A superficial study of the mold flora showed *A. ochraceus* and unidentified species of *Penicillia*. No attempt was made to determine the ochratoxin-producing capability of any of the isolates. Later at the same laboratory a more comprehensive study of the mold flora of green coffee (*133*) found both *A. ochraceus* and *P. viridicatum*. Ochratoxin was produced in culture by most isolates of *A. ochraceus* but by none of the isolates of *P. viridicatum*. Roasting of coffee destroys much of the ochratoxin in the bean (*132*).

Citrinin. Citrinin was originally isolated from *Penicillium citrinum* (*134*) as part of the monumental effort by Raistrick and his co-workers at the London School of Hygiene and Tropical Medicine to isolate and characterize the metabolic products of molds. Citrinin-producing isolates of *P. citrinum* have been obtained from yellow-colored rice of the type associated in Japan with toxic symptoms (*11*). However, the occurrence of citrinin as a contaminant of feedstuffs has been associated with *P. viridicatum* and always as a co-contaminant with ochratoxin. In the Canadian survey of moldy feedstuffs previously referred to (*42*), citrinin was found at 0.07–80 mg/kg levels in 13 of the 18 samples in which ochratoxin had been found. There was no consistent ratio of the two toxins. In the Danish survey of grains associated with swine nephropathy (*125*), citrinin was determined at 0.16, 1.0, and 2.0 mg/kg in three of the 22 samples of barley in which ochratoxin had been detected. Experimental beers made from malted barley with citrinin added at 1 mg/kg malt had no detectable citrinin (129). Barleys naturally contaminated with citrinin had inadequate germination for malting.

Penicillic Acid. Penicillic acid was first isolated from a mold culture in 1913 as part of a study of corn deterioration (*135*). The cycle was completed 60 years later when a newly developed analytical method was tested on samples of corn collected as part of an FDA survey of the 1972 crop (*136*). Penicillic acid was found in seven of 20 random samples assayed at 5–231 μg/kg (average 59 μg/kg). Since the fungi associated with the blue–green discoloration of corn known as blue eye were demonstrated producers of penicillic acid (*137*), the method was also tested on 48 samples of corn selected by USDA's Agricultural Marketing Service graders as having this discoloration. Penicillic acid was detected in all samples at 5–184 μg/kg (average 46 μg/kg). Dried bean samples, selected from a nationwide survey because a high proportion of seeds contained viable *Penicillium cyclopium,* were also assayed (*P. cyclopium* is one of the blue eye molds). Penicillic acid was found in five of 20 samples tested at 11–179 μg/kg (average 82 μg/kg).

In a study of mold species isolated from fermented sausage (*138*), penicillic acid was produced in synthetic culture by 44 of 421 isolates and by at least one isolate in seven of 18 identified species including some not previously recorded as producers of penicillic acid. However, when demonstrated penicillic acid producers were used to ferment sausage, no penicillic acid could be found (*139*). Penicillic acid added to sausage meat could be totally recovered if extracted immediately following addition, but after three days only 5% could be recovered. The loss was attributed to the formation of adducts with cysteine or glutathione in the meat. Similar observations have been made on the disappearance of penicillic acid added to wheat flour (*140*) with the same proposed mechanism of reaction. Intentionally formed adducts of penicillic acid with these compounds were markedly less toxic than the penicillic acid alone.

Patulin. The natural occurrence of patulin has been associated with *Penicillium expansum* rot in apples (*141, 142, 143*) and the invasion of soils and plant stubble by *Penicillium urticae* (*P. patulum*) (*144*). Both molds are common and highly competitive in their normal environments. Concentrations of patulin found in natural apple rots have been as high as 136 mg/kg of fruit (*143*). The first observation for patulin in commercial products was in a limited Canadian survey (*145*). Patulin was found at 1.0 mg/l. in one of 12 samples of apple juice. A 1971 survey of four cider mills in upper New York State showed that the presence of patulin in the apple juice was related to the inclusion of decayed apples with the fruit going into the press. Nine of 40 samples of juice from two mills that used up to 50% decayed apples had patulin levels of 20–45 mg/l. (*146*). Patulin has also been isolated from five of 21 samples of baked goods covered with a green mold identified as a *Penicillium* species (*147*).

Based on these observations, the U.S. FDA conducted a survey during fiscal 1973 of apple juice on the U.S. market. Patulin was detected in 37% of 136 samples at an average contamination level of 69 μg/l. (range 40–440 μg/l.). The possibility of patulin occurrence has been demonstrated in other fruits (peaches, pears, apricots, cherries) for which *P. expansum* is a common storage rot organism (*148*).

There are only a few natural substrates such as apple juice in which patulin has shown a reasonable stability (*140, 149*). Although patulin-producing strains of *P. expansum* have been used for ripening some types of fermented sausage, patulin is not detectable in the finished product (*150*) nor is there any detectable biological activity that could be related to patulin (*151*). The inactivation of patulin has been related to its ability to react with sulfhydryl compounds such as cysteine and glutathione (*141, 152*), similarly to penicillic acid. Alcoholic fermentation of a contaminated juice will also eliminate patulin (*152*).

Conclusion

Information on mycotoxin incidence should be interpreted cautiously. Incidence data can tell only what has happened in the past and applies only to that cross-section of the commodity represented by the sample. Unless information is included on how the contamination occurred, there is no basis for future projections. However, some idea of the past is needed to determine how much effort to put into the future. Often this effort consists in determining the magnitude of the toxicological risk from the levels of toxin encountered since reliable information on the effects of chronic human exposure to these toxins is practically nonexistent.

Literature Cited

1. Tanner, F. W., "The Microbiology of Foods," p. 669, Twin City Printing, Champaign, Ill., 1932.
2. Barger, G., "Ergot and Ergotism," p. 85, Gurney and Jackson, London, 1931.
3. Mayer, C. F., "Endemic Panmyelotoxicosis in the Russian Grain Belt," *Mil. Surg.* (1953) **113**, 295–315.
4. Bilay, V. I., "Mycotoxicoses of Man and Agricultural Animals," Kiev, 1960. Translation distributed by Office of Technical Services, U.S. Department of Commerce, Washington, D.C.
5. Shapovalov, M., *Phytopathology* (1917) **7**, 384–386.
6. Dounin, M., "The Fusariosis of Cereal Crops in Europian Russia in 1923," *Phytopathology* (1926) **16**, 305–308.
7. Saito, M., Tatsuno, T., "Toxins of *Fusarium nivale*," in "Microbial Toxins," Vol. 7, S. Kadis, A. Ciegler, S. J. Ajl, Eds., Academic, New York, 1971.
8. Bamburg, J. R., Strong, F. M., "12,13-Epoxytrichothecenes," in "Microbial Toxins," Vol. 7, S. Kadis, A. Ciegler, S. J. Ajl, Eds., Academic, New York, 1971.
9. Mirocha, C. J., Pathre, S., "Identification of the Toxic Principle in a Sample of Poaefusarin," *Appl. Microbiol.* (1973) **26**, 719–724.
10. Kinosita, R., Shikata, T., "On Toxic Moldy Rice," in "Mycotoxins in Foodstuffs," G. N. Wogan, Ed., MIT Press, Cambridge, Mass., 1965.
11. Saito, M., Enomoto, M., Tatsuno, T., "Yellowed Rice Toxins," in "Microbial Toxins," Vol. 6, A. Ciegler, S. Kadis, S. J. Ajl, Eds., Academic, New York, 1971.
12. Forgacs, J., Carll, W. T., "Mycotoxicoses," *Advan. Vet. Sci.* (1962) **7**, 273–382.
13. "Mycotoxicoses—Food-Borne Fungal Diseases," in "Animal Diseases," *Nutr. Rev.* (1962) **20**, 339–342.
14. Eppley, R. M., Bailey, W. J., "12,13-Epoxy-Δ^9-trichothecenes as the Probable Mycotoxins Responsible for Stachybotryotoxicosis," *Science* (1973) **181**, 758–760.
15. Christensen, J. J., Kernkamp, H. C. H., "Studies on the Toxicity of Blighted Barley to Swine," (Univ. of Minn.), *Agr. Exp. Sta. Tech. Bull.* (1936) 113.

16. Hoyman, W. G., "Concentration and Characterization of the Emetic Principle Present in Barley Infected with *Gibberella Saubinetii*," *Phytopathology* (1941) **31**, 871–885.
17. Tuite, J., Shaner, G., Rambo, G., Foster, J., Caldwell, R. W., "The *Gibberella* Ear Rot Epidemics of Corn in Indiana in 1965 and 1972," *Cereal Sci. Today* (1974) **19**, 238–241.
18. Prentice, N., Dickson, A. D., "Emetic Material Associated with *Fusarium* Species in Cereal Grains and Artificial Media," *Biotech. Bioeng.* (1968) **10**, 413–427.
19. Vesonder, R. F., Ciegler, A., Jensen, A. H., "Isolation of the Emetic Principle from *Fusarium*-Infected Corn," *Appl. Microbiol.* (1973) **25**, 1008–1010.
20. Ellison, R. A., Kotsonis, F. N., "T-2 Toxin as an Emetic Factor in Moldy Corn," *Appl. Microbiol.* (1973) **25**, 540–543.
21. Ueno, Y., Ishii, K., Sato, N., Ohtsubo, K., "Toxicological Approaches to the Metabolites of *Fusaria* VI. Vomiting Factor from Moldy Corn Infected with *Fusarium* Spp," *Jap. J. Exp. Med.* (1974) **44**, 123–127.
22. Bailey, W. S., Grotn, A. H., "The Relationship of Hepatitis-X of Dogs and Moldy Corn Poisoning of Swine," *J. Amer. Vet. Med. Ass.* (1959) **134**, 514–516.
23. Wilson, B. J., Teer, P. A., Barney, G. H., Blood, F. R., "Relationship of Aflatoxin to Epizootics of Toxic Hepatitis Among Animals in Southern United States," *Amer. J. Vet. Res.* (1967) **28**, 1217–1230.
24. Taylor, A., "The Toxicology of Sporidesmins and Other Epithiodioxopiperazines," in "Microbial Toxins," Vol. 7, S. Kadis, A. Ciegler, S. J. Ajl, Eds., Academic, New York, 1971.
25. Blount, W. P., "Turkey 'X' Disease," *Turkeys* (1961) **9**, 52.
26. Sargent, K., Carnaghan, R. B. A., "Groundnut Toxicity in Poultry: Experimental and Chemical Aspects," *Brit. Vet. J.* (1963) **119**, 178–184.
27. Lancaster, M. C., Jenkins, F. P., Philp, J. McL., Sargeant, K., Sheridan, A., O'Kelly, J., "Toxicity Associated with Certain Samples of Groundnuts," *Nature* (1961) **192**, 1095–1096.
28. Dickens, F., Jones, H. E. H., "The Carcinogenic Action of Aflatoxin After its Subcutaneous Injection in the Rat," *Brit. J. Cancer* (1963) **19**, 691–698.
29. Le Breton, E., Frayssinet, C., Boy, J., "Sur l'Apparition D'Hepatomes 'Spontanes' Chez le Rat Wistar. Role de la Toxine de l'*Aspergillus flavus*. Interet en pathologie humaine et cancerologie experimentale," *C.R. Acad. Sci.* (1962) **25**, 784–786.
30. "There's a Fungus Among Us (A Note on the Peanut Toxicity Problem)," World Health Organization Nutrition Document R.3/Add. 23, PAG-(WHO/FAO/UNICEF) Rome, 1962.
31. Salmon, W. D., Newberne, P. M., "Occurrence of Hepatomas in Rats Fed Diets Containing Peanut Meal as a Major Source of Protein," *Cancer Res.* (1963) **23**, 571–575.
32. "Official Methods of Analysis," 12th Ed., *Ass. Off. Anal. Chem.* (1975) Chapter 26.
33. Nesheim, S., "Analysis of Ochratoxins A and B and Their Esters in Barley, Using Partition and Thin Layer Chromatograph. I. Development of the Method, II. Collaborative Study," *J. Ass. Offic. Anal. Chem.* (1973) **56**, 817–826.
34. Scott, P. M., "Collaborative Study of a Chromatographic Method for Patulin in Apple Juice," *J. Ass. Offic. Anal. Chem.* (1974) **57**, 621–625.
35. Hald, B., Krogh, P., "Analysis and Chemical Confirmation of Citrinin in Barley," *J. Ass. Offic. Anal. Chem.* (1973) **56**, 1440–1443.
36. Thorpe, C. W., Johnson, R. L., "Analysis of Penicillic Acid by Gas-Liquid Chromatography," *J. Ass. Offic. Anal. Chem.* (1974) **57**, 861–865.

37. Eppley, R. M., "Screening Method for Zearalenone, Aflatoxin and Ochratoxin," *J. Ass. Offic. Anal. Chem.* (1968) **51**, 74–78.
38. Purchase, I. F. H., Van der Watt, J. J., "Carcinogenicity of Sterigmatocystin," *Food Cosmet. Toxicol.* (1970) **8**, 289–295.
39. van der Merwe, K. J., Fourie, L., Scott, de B., "On the Structure of the Aflatoxins," *Chem. Ind.* (1963) 1660–1661.
40. Stack, M. E., Rodricks, J. V., "Collaborative Study of the Quantitative Determination and Chemical Confirmation of Sterigmatocystin in Grains," *J. Ass. Offic. Anal. Chem.* (1973) **56**, 1123–1125.
41. Purchase, I. F. H., Goncalves, T., "Preliminary Results from Food Analyses in the Inhambane Area," in "Mycotoxins in Human Health," I. F. H. Purchase, Ed., pp. 263–269, Macmillan Press, London, 1971.
42. Scott, P. M., van Walbeek, W., Kennedy, B., Anyeti, D., "Mycotoxins (Ochratoxin A, Citrinin, and Sterigmatocystin) and Toxigenic Fungi in Grains and Other Agricultural Products," *J. Agr. Food Chem.* (1972) **20**, 1103–1109.
43. Purchase, I. F. H., Pretorius, M. E., "Sterigmatocystin in Coffee Beans," *J. Ass. Offic. Agr. Chem.* (1973) **56**, 225–226.
44. Hsu, I-C., Smalley, E. B., Strong, F. M., Ribelin, W. E., "Identification of T-2 Toxin in Moldy Corn Associated with a Lethal Toxicosis in Dairy Cattle," *Appl. Microbiol.* (1972) **24**, 684–690.
45. Hunter, J. H., "Growth and Aflatoxin Production in Shelled Corn by the *Aspergillus flavus* Group as Related to Relative Humidity and Temperature," Ph.D. Thesis, Purdue University, 1969.
46. "Report on a Surveillance Program—Aflatoxins in Consumer Peanut Products," FDA Bureau of Foods, 1973.
47. Whitaker, T. B., Dickens, J. W., "Variability of Aflatoxin Test Results," *J. Amer. Oil Chem. Soc.* (1974) **51**, 214–218.
48. Shank, R. C., Wogan, G. N., Gibson, J. B., Nondasuta, A., "Dietary Aflatoxins and Human Liver Cancer. II. Aflatoxins in Market Foods and Foodstuffs of Thailand and Hongkong," *Food Cosmet. Toxicol.* (1972) **10**, 61–69.
49. Campbell, T. C., Salamat, L., "Aflatoxin Ingestion and Excretion by Humans," in "Mycotoxins in Human Health," I. F. H. Purchase, Ed., Macmillan Press, London, 1971.
50. Campbell, T. C., Stoloff, L., "Implications of Mycotoxins for Human Health," *J. Agr. Food Chem.* (1974) **22**, 1006–1015.
51. Alpert, M. E., Hutt, M. S. R., Wogan, G. N., Davidson, C. S., "Association Between Aflatoxin Content of Food and Hepatoma Frequency in Uganda," *Cancer* (1971) **28**, 253–260.
52. Suzangar, M., Emani, A., Barnett, R., "Contamination of Pistachio Nuts with Aflatoxins While on the Trees and in Storage," *2nd Intern. IUPAC Symp. Mycotoxins Food, Pulawy, Poland, 1974*.
53. Mattei, J. A., California Almond Growers Exchange, personal communication, 1974.
54. Johnson, R. A., Diamond Walnut Growers, Inc., personal communication, 1974.
55. Jackson, E. W., Wolf, H., Sinnhuber, R. O., "The Relationship of Hepatoma in Rainbow Trout to Aflatoxin Contamination and Cottonseed Meal," *Cancer Res.* (1968) **28**, 987–991.
56. Whitten, M. E., "Occurrence of Aflatoxins in Cottonseed and Cottonseed Products," *Mycotoxin Res. Sem., Proc., Washington, D. C., June 8–9, 1967*, pp. 7–9, 1968.
57. Harper, G. A., National Cottonseed Products Assn., Inc., personal communication, 1974.
58. Whitten, M. E., USDA Agricultural Marketing Research Institute, Cereal and Oilseed Research, personal communication, 1974.

59. Simpson, M. E., Marsh, P. B., "The Geographical Distribution of *Aspergillus flavus* Boll Rot in the U.S. Cotton Crop of 1970," *Plant Dis. Rep.* (1971) **55**, 510–514.
60. Marsh, P. B., Simpson, M. E., Craig, G. O., Donoso, J., Ramey, H., Jr., "Occurrence of Aflatoxins in Cotton Seeds at Harvest in Relation to Location of Growth and Field Temperatures," *J. Environ. Qual.* (1973) **2**, 276–281.
61. Marsh, P. B., Bollenbacher, K., San Antonio, J. P., Merola, G. V., "Observations on Certain Fluorescent Spots in Raw Cotton Associated with the Growth of Micro-Organisms," *Text. Res. J.* (1955) **25**, 1007–1016.
62. Ashworth, L. J., Jr., McMeans, J. L., "Association of *Aspergillus flavus* and Aflatoxins with a Greenish Yellow Fluorescence of Cotton Seed," *Phytopathology* (1966) **56**, 1104–1105.
63. Whitten, M. E., "Screening Cottonseed for Aflatoxins," *J. Amer. Oil Chem. Soc.* (1969) **46**, 39–40.
64. Marsh, P. R., Simpson, M. E., Ferretti, R. J., Campbell, T. C., Donoso, J., "Relation of Aflatoxins in Cottonseeds at Harvest to Fluorescence in the Fiber," *J. Agr. Food Chem.* (1969) **17**, 462–467.
65. Marsh, P. B., Simpson, M. E., Ferretti, R. J., Merola, G. V., Donoso, J., Craig, G. O., Trucksess, M. W., Work, P. S., "Mechanism of Formation of a Fluorescence in Cotton Fiber Associated with Aflatoxins in the Seeds at Harvest," *J. Agr. Food Chem.* (1969) **17**, 468–472.
66. Ashworth, L. J., Jr., Rice, R. E., McMeans, J. L., Brown, C. M., "The Relationship of Insects to Infection of Cotton Bolls by *Aspergillus flavus*," *Phytopathology* (1971) **61**, 488–493.
67. Ashworth, L. J., Jr., McMeans, J. L., Brown, C. M., "Infection of Cotton by *Aspergillus flavus*: The Influence of Temperature and Aeration," *Phytopathology* (1968) **59**, 383–385.
68. Marsh, P. B., Simpson, M. E., Craig, G. O., Donoso, J., Ramey, H. H., Jr., "Occurrence of Aflatoxins in Cottonseeds at Harvest in Relation to Location of Growth and Field Temperatures," *J. Environ. Quality* (1973) **2**, 276–281.
69. Ashworth, L. J., Jr., McMeans, J. L., Houston, B. R., Whitten, M. E., Brown, C. M., "Mycoflora, Aflatoxins and Free Fatty Acids in California Cottonseed During 1967–1968," *J. Amer. Oil Chem. Soc.* (1971) **48**, 129–133.
70. Hald, B., Krogh, P., "Occurrence of Aflatoxin in Imported Cottonseed Products," *Nord. Vet.-Med.* (1970) **22**, 39–47.
71. Vedanayagam, H. S., Indulkar, A. S., Rao, S. R., "Aflatoxins and *Aspergillus flavus* Link in Indian Cottonseed," *Indian J. Exp. Biol.* (1971) **9**, 410–411.
72. Krogh, P., Hald, B., Korpinen, E.-L., "Occurrence of Aflatoxin in Groundnut and Copra Products Imported to Finland," *Nord. Vet.-Med.* (1970) **22**, 584–589.
73. Dwarakanath, C. T., Sreenivasamurthy, V., Parpia, H. A. B., "Aflatoxin in Indian Peanut Oil," *J. Food Sci. Technol. (Mysore)* (1969) **6**, 107–109.
74. Ling, K-H., Tung, C-M., Sheh, P., Wang, J-J., Tung, T-C., "Aflatoxin B_1 in Unrefined Peanut Oil and Peanut Products in Taiwan," *J. Formosan Med. Ass.* (1968) **67**, 309–313.
75. Parker, W. A., Melnick, D., "Absence of Aflatoxin from Refined Vegetable Oils," *J. Amer. Oil Chem. Soc.* (1966) **43**, 635–638.
76. Shotwell, O. L., Hesseltine, C. W., Burmeister, H. R., Kwolek, W. F., Shannon, G. M., Hall, H. H., "Survey of Cereal Grains and Soybeans for the Presence of Aflatoxin. II. Corn and Soybeans," *Cereal Chem.* (1969) **46**, 454–463.

77. Shotwell, O. L., Hesseltine, C. W., Goulden, M. L., Vandegraft, E. E., "Survey of Corn for Aflatoxin, Zearalenone, and Ochratoxin," *Cereal Chem.* (1970) **47**, 700–707.

78. Shotwell, O. L., Hesseltine, C. W., Vandegraft, E. E., Goulden, M. L., "Survey of Corn from Different Regions for Aflatoxin, Ochratoxin, and Zearalenone," *Cereal Sci. Today* (1971) **16**, 266–273.

79. Shotwell, O. L., Hesseltine, C. W., Goulden, M. L., "Incidence of Aflatoxin in Southern Corn, 1969–1970," *Cereal Sci. Today* (1973) **18**, 192–195.

80. Shotwell, O. L., Goulden, M. L., Hesseltine, C. W., "Aflatoxin Contamination: Association with Foreign Material and Characteristic Fluorescence in Damaged Corn Kernels," *Cereal Chem.* (1972) **49**, 458–465.

81. Velasco, J., "Detection of Aflatoxin Using Small Columns of Florisil," *J. Amer. Oil Chem. Soc.* (1973) **49**, 141–142.

82. Hunt, W. H., Liebe, E. B., Velasco, J., "Incidence of Aflatoxin in Corn and a Field Method for Aflatoxin Analysis," *Cereal Chem.*, submitted for publication, 1975.

83. Shotwell, O. L., Goulden, M. L., Hesseltine, C. W., "Aflatoxin: Distribution in Contaminated Corn," *Cereal Chem.* (1974) **51**, 492–499.

84. Shotwell, O. L., Goulden, M. L., Jepson, A. M., Kwolek, W. F., Hesseltine, C. W., "Aflatoxin Occurrence in White Corn Under Loan, 1971. III. Association with Bright Greenish-Yellow Fluorescence in Corn," *Cereal Chem.*, in press, 1975.

85. Lillehoj, E. B., Kwolek, W. F., Fennell, D. I., Milburn, M. S., "Bright Greenish-Yellow Fluorescence and Aflatoxin in Freshly Harvested High-Moisture Corn from Southern Illinois and Southeastern Missouri," *Cereal Chem.* (1975) **52**, 403–412.

86. Lillehoj, E. B., Kwolek, W. F., Shannon, G. M., Shotwell, O. L., Hesseltine, C. W., "Aflatoxin Occurrence in 1973 Field Corn: A Limited Survey in the Southeastern U.S.," *Cereal Chem.*, in press, 1975.

87. Knake, R. P., Deyoe, C. W., "Production of Aflatoxin by *Aspergillus parasiticus* in Maturing White Corn," *Poultry Sci.* (1973) **52**, 2049.

88. Rambo, G., Tuite, J., Crane, P., "Preharvest Inoculation and Infection of Dent Corn Ears with *Aspergillus flavus* and *A. parasiticus*," *Phytopathology* (1974) **64**, 797–800.

89. Ullola-Sosa, M., Schroeder, H. W., "Note on Aflatoxin Decomposition in the Process of Making Tortillas from Corn," *Cereal Chem.* (1969) **46**, 397–400.

90. Yahl, K. R., Watson, S. A., Smith, R. J., Barabolok, R., "Laboratory Wet Milling of Corn Containing High Levels of Aflatoxin and a Survey of Commercial Wet-Milling Products," *Cereal Chem.* (1971) **48**, 385–391.

91. Brekke, O. L., Peplinski, A. J., Nelson, G. E. N., Griffin, E. L., Jr., "Pilot-plant Dry Milling of Corn Containing Aflatoxin," *Cereal Chem.* (1975) **52**, 205–211.

92. Shotwell, O. L., Hesseltine, C. W., Burmeister, H. R., Kwolek, W. F., Shannon, G. M., Hall, H. H., "Survey of Cereal Grains and Soybeans for the Presence of Aflatoxin: I. Wheat, Grain Sorghum, and Oats," *Cereal Chem.* (1969) **46**, 446–454.

93. Shotwell, O. L., Goulden, M. L., Fennell, D. I., Hesseltine, C. W., "Survey of Wheat for Aflatoxin and Ochratoxin," *J. Agr. Food Chem.*, submitted for publication, 1975.

94. Shank, R. C., Gordon, J. E., Wogan, C. N., Nondasuta, A., Subhamani, B., "Dietary Aflatoxins and Human Liver Cancer. III. Field Survey of Rural Thai Families for Ingested Aflatoxins," *Food Cosmet. Toxicol.* (1972) **10**, 71–84.

48 MYCOTOXINS

95. Hesseltine, C. W., Shotwell, O. L., Ellis, J. J., Stubblefield, R. D., "Aflatoxin Formation by *Aspergillus flavus*," *Bacteriol. Rev.* (1966) **30**, 795–805.
96. Scott, P. M., Kennedy, B. P. C., "Analysis and Survey of Ground Black, White, and Capsicum Peppers for Aflatoxins," *J. Ass. Off. Anal. Chem.* (1973) **56**, 1452–1457.
97. Schuller, P. L., Ockuizen, Th., Werringloer, J., Marquardt, P., "Aflatoxin B_1 und Histamin in Wein," *Arzneim. Forsch.* (1967) **17**, 888–890.
98. Drawert, F., Barton, H., "Zun Nachweis von Aflatoxinen in Wein," *Z. Lebensm. Unters. Forsch.* (1974) **154**, 223–224.
99. Takahashi, D. M., "Thin Layer Chromatographic Determination of Aflatoxins in Wine," *J. Ass. Offic. Anal. Chem.* (1974) **57**, 875–879.
100. "Report on a Surveillance Program—Aflatoxins in Milk Products," FDA Bureau of Foods, 1973.
101. Purchase, I. F. H., Vorster, L. J., "Aflatoxin in Commercial Milk Samples," *S. Afr. Med. J.* (1968) **42**, 219.
102. Neumann-Kleinpaul, A., Terplan, G., "Zum Vorkommen von Aflatoxin M_1 in Trockenmilchprodukten," *Arch. Lebensmittelhyg.* (1972) **23**, 128–131.
103. Jung, M., Hanssen, E., "Uber das Vorkommen von Aflatoxin M_1 in Trockenmilcherzeugnissen," *Food Cosmet. Toxicol.* (1974) **12**, 131–138.
104. van der Linde, J. A., Frens, A. M., van Esch, C. J., "Experiments with Cows Fed Groundnut Meal Containing Aflatoxin," in "Mycotoxins in Foodstuffs," G. Wogan, Ed., pp. 247–249, MIT Press, Cambridge, Mass., 1965.
105. Polan, C. E., Hayes, J. R., Campbell, T. C., "Consumption and Fate of Aflatoxin B_1 by Lactating Cows," *J. Agr. Food Chem.* (1974) **22**, 635–638.
106. McKinney, J. D., Cavanagh, G. C., Bell, J. T., Hoversland, A. S., Nelson, D. M., Pearson, J., Selkirk, R. J., "Effects of Ammoniation on Aflatoxins in Rations Fed Lactating Cows," *J. Amer. Oil Chem. Soc.* (1973) **50**, 79–84.
107. Masri, M. S., Garcia, V. C., Page, J. R., "The Aflatoxin M Content of Milk from Cows Fed Known Amounts of Aflatoxin," *Vet. Rec.* (1969) **84**, 146–147.
108. Allcroft, R., Roberts, B. A., "Toxic Groundnut Meal: The Relationship Between Aflatoxin B_1 Intake by Cows and Excretion of Aflatoxin M_1 in Milk," *Vet. Rec.* (1968) **82**, 116–118.
109. Mirocha, C. J., Christensen, C. M., Nelson, G. H., "Estrogenic Metabolite Produced by *Fusarium graminearum* in Stored Corn," *Appl. Microbiol.* (1967) **15**, 497–503.
110. Caldwell, R. W., Tuite, J., Stob, M., Baldwin, R., "Zearalenone Production by *Fusarium* Species," *Appl. Microbiol.* (1970) **20**, 31–34.
111. Mirocha, C. J., Christensen, C. M., Nelson, G. H., "Biosynthesis of the Fungal Estrogen F-2 and a Naturally Occurring Derivative (F-3) by *Fusarium moniliforme*," *Appl. Microbiol.* (1969) **17**, 482–483.
112. Caldwell, R. W., Tuite, J., "Zearalenone Production in Field Corn in Indiana," *Phytopathology* (1970) **60**, 1696–1697.
113. Caldwell, R. W., Tuite, J., "Zearalenone in Freshly Harvested Corn," *Phytopathology* (1974) **64**, 752–753.
114. Koehler, B., "Fungus Growth in Shelled Corn as Affected by Moisture," *J. Agr. Res.* (1938) **56**, 291–307.
115. Mirocha, C. J., Christensen, C. M., Nelson, G. H., "F-2 (Zearalenone) Estrogenic Mycotoxin from *Fusarium*," in "Microbial Toxins," Vol. VII, S. Kadis, A. Ciegler, S. A. Ajl, Eds., pp. 107–138, Academic Press, New York, 1971.

116. Eppley, R. M., Stoloff, L., Trucksess, M. W., Chung, C. W., "Survey of Corn for Fusarium Toxins," *J. Ass. Offic. Anal. Chem.* (1974) **57**, 632–635.
117. Roine, K., Korpinen, E-L., Kallela, K., "Mycotoxicosis as a Probable Cause of Infertility in Dairy Cows," *Nord. Vet. Med.* (1971) **23**, 628–633.
118. Erikson, E., "Estrogenic Factors in Moldy Grain," *Nord. Vet. Med.* (1968) **20**, 396–401.
119. Jemmali, M., "Presence d'un Facteur Oestrogenique d'Origine Fongique la Zearalenone ou F-2, comme Contaminant Naturel, dans du Mais," *Ann. Microbiol. (Inst. Pasteur)* (1973) **124B**, 109–114.
120. Mirocha, C. J., Harrison, J., Nichols, A. A., McClintock, M., "Detection of a Fungal Estrogen (F-2) in Hay Associated with Infertility in Dairy Cattle," *Appl. Microbiol.* (1968) **16**, 797–798.
121. Bennett, G. A., Peplinski, A. J., Brekke, O. L., Jackson, L., Wischer, R., "Distribution of Zearalenone in Dry Milled Fractions of Contaminated Corn," *Cereal Chem.*, submitted for publication, 1975.
122. Scott, De B., "Toxigenic Fungi Isolated from Cereal and Legume Products," *Mycopath. Mycolog.* (1965) **25**, 213–222.
123. van der Merwe, K. J., Steyn, P. S., Fourie, L., Scott, De B., Theron, J. J., "Ochratoxin A, a Toxic Metabolite Produced by *Aspergillus ochraceus* Wilh," *Nature* (1965) **205**, 1112–1113.
124. van Walbeek, W., Scott, P. M., Harwig, J., Lawrence, J. W., "*Penicillium viridicatum* Westling: a New Source of Ochratoxin A," *Can. J. Microbiol.* (1969) **15**, 1281–1285.
125. Krogh, P., Hald, B., Pedersen, J., "Occurrence of Ochratoxin A and Citrinin in Cereals Associated with Mycotoxic Porcine Mephropathy," *Acta. Path. Microbiol. Scand.* (1973) **B81**, 689–695.
126. Harwig, J., Chen, Y.-K., "Some Conditions Favoring Production of Ochratoxin A and Citrinin by *Penicillium viridicatum* in Wheat and Barley," *Can. J. Plant Sci.* (1974) **54**, 17–22.
127. Shotwell, O. L., Hesseltine, C. W., Goulden, M. L., "Ochratoxin A: Occurrence as a Natural Contaminant of a Corn Sample," *Appl. Microbiol.* (1969) **17**, 765–766.
128. Krogh, P., Royal Veterinary and Agricultural University, Denmark, 1971, personal communication.
129. Krogh, P., Hald, B., Gjertsen, P., Myken, F., "Fate of Ochratoxin A and Citrinin During Malting and Brewing Experiments," *Appl. Microbiol.* (1974) **28**, 31–34.
130. Krogh, P., Hald, B., 1974, personal communication.
131. Hald, B., Krogh, P., Ochratoxin Residues in Bacon Pigs. Abstr. IUPAC-sponsored symp. "Control of Mycotoxins," Goeteborg, Sweden (1972) 18.
132. Levi, C. P., Trenk, H. L., Mohr, H. K., "Study of the Occurrence of Ochratoxin A in Green Coffee Beans," *J. Ass. Offic. Anal. Chem.* (1974) **57**, 866–870.
133. Trenk, H., General Foods Technical Center, 1974, personal communication.
134. Hetherington, A. C., Raistrick, H., "Biochemistry of Microorganisms XIV. Production and Chemical Constitution of a New Yellow Coloring Matter, Citrinin, Produced from Dextrose by *Penicillium citrinum* Thom," *Trans. Royal Soc. (London)* (1931) **B220**, 269–296.
135. Alsberg, C. L., Black, O. F., "Contributions to the Study of Maize Deterioration," *U.S. Dept. Agr., Bur. Plant Ind. Bull.* (1913) **270**, 7–48.
136. Thorpe, C. W., Johnson, R. L., "Analysis of Penicillic Acid by Gas–Liquid Chromatography," *J. Ass. Offic. Anal. Chem.* (1974) **57**, 861–865.

137. Ciegler, A., Kurtzman, C. P., "Penicillic Acid Production by Blue-Eye Fungi on Various Agricultural Commodities," *Appl. Microbiol.* (1970) **20**, 761–764.
138. Ciegler, A., Mintzlaff, H-J, Machnik, W., Leistner, L., "Untersuchungen uber das Toxinbidungsvermogen von Rohwursten Isolierter Schimmelpilze der Gattung *Penicillium*," *Fleischwirtschaft* (1972) **52**, 1311–1318.
139. Ciegler, A., Mintzlaff, H-J., Weisleder, D., Leistner, L., "Potential Production and Detoxification of Penicillic Acid in Mold-Fermented Sausage (Salami)," *Appl. Microbiol.* (1972) **24**, 114–119.
140. Scott, P. M., Somers, E., "Stability of Patulin and Penicillic Acid in Fruit Juices and Flour," *J. Agr. Food Chem.* (1968) **16**, 483–485.
141. Brian, P. W., Elson, G. W., Lowe, D., "Production of Patulin in Apple Fruits by *Penicillium expansum*," *Nature* (1956) **178**, 263–264.
142. Walker, J. R. L., "Inhibition of the Apple Phenolase System through Infection by *Penicillium expansum*," *Phytochemistry* (1969) **8**, 561–566.
143. Harwig, J., Chen, Y-K., Kennedy, B. P. C., Scott, P. M., "Occurrence of Patulin and Patulin-Producing Strains of *Penicillium expansum* in Natural Rots of Apple in Canada," *Can. Inst. Food Sci. Technol. J.* (1973) **6**, 22–25.
144. Norstadt, F. A., McCalla, T. M., "Microbially Induced Phytotoxicity in Stubble-Mulched Soil," *Soil Sci. Soc. Amer. Proc.* (1968) **32**, 241–245.
145. Scott, P. M., Miles, W. F., Toft, P., Dubé, J., "Occurrence of Patulin in Apple Juice," *J. Agr. Food Chem.* (1972) **20**, 450–451.
146. Wilson, D. M., 1974, private communication.
147. Reiss, J., "Nachweis von Patulin in Spontan Verschimmeltem Brot und Geback," *Naturwissenschaften* (1972) **59**, 37.
148. Buchanan, J. R., Sommer, N. F., Fortlage, R. J., Maxie, E. C., Mitchell, F. G., Hsieh, D. P. H., "Patulin from *Penicillium expansum* in Stone Fruits and Pears," *J. Amer. Soc. Hort. Sci.* (1974) **99**, 262–265.
149. Pohland, A. E., Allen, R., "Stability Studies with Patulin," *J. Ass. Offic. Anal. Chem.* (1970) **53**, 688–691.
150. Alperden, I., Mintzlaff, H-J., Tauchmann, F., Leistner, L., "Untersuchungen uber die Bildung des Mykotoxins Patulin in Rohwurst," *Fleischwirtschaft* (1973) **53**, 566–568.
151. Hofmann, K., Mintzlaff, H-J., Alperden, I., Leistner, L., "Untersuchung uber die Inaktivierung des Mykotoxins Patulin durch Sulfhydrylgruppen," *Fleischwirtschaft* (1971) **51**, 1534–1536.
152. Harwig, J., Scott, P. M., Kennedy, B. P. C., Chen, Y-K., "Disappearance of Patulin from Apple Juice Fermented by *Saccharomyces* spp," *J. Inst. Can. Sci. Technol. Aliment.* (1973) **6**, 45–46.

RECEIVED November 8, 1974.

The Role of Aflatoxin in Human Disease

R. C. SHANK[1]

Department of Nutrition and Food Science, Massachusetts Institute of Technology, Cambridge, Mass. 02139

Since the finding that aflatoxin B₁ is the most potent hepato-carcinogen known, several international studies have been conducted to determine to what extent this toxin is causally related to liver cancer in man. In areas of Uganda and Swaziland where the incidence of liver cancer is high, afla-toxin contamination of food crops is also high. Daily inges-tion of aflatoxins in Thailand and Kenya correlated well with liver cancer incidence. Mounting evidence relates aflatoxins to acute poisonings in children, especially Reye's syndrome in Thailand.

Much is known about the occurrence and toxicity of the aflatoxins. Aflatoxin B₁, the most common of the group in natural contamina-tion of foodstuffs, is the most potent hepatocarcinogen known for experi-mental animals. Obviously the ultimate question is what role if any aflatoxin plays in human disease.

Chronic Toxicity

The first study that associated aflatoxins in the food supply with the incidence of human liver cancer was done in Uganda by Alpert and co-workers (1). Of the 480 food samples collected from various areas of Uganda during 1966–1967, almost 4% contained more than 1 ppm total aflatoxins; this is regarded as heavy contamination. More important, there was a geographical distribution to the contamination which when compared with the distribution of liver cancer in Uganda suggested an association of the toxin and the disease.

Keen and Martin (2) measured the extent of aflatoxin contamination in peanuts collected from various areas in Swaziland and at the same

[1] Present address: Department of Community and Environmental Medicine, College of Medicine, University of California, Irvine, Calif. 92664.

time estimated the geographical distribution of liver cancer cases based on cancer registry data for 1964 to 1968. In areas where contamination of peanuts was high, the estimated incidence of liver cancer was high; in addition, inhabitants of the high liver cancer areas tended to eat more peanuts than those in other areas, increasing the likelihood of greater exposure to aflatoxin.

These two studies did not show how much aflatoxin was consumed. Initial reports on aflatoxin consumption came from Campbell and co-workers (3) who examined urine from Philippine children who had eaten contaminated peanut butter. Chemical analysis performed on peanut butter samples from 1967 to 1969 revealed that the local product had a median level of aflatoxins of 500 μg/kg. Children who consumed 60 g or more of such peanut butter excreted detectable levels of the aflatoxin metabolite, aflatoxin M_1.

Not until recently were there reports of epidemiologic studies on levels of aflatoxin consumed on a daily basis and the simultaneous incidence of hepatocellular carcinoma. One study was made in Thailand (4, 5, 6, 7, 8). Of the 2180 samples of foods and foodstuffs that were collected for almost two years from markets, mills, warehouses, distributors, farms, and homes throughout Thailand, 9% had aflatoxins, and peanuts, corn, millet, and dried chili peppers were contaminated most frequently. Toxin levels in foods destined for human consumption were as high as 772 μg/kg in dried fish, 966 μg/kg in dried chili peppers, 2700 μg/kg in corn, and more than 12,000 μg/kg in peanuts.

The market survey indicated a geographical distribution of aflatoxin contamination and served as a basis for designing a pilot study to measure simultaneously aflatoxin consumption and liver cancer incidence in two different populations. Three villages were selected in each of three areas of expected high, intermediate, and low toxin consumptions. In each village 16 households were selected randomly to serve as the dietary survey population; food prepared and eaten by these families was assayed for aflatoxins for three separate two-day intervals over 12 months. In central Thailand where aflatoxin contamination was shown high by the market survey, daily total aflatoxin consumption averaged 73–81 ng/kg body weight on a family basis; in western Thailand where the market survey indicated moderate contamination, the total aflatoxin consumption averaged 45–77 ng/kg body weight per day, and in the southern-most area (expected low contamination) the average was 5–8 ng/kg body weight per day.

Although the market survey indicated that peanuts, corn, and millet were high in toxin, these were not the important sources in the Thai diet. Peanuts in Thailand are a snack food and garnish, and corn and millet are only a small part of the diet. Although rice in markets and storage areas was relatively free of aflatoxins, it was a major source of toxin in the diet. Indirect evidence suggested that leftover foods were an appreciable source of dietary aflatoxins. The market survey did predict successfully, however, that foods containing garlic, dried chili peppers, or dried fish, common ingredients in Thai foods, would probably contain the toxins.

During the dietary survey, the incidence of primary liver cancer was also measured in western and southern-most Thailand. Investigation of all hospital and home deaths within a defined population of approximately 100,000 people per area continued for 12 months. Liver viscerotomy specimens were collected whenevr possible for histopathological examination and verification of diagnosis. The incidence of primary liver cancer in western Thailand was six new cases per year per 100,000 people, unadjusted for sex and age. In southern-most Thailand the incidence was 2/100,000/year; thus where aflatoxin consumption was high, incidence of liver cancer was also high. Note however that there is presumably a lag between aflatoxin consumption and tumor expression, and therefore it must be assumed that aflatoxin intakes measured in the Thailand survey were indicative of those of the liver cancer cases at the time their tumors were being induced. Although the amount of aflatoxin consumed may seem minute, the potency of aflatoxin B_1 must be remembered. Continuous exposure of aflatoxin B_1 to rats at a 1 μg/kg diet level results in a significant incidence of liver tumors. The highest daily aflatoxin B_1 intake measured in Thailand was 55 ng/kg body weight (*6*), comparable to a carcinogenic dose for the rat.

Further support that causally relates dietary aflatoxins to human liver cancer are the results from an extensive and careful epidemiological study carried out in Kenya from 1967 to 1970 by Peers and Linsell (*9*). The study was conducted in the Murang'a district (population 334,068, 16 years of age and older) on the eastern slopes of the Aberdare Mountains with three geographically distinct areas of high, intermediate, and low elevation. The amounts of aflatoxins contaminating the food supplies and the dietary loads of aflatoxins in these areas varied inversely with altitude. The incidence of liver cancer was determined through the cancer registry in the same general populations in which aflatoxin ingestion was measured. The data were plotted as incidence *vs.* log dose to yield a regression line with a correlation coefficient of 0.87 (for four degrees of freedom). The data obtained from Thailand are in excellent agreement with the Kenyan regression line.

Note that the 10,885 females over the age of 16 in the high elevation area had no cases of liver cancer within the 12-month study period even though the mean aflatoxin consumption was 3.46 ng/kg body weight; however this does not mean that this level of aflatoxin consumption is not carcinogenic. At that exposure the observed incidence of liver cancer was zero per 10,000 people in one year and should not be considered as the safe or no-effect level.

Acute Toxicity

Aflatoxins were discovered because of their acute toxicity; it is reasonable to assume that if these toxins are sufficiently prevalent in the human diet to be causally related to human liver cancer, there exists a potential for exposure to larger amounts for shorter periods resulting in an acute response. Three reports have associated aflatoxins with acute poisoning in man—specifically, rural children.

In 1967 Ling and co-workers (10) reported on an intoxication of 26 persons with three deaths in two Taiwan farming villages. The victims suffered edema of the lower extremities, abdominal pain, vomiting, and palpable liver but no fever. In three families of ten households, five households consumed moldy rice for periods up to three weeks and experienced the intoxication. Members of the same families living in the same compounds but in different houses consumed other rice and were unaffected. One or two samples of rice were taken from each of the affected families and assayed for aflatoxin B_1; in only two samples, both from the same family, was the toxin found at approximately 200 μg/kg. Neither sex nor age governed the illness, but all three deaths were children aged four, five, and six years. One child died 6½ hrs after the onset of illness, another 3½ days after, and the third several days after.

Another report (11) of suspected aflatoxin poisoning involved a 15-year old African (Uganda) boy with a history of four days of abdominal pain and swelling. Upon admission to the hospital he had edema of both legs, a palpable tender liver, and no fever, symptoms closely resembling the Taiwan cases. He was treated for heart failure, but his condition worsened, and he died two days after admission. The autopsy revealed pulmonary edema, a flabby heart, and diffuse necrosis of the liver; there was congestion and edema of the lung, interstitial edema of the heart, and centrilobular necrosis and mild fatty changes in the liver. Two siblings were also ill at the same time but recovered. The children's diet consisted principally of cassava, beans, fish, and meat. Analysis of the cassava sampled in the home revealed mold infestation and an aflatoxin concentration of 1.7 mg/kg; presumably this level, based on monkey data (12), could be fatal if the boy ate cassava for a few weeks.

The most incriminating evidence comes from Thailand (13, 14). Reye's syndrome which occurs in epidemic proportions in northeastern Thailand (15) is a children's disease characterized by a short prodrome, vomiting, hypoglycemia, convulsions, hyperammoniemia, coma, and usually death. Histopathologic examination reveals severe cerebral edema and extensive fatty accumulation in hepatocytes, renal tubular epithelium, and myocardial fibers.

Although attempts to associate a virus with the Thai cases have not been successful (16), a case did occur which suggested a mycotoxin etiology (13). A three-year-old Thai boy had been ill for 12 hrs with fever, vomiting, coma, and convulsions. He was admitted to a hospital where examination showed severe hypoglycemia—24 mg/100 ml. Six hours later the child died, and the diagnosis of Reye's syndrome was confirmed by autopsy and histopathology. A visit to the boy's village home revealed that for two days prior to the onset of illness, the child had eaten only leftover cooked rice stored without refrigeration. The rice was moldy but organoleptically appealing; it assayed at more than 10 mg total aflatoxins/kg.

Since the rodent does not respond to aflatoxin in any way similar to Reye's syndrome, acute aflatoxicosis was re-examined in the macaque monkey and was strikingly similar to the human disease (13). Tissue analysis from monkeys in this test demonstrated recoverable aflatoxin B_1 from brain, liver, kidney, heart, bile, and blood up to six days after single oral administration of the toxin (17). This finding prompted similar analyses on autopsy specimens from Thai Reye's syndrome cases (14). Aflatoxin B_1 was found in one or more specimens from 22 of the 23 cases studied; in two instances the human tissue levels were comparable with those in the monkeys given nearly an LD_{50} dose of aflatoxin.

Becroft and Webster (18) found aflatoxin in two cases of Reye's syndrome in New Zealand, and Dvorackova (19) found the toxin in six cases in Czechoslovakia. However, we examined autopsy specimens from five cases in the United States and have not detected aflatoxin B_1 or any of its chloroform-soluble metabolites. Doris Collins (20) recognized intranuclear inclusions in pancreatic acinar cells in four New York and Massachusetts cases of Reye's syndrome and notes their similarity to such inclusions seen in macaques acutely poisoned with aflatoxin B_1 (13). These data do not establish aflatoxins as the causative agents in Reye's syndrome, but they strongly suggest that these mycotoxins should be considered as at least one factor in the genesis of the disease.

There may be an association between Reye's syndrome and liver cancer in Thailand. Reye's syndrome occurs most frequently in northeast Thailand, and, although the liver cancer rate has not been measured directly in that area, a review of hospital records covering all provinces of Thailand indicated that the northeast had the greatest number of reported cases of liver cancer per capita. However, in many instances these cases were not proved by histopathology (7), and liver parasitism, especially opisthorciasis, was also frequently reported in this area. It may be that Reye's syndrome in Thailand, as a manifestation of acute aflatoxicosis, identifies a population at increased risk for liver cancer; indeed not only greater exposure is suggested, but survivors of the acute disease may have an especially high risk for liver cancer. This possible association should be tested epidemiologically.

To complete this survey of evidence implicating aflatoxins in human disease, it is necessary to consider Indian childhood cirrhosis. This is a disease marked by infiltration of hepatocytes with neutral fat leading to degeneration, fibrosis, and hepatomegaly. In advanced stages it proceeds to jaundice, ascites, and hepatic coma. Presumptive tests indicated aflatoxin B_1 in peanuts and peanut products eaten by children with this disease and in a few samples of human milk and urine from mothers of patients (21). Kwashiorkor cases that were fed protein supplements (derived from peanuts contaminated with aflatoxins, 300 μg/kg supplement) developed central and periportal fat accumulation, fibrosis, and cirrhosis of the liver (22). More epidemiological studies are needed to assess the role of aflatoxins in Indian childhood cirrhosis.

Summary

Considerable indirect evidence suggests that the aflatoxins play a role in the etiology of primary cancer of the liver in human populations of Africa and Southeast Asia where mold damage to foods and foodstuffs is frequent. Further epidemiological studies may support this suggestion by increasing statistical significance of the data, but they are unlikely to provide a more direct association than has already been established.

Diets contaminated with aflatoxin are likely to contain other mycotoxins and food-borne toxicants, but no such agents are known which approach, even remotely, the carcinogenic potency of aflatoxin (as demonstrated in the rat and trout). For this reason primary focus on aflatoxin B_1 seems justified but does not exclude the possibility that other factors such as dietary ones also may contribute to this disease.

In addition to the chronic effects of aflatoxin consumption, circumstantial evidence suggests that this mold metabolite may be a factor in the etiology of Reye's syndrome at least as it occurs in Thailand. An epidemiological study should be carried out to evaluate more fully the role of aflatoxins in Reye's syndrome.

Literature Cited

1. Alpert, M. E., Hutt, M. S. R., Wogan, G. N., Davidson, C. S., *Cancer Res.* (1971) **28**, 253.
2. Keen, P., Martin, P., *Trop. Geogr. Med.* (1971) **23**, 35.
3. Campbell, T. C., Caedo, J. P., Jr., Bulatao-Jayme, J., Salamat, L., Engel, R. W., *Nature* (1970) **227**, 403.

4. Shank, R. C., Wogan, G. N., Gibson, J. B., *Food Cosmet. Toxicol.* (1972) **10**, 51.
5. Shank, R. C., Wogan, G. N., Gibson, J. B., Nondasuta, A., *Food Cosmet. Toxicol.* (1972) **10**, 61.
6. Shank, R. C., Gordon, J. E., Wogan, G. N., Nondasuta, A., Subhamani, B., *Food Cosmet. Toxicol.* (1972) **10**, 71.
7. Shank, R. C., Bhamarapravati, N., Gordon, J. E., Wogan, G. N., *Food Cosmet. Toxicol.* (1972) **10**, 171.
8. Shank, R. C., Siddhichai, P., Subhamani, B., Bhamarapravati, N., Gordon, J. E., Wogan, G. N., *Food Cosmet. Toxicol.* (1972) **10**, 181.
9. Peers, F. G., Linsell, C. A., *Brit. J. Cancer* (1973) **27**, 473.
10. Ling, K.-H., Wang, J.-J., Wu, R., Tung, T.-C., Lin, C.-K., Lin, S.-S., Lin, T.-M., *J. Formosan Med. Ass.* (1967) **66**, 517.
11. Serck-Hanssen, A., *Arch. Environ. Health* (1970) **20**, 729.
12. Alpert, E., Serck-Hanssen, A., Rajagopolan, B., *Arch. Environ. Health* (1970) **20**, 723.
13. Bourgeois, C. H., Shank, R. C., Grossman, R. A., Johnsen, D. O., Wooding, W. L., Chandavimol, P., *Lab. Invest.* (1971) **24**, 206.
14. Shank, R. C., Bourgeois, C. H., Keschamras, N., Chandavimol, P., *Food Cosmet. Toxicol.* (1971) **9**, 501.
15. Bourgeois, C., Olson, L., Comer, D., Evans, H., Keschamras, N., Cotton, R., Grossman, R., Smith, T., *Amer. J. Clin. Pathol.* (1971) **56**, 558.
16. Olson, L., Bourgeois, C. H., Cotton, R., Harikul, S., Grossman, R., Smith, T., *Pediatrics* (1971) **47**, 707.
17. Shank, R. C., Johnsen, D. O., Tanticharoenyos, P., Wooding, W. L., Bourgeois, C. H., *Toxicol. Appl. Pharmacol.* (1971) **20**, 227.
18. Becroft, D. M. O., Webster, D. R., *Brit. Med. J.* (1972) **4**, 117.
19. Dvorackova, Ivana, private communication.
20. Collins, D. N., *Lab. Invest.* (1974) **30**, 333.
21. Robinson, P., *Clin. Pediatrics* (1967) **6**, 57.
22. Amla, I., Kamala, C. S., Gopalakrishna, G. S., Jayaraj, A. P., Sreenivasamurthy, V., Parpia, H. A. B., *Amer. J. Clin. Nutr.* (1971) **24**, 609.

RECEIVED November 8, 1974.

4

Chemical Methods Investigated for Detoxifying Aflatoxins in Foods and Feeds

ALFRED C. BECKWITH, RONALD F. VESONDER, and ALEX CIEGLER

Northern Regional Research Laboratory, Agricultural Research Service, U.S. Department of Agriculture, Peoria, Ill. 61614

Refined edible vegetable oils are dependably free of aflatoxins because the alkaline washes and bleaching agents used in the oil processing are among the chemical systems that remove or destroy aflatoxin. Currently, ammonia in conjunction with elevated temperatures or pressures, or both, as well as elevated moisture levels offers the best way to detoxify agricultural seed commodities for feed. Research at the Northern Laboratory has shown that ammoniation of contaminated whole corn reduces aflatoxin B_1 to a chemically nondetectable level and that the ammoniation products are nontoxic to ducklings and chickens. Using radio labelled aflatoxin B_1 to spike white corn meals we showed that ammoniation at ambient temperature induces the covalent binding of B_1 or B_1 degradative products primarily to corn proteins and water-soluble components.

S everal methods have been used to detoxify the aflatoxin in agricultural commodities. Since publication of a review of these methods (1), many studies of the ability of certain chemicals to destroy aflatoxins have been undertaken (2). Any chemical detoxification must reduce the mycotoxin level to within limits set by proper regulatory agencies, must have no toxic residues, and should not decrease the nutritive value of the treated commodity. These restrictions as well as simple economic considerations have narrowed the types of chemical agents likely to achieve significance in a commercially scaled detoxification process. Chemicals having good promise in this regard can be classified simply as oxidizing agents, acid, and bases. In this review the authors try to present as much chemistry as possible relating to toxin destruction as well as results of biological assays which are not yet complete. These assays establish the overall effectiveness of any particular chemical process.

Oxidizing Agents

There are several oxidation-reduction systems that destroy the biological activity of aflatoxin B_1 and G_1 but not B_2 and G_2 (*3*). Of oxidizing systems that destroy all the aflatoxin only hydrogen peroxide has shown promise to detoxify foods and feeds (*4, 5*). Sreenivasamurthy *et al.* (*4*) treated aqueous suspensions of peanut meals containing 90 ppm aflatoxin with 6% solutions of hydrogen peroxide at pH 9.5 for 30 min at 80°C. The treatment destroyed 97% of the toxin, and the treated meals were shown to be nontoxic to ducklings. When added to wheat and chick pea flour diets, the treated peanut cake did not change the PER values of flours fed to weanling albino rats.

Researchers at the Southern Regional Research Center, USDA (*6*), compared the ability of ozone, oxygen, and air to reduce the level of aflatoxin in contaminated cottonseed and peanut meals. Heating the meals which contained 22% moisture for 2 hr at 100°C in air and oxygen reduced the toxin level by 67–76%. Under similar conditions ozonized air completely destroyed aflatoxin B_1 and G_1 in one hr. Unfortunately this treatment did not reduce the B_2 level. Ozone treatment also decreased the amount of available lysine as well as the PER values for the meals (*7*).

From accumulated chemical evidence it seems clear that the terminal double bond in the dihydrofurofuran ring of B_1 (Figure 1) is susceptible to attack by reactive forms of oxygen. In 1970 Schoental (*8*) postulated that the biological activity of B_1 entailed an epoxidation of this double bond. The work of Garner et al. (*9*) has shown that oxygen is needed before liver microsomes can convert B_1 to a reactive product. More recently Swenson and coworkers (*10*) proposed a mechanism involving oxygen to explain the *in vitro* binding of B_1 to RNA by liver microsomes.

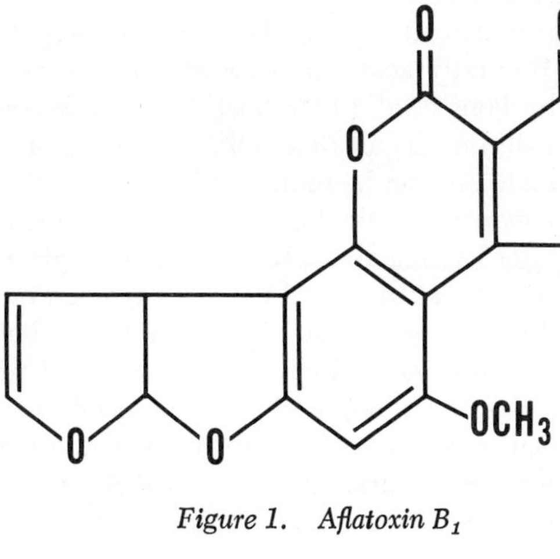

Figure 1. Aflatoxin B_1

The binding site in the B_1 molecule was at the terminal double bond. Mild acid hydrolysis of the complex produced the dihydroxy derivative of B_1. These workers also synthesized the dihydroxy derivative by the reaction of B_1 with osmium tetroxide followed by hydrolysis of the osmic acid ester.

Since aflatoxins G_1 and M_1 also contain the reactive double bond found in B_1, these two toxins might be expected to undergo a similar sequence of reactions as noted for B_1. However aflatoxins B_2, G_2, and M_2 lack the reactive double bond and yet are destroyed by hydrogen peroxide. Knowledge of this more general oxidative degradation is not available.

In closing the discussion of oxidizing agents it is of historical note to point out that hydrogen peroxide, ozone, oxygen, or air have been used occasionally in the refinement of edible oils and fats (11). While processing steps prior to those using oxidizing agents probably remove practically all of any possible toxin contamination from oils, the use of an oxidizing agent should destroy any remaining aflatoxins.

Acids

The ability of aqueous solutions of strong acids to destroy the biological activity of aflatoxins B_1 and G_1 has long been known to involve the catalytic addition of water to the terminal double bond in the furofuran ring system (12, 13, 14, 15). The hemiacetals formed by the water addition are commonly referred to as aflatoxins B_{2a} and G_{2a}. In 1966 Dutton and Heathcoate (16) reported the isolation of B_{2a} from culture media of *A. flavis*, and later Ciegler and Peterson (17) noted that B_1 could be converted to B_{2a} by acid-producing molds. In alkaline media B_{2a} readily undergoes a reversible ring opening which leads to the formation of a phenolic dialdehyde (13, 18).

The use of acids as detoxifying agents has a definite potential in the recovery process of free fatty acids from commercial soapstock preparation as pointed out by Pons et al. (19). Soapstock can become contaminated with aflatoxins during the alkaline refining process of oils and fats. Details of the acid treatment can be found in the just mentioned citation. These workers also conducted a kinetic study of the conversion of B_1 to B_{2a} and G_1 to G_{2a}. After heating at 100°C for 10 min at pH 1, 95% of B_1 is converted to B_{2a}, whereas at pH 3 and the same temperature 7 hr were needed to achieve the same extent of conversion (19). Pohland et al. (13) noted earlier that moderately high concentrations of mineral acids and elevated temperatures were required to obtain good yields of B_{2a}.

It is not likely that aqueous acid solutions will find a general use in detoxifying large quantities of agricultural commodities since moderately drastic conditions are needed by bring about the conversion of B_1 and G_1

to their water addition products; furthermore the B_2 and G_2 toxins would be relatively little affected by such treatment. Lindenfelser and Ciegler (*20*) reported that acids produced during the ensilage of corn did not bring about any inactivation of B_1 toxin.

Bases

The use of inorganic and organic bases affords an efficient and relatively inexpensive means to achieve aflatoxin destruction or removal from large quantities of contaminated agricultural commodities. The refinement of edible oils is a classic example of the use of bases under conditions that would destroy or remove aflatoxins.

Crude oils are generally washed with 0.3–8.3N sodium hydroxide solutions. This is done primarily to remove gums, free fatty acids, and base-soluble pigments from the oil (*11*). The alkaline treatment is followed by water washes and a bleaching process with special clays at elevated temperature to reduce pigment content further. As noted in the review by Dollear (*1*), any aflatoxin present in the crude oil is reduced to a low level (less than 1 μg/kg) in the standard refining process.

Finely divided calcium hydroxide has been used successfully by Espoy (*21*) to reduce aflatoxin levels in pelletized copra, peanut, and cottonseed meals. A mean particle size of 50 μ or less for the hydroxide is essential in this treatment.

With stored cereal and seed crops aflatoxins can occasionally be found randomly localized throughout the lot. To combat this problem researchers focused on volatile bases, particularly methylamine and ammonia.

Recent investigation by Kiermeier and Ruffer (*22*) have shown that toxic products are formed when aflatoxin B_1 is treated with diethanolamine; however when treated with concentrated solutions of ammonium hydroxide, acetone insoluble B_1 products were found to be nontoxic to chick embryos by Vesonder et al. (*23*).

While studying the efficacy of several reagents Dollear et al. (*7*) noted that 1.25% methylamine added to peanut meals that have 30% moisture reduced the total aflatoxin content to less than 5 μg/kg when the treated meals were heated for 90 min at 100°C in a Groen reactor. (Mention of firm names or trade products does not imply that they are endorsed or recommended by the U.S. Department of Agriculture over other firms or similar products not mentioned.) These workers found that available lysine was lowered and PER values were reduced in the treated meals. Mann and co-workers (*24*) again using methylamine, but with contaminated cottonseed meal, obtained good destruction of total toxin. In this instance aflatoxin reduction was enhanced in the presence of 1% sodium hydroxide. The methylamine treatment did not lower PER values for the cottonseed meals but did produce a temporary nontoxic liver enlargement in rats. Unfortunately other adverse biological findings in rats reported by these workers as well as economic considerations will possibly preclude the use of methylamine as a general detoxicant for animal feeds.

Ammonia as a detoxifying agent has been used as the anhydrous gas at elevated temperatures and pressures to bring about 95–98% reductions in total aflatoxin contents of peanut meals (7, 25). This level of reduction indicates almost complete destruction of B_1 and G_1 or to values less than 5 μg/kg. Likewise a similar treatment of cottonseed meals was as effective in reducing total toxin content (24, 26). Other reported findings in these citations show that PER values for treated meals are lowered, and chemical composition of the meals is altered. Ammoniated cottonseed meals have been fed to lactating cows, and the milk from these cows examined for aflatoxin M_1, a metabolic product of B_1 (27). Results from this cooperative research showed that the milk contained very low to chemically nondetectable amounts of M_1 toxin. No residual toxins could be detected in any tissues examined for the anmials fed the treated meal, thus providing good evidence of the effectiveness of ammonia as a detoxicant for ruminant feeds. Ammoniated cottonseed meals have also been used successfully in poultry diets (28).

Aflatoxin contamination is not peculiar to peanuts and cottonseeds; it has been found in corn which is used chiefly as an animal and poultry feed (29). Currently is progress at the North Central Region of USDA are intensive investigations concerning the use of ammonia as a means of detoxifying contaminated corn. Aside from preliminary findings most of the work done is this region is unpublished. As reported by Lancaster (30), engineers at the Northern Regional Research Laboratory applied concentrated ammonium hydroxide to corn samples to bring the ammonia as NH_3 to 0.5–2.0 g/kg of corn. The treated corn held in sealed containers is maintained at 25°–50°C for periods ranging from a few days to several weeks. This method of ammonia treatment can reduce B_1 content to a nondetectable level in most cases. Reporting the results of a private communication from fellow workers, Ciegler (31) cited a specific example of this treatment. Yellow dent corn initially containing 1200 μg/kg B_1 and 120 μg/kg B_2 was treated with 1.5% ammonia for 8 days at 26°–47°C; the B_1 content was reduced to 15 μg/kg, and B_2 was reduced to about 1 μg/kg. The authors point out on the basis of personal knowledge that all biological tests with ducklings, chickens, and currently with rainbow trout show encouraging results, indicating that ammonia is also suitable for detoxifying corn even though it is used under reaction conditions different from those employed with peanuts and cottonseeds. However the treatment cannot be recommended for use until biological testing is completed and FDA clearance is obtained.

The authors have been interested primarily in the chemistry of B_1 destruction by ammonia (23, 32). The common aflatoxins are substituted coumarin derivatives and as such are aromatic lactones. Wogan (33) noted from accumulated evidence that the lactone function is also partly responsible for aflatoxin biological activity. As lactones, the initial action of a base on these toxins is to convert them to the salts of their corresponding o-coumaric acid derivatives (34). This conversion to salts changes toxin solubility which is used in crude oil refinement.

Recently Lee and associates (35) reported a lactone ring opening in B_1 when the toxin was heated at 100°C in a Parr bomb with concentrated ammonium hydroxide. Under these drastic conditions the reaction proceeded through a decarboxylation step to yield a new B_1 derivative (aflatoxin D_1) with a molecular weight of 286. According to Coomes et al. (36) the lactone ring of B_1 is opened merely upon refluxing in water, and spectral evidence is given for this ring opening. Heat and pressure are not needed for ammonium hydroxide ring opening as shown in Figure 2. The molar absorbance for B_1 in methanol at 363 nm is 22,400. In concentrated ammonium hydroxide the authors (23) noted that the position of the maxima does not change, but the molar absorbance is reduced to 13,400. When the basic solution is taken to dryness and redissolved in water, the ultraviolet spectrum has a very broad band with a maximum near 325 nm. In accordance with the interpretation of Coomes et al. (36) this spectrum in water indicates the presence of free acid and ammonium

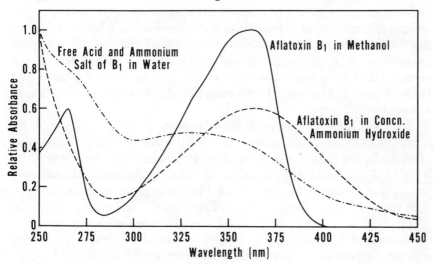

Figure 2.   Relative ultraviolet absorbance (300–400 nm) for B_1 in various solvents

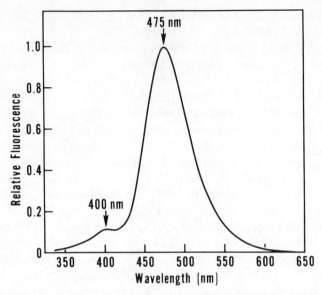

Figure 3.   Relative fluorescence of B_1 in ammonium hydroxide solution

salt. The spectrum for B_1 in ammonium hydroxide (Figure 2) extends beyond 400 nm in contrast to the B_1 spectrum in methanol. This extension of absorbance beyond 400 nm could suggest the formation of a new absorbance band. The results shown in Figure 3 also indicate the existence of a new absorbance band. When excited with 400 nm radiation, B_1 in ammonium hydroxide fluoresces with an emission maxima at 475 nm. The authors are unaware of any report of B_1 fluorescence in a basic media, but this fluorescence has been observed in model solid reaction systems at our Laboratory (32). Although the authors cannot state definitely that the hemiacetal of B_1 is formed in basic media, it is interesting to note that Pohland et al. (13) observed an intense absorbance band with maxima at 404 nm for B_{2a}.

A very brief summary of the chemistry of B_1 detoxification by ammonia in contaminated corn appears in Figure 4. Using ^{14}C labelled aflatoxin B_1 the authors (32) found that ammonia treatment eventually leads to the covalent binding of B_1 to corn components, primarily the protein and water-soluble constituents. In the upper portion of Figure 4, B_1 is presented as a resonance form of the ionized acid after lactone ring opening. This form better demonstrates the possibility for reversible electrostatic and/or hydrogen bond interaction with substrates. Prolonged exposure to base in the heterogenous reaction media eventually leads to chemical modification of the difuran ring segment of the toxin and subsequently to covalent attachment to toxin to substrate. As shown schematically in Figure 4, acidification of the reaction media leaves the B_1 chromophore chemically bonded to corn substrate. Finally, based upon a mathematical analysis of data available (37), the simple scheme shown at the bottom of Figure 4 appears adequate to develop a description for the time- and temperature-dependent destruction of B_1. Base and moisture are generally in excess and therefore not specifically indicated in this scheme. The quantity B represents B_1 in the alkaline reaction media, and S represents the corn substrate. Integration of the appropriate rate expression obtained with this scheme yields Equation 1.

$$\frac{B_1 \text{ (at time } t \text{ after acidification)}}{B_1 \text{ (present initially)}} = \alpha + (1 - \alpha)e^{-kt} \qquad (1)$$

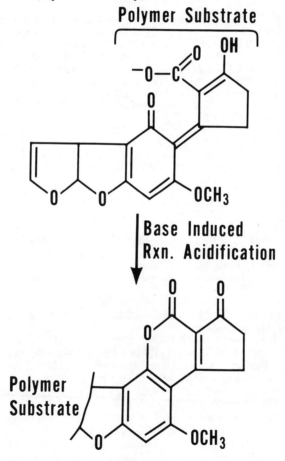

$$B + S \rightleftharpoons SB \longrightarrow P$$

Figure 4. *Proposed sequences for B_1 destruction in corn by ammonia*

In relation to the scheme in Figure 4 the quantity α in Equation 1 has the definition $\alpha = 1/[1 + K_{ASSOC} \cdot S]$ and represents a plateau value to which the relative B_1 level is reduced. As the temperature increases, α rapidly approaches zero to represent the chemically nondectable B_1 level. Also, as the temperature is raised the time required to achieve this level decreases. Equation 1 could have a more general application than indicated here. Within the analytical error for aflatoxin content, Equation 1 might adequately describe the extent of toxin reduction noticed by others —e.g., the results given by Dwarakanath et al. (6) and by Cater et al. (5).

Literature Cited

1. Dollear, F. G., "Detoxification of Aflatoxins in Foods and Feeds," in "Afla-toxin-Scientific Background, Control, and Implications," Chapter XIII (L. A. Goldblatt, Ed.), pp. 359-391, Academic, New York, 1969.
2. Goldblatt, L. A., *J. Am. Oil Chem. Soc.* (1971) **48**, 605.
3. Trager, W., Stoloff, L., *J. Agric. Food Chem.* (1967) **15**, 679.
4. Sreenivasamurthy, V., Parpia, H. A. B., Srikanta, S., Shankarmurti, A., *J. Assoc. Off. Anal. Chem.* (1967) **50**, 350.
5. Cater, C. M., Rhee, K. C., Hagenmaier, R. D., Mattil, K. F., *J. Am. Oil Chem. Soc.* (1974) **51**, 137.
6. Dwarakanath, C. T., Rayner, E. T., Mann, G. E., Dollear, F. G., *J. Am. Oil Chem. Soc.* (1968) **45**, 93.
7. Dollear, F. G., Mann, G. E., Codifer, L. P., Jr., Gardner, H. K., Jr., Koltun, S. P., Viv, H. L. E., *J. Am. Oil Chem. Soc.* (1968) **45**, 862.
8. Schoental, R., *Nature* (1970) **227**, 401.
9. Garner, R. C., Miller, E. C., Miller, J. A., Garner, J. V., Hanson, R. S., *Biochem. Biophys. Res. Commun.* (1971) **45**, 774.
10. Swenson, D. H., Miller, J. A., Miller, E. C., *Biochem. Biophys. Res. Commun.* (1973) **53**, 1260.
11. Andersen, A. J. C., "Refining of Oils and Fats for Edible Purposes," (P. N. Williams, Ed.), 2nd ed., Pergamon, New York, 1962.
12. Andrellos, P. J., Reid, G. R., *J. Assoc. Off. Anal. Chem.* (1964) **47**, 801.
13. Pohland, A. E., Cushmac, M. E., Andrellos, P. J., *J. Assoc. Off. Anal. Chem.* (1968) **51**, 907.
14. Dutton, M. F., Heathcote, J. G., *Chem. Ind.* (1968) 418.
15. Verrett, M. J., Marliac, J. P., McLaughlin, J., Jr., *J. Assoc. Off. Anal. Chem.* (1964) **47**, 1003.
16. Dutton, M. F., Heathcote, J. G., *Biochem. J.* (1966) **101**, 21P.
17. Ciegler, A., Peterson, R. E., *Appl. Microbiol.* (1968) **16**, 665.
18. Büchi, G., Foulker, D. M., Kurouo, M., Mitchell, G. F., Schneider, S. R., *J. Am. Chem. Soc.* (1967) **89**, 6745.
19. Pons, W. A., Jr., Cucullu, A. F., Lee, L. S., Janssen, H. J., Goldblatt, L. A., *J. Am. Oil Chem. Soc.* (1972) **49**, 124.
20. Lindenfelser, L. A., Ciegler, A., *J. Agric. Food Chem.* (1970) **18**, 640.
21. Espoy, H. M., U.S. Patent 3,689,275 (1972).
22. Kiermeier, F., Ruffer, L., *Z. Lebensm. Unters. Forsch.* (1974) **155**, 129.
23. Vesonder, R. F., Beckwith, A. C., Ciegler, A., Dimler, R. J., *J. Agric. Food Chem.* (1975) **23**, 242.
24. Mann, G. E., Gardner, H. K., Jr., Booth, A. N., Gumbmann, M. R., *J. Agric. Food Chem.* (1971) **19**, 1155.
25. Masri, M. S., Vix, H. L. E., Goldblatt, L. A., U.S. Patent 3,429,709 (1969).

26. Gardner, H. K., Jr., Koltun, S. P., Dollear, F. G., Rayner, E. T., *J. Am. Oil Chem. Soc.* (1971) **48**, 70.
27. McKinney, J. D., Cavanagh, G. C., Bell, J. T., Hoversland, A. S., Nelson, D. M., Pearson, J., Selkirk, R. J., *J. Am. Oil Chem. Soc.* (1973) **50**, 79.
28. Reid, R.L., *Feedstuffs* (1972) **44** (46), 42.
29. Shotwell, O. L., Hesseltine, C. W., Goulden, M. L., *Cereal Sci. Today* (1973) **18**, 192.
30. Lancaster, E. B., "Chemical Detoxification of Aflatoxin Contaminated Corn." Presented before the 13th Annual Corn Dry Milling Conference, June 14-15, 1972, Peoria, Ill.
31. Ciegler A., "Aflatoxin Removal or Inactivation in Selected Commodities." Presented before the North Carolina Nutrition Conference, Dec. 5-6, 1973, Raleigh, N.C.
32. Beckwith, A. C., Vesonder, R. F., Ciegler, A., *J. Agric. Food Chem.* (1975) **23**, 582.
33. Wogan, G. N., "Aflatoxin Carcinogenesis," in "Methods in Cancer Research," (H. Busch, Ed.), Chapter VII, pp. 309-344, Academic, New York, 1973.
34. Parker, W. A., Melnich, D., *J. Am. Oil Chem. Soc.* (1966) **43**, 635.
35. Lee, L. S., Stanley, J. B., Cucullu, A. F., Pons, W. A., Jr., Goldblatt, L. A., *J. Assoc. Off. Anal. Chem.* (1974) **57**, 626.
36. Coomes, T. J., Crowther, P. C., Feuell, A. J., Francis, B. J., *Nature* (1966) **209**, 406.
37. Brekke, O. L., Lancaster, E. B., Northern Regional Research Center, 1973, private communication.

RECEIVED November 8, 1974.

5

Aspergillus Toxins Other Than Aflatoxin

RICHARD J. COLE

National Peanut Research Laboratory, U.S. Department of Agriculture, P.O. Box 637, Dawson, Ga. 31742

Available physical, chemical, and biological data are presented for all known Aspergillus *mycotoxins other than the aflatoxins with emphasis on the chemistry of those that are of major interest. Included in this latter category are the ochratoxins, the sterigmatocystins, and the aspergillic acid group. Other* Aspergillus *mycotoxins presented in less detail are kojic acid, austamide, ascladiol, terreic acid, viriditoxin, cytochalasin E, maltoryzine, 3-nitropropanoic acid, oxalic acid, helvolic acid, gliotoxin, fumigatin, fumagillin, terrein, spinulosin, and butenolide.*

Members of the genus *Aspergillus* represent some of the most prevalent mycotoxin-producing fungi associated with feed and food materials. The known mycotoxins of *Aspergillus spp.*, other than aflatoxins, are presented in this review. Major emphasis is on the chemistry of those *Aspergillus* toxins currently recognized to be of major interest, including the ochratoxins, the sterigmatocystins, and aspergillic acid. All *Aspergillus* toxins, until proved otherwise, are considered potentially hazardous to animal health.

Ochratoxins

The ochratoxins comprise a group of chemically related metabolites isolated originally from culture extracts of *Aspergillus ochraceus* (*1, 2*) and subsequently from other *Aspergillus spp.* (*3*) and from *Penicillium viridicatum* (*4, 5*). The achratoxins contain a 3,4-dihydro-3-methylisocoumarin moiety linked through a carboxyl group to L-β-phenylalanine by a secondary amide bond. The most toxic derivatives, ochratoxins A (Structure Ia) and C (Structure Ic) contain a chlorine atom at position 5 (*6, 7, 8*). Ochratoxin B (Structure Ib), which differs from ochratoxin A

Structure I.   *Ochratoxins*
Ia: $R = H$, $R_t = Cl$, $R_2 = H$
Ib: $R = H$, $R_t = H$, $R_2 = H$
Ic: $R = C_2H_5$, $R_t = Cl$, $R_2 = H$
Id: $R = H$, $R_t = Cl$, $R_2 = OH$

by the absence of chlorine at position 5, was considerably less toxic (*6, 8, 9*). Chu et al. (*10*) postulated that the chlorine atoms on ochratoxins A and C play an indirect role in toxicity. They presented a direct correlation between the dissociation constants for the phenolic hydroxyl groups on the ochratoxins and their acute toxicity. They suggested that the phenolic hydroxyl group in the dissociated form was necessary for toxicity and that the chlorine atom may have a direct effect on the dissociation of the phenolic hydroxyl groups in ochratoxins A and C, rendering them toxic. They further noted that the acid dissociation constant of ochratoxin B was one-tenth as large as ochratoxin A, and the toxicity of ochratoxin B was correspondingly about one-tenth that of ochratoxin A (*9*).

Data on the toxicity of the recently reported 4-hydroxyochratoxin A (Structure Id) were not presented in detail, but the toxin was reported to be non-lethal to rats at 40 mg/kg (intraperitoneal) (*5*). Ochratoxin A was lethal to all rats tested at this dosage level.

The chemical structures of the ochratoxins were elucidated by South African scientists (*1, 2, 6*) and subsequently proved by synthesis (*11*). Acid hydrolysis of ochratoxin A gave L-β-phenylalanine and 7-carboxy-5-chloro-3,4-dihydro-8-hydroxy-3-methylisocoumarin. Support for a secondary amide was presented by the IR spectrum which showed a typical amide I band at 1678 cm^{-1} (C=O stretchin) and amide II band at 1535 cm^{-1} (N–H bending) and at 3380 cm^{-1} (N–H stretching). Carboxyl group absorptions appeared at 1723 cm^{-1} (C=O stretching), and a broad band appeared between 2500 and 3000 cm^{-1} (O–H stretching). The lactone function was observed at 1678 cm^{-1} (shifted to lower frequency because of intramolecular H bonding with the 8 hydroxyl group) and at 1132 cm^{-1} (C–O–C stretching).

The uv spectrum of ochratoxin A showed λ_{max}^{EtOH} 215 ($\epsilon = 36{,}800$) and 333 nm ($\epsilon = 6400$); ochratoxin B had the same uv spectrum with the exception of a hypsochromatic shift of the long wave length band (λ_{max}^{EtOH} 218, $\epsilon = 37{,}200$ and 318 nm, $\epsilon = 6900$) (*2*).

The high resolution mass spectrum of ochratoxin A showed m/e 403.08187 with a calculated elemental composition of $C_{20}H_{18}ClNO_6$ and, in accordance with the calculated formula, an isotope peak at m/e 405 (*2*). A protonated molecular ion peak at nominal mass 404 was observed in the low resolution mass spectrum of ochratoxin A after chemical ionization with isobutane.

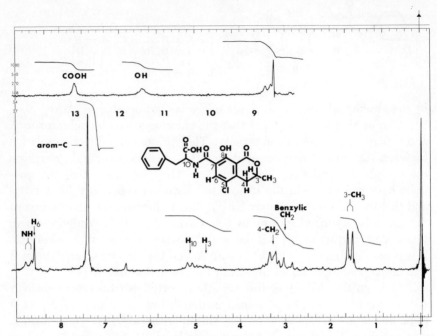

*Figure 1. Sixty MHz proton magnet resonance spectrum of ochratoxin in chloroform-*d *solution*

The proton magnetic resonance spectrum of ochratoxin A (Figure 1) consisted of an ABX system in the 3,4-dihydroisocoumarin moiety. The signals for the secondary methyl at position 3 resonated at δ 1.54 as a doublet (J = 7.0 Hz). Included in this system were the methylene protons at position 4 which resonated at δ 3.2 (complex signal) and the methine proton at position 3 which resonated at approximately δ 4.75 (complex signal). These signals are similar to those observed for the same 3,4-dihydroisocoumarin system in mellein (Structure II) (12): the methine proton (position 3) appeared as a sextet at δ 4.50 (J = 7.0 Hz). Strongly coupled to the methine proton were the secondary methyl (position 3) which resonated at δ 1.50 as a doublet (J = 7.0 Hz) and the methylene protons (position 4) which resonated at δ 2.83 as a doublet (J = 7.0 Hz). (These three values were incorrectly reported as 3.0 Hz.) Nearly superimposed on the methylene protons (δ 3.20) of ochratoxin A was a complex two-proton signal assigned to the benzylic methylene protons, and nearly superimposed on the methine signal (δ 4.55) was a

Structure II.
Mellein

complex signal (δ 5.02) assigned to the methine proton positioned next to the amide nitrogen. The single aromatic proton of the dihydroisocoumarin moiety resonated at δ 8.60 as a singlet; the five aromatic protons of phenylalanine resonated at δ 7.40 as a singlet. The carboxyl proton was observed at δ 13.00 and the hydroxyl protein at δ 11.61. The extreme downfield position of the latter was typical of an H-bonded OH group. This same extreme downfield position was reported for the H-bonded dihydroisocoumarin OH protons of mellein and 4-hydroxymellein (δ = 11.03 and 11.03) (*12*). The amide proton on ochratoxin A resonated at δ 8.75 as a doublet (*J* = 8.0 Hz). The NMR spectrum of ochratoxin B contained similar chemical shifts but differed from ochratoxin A by the presence of two ortho-coupled aromatic protons (located on positions 5 and 6) resonating at δ 8.22 and 7.05 (*J* = 8.0 Hz) (*2*).

The ^{13}C-NMR (off center resonance decoupling spectrum) of dimethylisocoumarin carboxylate as presented by Maebayashi et al. (*13*) is shown in Figure 2. The two signals occurring at lowest field, 31.56 and 27.65 ppm downfield from CS_2, were assigned to carbonyl carbons 1 and 11 respectively. The chemical shifts between 71.08 and 49.12 ppm were assigned to the aromatic carbons with the signal for the aromatic carbon C-6 easily recognized from the off resonance decoupling spectrum. The two methoxy carbons were located at 128.19 and 139.80 ppm. The methylene carbon at C-4 was observed at 158.66 ppm; the tertiary methyl (C-10) on position 3 of the dihydroisocoumarin moiety was at 171.95 ppm. The methine carbon (C-3) was assigned to the chemical shift at 118.79 ppm.

The most recent ochratoxin-type compound reported was 4-hydroxyochratoxin A (Structure Id) (*5*) from *Penicillium viridicatum*. Characteristic differences between the NMR spectra of ochratoxin A and 4-hydroxyochratoxin A were in the dihydroisocoumarin moiety. An AMY_3

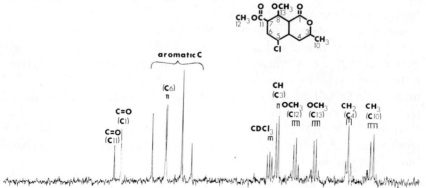

Figure 2. ^{13}C—*off center resonance decoupling spectrum of dimethylisocoumarin carborylate in chloroform-d solution*

system in the 3,4 positioned area was evident in the NMR spectrum of 4-hydroxyochratoxin A whereas ochratoxin A had an ABX system in this region. The AMY_3 system consisted of the following: a secondary methyl at position 3 which appeared as a doublet at δ 1.68 ($J = 7.0$ Hz), the methine proton at position 3 which resonated as a quaretet of doublets at δ 4.80 ($J = 2, 7$ Hz), and the methine proton on position 4 which resonated as a doublet at δ 5.11 ($J = 2$ Hz).

The biosynthesis of the ochratoxins has been studied with the aid of ^{14}C- and ^{13}C-labeled precursors. It has been demonstrated that phenylalanine was incorporated directly into the ochratoxins (13, 14, 15), and it was presumed that the biosynthesis of phenylalanine occurred in the usual manner—i.e., via the shikimic acid pathway. Searcy et al. (14) reported that their data were consistent with the hypothesis that the major portion of the isocoumarin moiety of ochratoxin A was synthesized via acetate condensation with most of the ^{14}C-label from supplemented [2-^{14}C] sodium acetate located in carbons 2, 4, and 6 (Structure III).

Structure III.   Ochratoxin A

(The numbering system of the isocoumarin nucleus introduced by Searcy et al. (14) is retained to facilitate discussion.) They observed little or no radioactivity in carbons 1, 3, 5. 9, 10, or 11 of the isocoumarin moiety. They concluded that the absence of radioactivity in carbon 10 suggested that it was not derived from acetate. In similar studies, Steyn and Holzapfel (15) reported that the isocoumarin acid moiety was derived from five acetate units by head-to-tail condensation, and they concluded, therefore, that carbons 9 and 10 were also derived from acetate. They suggested that the absence of appreciable radioactivity observed by Searcy et al. (14) in carbons 9 and 10 may have arisen from a low yield of acetate from degradation experiments and from the reliance on total radioactivity rather than on specific radioactivity. They also established with the aid of methionine-S-$^{14}CH_3$ that the source of the carboxyl carbon at position 4 was via transmethylation probably from S-adenosylmethionine. More recently Maebayashi et al. (13) using ^{13}C-NMR studies confirmed the participation of sodium formate-^{13}C in the formation of the carboxyl function at position 4.

These studies strongly suggested that the isocoumarin acid was derived via the acetate–malonate pathway with the exception of the carboxyl function at C_4 which was derived from the C_1 pool. The point in the biosynthesis of ochratoxin A at which the chlorine atom was incorporated was not determined. It was assumed that phenylalanine was formed via the shikimic acid pathway.

Sterigmatocystins

The sterigmatocystins are a group of closely related fungal metabolites characterized by a xanthone nucleus fused to a dihydrodifurano or a tetrahydrodifurano moiety. The most economically important member of the group is sterigmatocystin (Structure IVa) from *Aspergillus versicolor* (*16*), *A. nidulans*, *A. rugulosus*, and *Bipoloris sp.* (*17*), other members include aspertoxin (3-hydroxy-6,7-dimethoxydifuroxanthone) (Structure IVb), (*18, 19, 20*), O-methylsterigmatocystin (Structure IVc) (*21*) and dihydro-O-methylsterigmatocystin (Structure Va) (*22*), from *Aspergillus flavus;* 5-methoxysterigmatocystin (Structure IVd) (*23*),

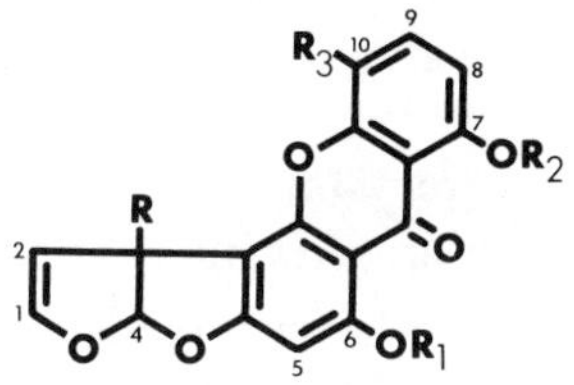

Structure IV. Sterigmato-
cystins
IVa: R = H, R₁ = CH₃, R₂ = H, R₃ = H
IVb: R = OH, R₁ = CH₃, R₂ = CH₃, R₃ = H
IVc: R = H, R₁ = CH₃, R₂ = CH₃, R₃ = H
IVd: R = H, R₁ = CH₃, R₂ = H, R₃ = OCH₃
IVe: R = H, R₁ = H, R₂ = H, R₃ = H

6-demethylsterigmatosystin (Structure IVe) (*24*), dihydrosterigmatocystin (Structure Vb) (*25*), and dihydrodemethylsterigmatocystin (Structure Vc) (*25*) from *Aspergillus versicolor*. The major differences among the various sterigmatocystins are the presence or absence of unsaturation in the difurano ring system (similar to aflatoxins B_1 and B_2) and in the substitution pattern on positions 6, 7, and 10 of the xanthone ring system and/or position 3 of the difurano system.

Englebrecht and Altenkirk (*26*) studied the toxicity of sterigmatocystin analogs on primary cell cultures. They concluded that compounds containing the $\Delta^{1,2}$-furobenzofuran-ring system (Structure IV) were more toxic than those containing a saturated furobenzofuran-ring system (Structure V). The carcinogenicity of sterigmatocystin has been well docu-

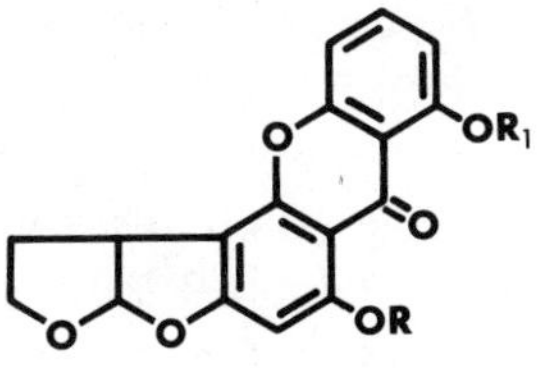

Structure V. Sterigma-
tocystins
Va: R = CH₃, R₁ = CH₃
Vb: R = CH₃, R₁ = H
Vc: R = H, R₁ = H

mented (27, 28, 29). Engelbrecht and Altenkirk (26) further suggested that a carbonyl group unsaturated in the α,β position and an unsaturated bond in the $\Delta^{1,2}$-position are required for carcinogenicity. Also a methoxy group at position 6 enhanced toxicity of these compounds, and a methoxy group at position 7 decreased toxicity. Holzapfel et al. (17), in studies on the acute toxicity of sterigmatocystin to albino rats, reported LD_{50} values of 120–166 mg/kg (per os) and 60–65 mg/kg (IP).

Bullock et al. (16) elucidated the chemical structure of sterigmatocystin. Sterigmatocystin is a pale yellow crystalline compound with a melting point of 246°C (dec) (30). Its uv spectrum showed λ_{max}^{EtOH} 208, 235, 249, and 329 nm (log ϵ 4.28, 4.39, 4.44, and 4.12, respectively) (16). The uv spectrum agreed with spectra of many other hydroxylated and/or methoxylated xanthones (30). The most characteristic features of the infrared (ir) spectrum of sterigmatocystin were 3450 cm^{-1} (OH), 1650 cm^{-1} (γ-pyrone), 1627 cm^{-1}, 1610 cm^{-1}, and 1590 cm^{-1} (phenyl) (16).

The high resolution mass spectrum of sterigmatocystin showed m/e 324.0627 which analyzed for $C_{18}H_{11}O_6$. The most prominent peak in the chemical-ionization mass spectrum was at nominal mass m/e 325 with no prominent fragment ions.

The proton NMR spectrum of sterigmatocystin consisted of chemical shifts for two different systems: the dihydrodifurano system and the xanthone system. Coupling between the three nonequivalent protons of the xanthone system, H_8, H_9, and H_{10}, gave rise to an ABX spectrum in which $J_{AX} = J_{BX} = 8.1$ Hz (Figure 3). The X portion of this spectrum consisted of a triplet at δ 7.64 ($J = 8.1$ Hz). The AB portion of the spectrum was complicated by the H_4 proton of the dihydrodifurano ring system which resonated in the same area (superimposed on chemical shifts for H_8 and H_{10} between δ 6.7–7.0) (Figure 3). However, Bullock et al. (16) observed a coupling constant of 2 Hz in a complex group corresponding to the chemical shifts of the H_8 and H_{10} protons (about δ 6.8; $J_{AB} = 2$ Hz) of sterigmatocystin. Rodricks et al. (19) reported that the corresponding AB portion of the ABX system (xanthone protons) in aspertoxin acetate was not entirely discernible, but three doublets were observed with a coupling constant of 1 Hz (δ 6.98 and 6.78; $J_{AB} = 1$ Hz) in the region of the H_8 and H_{10} protons. The remaining doublet was superimposed on the acetal proton (H_4) of the dihydrodifurano system. Therefore, analysis of the ABX system of aspertoxin acetate was $J_{AX} = J_{BX} = 8.0$ Hz (ortho substituted) and $J_{AB} = 1$ Hz (meta substituted) (19).

NMR analysis of the corresponding protons in the spectrum of di-hydro-o-methylsterigmatocystin (22) provided a more discernible view of the xanthone protons since the acetal proton (doublet δ 6.5, $J = 6.0$ Hz) was not superimposed on the chemical shifts of protons H_8 and H_{10} of the

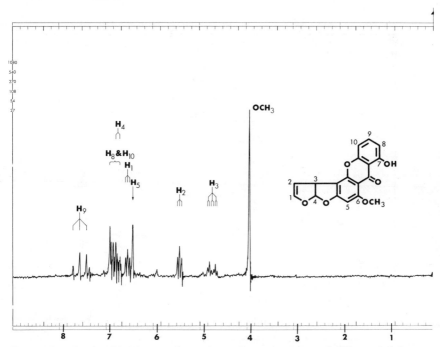

*Figure 3. Proton NMR spectrum of sterigmatocystin in cloroform-*d *solution*

xanthone system. It can be readily observed from this spectrum (Figure 4) that the X portion of the spectrum (H_9 proton) again appeared as a di-ortho triplet at δ 7.57 ($J = 8.0$ Hz); the AB portion (H_8 and H_{10}) resonated as two ortho-meta doublet of doublets at δ 7.0 and 6.8, respectively ($J = 8.0$ Hz and 1.0 Hz). The values for $J_{AX} = J_{BX} = 8.0$ Hz and $J_{AB} = 1.0$ Hz also agree with *J*-ortho and *J*-meta for benzenoid systems.

The NMR spectrum of sterigmatocystin also contained the typical chemical shifts for protons of a dihydrodifurano system similar to those observed for the corresponding protons in aflatoxin B_1 (*31, 33*) (Figure 3): H_1 = triplet, δ 6.62 ($J = 2.5$ Hz); H_2 = triplet, δ 5.50 ($J = 2.5$ Hz); H_3 = triplets of doublet, δ 4.81 ($J = 2.5$ and 7.0 Hz); H_4 = doublet, ca. δ 6.85 ($J = 7$ Hz). The noncoupled aromatic proton, H_5, resonated at δ 6.50 as a singlet, and the methoxy protons at position 6 were observed at δ 4.00 (Figure 3) (*16*).

The structural analysis of the *p*-bromobenzoate derivative of sterigmatocystin by x-ray diffraction (*33*) agreed with the structure of sterigmatocystin proposed by Bullock et al. (*16*). The structural assignment of sterigmatocystin was verified further through total synthesis (±)-*O*-methylsterigmatocystin (*34*) and by the conversion of *O*-methyldihydrosterigmatocystin into dihydroaspertoxin by treating it with methanolic alkali and then with lead tetraacetate and dilute alkaline hydrolysis (*1*).

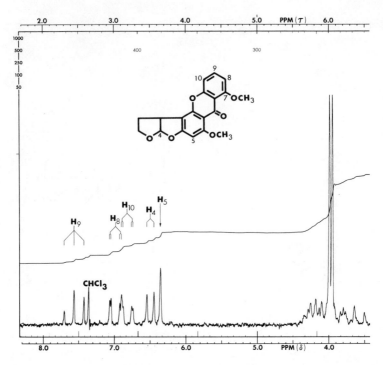

Figure 4.   Proton NMR spectrum of dihydro-O-methylsterigmato-
cystin in chloroform-d solution

Holker and Mulheirn (35) studied the biosynthesis of sterigmatocystin by degradation of ^{14}C-labeled toxin produced by *Aspergillus versicolor*
from [1-^{14}C] acetate. They reported that the distribution of radioactivity
indicated that the xanthone ring system in sterigmatocystin probably
originated via the acetate–malonate pathway and that the 4-carbon bisfuran moiety also seemed to arise from head-to-tail condensation of two
acetate units with the C—C bond joining the xanthone and bisfuran
moieties derived from acetate methyl groups. They also observed that
the level of radioactivity in the bisfuran moiety was significantly lower
than that in the xanthone system. From the above observations Holker
and Mulheirn (35) suggested that sterigmatocystin was derived from two
separate ketide units combined in an unknown fashion.

Since sterigmatocystins, versicolorins, and aflatoxins all contain the
furobenzofuran ring system, it has been speculated that they have a
common biogenetic pathway or that the aflatoxins may be derived from
sterigmatocystin and/or versicolorin type precursors (32, 35, 36, 37).
Recent evidence partially supported these hypotheses. Hsieh et al. (38)
demonstrated that ^{14}C-sterigmatocystin was efficiently converted to aflatoxin B_1 by the resting mycelium of *Aspergillus paraciticus*. Their results

indicated a biosynthetic pathway leading from 5-hydroxysterigmatocystin to sterigmatocystin and then to aflatoxin B_1. Schroeder et al. (*39*) reported that an orange versicolorin-type pigment, tentatively identified as versiconal acetate, accumulated in cultures of *Aspergillus flavus* with a concomitant reduction in aflatoxin production as a result of the inhibitory action of the insecticide dichlorvos.

Aspergillic Acid

Aspergillic acid (Structure VI), first of a number of closely related pyrazine metabolites reported, was discovered and named by White (*40*) and White and Hill (*41*). As with many other mycotoxins, aspergillic acid was originally discovered because of its antibiotic properties. Aspergillic acid and its analogs are major metabolites of certain strains of *A. flavus* and other *Aspergillus* spp.

Aspergillic acid is acutely toxic to mice (100–150 mg/kg, ip) but has no chronic effects at sublethal dosages (*41*). The analogs of aspergillic acid showed ranges of toxicity from near zero to toxicity equaling that for aspergillic acid (*42, 43, 44*). Toxicity appeared to be related to the hydroxamic acid functionality, and little effect on toxicity was observed for differences in the 3 and 6 positioned side-chain substituents.

MacDonald (*45, 46*) in studies with DL-leucine-^{14}C and L-isoleucine-^{14}C showed that *Aspergillus flavus* synthesized aspergillic acid and hydroxyaspergillic acid (Structure VII) from one molecule of leucine plus one molecule of isoleucine. This conclusion was based on the fact that aspergillic acid from medium supplemented with L-isoleucine-^{14}C had most of the radioactivity in the isoleucine moiety and only a small amount in the leucine moiety. The opposite was found when aspergillic acid was produced in medium supplemented with DL-leucine-[14]C. Data were similar from studies on the biosynthesis of hydroxyaspergillic acid. In another study aspergillic acid-^{14}C was converted to hydroxyaspergillic acid-^{14}C, but the reverse was not true. Also, in the early stages of growth of *A. flavus*, more aspergillic acid than hydroxyaspergillic acid was present in the medium, but in the later stages, hydroxyaspergillic acid predominated. The above findings support the hypothesis that hydroxyaspergillic acid is produced irreversibly from aspergillic acid.

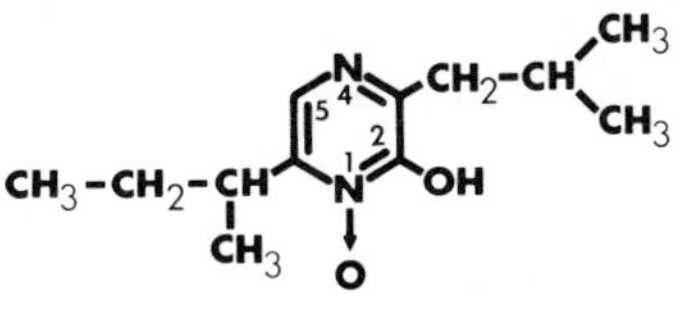

Structure VI. Aspergillic Acid

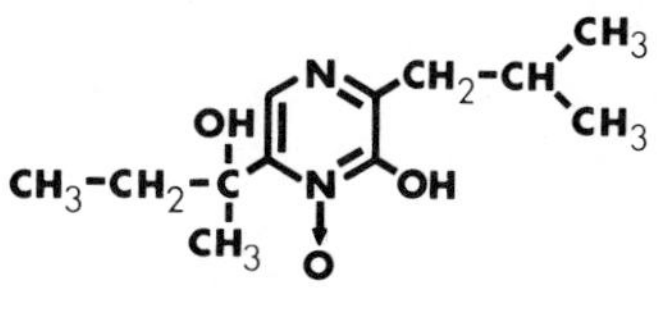

Structure VII. Hydroxyaspergillic Acid

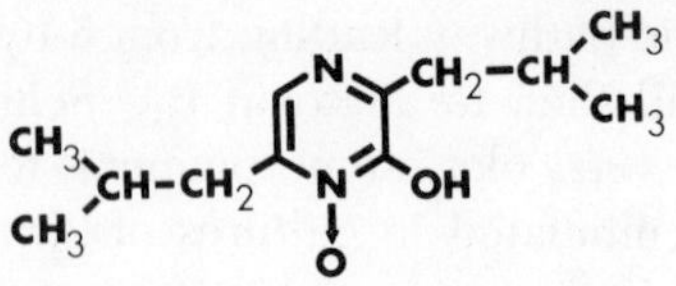

Structure VIII. Neoaspergillic
Acid

In later studies using radioisotopes, Micetich and MacDonald (47)
showed that neoaspergillic acid (Structure VIII) was biosynthesized from
two molecules of leucine. Results also strongly suggested that the sequence in the biosynthesis of neoaspergillic acid was (2) leucine →
flavacol (Structure IX) → neoaspergillic acid → neohydroxyaspergillic
acid (Structure X).

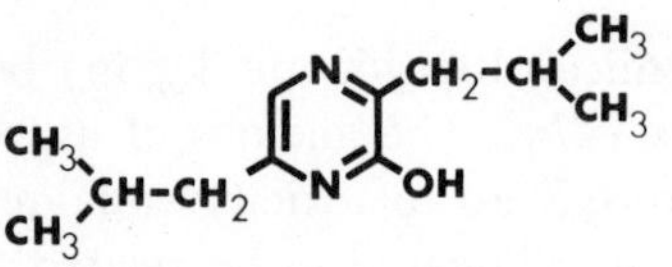

Stucture IX. Flavacol

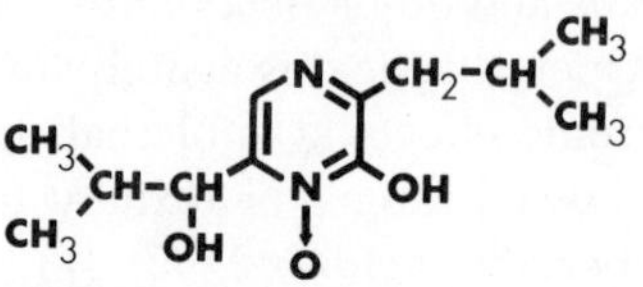

Structure X. Neohydroxyaspergillic Acid

Elucidation of the chemical structure of aspergillic acid ($C_{12}H_{20}N_2O_2$)
(Structure VI) primarily arose from the work of Dutcher (48, 49)
and Dutcher and Wintersteiner (50) along with subsequent studies by
other investigators which eventually revised the nature of the side chains
and established their location on the pyrazine ring (51, 52, 53, 54).

Principle chemical features of aspergillic acid are pyrazine ring,
cyclic hydroxamic acid, sec-butyl and isobutyl moieties. The various
analogs of aspergillic acid differ from each other primarily in the nature
of the side-chain substituents on positions 3 and 6. Aspergillic acid and
most analogs can exist in either the hydroxamic acid form (2-hydroxy-
pyrazine-1-oxide) or the 1-hydroxy-2-pyrazinone form (Structure XI).

The uv spectrum of aspergillic acid was λ_{max}^{EtOH} 328 (ϵ = 8500)
and 235 nm (ϵ = 10,500) and λ_{max} 336 nm (ϵ = 10,800) in 0.05M phosphate buffer, pH 7.3. The ir spectrum showed absorptions at 3120, 2940,

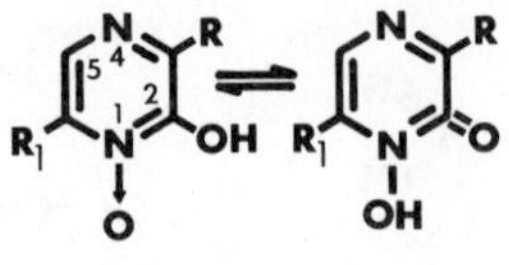

Structure XI. $A \rightleftharpoons B$
Aspergillic Acid Nu-
cleus

2850, 2800–2250 (broad), 2040 (absent in chloroform solution), 1640, 1585, 1150, and 710 cm⁻¹ (*48*).

The NMR spectrum of aspergillic acid taken in trifluoroacetic acid solution with tetramethylsilane as internal reference showed the following recognizable features: a chemical shift resonating at δ 7.83 for a single proton was assigned to the aromatic proton on position 5 (Structure VI); the methylene protons attached to C-3 resonated as a doublet (*J* = 8.0 Hz) at δ 3.12; the methine proton in the *sec*-butyl side chain attached to C-6 was observed at δ 3.73 (multiplet), and the four methyl groups on the *sec*- and isobutyl side chains were at δ 1.02 and δ 1.51 (*β*-methyl on the *sec*-butyl side chain was presumably superimposed on gem-dimethyl doublet) (*47*). The 3 proton doublet at δ 1.51 (*J* = 6 Hz) was assigned to the methyl group on the *sec*-butyl side chain (position 6) and apparently showed virtual coupling to the adjacent methine proton which was in turn coupled to the adjacent methylene protons.

Kojic Acid

Kojic acid [5-hydroxy-2-(hydroxymethyl)-4*H*-pyran-4-one] (Structure XII), a relatively common metabolite of *Aspergillus* spp. and in

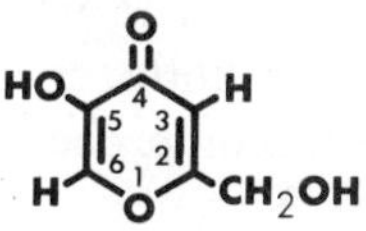

Structure XII.
Kojic Acid

particular of *A. flavus*, was first discovered by Saito (*55*). Yabuta (*56*) studied the chemistry of kojic acid and was mainly responsible for elucidating its chemical structure.

Early work on kojic acid was no doubt related to its antimicrobial properties. Considerable emphasis remained on the potential usefulness of kojic acid in spite of reports of its toxicity to animals. Thus, kojic acid has been the target of extensive chemical research (Data sheet No. 502, Charles Pfizer and Co.).

Although kojic acid has not been directly implicated in natural outbreaks of mycotoxicosis, it remains a potential problem in view of the large number of microorganisms capable of producing large amounts of it. The LD$_{50}$ of kojic acid in 17 g mice was 30 mg ip injection (*57*). Kojic acid also showed toxicity in plant cells at $10^{-1}M$ (*58*).

Kojic acid is characterized by a γ-pyrone nucleus substituted on posiations 2 and 5 with a hydroxymethyl and a hydroxy group. Its uv spectrum showed λ_{max}^{EtOH} 268 nm ($\epsilon = 8000$) and 216 nm ($\epsilon = 11,000$).

The infrared spectrum of kojic acid shows typical γ-pyrone absroptions—i.e., C=O stretching frequency at 1765 cm^{-1} and νc=c stretching frequencies at 1620 cm^{-1} and 1588 cm^{-1}. Other significant absorptions occurred at 3285 (OH), 1350, 1285, 1230, 1142, 1085, 990, 944, and 865 cm^{-1}.

The NMR spectrum of kojic acid, taken in D$_2$O solution, exhibited chemical shifts for a two-proton signal at δ 4.54 (singlet, 2-hydroxymethyl group) and one-proton singlets at δ 6.59 and δ 8.10 for the protons on positions 3 and 6. Signals for the two OH protons were not observed because of chemical exchange with D$_2$O. A chemical shift resonating at δ 4.69 was assigned to HDO (59).

In spite of extensive research on the biosynthesis of kojic acid, its mode of formation was dubious. The work of Arnstein and Bentley (60, 61, 62, 63, 64), in a series of elegant experiments using ^{14}C-labeled precursors with subsequent degradation of the products, provided strong evidence that kojic acid was formed directly from the oxidation of D-glucose. They suggested that D-glucose could be oxidized to 3-ketogluconic acid lactone which could in turn take two possible pathways to kojic acid. Both pathways involve enzymatic dehydration and reduction from 3-ketogluconic acid lactone to form kojic acid. Further support for these pathways was provided when it was experimentally shown that gluconic acid and gluconolactone both serve as precursors for kojic acid biosynthesis (64). An excellent comprehensive review of kojic acid has been prepared by Beelik (65).

Austamide

Steyn (66, 67) recently reported on the chemical structures of five new diketopiperazine compounds isolated from cultures of *Aspergillus ustus*. Austamide (Structure XIII) and 12,13-dihydroaustamide are characterized by a basic Ψ-indoxyl moiety substituted on position two with a seven-membered spiran ring system and containing in addition diketopiperazine and proline moieties. The uv spectra of both compounds showed typical Ψ-indoxyl chromophores (λ_{max}^{EtOH} 234, 256, and 392 nm).

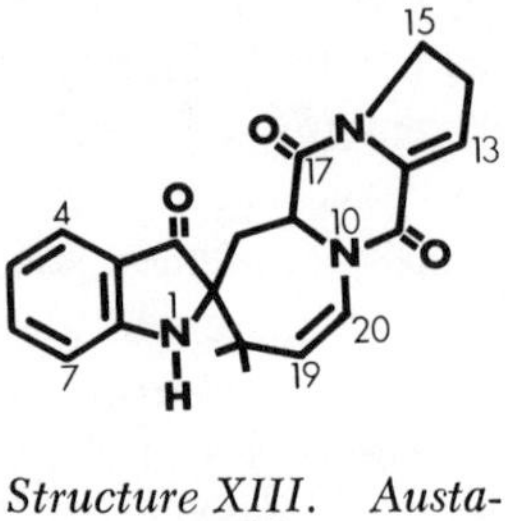

Structure XIII.   Austamide

Austamide contained additional UV absorptions (λ_{max}^{EtOH} 268 and 282 nm) attributed to the enamide chromophore (*66, 67*).

The ir spectrum of austamide showed 3420 cm^{-1} (NH group), 1700 cm^{-1} (Ψ-indoxyl C=O), and 1680 cm^{-1} and 1650 cm^{-1} (diketopiperazine C=O groups). Dihydroaustamide had similar ir absorption for the major functional groups. Mass spectral analysis of austamide showed a molecular ion peak (m*) at m/e 363 which analyzed for $C_{21}H_{21}N_3O_3$. The base peak appeared at m/e 203 ($C_{11}H_{11}N_2O_2$) which resulted from cleavage of the spiran ring to form an alicyclic fragment at m/e 218 ($C_{12}H_{14}N_2O_2$) followed by a loss of a methyl group. Dihydroaustamide showed a m* peak at m/e 365 with a corresponding fragment representing the alicyclic part of the molecule at m/e 220 (*67*).

Characteristic features of the NMR spectrum of austamide were chemical shifts for two nonequivalent geminal methyl groups resonating at δ 1.38 (singlet) and δ 0.88 (singlet); the olefinic protons located on the other part of the isoprene unit appeared at δ 4.89 (doublet) and at δ 6.82 (doublet) (J_{AB} = 10 Hz). The nonequivalent methylene protons at position 3 resonated at δ 3.06 (equitorial quartet) and δ 2.10 (axial quartet) as part of an ABX system with J_{AB} = 14, J_{AX} = 5, and J_{BX} = 12 Hz. The X portion consisted of the methine proton on the diketopiperazine moiety resonating at δ 4.99 as a pair of doublets (J_{AX} = 5; J_{BX} = 12 Hz).

The protons in the proline ring comprised an A_2M_2X system. The methylene protons adjacent to the proline nitrogen appeared as two overlapping triplets at δ 3.85 (J = 9, 9 Hz); the chemical shifts for the two protons at position 19 resonated as a sextet at δ 2.40 (J = 3, 9, 9 Hz). The aromatic protons on the indoxyl nucleus were observed between δ 7.7 and δ 6.6, and the NH proton (D_2O exchangeable) was observed at δ 4.73 as a broad signal. The NMR spectrum of dihydroaustamide was similar except that the olefinic triplet at δ 6.26 was absent and a proton (position 12) appeared at δ 4.18; chemical shifts for the proline protons became more complex.

The other three diketopiperazines consisted of closely related 2,3-disubstituted indoles. The major compound of this group, prolyl-2-(1',1'-dimethylallyltryptophyldiketopiperazine [$C_{21}H_{25}N_3O_2$] (Structure XIV) will serve as a model for discussion. It had typical UV absorption for 2,3-disubstituted indole (λ_{max}^{EtOH} 225, 275, 283, and 291 nm; log ϵ 4.51, 3.85, 3.91, and 3.85). The ir showed characteristic NH absorption at 3480, 3460, and 3365 cm^{-1}. The amide I bands occurred at 1685 (weak sh) and 1670 cm^{-1}. Absence of an amide II band supported the presence of a diketopiperazine system.

The mass spectrum of Structure XIV had a m* peak at m/e 351 and one prominent peak at m/e 198 (base peak) resulting from cleavage of the bond between carbons 8 and 9. The NMR spectrum showed chemical shifts for two D_2O exchangeable proton singlets at δ 8.75 and δ 5.72 arising from the NH protons. The four aromatic protons appeared as a multiplet between δ 7.52–6.95; the gem-dimethyl protons were located at δ 1.50 as a six-proton singlet. The three exocyclic protons on positions 19 and 20 comprised a AA^1X system with the X part (H on position 19) at δ 6.10 ($J_{AX} = 18.0$ Hz; $J_{A^1X} = 9$ Hz) and the AA^1 part at δ 5.08 ($J_{AX} = 18.0$ Hz; $J_{A^1A^1} = 9$ Hz).

The 3 protons at positions 8 and 9 resonated as an ABX system at δ 4.44 (H on position 9 = X part; $J_{AX} = 4$; $J_{BX} = 11.0$ Hz), δ 3.75 (H_A) ($J_{AB} = 15.5$; $J_{AX} = 4$ Hz), and δ 3.17 (H_B) ($J_{AB} = 15.5$; $J_{BX} = 11.0$ Hz). A signal arising from the methine proton at position 12 was observed as a triplet at δ 4.05 ($J = 7$ Hz). The protons on position 15 were located at δ 3.66, and the other four protons of the proline ring were between δ 2.4 and 1.8 as a multiplet.

Austamide (Structure XIII) was reported as toxic to ducklings, but no specific toxicological data have been reported (66). Although no data concerning biosynthesis of the diketopiperazines were available, the amino acids, tryptophan and proline, might be involved.

Ascladiol

A patulin-producing strain of *Aspergillus clavatus* isolated from wheat flour (68) produced a new mycotoxin named ascladiol (Structure XV). Ascladiol ($C_7H_8O_4$), a metabolite closely related to patulin, was

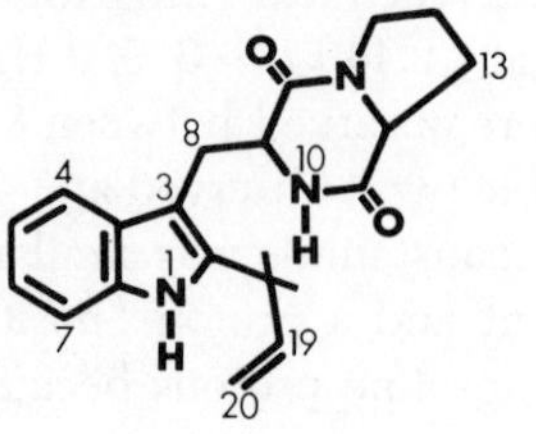

Structure XIV. Diketo-
piperazine

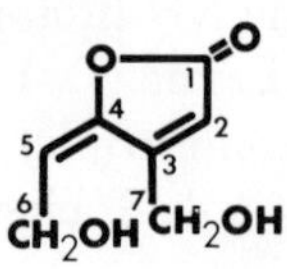

Structure XV.
Ascladiol

only one-fourth as acutely toxic to mice as patulin. Major absorption bands in the ir spectrum were 1735 cm^{-1} and 1750 cm^{-1} (supporting five-membered lactone ring system) and 3300 cm^{-1} (OH) (68). The uv spectrum showed λ_{max}^{EtOH} 271 nm.

The proton magnetic resonance spectrum taken in acetone-d_6 solution showed resonances for two methine protons at δ 6.29 (multiplet; C-2) and δ 5.87 (quartet; C-5). The two pair of methylene protons located on C-6 and C-7 were positioned at δ 4.74 and δ 4.30. Superimposed on the methylene protons at δ 4.74 were two D_2O exchangeable protons assigned to the OH protons on C-6 and C-7 (68).

Terreic Acid

The antibiotic terreic acid (Structure XVI) was first discovered by Wilkins and Harris (69). Its utility was negated because in vivo tests showed that it was highly toxic to mammals (70). Intravenous injection of terreic acid to mice showed an LD_{50} of 71–119 mg/kg (70).

The chemical structure of terreic acid was proposed by Sheehan et al. (71) as 2,3-epoxy-6-hydroxytoluquinone (Structure XVI). The structure assignment was based on comparisons of the NMR spectra of terreic acid and 2,3-epoxy-1,4-naphthoquinone (Structure XVII) together with physical data and chemical transformation products.

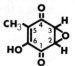

Structure XVI.   Structure XVII.
Terreic Acid   Naphthoquinone

The ir spectrum of terreic acid had sharp absorptions at 3300, 1655, and 1629 cm^{-1} compatible with the presence of an enolized 1,2,4-triketone system. Additional strong absorptions were 1690, 1380 (CH$_3$), 1370, 1350, 1305, 1200, 1135, 1035, and 760 cm^{-1} (71). The uv spectrum had maxima at 214 (log ϵ 4.03) and 316 nm (log ϵ 3.88); the latter absorption shifted to 304 nm in an acid solution. A similar shift to 304 nm was observed when it was converted to the methyl ether derivative.

The chemical shifts for terreic acid analyzed in chloroform-d solution were reported relative to the OH absorption of water. The NMR spectrum had three distinguishable resonances attributed to the methyl group (+ 107 Hz), the two epoxide protons (+ 30 Hz), and the OH proton (− 93 Hz). The epoxide protons of 5,6-epoxy-3-hydroxytoluquinone (+ 32 Hz) and terreic acid were similarly positioned (71).

Viriditoxin

Viriditoxin was isolated from mycelia of a toxigenic strain of *Aspergillus veri-nudans* found during routine screening for toxigenic fungi (72, 73). Viriditoxin was shown to be a symmetrical dimer with Structure XVIII. Elemental and mass spectral analyses established the molecular

Structure XVIII. Viriditoxin

weight as 662 with a molecular formula of $C_{34}H_{30}O_{14}$. The toxin in ethanol solution showed uv absorption at λ_{max} 266 and 380 nm (73).

Significant carbonyl absorptions in the ir spectrum were 1740 cm^{-1} (ester) and 1635 cm^{-1}. The latter absorption shifted to 1720 after acetylation which suggested a hydrogen-bonded lactone. Further support arose from the NMR spectrum which showed a D_2O exchangeable proton at δ 13.70. This extreme downfield position is typical of a hydrogen-bonded OH group. A chemical shift for an additional OH proton appeared at δ 9.72. Two methoxy resonances were at δ 3.66 and δ 3.74. Chemical shifts in the aromatic region (singlets at δ 6.24 and 6.78) were assigned to the two meta-positioned aromatic protons on the napthalene ring system. The methylene protons in the lactone ring and the exocyclic methylene protons were coupled with the adjacent methine proton. The methine proton resonated as a multiplet at δ 4.96, and the methylene protons partially overlapped at δ 2.76 (multiplet) and δ 2.81 (doublet). Viriditoxin had an LD$_{50}$ of 2.8 mg/kg (ip) in 20 g mice. No biosynthetic data were given for viriditoxin.

Cytochalasin E

A recent report implicated cytochalasin E from *Aspergillus clavatus* to human mortality from ingestion of mold-damaged rice (74, 75). Cytochalasin E (Structure XIX) contained mono-substituted aromatic, secondary amide, epoxide, ketone, and alkyl vinyl carbonate moieties (75). Its ir spectrum showed major absorptions at 3475 cm^{-1} (OH, NH), 1765 cm^{-1}, 1660 cm^{-1}, and 1720 cm^{-1}.

Proton chemical shifts for cytochalasin E were assigned as follows: two exchangeable protons appeared at δ 6.93 (NH proton on C-2) and δ 4.1 (OH proton on C-15); the aromatic protons occurred as a multiplet at δ 7.1. Resonances for 4 methyl groups were observed at δ 1.0 (doublet, $J = 6$ Hz; C-5), δ 1.2 (singlet; C-6), δ 1.13 (doublet, $J = 6$ Hz; C-13), and δ 1.4 (singlet; C-15). Two strongly coupled protons resonated at δ 5.45 (doublet) and δ 6.25 (doublet, $J = 11$ Hz). These were assigned to the protons located on C-16 and C-17 (75).

The corrected structure and stereochemistry were obtained via single crystal x-ray diffraction analysis (75). Cytochalasin E reportedly killed rats within a few hours after dosing. The LD$_{50}$ values were 2.6 mg/kg (ip) and 9.1 mg/kg (oral) (75).

Maltoryzine

Two cases of feed poisoning in dairy cattle were traced to malt sprout contaminated with a toxigenic strain of *Aspergillus oryzae* var. *microsporis*

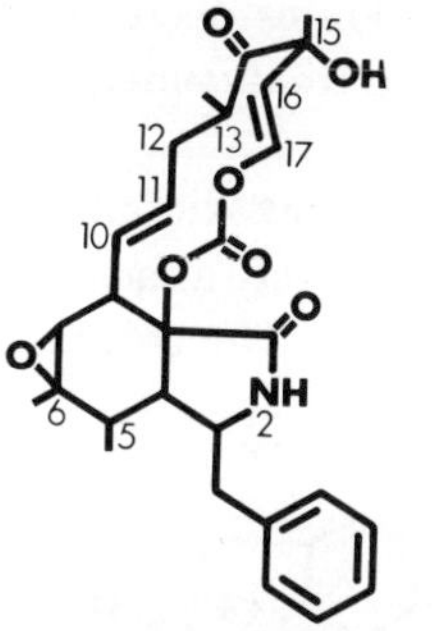

Structure XIX.
Cytochalasin E

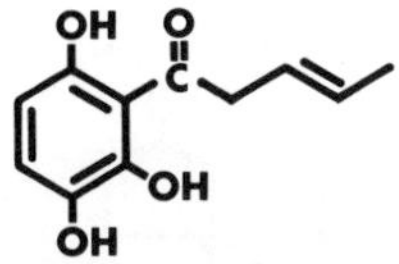

Structure XX.
Maltoryzine

(76). The toxin was named maltoryzine ($C_{11}H_{14}O_4$) (Structure XX) (77). Maltoryzine had an LD_{50} of 3 mg/kg (ip) in mice.

The uv spectrum of this toxin was λ_{max} 220 (log ϵ 4.1), 280 (log ϵ 3.1), and 320 nm (log ϵ 2.1). The IR spectrum of maltoryzine supported OH (3300 cm^{-1}), ketone (1700 cm^{-1}), and aromatic moieties (1600 and 1500 cm^{-1}). The chemical structure of maltoryzine was deduced from chemical degradation studies of the trimethoxy derivative of maltoryzine (77).

Other Toxins of Aspergillus Spp.

The following is a brief survey of other toxic *Aspergillus* metabolites. Bush et al. (78) isolated and identified 3-nitropropanoic acid (Structure XXI) from toxic extracts of *A. flavus* cultures. 3-Nitropropanoic acid has also been reported as a metabolite of *A. oryzae*. In both cases, it occurred together with pyrazine compounds which may suggest a role in the nitrification pathway.

Oxalic acid (Structure XXII) is a metabolic product of several fungi including *A. flavus, A. glaucus, A. luchuensis,* and *A. niger*. The toxicological properties of oxalic acid may rely on the presence of large quantities in contaminated feed supplies or on synergistic effects with other metabolites functioning in concert. Unfortunately, fundamental information

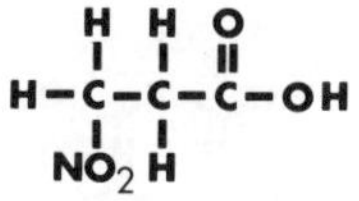

Structure XXI.
β-Nitropropanoic Acid

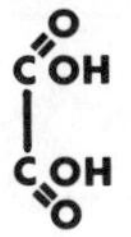

Structure XXII.
Oxalic Acid

relative to the synergistic effects of fungal metabolites occuring naturally is minimal or lacking although it is recognized that synergism occurs naturally.

Helvolic acid (fumigacin) (Structure XXIII), a toxic antibiotic produced by some isolates of A. *fumigatus*, was reported almost simultaneously by Waksman et al. (*79*) and Chain et al. (*80*). The correct chemical

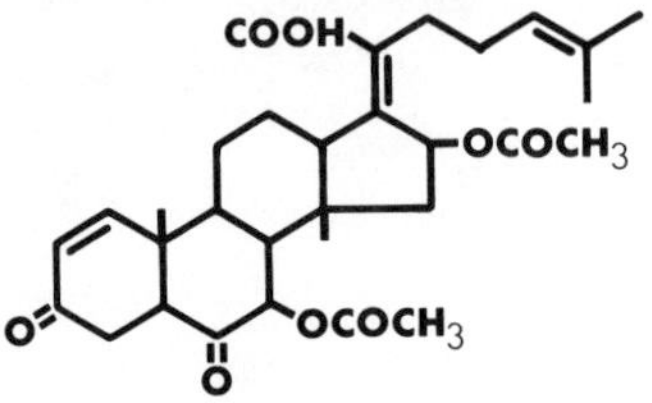

Structure XXIII.
Helvolic Acid

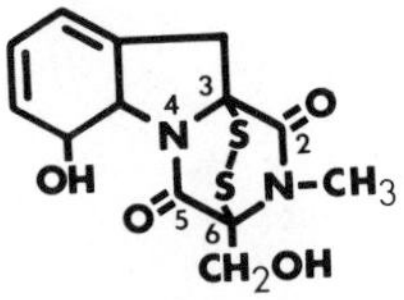

Structure XXIV.
Gliotoxin

structure of helvolic acid was determined by chemical and physical considerations and proton magnetic resonance studies (*81*).

Gliotoxin ($C_{13}H_{14}N_2O_4S_2$) (Structure XXIV), an antibiotic first reported from *Gliocladium frimbriatum* (*82*), is a metabolic product of several fungi including *Aspergillus fumigatus* (*83*), A. *chevalieri* (*84*), and A. *Terreus* (*85, 86*). Gliotoxin is characterized by a disulfide bridge across a diketopiperazine ring system. The basic structure is a 3,6-epidithio-2,5-dioxopiperazine moiety. Although several other epipolythiodioxopiperazines occur naturally (*87*), only gliotoxin and acetylaranatin (Structure XXV) (*86*) have been reported as metabolites of *Aspergillus* sp.

In addition to potent antibiotic properties, gliotoxin was acutely toxic to rabbits ($LD_{50} = 45$ mg/kg), mice ($LD_{50} = 50$ mg/kg), and rats ($LD_{50} = 50$–65 mg/kg) (*88*); at sublethal doses the animals had kidney lesions. A comprehensive review of the biosynthesis of epipolythiodioxopiperazines was presented by Taylor (*87*).

Other toxigenic metabolites of A. *fumigatus* are fumigatin (Structure XXVI) (*89*), fumagillin (Structure XXVII) (*90*), Terrein (Structure XXVIII) (*91, 92, 93, 94*), and spinulosin (Structure XXIX) (*88*). Ojima

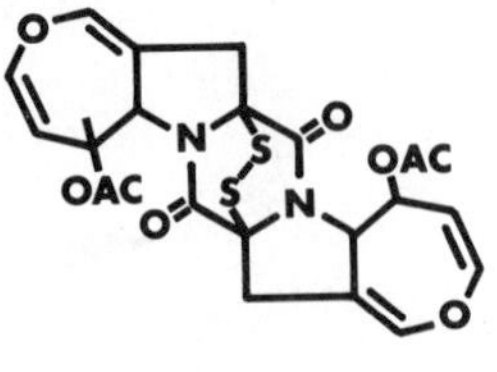

Structure XXV.
Acetylaranatin

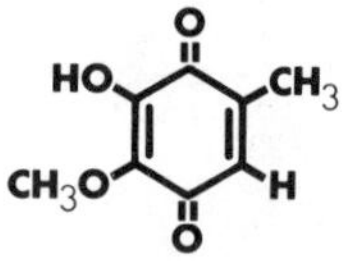

Structure XXVI.
Fumigatin

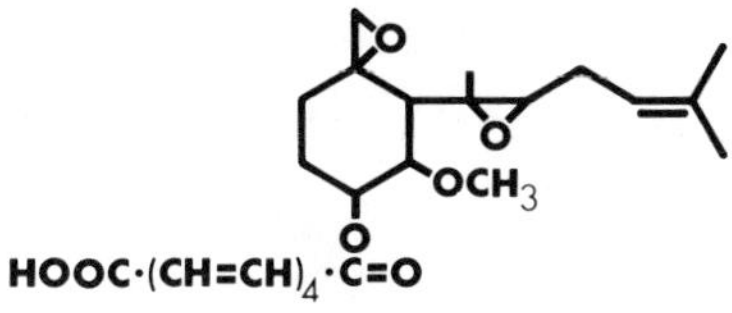

Structure XXVII.
Fumagillin

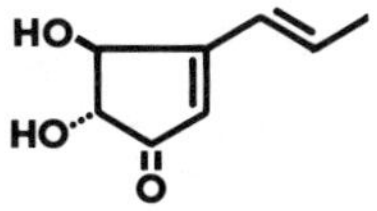

Structure XXVIII.
Terrein

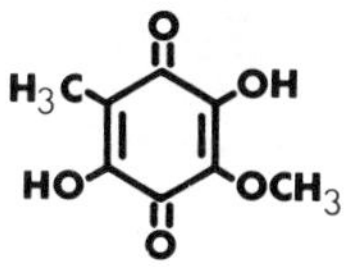

Structure XXIX.
Spinulosin

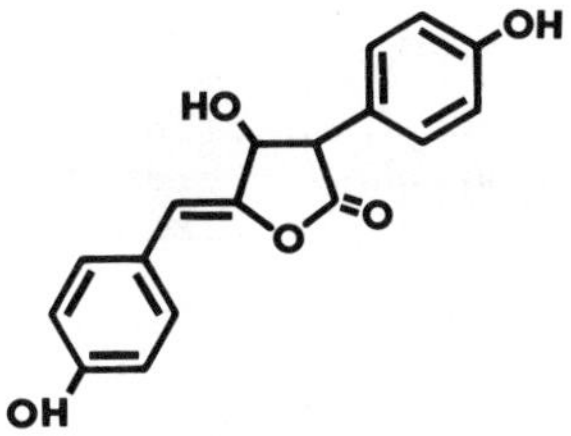

Structure XXX.
Butenolide

et al. (95) recently reported the identity of a new butenolide (Structure XXX) from culture filtrates of *A. terreus*. They also found six other closely related metabolites associated with this compound. Information not presented in this review is provided in Ref. 96.

Literature Cited

1. Hutchison, R. D., Hozapfel, C. W., *Tetrahedron* (1971) **27**, 426.
2. Van Der Merwe, K. J., Steyn, P. S., Fourie, L., *J. Chem. Soc., B* (1965) 7083.
3. Hesseltine, C. W., Vandergraft, E. E., Fennell, D. I., Smith, M. L., Shotwell, O. L., *Mycologia* (1972) **64**, 539.
4. Van Walbeek, W., Scott, P. M., Harwig, J., Lawrence, J. W., *Can. J. Microbiol.* (1969) **15**, 1281.
5. Hutchison, R. D., Steyn, P. S., Thompson, D. L., *Tetrahedron Lett.* (1971) **43**, 4033.
6. Steyn, P. S., Holzapfel, C. W., *J. S. Africa Chem. Inst., A* (1967) **20**, 186.
7. Purchase, I. F. H., Theron, J. J., *Food Cosmet. Toxicol.* (1968) **6**, 479.
8. Chu, F. S., Chang, C. C., *J. Amer. Off. Anal. Chem.* (1971) **54**, 1032.
9. Peckham, J. C., Doupnik, B., Jones, O. H., *Appl. Microbiol.* (1971) **21**, 492.
10. Chu, F. S., Noh, I., Chang, C. C., *Life Sci.* (1972) **11**, 503.
11. Steyn, P. S., Holsapfel, C. W., *Tetrahedron, B* (1967) **23**, 4449.
12. Cole, R. J., Moore, J. H., Davis, N. D., Kirksey, J. W., Diener, U. L., *J. Agr. Food Chem.* (1971) **19**, 909.
13. Maebayashi, Y., Miyaki, K., Yamazaki, M., *Chem. Pharm. Bull.* (1972) **152**, 149.
14. Searcy, J. W., Davis, N. D., Diener, U. L., *Appl. Microbiol.* (1969) **18**, 622.
15. Steyn, P. S., Holzapfel, C. W., *Phytochemistry* (1970) **9**, 1977.
16. Bullock, E., Roberts, J. C., Underwood, J. G., *J. Chem. Soc.* (1962) 4179.
17. Holzapfel, C. W., Purchase, I. F. H., Steyn, P. S., Gouws, L., *S. Afr. Med. J.* (1966) **40**, 1100.

18. Rodricks, J. V., Henery-Logan, K. R., Campbell, A. D., Stoloff, L., Verrett, M. J., *Nature, A* (1968) **217,** 688.
19. Rodricks, J. V., Lustig, E., Campbell, A. D., Stoloff, L., *Tetrahedron Lett., B* (1968) **25,** 2975.
20. Waiss, A. C., Jr., Wiley, M., Black, D. R., Lundin, R. E., *Tetrahedron Lett.* (1968) **28,** 3207.
21. Burkhardt, H. J., Forgacs, J., *Tetrahedron* (1968) **24,** 717.
22. Cole, R. J., Kirksey, J. W., *Tetrahedron Lett.* (1970) **35,** 3109.
23. Holker, J. S. E., Kagal, S. A., *Chem. Commun.* (1968) 1574.
24. Elsworthy, G. C., Holker, J. S. E., McKeown, J. M., Robinson, J. B., Mulheirn, L. J., *Chem. Commun.* (1970) 1069.
25. Hatsuda, Y., Hamasaki, T., Ishida, M., Matsui, K., Hara, S., *Agr. Biol. Chem., Japan* (1972) **36,** 521.
26. Englebrecht, J. C., Altenkirk, B., *J. Nat. Cancer Inst.* (1972) **48,** 1647.
27. Dickens, F., Jones, H. E. H., Waynforth, H. B., *Brit. J. Cancer* (1966) **20,** 134.
28. Purchase, I. F. H., Van Der Watt, J. J., *Food Cosmet. Toxicol.* (1968) **6,** 555.
29. Purchase, I. F. H., Van Der Watt, J. J., *Food Cosmet. Toxicol.* (1970) **8,** 289.
30. Davies, J. E., Kirkaldy, D., Roberts, J. C., *J. Chem. Soc.* (1960) 2169.
31. Asao, T., Buchi, G., Abdel-Kader, M. M., Chang, S. B., Wick, E. L., Wogan, G. N., *J. Amer. Chem. Soc.* (1965) **87,** 885.
32. Rodricks, J. V., *J. Agr. Food Chem.* (1969) **17,** 457.
33. Tanaka, N., Katsube, Y., Hatsuda, Y., Hamasaki, T., Ishida, M., *Chem. Soc., Japan* (1970) **43,** 3635.
34. Rance, M. J., Roberts, J. C., *Tetrahedron Lett.* (1969) 277.
35. Holker, J. S. E., Mulheirn, L. J., *Chem. Commun.* (1968) **24,** 1576.
36. Holker, J. S. E., Underwood, J. G., *Chem. Ind.* (1964).
37. Biollaz, M., Buchi, G., Milne, G., *J. Amer. Chem. Soc.* (1970) **92,** 1035.
38. Hsieh, D. P. H., Lin, M. T., Yao, R. C., *Biochem. Biophys. Res. Commun.* (1973) **52,** 992.
39. Schroeder, H. W., Cole, R. J., Grigsby, R. D., Hein, H., Jr., *Appl. Microbiol.* (1974) **27,** 394.
40. White, E. C., *Science* (1940) **92,** 127.
41. White, E. C., Hill, J. H., *J. Bacteriol.* (1943) **45,** 433.
42. MacDonald, J. C., *Can. J. Biochem.* (1973) **51,** 1311.
43. Sasaki, M., Asao, Y., Yokotsuka, T., *Nippon Nogei Kagaku Kaishi* (1968) **42,** 351.
44. Yokotsuka, T., Asao, Y., Sasaki, M., *Nippon Nogei Kagaku Kaishi* (1968) **42,** 346.
45. MacDonald, J. C., *J. Biol. Chem.* (1961) **236,** 512.
46. MacDonald, J. C., *J. Biol. Chem.* (1962) **237,** 1977.
47. Micetich, R. G., MacDonald, J. C., *J. Biol. Chem.* (1964) **240,** 1692.
48. Dutcher, J. D., *J. Biol. Chem.* (1947) **171,** 321.
49. Dutcher, J. D., *J. Biol. Chem.* (1958) **232,** 785.
50. Dutcher, J. D., Wintersteiner, O., *J. Biol. Chem.* (1944) **155,** 359.
51. Newbold, G. T., Spring, F. S., *J. Chem. Soc.* (1947) 373.
52. Dunn, G., Gallagher, J. J., Newbold, G. T., Spring, F. S., *J. Chem. Soc., A* (1949) 126.
53. Dunn, G., Newbold, G. T., Spring, F. S., *J. Chem. Soc., B* (1949) 131.
54. Newbold, G. T., Sharp, W., Spring, F. S., *J. Chem. Soc.* (1951) 2679.
55. Saito, K., *Botan. Mag., Tokyo* (1907) **21,** 7.
56. Yabuta, T., *J. Chem. Soc.* (1924) **125,** 575.
57. Morton, H. E., Kocholaty, W., Junowics–Kocholaty, R., Kelner, A., *J. Bacteriol.* (1945) **50,** 579.
58. Gaumann, E., von Arx, A., *Ber. Schweiz. Botan. Ges.* (1947) **57,** 174.

59. Bhacca, N. S., Johnson, L. F., Shoolery, J. N., "High Resolution NMR Spectra Catalog," Vol. 2, Varian Associates, 1963.
60. Arnstein, H. R. V., Bentley, R., *J. Chem. Soc.* (1951) 3436.
61. Arnstein, H. R. V., Bentley, R., *Biochem. J., A* (1953) 54, 493.
62. Arnstein, H. R. V., Bentley, R., *Biochem. J., B* (1953) 54, 508.
63. Arnstein, H. R. V., Bentley, R., *Biochem. J., C* (1953) 54, 517.
64. Arnstein, H. R. V., Bentley, R., *Biochem. J.* (1956) 62, 403.
65. Beelik, A., *Advan. Carbohydrate Chem.* (1944) Vol. XI.
66. Steyn, P. S., *Tetrahedron Lett.* (1971) 36, 3331.
67. Steyn, P. S., *Tetrahedron* (1973) 29, 107.
68. Suzuki, T., Takeda, M., Tanabe, H., *Chem. Pharm. Bull.* (1971) 19, 1786.
69. Wilkins, W. H., Harris, G. C. M., *Brit. J. Exp. Path.* (1942) 23, 166.
70. Kaplan, M. A., Hooper, I. R., Heinemann, B., *Antibiot. Chemotherapy* (1954) 4, 746.
71. Sheehan, J. C., Lawson, W. B., Gaul, R. J., *J. Amer. Chem. Soc.* (1958) 80, 5536.
72. Weisleder, D., Lillehoj, E. B., *Tetrahedron Lett.* (1971) 48, 4706.
73. Lillehoj, E. B., Ciegler, A., *Can. J. Microbiol.* (1972) 18, 193.
74. Glinsukon, T., Shank, R. C., *Toxicol. Appl. Pharmacol.* (1972) 22, 331.
75. Buchi, G., Kitaura, Y., Yaun, S., Wright, H. E., Clardy, J., Demain, A. L., Glinsukon, T., Hunt, N., Wogan, G. N., *J. Amer. Chem. Soc.* (1973) 95, 5423.
76. Iizuka, H., Iida, M., *J. Gen. Appl. Microbiol.* (1958) 4, 133.
77. Iizuka, H., Iida, M., *Nature* (1962) 196, 681.
78. Bush, M. T., Touster, O., Brockman, J. E., *J. Biol. Chem.* (1951) 188, 685.
79. Waksman, S. A., Horning, E., Spencer, E. L., *J. Bacteriol.* (1943) 45, 233.
80. Chain, E., Florey, H. W., Jennings, M. A., Williams, T. I., *Brit. J. Exp. Pathol.* (1943) 24, 108.
81. Okuda, S., Iwasaki, N., Tsuda, K., Sano, Y., Hata, T., Udagawa, S., Nakayama, Y., Yamaguchi, H., *Chem. Pharm. Bull.* (1964) 12, 121.
82. Weindling, R., Emerson, O., *Phyto. Path.* (1936) 26, 1068.
83. Menzel, A. E. O., Wintersteiner, O., Hoogerheide, J. C., *J. Biol. Chem.* (1944) 152, 419.
84. Wilkinson, S., Spilsbury, J. F., *Nature* (1965) 206, 619.
85. Miller, P. A., Milstrey, K. P., Trown, P. W., *Science, A* (1968) 159, 431.
86. Miller, P. A., Trown, P. W., Fulmor, W., Morton, G. O., Karliner, J., *Biochem. Biophys. Res. Commun., B* (1968) 33, 219.
87. Taylor, A., in "Microbiological Toxins," Vol. VII, S. Kadis, A. Ciegler, S. J. Ajl, Eds., p. 293, Academic Press, New York, 1971.
88. Johnson, J. R., Bruce, W. F., Dutcher, J. D., *J. Amer. Chem. Soc.* (1943) 65, 2005.
89. Anslow, W. K., Raistrick, H., *Biochem. J.* (1938) 32, 687.
90. Eble, T. E., Hanson, F. R., *Antibiot. Chemotherapy* (1951) 1, 54.
91. Raistrick, H., Smith, G., *Biochem. J.* (1935) 29, 606.
92. Grove, J. F., *J. Chem. Soc.* (1954) 4693.
93. Barton, D. H. R., Miller, E., *J. Chem. Soc.* (1955) 1028.
94. Birch, A. J., Cassera, A., Jones, A. R., *Chem. Commun.* (1965) 167.
95. Ojima, N., Takenaka, S., Seto, S., *Phytochemistry* (1973) 12, 2527.
96. Wilson, B. J., "Microbiological Toxins," Vol. 6, Chap. 3, Academic, New York, 1971.

RECEIVED November 8, 1974.

6

Patulin and Penicillic Acid

DAVID M. WILSON

Department of Plant Pathology, University of Georgia, College of Agriculture
Experiment Stations, Coastal Plain Station, Tifton, Ga. 31794

The mycotoxins patulin (4-hydroxy-4H-furo[3,2-c]pyran-2(6H)-one) and penicillic acid (3-methoxy-5-methyl-4-oxo-2,5-hexadienoic acid) are metabolites of several fungi, primarily species of Aspergillus *and* Penicillium. *Their chemical and physical properties and biosynthesis are discussed. Recent work on analytical methods, reports of natural occurrence, and stability in foods and feeds are emphasized. Both patulin and penicillic acid inhibit DNA, RNA, protein synthesis, and some enzymes containing SH groups. The precise mode of toxic action remains uncertain. Since both patulin and penicillic acid are toxic and have been implicated in carcinogenesis and since patulin causes mutations in yeasts, they are potentially dangerous. The biological effects of orally ingested patulin and penicillic acid need further study to assess their potential health hazard.*

Once upon a time gasoline was a nuisance and the problem was how to get rid of it; once upon a time moulds were a nuisance and the problem was how to get rid of them. Not so today. Since the epoch-making purification of penicillin . . . by Florey and his associates . . . the search for therapeutic agents from moulds has crossed oceans and continents. At the London School of Hygiene and Tropical Medicine in London, England, Professor Harold Raistrick and his associates . . . have assiduously isolated, purified, and established the structure of a number of therapeutically active compounds from various moulds. Their most recent and most interesting derivative from moulds is "patuline" which is obtained from the mould *Penicillium patulum* Bainier, and which holds promise of therapeutic activity against the common cold (*1*).

Patulin was soon found almost useless in curing the common cold (*2*) and was too toxic for use as an antimicrobial agent. Therefore interest has now shifted to the toxic properties of patulin and its relation to the potential contamination of foods and feeds.

The structure of patulin (4-hydroxy-4*H*-furo[3,2-*c*]pyran-2(6*H*)-one) was determined by Woodward and Singh (*3, 4*) (*see* Figure 1). Patulin

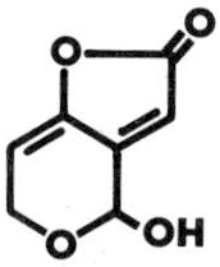

Figure 1.   Structure of patulin

has been isolated under various names: clavicin, clavitin, claviformin, expansin, leucopin, mycoin c, penicidin, and tercinin (*5*). It has been isolated from the following fungi: *Penicillium urticae* (*6*) [*P. patulum* (*7*) and perhaps synonymous *P. griseo-fulvum* (*8*)], *P. expansum* (*9*) [*P. leucopus* (*10*)], *P. granulatum* [*P. divergens* (*11*)], *P. lanosum* (*12*), *P. claviforme* (*13*), *P. melinii* (*14*), *P. novae-zeelandiae* (*14*), *P. cyclopium* (*15*), *P. lapidosum* (*16*), *P. equinum* (*14*), *Aspergillus clavatus* (*17*), *A. giganteus* (*18*), *A. terreus* (*6*), and *Byssochlamys nivea* (*19*) [*Gymnoascus* sp. (*20*)].

Penicillic acid ($C_8H_{10}O_4$), 3-methoxy-5-methyl-4-oxo-2,5-hexadienoic acid, was first isolated from *P. puberulum* by Alsberg and Black (*21*) who named the compound and found it toxic to mice. They also found that although *P. stoloniferum* produced mycophenolic acid ($C_{17}H_{20}O_6$), it did not produce penicillic acid. Birkinshaw (*22*) showed that the structure of penicillic acid was γ-keto-β-methoxy-δ-methylene-Δ^a-hexanoic acid or the corresponding γ-hydroxy lactone (*see* Figure 2). Penicillic acid has

Figure 2.   Structure of penicillic acid

been isolated from the following fungi: *Penicillium lividum* (*23*), *P. puberulum* (*21*), *P. griseum* (*23*), *P. simplicissimum* (*24*), *P. cyclopium* (*22*), *P. thomii* (*25*), *P. roqueforti* [*P. suavolens* (*25*)], *P. martensii* (*26*), *P. fenelliae* (*27*), *P. aurantio-virens* (*28*), *P. janthinellum* (*29*), *P. viridi-catum* (*29*), *P. palitans* (*30*), *P. baarnense* (*31*), *P. madriti* (*32*), *P. lilacinum* (*12*), *P. canescens* (*12*), *P. chrysogenum* (*21*), *P. olivino-viride* (*33*), *Aspergillus ochraceus* (*20*), *A. sulphureus* (*34*), *A. Melleus* (*35*)

[A. quercinus (34)], A. sclerotiorum (36), A. alliaceus (36), A. ostianus (36), and Paecilomyces ehrlichii (23).

Chemical and Physical Properties

Patulin. Patulin has an empirical formula of $C_7H_6O_4$, a molecular weight of 154, and a melting point of 110°–112°C. Patulin has an optically active carbon atom; however the racemic mixture occurs naturally. The crystals are large monoclinic tables (001). The plane of the optic axes is inclined at approximately 20° to the normal to (001) (γ is parallel to b). The unit cell dimensions are: $a = 12.42$, $b = 9.47$, $c = 7.78$ A ($\beta = 46.7°$). The density is 1.528 ± .003, and the space group is $P2_1/a$, $Z = 4$ (37).

Patulin is soluble in water, alcohol, acetone, ethyl acetate, and chloroform, slightly soluble in ethyl ether and benzene, and insoluble in petroleum ether. It decomposes slowly in water and methanol, but it is stable in benzene, chloroform, and methylene chloride (38). Patulin is not stable as a thin film from an evaporated solution (39).

The ir spectrum of patulin has major bands at 1768, 1745 (shoulder), and 3390 cm^{-1} in nujol mull (40); in hexachlorobutadiene mull there is a broad OH band at 3360 cm^{-1}, and in KBr disks there are bands at 1030, 1160, 1200, 1740, and 1765 cm^{-1} (41, 42). Patulin has a single uv absorption maximum at about 276 nm (43). Scott (44) presented the reported extinction coefficients in detail. The proton NMR spectrum in CDCl$_3$ exhibits chemical shifts at $\delta = 5.97$ (3P, complex), δ 4.73 (1P, doublet of doublets, A part of ABX system, $J_{AB} = 17$ cps), δ 4.40 (1P, doublet of doublets, B part of ABX system, $J_{AB} = 17$ cps), and δ 3.46 (1P, doublet, $J = 5$ cps) (44). The mass spectrum of patulin was reported by Scott et al. (45); the mass spectrum of the trimethylsilyl ether was reported by Scott (44). Scott and Yalpani (46) proposed structures for seven principal fragment ions of deuterated patulin with $m/e = 138, 128, 111, 99, 83, 72,$ and 56.

Patulin forms acetyl, 2,4-dinitrophenylhydrazone, phenylhydrazone, semicarbazone, oxime, and methyl ether derivatives. It reduces Fehlings reagent, potassium permanganate, and ammoniacal silver nitrate (43, 47, 48). Reduction with sodium borohydride yields ascladiol, a less toxic mycotoxin isolated from A. clavatus (49). Hydrogenation gives desoxy-patulinic acid which has been isolated from P. urticae [P. patulum] (50). Patulin was synthesized by Woodward and Singh (51); patulin oxime was synthesized starting from acetylenic compounds (52). For a detailed review of patulin synthesis see Korzybyski et al. (53).

Penicillic Acid. Penicillic acid, $C_8H_{10}O_4$, has a molecular weight of 170, a melting point of 84°–87°C (hydrated, 58°–64°C), and a neutralization equivalent of 169 (*25*). The K_a is 1.26×10^{-6} at 25°C in aqueous solution (*54*). Penicillic acid is slightly soluble in cold water, soluble in hot water, alcohol, ether, benzene, chloroform, and ethyl acetate and is insoluble in hexane and petroleum ether.

Penicillic acid absorbs Br_2, reduces Fehlings solution when heated, reduces ammoniacal silver nitrate, turns yellow in alkaline solution and deep red upon exposure to ammonia, and turns $FeCl_3$ brown red (*21, 22, 55*). Penicillic acid has a tendency to self-associate strongly in solution (*56*). The hydrogenated derivative dihydropenicillic acid was isolated from an unidentified fungus (*57*). The ammoniated derivative is fluorescent with excitation maxima at 350 nm and emission maxima at 440 nm (*58*).

The infrared spectrum has bands at 3270, 1728, 1643, 1352, 1223, 909, and 811 cm^{-1} in KBr (*57*). Kovac and Solcaniova (*56*) give solution ir bands for penicillin acid in carbon tetrachloride and chloroform. The uv absorption maximum is at 227 nm in H_2O, 225 nm in 76% ethanol, 224 nm in ethanol, 221 nm in methanol, and shifts to 224 nm in 0.02*N* HCl and 293 nm in 0.02*N* NaOH (*27, 56, 57, 59*). The uv absorption maximum for penicillic acid acetate is at 229 nm in ethanol and for methyl penicillate is at 224 nm in ethanol (*56*).

The proton NMR spectrum of penicillic acid in deuterated benzene exhibits chemical shifts for a 3-proton signal at δ 1.72 and δ 3.14 and for a 1-proton signal at δ 419, δ 4.91, δ 5.02, and δ 5.62 (*27*). Kobayashi et al. (*33*) determined the NMR spectrum in $CDCl_3$ and DMSO-d^6. The mass spectrum can be found in Ciegler and Kurtzman (*30*) and Suzuki et al. (*60*). Van Eijk (*27*) discussed possible structures for four principal fragment ions in the mass spectrum of pencillic acid but could not distinguish between the free acid and lactone tautomers. Penicillic acid and dihydropenicillic acid were synthesized by Raphael (*55, 64, 65*).

The tautomerism of penicillic acid has been studied using uv absorption spectroscopy (*31, 61, 62, 63*). Ford et al. (*61*) stated that uv spectral measurements have doubtful value in determining the cyclic or open chain form and could not adequately define the equilibrium between the cyclic and open chain forms using ir spectroscopy. Using mass spectroscopy, van Eijk (*27*) could not distinguish between the cyclic and open chain forms on the basis of possible structures of the ion fragments. The equilibrium and existence of the open chain and cyclic tautomers in various solutions warrants further investigation.

Biosynthesis

Patulin. Bu'Lock et al. (*66*) who studied conditions favoring patulin biosynthesis described two physiological phases in *P. urticae:* in the first phase (trophophase) mycelial N, P, RNA, and SH reach maximum values; in the second phase (idiophase) these values are reduced, and patulin and other secondary metabolites from 6-methylsalicylic acid appear. Bassett and Tanenbaum first proposed a scheme for patulin biosynthesis using known metabolic products of *P. urticae* (*67, 68, 69*). Patulin was derived from ^{14}C-labeled 6-methylsalicylic acid (*70*). The 6-methylsalicylic acid was derived from glucose or acetate with acetyl coenzyme A playing an important role (*71*) as did malonate, presumably in the form of malonyl coenzyme A (*72*).

Bu'Lock et al. (*73*) discussed the enzymes that may regulate patulin biosynthesis. Two of the enzymes required for the conversion of 6-methyl-salicylic acid to patulin are 6-methylsalicylic acid decarboxylase (*74*) and *m*-hydroxybenzyl alcohol dehydrogenase (*75*). Also Arihood and Light (*76*) reported that 6-methylsalicylic acid synthesis was inhibited by 6-methylsalicylic acid and some structural analogues of this compound.

Forrester and Gaucher (*77*) described the major pathway for patulin biosynthesis starting with acetyl Co-A + 3 malonyl Co-A → 6-methyl-salicylic acid → *m*-cresol → *m*-hydroxybenzyl alcohol → *m*-hydroxybenz-aldehyde → gentisaldehyde → pre-patulin → patulin. Scott *et al.* (*78*) proposed another pathway leading directly from *m*-hydroxybenzaldehyde through an intermediate to patulin (Figure 3).

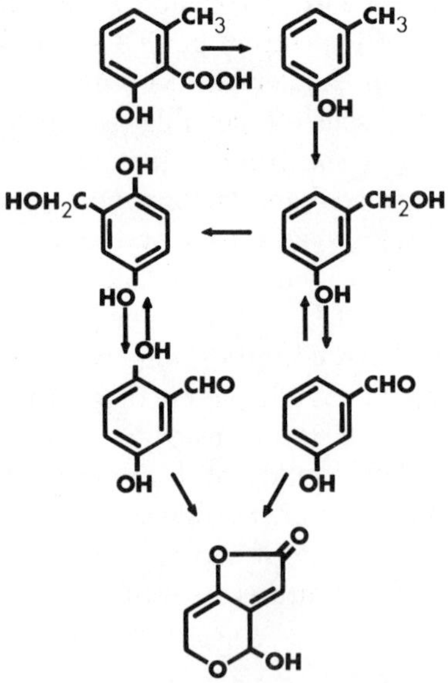

Bioorganic Chemistry

Figure 3. Proposed biosynthetic pathways from 6-methylsalicyclic acid to patulin (78)

Penicillic Acid. Birch et al. (*79*) suggested that in *P. cyclopium* penicillic acid was formed when four acetate units condensed to form orsellinic acid followed by ring cleavage and decarboxylation to yield penicillic acid. Mosbach (*80*) demonstrated a similar sequence in *P. baarense* as did Birkinshaw and Gowland (*32*) in *P. madriti.* Bentley and Keil (*81, 82*) showed that orsellinic acid was formed in *P. cyclopium* when one acetyl coenzyme A unit condensed with three malonyl coenzyme A units which subsequently lost three molecules of CO_2 forming orsellinic acid and which underwent ring cleavage and decarboxylation to yield penicillic acid (Figure 4). Ciegler et al. (*83*) reviewed the biosynthesis of penicillic acid in more detail.

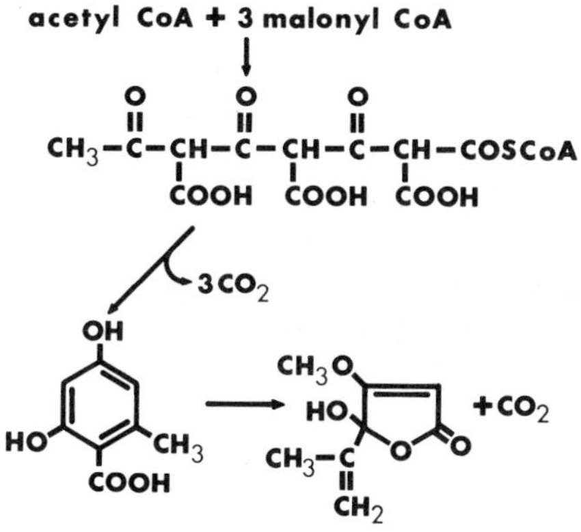

Journal of Biological Proceedings
of the Chemical Society

Figure 4. Intermediates in the biosynthesis of penicillic acid (81, 82)

Toxicity

Patulin. Patulin is a wide-spectrum biocide. It is toxic to many bacteria, protozoa, fungi, mammals, and plants and inactivates some viruses. For a detailed discussion of patulin toxicity, *see* reviews by Korzybski et al. (*53*), Enomoto and Satio (*84*), Scott (*44*) for toxicity details, and Broom et al. (*85*) for the pharmacology of patulin. However a brief consideration of the toxicity of patulin to farm animals and plants is important in relation to its natural occurrence. Patulin has been isolated from soils where phytotoxicity is observed. It contributes to the phytotoxicity of stubble-mulched soils (*89*) and to the soil sickness problem in apple nurseries (*90*).

There is only indirect evidence that patulin may be associated with animal diseases caused by mycotoxin contaminated feed. Ukai et al.

(86) obtained patulin from a *Penicillium* sp. that had been isolated from a malt feed associated with the death of several cattle in Japan. A toxic *A. clavatus* was isolated from a malt causing a feeding problem (87); patulin may have been responsible. Recently, the LD_{50} from oral administration of patulin for white Leghorn cockrels was 170 mg/kg (88)— demonstrating moderate toxicity.

Chronic and sub-acute feeding study trials are needed before the impact of patulin on farm animals and humans is known. The effects of patulin on the intestinal microflora need to be examined as well as the possibility of patulin and other compounds acting together to give a synergistic toxic reaction.

Penicillic Acid. Alsberg and Black (21) found that penicillic acid was lethal to mice at a subcutaneous injection of *ca.* 200–300 mg/kg. The antimicrobial activity was studied by Oxford et al.; gram-negative bacteria were affected more than gram-positive bacteria by penicillic acid (91, 92). However, heart broth was used in these experiments, and Oxford (93) later found that penicillic acid lost bacteriostatic power if a broth medium was used.

The pharmacology of penicillic acid was discussed by Murnaghan (94). The LD_{50} of penicillic acid was 110 mg/kg for mice by subcutaneous injection and 250 mg/kg by intravenous injection (94). No characteristic features were found post mortem. For rabbits the minimal lethal dose ranged from 100–200 mg/kg administered subcutaneously (95). With peroval administration of penicillic acid, up to 715 mg/kg body weight for 8 days was tolerated by white mice without recognizable detriment (95). Hall et al. (96) showed that penicillic acid had antiphage activity against free bacteriophage particles. The possible antitumor and antiviral properties of penicillic acid are discussed by Suzuki et al. (60).

The toxicity of penicillic acid and patulin in cultured cells was studied by Natori et al. (97), Umeda (98), and Kawasaki et al. (99). With HeLa cells, penicillic acid at 10 μg/ml produced an increase of mitotic cells and enlargement of interphasic cells. Enlarged interphasic cells contained large nuclei with dotty chromatin and irregular and larger nucleoli. Pleomorphism was relatively marked (97). The action of penicillic acid on HeLa cells was slow, and the accumulation of metaphasic cells was prominent, accompanied by elongation of the whole cell cycle (99).

Stability and Mode of Action

The stability of patulin and penicillic acid at the pH of interest and the reaction with cellular or medium constituents are important in considering the mode of action of these mycotoxins. Patulin, but not penicillic acid, loses its biological activity in alkaline conditions. Both patulin and penicillic acid are capable of reacting with sulfhydryl groups or amino groups, and the adducts seem to have little biological activity. Thus it is necessary to determine the stability under any set of experimental conditions in order to evaluate data properly concerning the mode of action of these mycotoxins. Also in determining the mode of action of patulin and penicillic acid, the mycotoxin concentration and time of the measured effect is critical to distinguish between primary and secondary effects.

Heatley and Philpot (*100*) found that penicillic acid was stable when heated to 100°C at pHs 2.0 and 9.5. Thus the effects of pH on detoxification of penicillic acid are probably minimal. Patulin on the other hand was stable at pH 2.0 and unstable at pH 9.5 (*100*). The decomposition of patulin produced in the culture medium by patulin producers probably arose from pH changes (*101*). Patulin was stable in McIlvaine buffer solutions at pH 3.3–6.3; at pH 6.3 slow inactivation occurred (*102*). Lovett and Peeler (*103*) determined the thermal destruction kinetics of patulin in McIlvaines' buffer of pH 3.5, 4.5, and 5.5 heated to 105°–125°C. Patulin was resistant to thermal destruction at all pHs. However, the thermal destruction parameters increased as the pH decreased.

Patulin is moderately stable at 22°C in apple and grape juice but not in orange juice or flour (*104*). Heating the juices to 80°C for short periods did not completely destroy patulin. It was stable in dry corn but unstable in wet corn, wheat, sorghum, or aqueous solutions containing SO_2 (*38, 105*). These studies were done at room tempreature; further studies on the production and stability of patulin and penicillic acid are needed at different moisture and temperature levels.

Penicillic acid was also moderately stable at 22°C in apple and grape juice but not in orange juice, whole wheat, or bleached flour (*104*). Heating the juices for short periods to 80°C did not completely destroy the penicillic acid. Penicillic acid was moderately stable in wet corn at 0°–15°C and less stable at 20°C. In general, commodities with high protein content (peanuts, soybeans, and cottonseed) either did not support penicillic acid synthesis or penicillic acid was not stable in them (*30, 59*).

Patulin was stable in acid soils and sand. It was more stable in heat-treated soil at pH 7.2 than in untreated soil, indicating that biological activity caused inactivation (*102*). Patulin was much more stable in soil containing molds that produced patulin than in garden soil with a neutral pH (*106*).

One of the first suggested mechanisms of the action of patulin was that it reacted with SH groups of enzymes and exerted its antibiotic activity in this way. Patulin and penicillic acid can react with free SH groups as well as NH_2 groups under the proper conditions. Oxford (93) demonstrated that at pH 7.0 penicillic acid solution reacted with some primary amines and amino acids in a medium kept at 37°C for several days. Geiger and Conn (107) found that cysteine and thioglycolate did not give a positive nitroprusside reaction with an excess of patulin or penicillic acid. These reaction products had no observed toxic properties. Thiosulfate inactivated patulin only. Dickens and Cooke (108) reported that patulin and penicillic acid reacted rapidly with cysteine. Goodman and Hiatt (109) and Andraud et al. (110) found that enzymic SH groups reacted with patulin.

Ashoor and Chu (111) found inhibition constants of alcohol dehydrogenase for patulin at $5.0 \times 10^{-5}M$ and for penicillic acid at $1.1 \times 10^{-4}M$ where non-competitive inhibition was observed and inhibition constants of lactic dehydrogenase for patulin at $6.2 \times 10^{-6}M$ and penicillic acid at $7.2 \times 10^{-5}M$ where competitive inhibition was observed. Cysteine reversed the effect on lactic dehydrogenase but not on alcohol dehydrogenase. Gottlieb and Singh (112) observed succinate oxidase and dehydrogenase inhibition at high concentration of patulin, $5 \times 10^{-2}M$.

Ciegler et al. (29) found that arginine, histidine, and lysine reacted with penicillic acid. The reaction between lysine and histidine and penicillic acid went to competion in nine days at pH 7.0. The reaction between penicillic acid and glutathione or cysteine was essentially complete in 7 hrs at pH 5, 6, or 7. The reaction products between glutathione or cysteine and penicillic acid were identified as an addition to the isolated double bond rather than the conjugated double bond (Figure 5).

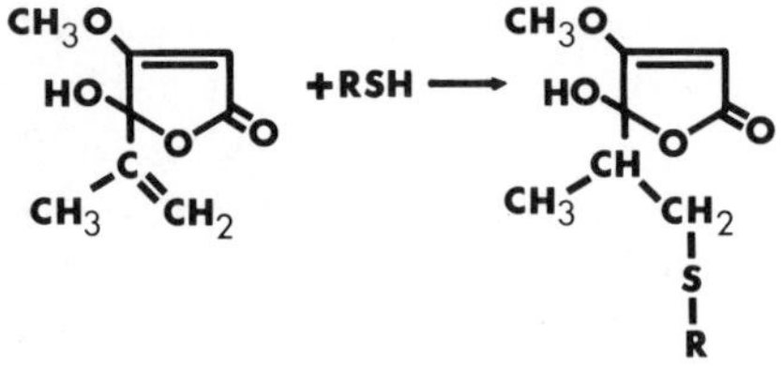

Applied Microbiology

Figure 5. Reaction between penicillic acid and RSH when RSH is cysteine or glutathione (29)

Hofmann et al. (113) observed faster reaction rates with patulin and sulfhydryl groups at pH 7.4 than at pH 5.0. They postulated that the addition of RSH could occur in several ways, but the reaction products were not isolated and identified. If the addition were at the 3 and 7 position with a shift in the double bond, the lactone ring might be less stable and more liable to hydrolysis, explaining the loss of biological activity (Figure 6).

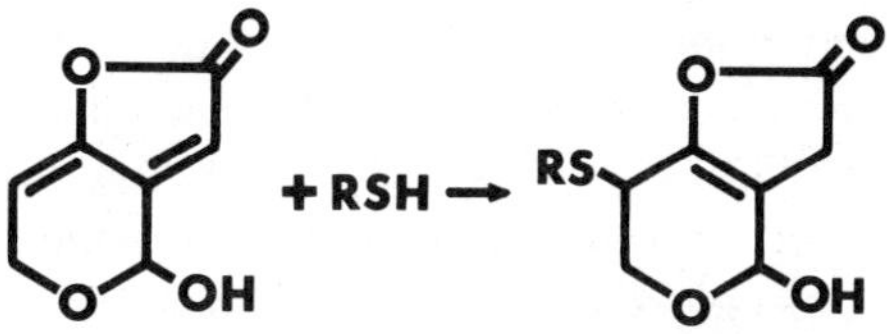

Figure 6.   One possible reaction between patulin and RSH

The reaction of sulfhydryl groups with β-propiolactone was studied by Dickens and Jones (*114*). They isolated S-2-carboxylethyl-L-cysteine as the major product when cysteine and β-propiolactone reacted in neutral solution. In the presence of β-propiolactone and heat-inactivated liver supernatant, no free acid was produced presumably because the β-propiolactone reacted with the denatured proteins (*115*). Compounds with α,β-unsaturation may react with SH groups attached to primary carbon atoms but probably not with those attached to tertiary carbon atoms (*116*). Jones and Young (*117*) found that the biologically active lactone (4-hydroxypent-2-enoic acid lactone) reacted with primary amines to yield an unstable Michael addition product whereas inactive lactones such as 4-hydroxypent-3-enoic acid lactone gave rise to amide derivatives. Further studies by Jones and Young (*118*) revealed that carcinogenic lactones such as 4-hydroxypent-2-enoic acid lactone underwent Michael addition with RSH which then gave rise to the S-alkylated derivative.

The reactions of patulin and penicillic acid with sulfhydryl and amino groups need to be studied in more detail, and the toxicity of the derivatives should be determined. In 1961 Dickens and Jones (*114*) reported that patulin and penicillic acid produced malignant tumors when administered subcutaneously to rats. All of the carcinogenically active lactones possessed either α,β-unsaturation, an external unsaturated bond at position 4, or both (*119, 120, 121*). Because both patulin and penicillic acid are quite reactive, oral feeding studies are needed to interpret properly their potential health hazard. Since the reaction product of β-propiolactone and cysteine, S-2-carboxyethyl-L-cysteine, had weak carcinogenic properties, the reaction products of penicillic acid and patulin with RSH should be evaluated for carcinogenic properties.

Some of patulin's other effects on biological systems are interesting in relation to defining primary and secondary effects, but the list is not intended to be inclusive. These include effects on cation transfer in human erythrocytes where patulin inhibited K^+ transfer at $10^{-3}M$ (122). At high concentrations $10^{-2}M$ patulin inhibited succinate oxidase and succinate dehydrogenase (112). Withers (123) found that patulin at $3.5 \times 10^{-6}M$ induced abnormal metaphases and a high percentage of polyploid cells in human chromosomes. Studying the effect of penicillic acid on mitosis, Gorini et al. (124) concluded that penicillic acid not only had a statmokinetic action but also a partial interkinetic blocking action in the megaloblasts of chicken embryos. No toxicity was associated with ^{14}C activity in eggs laid by hens fed patulin ^{14}C ($125, 126$). Austin et al. ($127, 128$) reported that patulin induced serotypic transformations in *Paramecium aurelia* that may in fact be mutations.

Petite mutants of *Saccharomyces cerevisiae* were induced by patulin. Exposure during the exponential phase produced a higher mutation frequency than during the stationary phase (129). Harwig et al. (130) found that *S. cerevisiae* fermentation of apple juice was not inhibited by similar concentrations of patulin and that the patulin disappeared during the fermentation process. The difference in the pH of the medium and of the apple juice may be important in these different observations.

Using cell culture systems Umeda (98) demonstrated that similar concentrations of patulin or penicllic acid damaged liver, kidney, lung, and HeLa cells. However penicillic acid was less cytotoxic than patulin. In HeLa cells penicillic acid acted slowly, and accumulation of metaphasic cells was prominent. Patulin acted rapidly and directly, stopping the whole cell cycle (99). At 100 μg/ml of penicillic acid and 3.2 μg/ml of patulin, DNA synthesis was almost entirely depressed, but RNA and protein synthesis was only partially depressed. Schaeffer et al. (131) found a depression of RNA synthesis within 20 min and a depression of protein synthesis within 60 min in Chang liver cells treated with 2.5 μg/ml of patulin. The rRNA species were more inhibited than the nonmethylated species; however both synthesis and maturation of the RNA precursor species occurred. This leads to the speculation that the inhibition in RNA biosynthesis most likely occurred at transcription from DNA rather than at maturation from precursor species (131). Recovery occurred after 6 hr of treatment of HeLa cells with penicillic acid, but no recovery was observed after 1 hr with patulin (99). Chang liver cells did not recover after a 20 min treatment with 2.5 μg/ml of patulin (131). Prior to these observations Hewitt et al. (132) observed a decrease in RNA content in patulin treated cauliflower leaf tissue. Patulin and penicillic acid at high concentrations induced breaks in HeLa cell DNA after a 1-hr incubation in both alkaline and neutral sucrose gradients (133).

Patulin and penicillic acid are both capable of interacting with SH groups of enzymes and are more inhibitory to some thiol enzymes than others. However with the exception of the work by Ashoor and Chu (*111*) the effective concentrations are probably too high to be primary effects. The inhibition of protein, RNA, and DNA syntheses occurs soon after intoxication of cell cultures, indicating a primary effect. Respiration seems to be inhibited only at high concentrations, and the effects on respiration are probably secondary. The precise mode of action is still not certain; indeed patulin and penicillic acid may have multiple effects in the cytoplasm.

Analysis

Patulin. Patulin has been detected in several ways including paper, thin layer, gas, and liquid chromatography. Patulin was detected on paper chromatograms by spraying with phenylhydrazine and alkali (*101*). The yellow spot visible after reaction with phenylhydrazine has been used for patulin detection in thin layer chromatography (*45, 104*). Scott (*44*) discussed in detail the solvent systems and spray reagents that have been used to detect patulin on paper and thin layer chromatograms.

Thin layer chromatography has been used extensively to estimate patulin in foods and feeds. Scott and Somers (*104*) extracted patulin with ethyl acetate, dried the extract with calcium sulfate, and eluted the patulin from a silica gel column with ethyl acetate. The patulin was detected after spraying with ammonia and phenylhydrazine hydrochloride and heating; the detection limit was 0.02–0.05 μg patulin (*39*). Using a *p*-anisaldehyde spray reagent containing ethanol, acetic acid, and H_2SO_4, the detction limit was 0.1 μg patulin (*134*). Reiss (*135, 136*) used *o*-dianisidine (saturated in glacial acetic acid) to detect 0.02 μg of patulin and *N*-methylbenzthiazolone-2-hydrazone (Besthorns hydrazone) to detect 0.06 μg patulin.

Acetonitrile–hexane ($4 + 1$) was used to extract patulin from corn, wheat, rye, oats, and sorghum. The acetonitrile phase was evaporated, and preparative TLC was used for preliminary purification. The patulin concentration was estimated using TLC plates containing a 254 nm fluorescent indicator. The limit of detection in corn was about 40 μg/kg (*38*).

Acetonitrile–hexane (100:45) was used to extract patulin from meat and meat products (*137*). The acetonitrile phase was passed through a celite 545 column. The patulin content was estimated using diphenylbor(in)ic acid giving a detection limit of 500 μg/kg. A similar detection limit, 400–1000 μg/kg of patulin in grains, was reported by Stoloff et al. (*138*) using a multimycotoxin detection method.

Ethyl acetate was an efficient solvent of patulin in apple juice (*39, 139*). The apple juice was extracted with ethyl acetate, the dried ethyl acetate was passed through a silicagel column using benzene–ethyl acetate (75 + 25) as the eluting solvent. Patulin was detected by TLC with 3-methyl-2-benzothiazolinone hydrochloride as a spray reagent; the detection limit was 0.01 μg patulin.

Patulin was detected in apple juice using gas chromatography after an initial preparative TLC purification (45). Pohland et al. (140) prepared the silyl ether, actate, and chloroacetate derivative of patulin and used GLC analysis of the chloroacetate derivative to detect 0.7 μg/ml of patulin in apple juice. Suzuki et al. (141), Pero and Harvan (142), and Pero et al. (143) developed methods for GLC analysis of the silyl ether and trimethylsilyl derivatives of patulin.

One liquid chromatographic method to determine patulin in apple juice has been reported (144). The initial extraction and column cleanup were essentially the same as that used by Scott (139). The patulin eluate was evaporated to dryness and immediately dissolved in a small volume of ethyl acetate containing β-methylumbelliferone as an internal standard. The patulin was separated using isooctane/methylene chloride/methanol (84 + 15 + 1) on Zorbax-sil silica with a flow of ca. 0.5 ml/min. The peak was collected for TLC confirmation or GC–MS determination of the acetate derivative.

The major problem with any method that estimates patulin or penicillic acid is not how to extract it but when to extract it. For example in canned apple juice an interferring substance was rapidly formed when exposed to air (139); in freshly pressed, unclarified juice only 50–60% of the patulin was recovered after overnight storage in a refrigerator (145). In meat and bread patulin occurs only temporarily during fermentation or molding (146, 147).

Penicillic Acid. Penicillic acid has been detected using bioassay, colorimetric, thin layer chromatographic, and gas chromatographic methods. Penicillic acid was non-toxic to zebra fish larvae at 5 μg/ml (148), and brine shrimp larvae were moderately sensitive to 10–20μg/disc (149). Betina (150) detected penicillic acid on paper chromatograms by noting the toxicity to *Bacillus subtillis* on the chromatogram.

Hydroxylamine reacted with penicillic acid to give a red color. At 530 nm, Beers law held true for 80–1000 mg/ml of penicillic acid (151). Another colorimetric method used the reddish-purple complex of ammonia with penicillic acid (81). Ethyl acetate (104), ethyl acetate–water (7:1) (141), chloroform-methanol (90:10) (59), chloroform-methanol (70:30) (36), and chloroform (29, 152) have extracted penicillic acid from various substances.

Several methods have been used for preliminary purification. Scott and Somers (104) dried the ethyl acetate extract with calcium sulfate and eluted the pencillic acid with ethyl acetate by passing it through a silica gel column. Pero et al. (143) used preparative thin layer chromatography for preliminary purification. Thorpe and Johnson (*153*) partitioned the penicillic acid with 3% sodium bicarbonate followed by acidification and extraction with ethyl acetate. The penicillic acid solution was passed through a silica gel column using hexane–ethyl acetate–formic acid (750 + 250 + 1) as the eluting solvent.

Penicillic acid has been detected on thin layer chromatograms because it fluoresces after exposure to ammonia (*59*); it gives a yellow fluorescence with ammonia and phenylhydrazine (*104*) and a green color with *p*-anisaldehyde (*134*).

The trimethylsilyl ether of pencillic acid was preferred for gas chromatography by Suzuki et al. (*141*) over the acetate which formed slowly and the trifluoroacetate which always gave two peaks. Pero et al. (*143*) and Pero and Harvan (*142*) described conditions for gas chromatographic detection of penicillic acid and the trimethylsilyl ether. The trimethylsilyl ether was used to detect penicillic acid in moldy tobacco (*152*). Thorpe and Johnson (*153*) successfully obtained the trifluoroacetate of penicillic acid for gas chromatographic detection in corn and beans and presented a confirmation method using gas chromatography–mass spectrometry.

Natural Occurrence

Patulin. Patulin was implicated in the mass deaths of over 100 cows that were intoxicated by dry malt feed. Patulin was obtained from *Penicillium urticae* that was subsequently isolated from the feed (*86*). Patulin may have been either the cause of the intoxication, or it may have been present in sublethal amounts that acted in association with other toxic substances. Male culms intoxication of cattle associated with moldy feed may be caused by patulin since the disease is associated with *A. clavatus* invasion of the feed. Apparently the toxic principal has not been identified (*87*).

Penicillium expansum causes a storage rot of apples, pears, and cherries. Brian et al. (*154*) identified patulin in decayed apple juice by its antimicrobial spectrum. Walker (*155*) used paper chromatography to detect patulin in apple juice by its ultraviolet quenching at 254 nm. Patulin was found in commercially available apple juice in Canada and the United States by Scott et al. (*45*) and Wilson and Nuovo (*145*). A limited survey of cider mills (*145*) revealed that patulin contamination depended on the proportion of decayed apples used in making fresh apple cider. Beer (*156*) found that patulin was present in fresh cider from unsound fruit; patulin was not detected in fresh cider made from undecayed apples. After inoculating apples with *P. expansum* Harwig *et al.* (*157*) found up to 250 μg/ml patulin per decayed apple in the expressed juice, and Wilson and Nuovo (*145*) found up to 146 μg patulin/ml expressed juice. Less than 11% of the isolates of *P. expansum* produced over 100 μg/ml of expressed juice in inoculated apples (*145*). Similar concentrations of patulin were found in lesions of pears and stone fruits decayed by *P. expansum* (*158*).

Patulin has been reported in spontaneously molded bread (*147, 159*) and was temporarily present during the ripening of fermented sausage (*146*). The stability of patulin at different temperatures and conditions should be studied in more detail. This is evident when one compares the studies on penicillic acid production in corn with the few studies on patulin production in various commodities. Patulin has also been isolated from soil and wheat straw residues where there is a phytotoxic problem associated with stubble mulching (*160*). The levels of patulin recovered are high enough to leave little doubt that patulin is a factor in this phytotoxicity.

Penicillic Acid. Penicillic acid has been found in moldy tobacco from commercial storage (*152*) and in moldy corn and beans (*153*). Kurtzman and Ciegler (*59*) reported that *P. martensii* molded high-moisture corn at 1°C. They isolated high levels of penicillic acid from artificially inoculated corn incubated at temperatures between 1° and 15°C. The penicillic acid disappeared within 45 days at higher temperatures. Several other species of *Penicillium* that cause blue-eyed disease of corn were capable of penicillic acid synthesis on several commodities. Peanuts, soybeans, and cottonseeds did not accumulate penicillic acid when inoculated with fungi capable of penicillic acid synthesis (*30*). Lillehoj et al. (*161*) found that atmospheres enriched with 60% CO_2 reduced penicillic acid accumulation below detectable levels when high-moisture corn was inoculated with *P. martensii* and was stored at 5°C.

A combination of low temperatures (15° or 22°C) and low moisture favored the production of penicillic acid in autoclaved poultry feed inoculated with *A. ochraceus* (*162*). Ciegler et al. (*29*) and Fielder (*163*) did not find penicillic acid in meat products overgrown with *Penicillia*.

Outlook

Both patulin and penicillic acid should be considered as potentially dangerous mycotoxins since both are toxic and both have been implicated in carcinogenesis. Patulin also causes mutations in yeast. The carcinogenic properties and other chronic effects need further evaluation to assess properly their importance when ingested orally.

Both mycotoxins are probably prevalent in the environment and are produced by several fungi capable of decaying food or feed. The natural occurrence and stability of either compound in foods and feeds at different moisture levels and temperatures have not been well studied; we can only assume their presence and stability in moldy foods if a fungus that produces either mycotoxin is associated with the decay.

The reactions and biological activity of adducts of patulin and penicillic acid with SH groups and NH_2 groups need further study for us to understand how detoxification occurs and if the presence of the adducts in food and feed should cause concern. The question of the tautomerism of penicillic acid is interesting and could be better understood. Both patulin and penicillic acid may be useful as models of anti-viral compounds. Perhaps suitable derivatives can be made that will help us understand or help us control virus-caused disorders.

Acknowledgments

The assistance of Martha Girardeau, William Tabor, and Theodosia Flowers in the literature retrieval is acknowledged with gratitude.

Literature Cited

1. Boyd, E. M., *Can. Med. Assoc. J.* (1944) **50**, 159.
2. Stansfield, J. M., Francis, A. E., Stuart-Harris, C. H., *Lancet* (1944) **2**, 370.
3. Woodward, R. B., Singh, G., *J. Amer. Chem. Soc.* (1949) **71**, 758.
4. Woodward, R. B., Singh, G., *Experientia* (1950) **6**, 238.
5. Singh, J., Patulin, in "Antibiotics I., Mechanism of Action," Gottleib, D. and Shaw, P. D., Eds., pp. 621-630, Springer-Verlag, Berlin, 1967.
6. Kent, J., Heatley, N. G., *Nature* (1945) **156**, 295.
7. Birkinshaw, J. H., Michael, S. E., Braken, A., Raistrick, H., *Lancet* (1943) **245**, 625.
8. Simonart, P., de Lathouwer, R., *Zentralbl. Bacteriol. Parasitenk. Abt II* (1956-57) **110**, 107.
10. Umezawa, H., Mizuhara, Y., Uekane, K., Hagiwara, M., *Jap. Med. J.* (1948) **1**, 97.
11. Barta, J., Mécir, R., *Experientia* (1948) **4**, 277.
12. Karchenko, S. M., *Mikrobiol. Zh. Akad.-Nauk Ukr.* (1970) **32**, 115.
13. Chain, E., Florey, H. W., Jennings, M. A., *Brit. J. Exp. Pathol.* (1942) **23**, 202.
14. Abraham, E. P., Florey, H. W., "Substances Produced by Fungi Imperfecti and Ascomycetes," in "Antibiotics," Vol. I, Florey, H. W., Chain, E., Heatley, N. G., Jennings, M. A., Sanders, A. G., Abraham, E. P., and Florey, M. E., Eds., pp. 273-355, Oxford University, London, 1949.
15. Efimenko, O. M., Yakimov, P. A., *Trudy Leningrad. Khim-Farmakol Inst.* (1960) **9**, 88.
16. Myrchink, T. G., *Antibiotiki (USSR)* (1967) **12**, 762.
17. Waksman, S. A., Horning, E. S., Spencer, E. L., *Science* (1942) **96**, 202.
18. Florey, H. W., Jennings, M. A., Philpot, F. J., *Nature* (1944) **153**, 139.
19. Kuehn, H. H., *Mycologia* (1958) **50**, 417.
20. Karow, E. O., Foster, J. W., *Science* (1944) **99**, 265.

21. Alsberg, C. L., Black, O. F., *U.S. Dept. Agr., Bur. Plant Ind. Bull.,* **270,** 1913.
22. Birkinshaw, J. H., Oxford, A. E., Raistrick, H., *Biochem. J.* (1936) **30,** 394.
23. Gorbach, von G., Friedrich, W., *Osterr. Chem.-Ztg.* (1949) **50,** 93.
24. Betina, V., Gašparíková, E., Nemec, P., *Biologia* (1969) **24,** 482.
25. Karow, E. O., Woodruff, H. B., Foster, J. W., *Arch. Biochem. Biophys.* (1944) **5,** 279.
26. Wirth, J. C., Gilmore, T. E., Noval, J. J., *Arch. Biochem. Biophys.* (1956) **63,** 452.
27. Van Eijk, G. W., Antonie van Leeuwenhoek, *J. Microbiol. Serol.* (1969) **35,** 497.
28. Wirth, J., Klosek, R., *Phytochemistry* (1972) **11,** 2615.
29. Ciegler, A., Mintzlaff, H. J., Weisleder, D., Leistner, L., *Appl. Microbiol.* (1972) **24,** 114.
30. Ciegler, A., Kurtzman, C. P., *Appl. Microbiol.* (1970) **20,** 761.
31. Burton, H. S., *Brit. J. Exp. Pathol.* (1949) **30,** 151.
32. Birkinshaw, J. H., Gowland, A., *Biochem. J.* (1962) **84,** 342.
33. Kobayashi, H., Tsunoda, H., Tatsuno, T., *Chem. Pharmacol. Bull. (Tokyo)* (1971) **19,** 839.
34. Gill-Carey, D., *Brit. J. Exp. Pathol.* (1949) **30,** 119.
35. Burton, H. S., *Nature* (1950) **165,** 274.
36. Ciegler, A., *Can. J. Microbiol.* (1972) **18,** 631.
37. Chain, E., Florey, H. W., Jennings, M. A., Crowfoot, D., Low, B., *Lancet* (1944) **I,** 112.
38. Pohland, A. E., Allen, R., *J. Assoc. Offic. Anal. Chem.* (1970) **53,** 686.
39. Scott, P. M., Kennedy, B. P. C., *J. Assoc. Offic. Anal. Chem.* (1973) **56,** 813.
40. Grove, J. F., *J. Chem. Soc.* (1951) 883.
41. Lalau-Keraly, F., Nivière, P., Tronche, P., *C.R.* (1965) **261,** 4028.
42. Schepartz, A. I., Fleischman, R. A., Cisle, J. H., *J. Chromatogr.* (1972) **69,** 411.
43. Katzman, P. A., Hays, E. E., Cain, C. K., van Wyk, J. J., Reithel, F. J., Thayer, S. A., Doisy, E. A., Gaby, W. L., Carroll, C. J., Muir, R. D., Jones, L. R., Wade, N. J., *J. Biol. Chem.* (1944) **154,** 475.
44. Scott, P. M., Patulin in "Mycotoxins," I. F. H. Purchase, Ed., Elsevier Sci. Pub. Co., Amsterdam, in press.
45. Scott, P. M., Miles, W. F., Tóft, P., Dubé, J. G., *J. Agr. Food Chem.* (1972) **20,** 450.
46. Scott, A. I., Yalpani, M., *Chem. Commun. (J. Chem. Soc., Sect. D)* (1967) **18,** 945.
47. Raistrick, H., Birkinshaw, J. H., Braken, A., Michael, S. E., *Lancet* (1943) 625.
48. Bergel, F., Morrison, A. L., Moss, A. R., Klein, R., Rinderknecht, H., Ward, J. L., *Nature* (1943) **152,** 750.
49. Suzuki, T., Takeda, M., Tanabe, H., *Chem. Pharm. Bull. (Tokyo)* (1971) **19,** 1786.
50. Scott, P. M., Kennedy, B., van Walbeek, W., *Experientia* (1972) **28,** 1252.
51. Woodward, R. B., Singh, G., *J. Amer. Chem. Soc.* (1950) **72,** 1428.
52. Serratosa, F., *Tetrahedron* (1961) **16,** 185.
53. Korzybski, T., Kowszyk-Gindifer, Z., Kurylowicz, W., "Antibiotics Origin, Nature and Properties," Vol. II, pp. 1223-1230, Pergamon, New York, 1967.
54. Page, J. E., Robinson, F. A., *J. Chem. Soc.* (1943) 133.
55. Raphael, R. A., *J. Chem. Soc.* (1947) 805.
56. Kovac, S., Solcaniova, E., Eglinton, G., *Tetrahedron* (1969) **25,** 3617.

57. Sassa, T., Hayakara, S., Ikeda, M., Miura, Y., *Agr. Biol. Chem. (Tokyo)* (1971) **35**, 2130.
58. Ciegler, A., Kurtzman, C. P., *J. Chromatogr.* (1970) **51**, 511.
59. Kurtzman, C. P., Ciegler, A., *Appl. Microbiol.* (1970) **20**, 204.
60. Suzuki, S., Kimura, T., Saito, F., Ando, K., *Agr. Biol. Chem.* (1971) **35**, 287.
61. Ford, J. H., Johnson, A. R., Hinman, J. W., *J. Amer. Chem. Soc.* (1950) **72**, 4529.
62. Shaw, E., *J. Amer. Chem. Soc.* (1946) **68**, 2510.
63. Szilágyi, I., Vályi-Nagy, T., Galambos, G., *Microchim. Ichnoanal. Acta* (1963) **5-6**, 864.
64. Raphael, R. A., *J. Chem. Soc.* (1948) 1508.
65. Raphael, R. A., *Roy. Inst. Chem. Lectures.* Monographs and Reports (1950) **3**, 18.
66. Bu'Lock, J. D., Hamilton, D., Hulme, M. A., Powell, A. J., Smalley, H. M., Shepherd, D., Smith, G. N., *Can. J. Microbiol.* (1965) **11**, 765.
67. Bassett, E. W., Tanenbaum, S. W., *Experientia* (1958) **14**, 38.
68. Tanenbaum, S. W., Bassett, E. W., *Biochim. Biophys. Acta* (1958) **28**, 21.
69. Tanenbaum, S. W., Bassett, E. W., *J. Biol. Chem.* (1959) **234**, 1861.
70. Bu'Lock, J. D., Ryan, A. J., *Proc. Chem. Soc.* (1958) 222.
71. Bassett, E. W., Tanenbaum, S. W., *Biochim. Biophys. Acta* (1960) **40**, 535.
72. Bu'Lock, J. D., Smalley, H. M., *Proc. Chem. Soc.* (1961) 209.
73. Bu'Lock, J. D., Shepherd, D., Winstanley, D. J., *Can. J. Microbiol.* (1969) **15**, 279.
74. Light, R. J., *Biochim. Biophys. Acta* (1969) **191**, 430.
75. Forrester, P. I., Gaucher, G. M., *Biochemistry* (1972) **11**, 1108.
76. Arihood, S., Light, R. J., *Nature* (1966) **210**, 629.
77. Forrester, P. I., Gaucher, G. M., *Biochemistry* (1972) **11**, 1102.
78. Scott, A. I., Zamir, L., Phillips, G. T., Yalpani, M., *Bioorg. Chem.* (1973) **2**, 124.
79. Birch, A. J., Blance, G. E., Smith, H., *Proc. Chem. Soc.* (1958) 4582.
80. Mosbach, K., *Acta Chem. Scand.* (1960) **14**, 457.
81. Bentley, R., Keil, J. G., *J. Biol. Chem.* (1962) **237**, 867.
82. Bentley, R., Keil, J. G., *Proc. Chem. Soc.* (1961) 111.
83. Ciegler, A., Detroy, R. W., Lillehoj, E. B., "Patulin, Penicillic Acid and Other Carcinogenic Lactones," in "Microbial Toxins," Vol. 6, Ciegler, A., Kadis, S., Ajl, S. J., Eds., pp. 409–434, Academic, New York, 1971.
84. Enomoto, M., Saito, M., *Annu. Rev. Microbiol.* (1972) **26**, 279.
85. Broom, W. A., Bülbring, E., Chapman, C. J., Hampton, J. W. F., Thomson, A. M., Ungar, J., Wein, R., Woolfe, G., *Brit. J. Exp. Pathol.* (1944) **25**, 195.
86. Ukai, T., Yamamoto, Y., Yamamoto, T., *J. Pharm. Soc. Japan* (1954) **74**, 450.
87. Schultz, V. J., Motz, R., *Monatsh. Veterinaermed.* (1973) **28**, 790.
88. Lovett, J., *Poultry Sci.* (1972) **51**, 2097.
89. McCalla, T. M., Guenzi, W. D., Norstadt, F. A., *Z. Allg. Mikrobiol.* (1963) **3**, 202.
90. Borner, H., *Phytopathol. Z.* (1963) **49**, 1.
91. Oxford, A. E., *Chem. Ind.* (1942) 48.
92. Oxford, A. E., Raistrick, H., Smith, G., *Chem. Ind.* (1942) 22.
93. Oxford, A. E., *Biochem. J.* (1942) **36**, 438.
94. Murnaghan, M. F., *J. Pharmacol.* (1946) **88**, 119.
95. Zeller, A., Matthes, T., *Deut. Gesuntheitsw. (Berlin)* (1946) **1**, 499.
96. Hall, E. A., Kavanagh, F., Asheshov, I. N., *Antibiot. Chemother.* (1951) **1**, 369.

97. Natori, S., Sakaki, S., Kurata, H., Udagawa, S., Ichinoe, M., Saito, M., Umeda, M., *Chem. Pharm. Bull. (Tokyo)* (1970) **18**, 2259.
98. Umeda, M., *Jap. J. Exp. Med.* (1971) **41**, 195.
99. Kawasaki, I., Oki, T., Umeda, M., Saito, M., *Jap. J. Exp. Med.* (1972) **42**, 327.
100. Heatley, N. G., Philpot, F. J., *J. Gen. Microbiol.* (1947) **1**, 232.
101. Yamamoto, T., *J. Pharm. Soc., Jap.* (1956) **76**, 1419.
102. Jeffreys, E. G., *J. Gen. Microbiol.* (1952) **7**,295.
103. Lovett, J., Peeler, J. T., *J. Food Sci.* (1973) **38**, 1094.
104. Scott, P. M., Somers, E., *J. Agr. Food Chem.* (1968) **16**, 483.
105. Pohland, A. E., Allen, R., *J. Ass. Off. Anal. Chem.* (1970) **53**, 688.
106. *Proc. Intern. Botan. Congr., Stockholm, 1950,* **7**, 448 (1954).
107. Geiger, W. B., Conn, J. E., *J. Amer. Chem. Soc.* (1945) **67**, 112.
108. Dickens, F., Cooke, J., *Brit. J. Cancer* (1965) **19**, 404.
109. Goodman, I., Hiatt, R. B., *Biochem. Pharmacol.* (1964) **13**, 871.
110. Andraud, G., Couquelet, J., Tronche, P., Dorel, M., *Ann. Biol. Clin. (Paris)* (1966) **24**, 469.
111. Ashoor, S. H., Chu, F. S., *Food Cosmet. Toxicol.* (1973) **11**, 617.
112. Gottlieb, D., Singh, J., *Riv. Patol. Veg.* (1964) **4**, 455.
113. Hofman, K., Mintzlaff, H. J., Alperden, I., Leistner, L., *Fleischwirtschaft* (1971) **51**, 1534.
114. Dickens, F., Jones, H. E. H., *Brit. J. Cancer* (1961) **15**, 85.
115. Al-Kassab, S., Davis, W., Boyland, E., *Brit. Emp. Cancer Campgn., 40th Annual Report* (1962) 59.
116. Friedman, M., Cavins, J. F., Wall, J. S., *J. Amer. Chem. Soc.* (1965) **87**, 3672.
117. Jones, J. B., Young, J. M., *Can. J. Chem.* (1966) **44**, 1059.
118. Jones, J. B., Young, J. M., *J. Med. Chem.* (1968) **11**, 1176.
119. Dickens, F., *Essays Exp. Biol.* (1962) 107.
120. Dickens, F., Jones, H. E. H., *Brit. J. Cancer* (1963) **17**, 100.
121. Dickens, F., Jones, H. E. H., *Brit. J. Cancer* (1965) **19**, 392.
122. Kahn, Jr., J. B., *J. Pharmacol. Exp. Ther.* (1957) **121**, 234.
123. Withers, R. F. J., "Mech. Mutat. Inducing Factors, Proc. Symp. (1966) 359.
124. Gorini, P., Rondanelli, R., Moratti, R., Gerna, G., Dionisi, D., *Giorn. Ital. Chemioterap.* (1967) **14**, 7.
125. Lovett, J., *Bacteriol. Proc., A* (1970) 92.
126. Lovett, J., *Abs. Annu. Meetg. Amer. Soc. Microbiol.* (1972), E 99, 17.
127. Austin, M. L., Pasternak, J., Rudman, B. M., *Exp. Cell Res.* (1967) **45**, 289.
128. Austin, M. L., Pasternak, J., Rudman, B. M., *Exp. Cell Res.* (1967) **45**, 306.
129. Mayer, V. W., Legator, M. S., *J. Agr. Food Chem.* (1969) **17**, 454.
130. Harwig, J., Scott, P. M., Kennedy, B. P. C., Chen, Y. K., *Can. Inst. Food Technol. J.* (1973) **6**, 45.
131. Schaeffer, W. I., Smith, N. E., Payne, P. A., Wilson, D. M., in press.
132. Hewitt, E. J., Notton, B. A., Afridi, M. M. R. K., *Plant Cell Physiol. (Tokyo)* (1967) **8**, 385.
133. Umeda, M., Yamamoto, T., Saito, M., *Jap. J. Exp. Med.* (1972) **42**, 527.
134. Scott, P. M., Lawrence, J. W., van Walbeek, W., *Appl. Microbiol.* (1970) **20**, 839.
135. Reiss, J., *Chromatographia* (1971) **4**, 576.
136. Reiss, J., *J. Chromatogr.* (1973) **86**, 190.
137. Tauchmann, F., Tóth, L., Leistner, L., *Fleischwirtschaft* (1971) **51**, 1079.
138. Stoloff, L., Nesheim, S., Yin, L., Rodricks, J. V., Stack, M., Campbell, A. D., *J. Ass. Off. Anal. Chem.* (1971) **54**, 91.

139. Scott, P. M., *J. Ass. Off. Anal. Chem.* (1974) **57**, 621.
140. Pohland, A. E., Sanders, K., Thorpe, C. W., *J. Ass. Off. Anal. Chem.* (1970) **53**, 692.
141. Suzuki, T., Takeda, M., Tanabe, H., *Shokuhin Eiseigaku Zasshi* (1971) **12**, 495.
142. Pero, R. W., Harvan, D., *J. Chromatogr.* (1973) **80**, 255.
143. Pero, R. W., Harvan, D., Owens, R. G., Snow, J. P., *J. Chromatogr.* (1972) **65**, 501.
144. Ware, G. M., Thorpe, C. W., Pohland, A. E., *J. Ass. Off. Anal. Chem.* (1974) **57**, 1113.
145. Wilson, D. M., Nuovo, G. J., *Appl. Microbiol.* (1973) **26**, 124.
146. Alperden, I., Mintzlaff, H. J., Tauchmann, F., Leistner, L., *Fleischwirtschaft* (1973) **53**, 566.
147. Reiss, J., *Chem. Mikrobiol., Technol. Lebensm.* (1973) **2**, 171.
148. Abedi, Z. H., Scott, P. M., *J. Ass. Off. Anal. Chem.* (1969) **52**, 963.
149. Harwig, J., Scott, P. M., *Appl. Microbiol.* (1971) **21**, 1011.
150. Betina, V., *J. Chromatogr.* (1964) **15**, 379.
151. Sternberg, M., *Acad. Rep. Pop. Rom. Studii Cer. Chim.* (1956) **4**, 315.
152. Snow, J. P., Lucas, G. B., Harvan, D., Pero, R. W., Owens, R. G., *Appl. Microbiol.* (1972) **24**, 34.
153. Thorpe, C. W., Johnson, R. L., *J. Ass. Off. Anal. Chem.* (1974) **57**, 861.
154. Brian, P. W., Elson, G. W., Lowe, D., *Nature* (1956) **178**, 263.
155. Walker, J. R. L., *Phytochemistry* (1969) **8**, 561.
156. Beer, S. V., *Proc. N.Y. St. Hort. Soc.* (1974) **119**, 165.
157. Harwig, J., Chen, Y. K., Kennedy, B. P. C., Scott, P. M., *Can. Inst. Food Technol. J.* (1973) **6**, 22.
158. Buchanan, J. R., Sommer, N. F., Fortlage, R. J., Maxie, E. C., Mitchell, F. G., Hseih, D. P. H., *J. Amer. Soc. Hort. Sci.* (1974) **99**, 262.
159. Reiss, J., *Naturwissenschaften* (1972) **59**, 37.
160. Norstadt, F. A., McCalla, T. M., *Soil Sci.* (1969) **107**, 188.
161. Lillehoj, E. B., Milburn, M. S., Ciegler, A., *Appl. Microbiol.* (1972) **24**, 198.
162. Bacon, C. W., Sweeney, J. G., Robbins, J. D., Burdick, D., *Appl. Microbiol.* (1973) **26**, 155.
163. Fiedler, von H., *Arch. Lebensmittelhyg.* (1973) **8**, 180.

RECEIVED November 8, 1974.

7

Metabolites of Various *Penicillium* Species Encountered on Foods

A. E. POHLAND and P. MISLIVEC

Bureau of Foods, Food and Drug Administration, Washington, D. C. 20204

The number of species in the genus Penicillium *which have been shown to produce toxic metabolites is great. A survey of the literature concerning the frequency of occurrence of* Penicillium *species on foods and feeds has been made, and 13 species have been identified as common contaminants of foods and feeds. The chemistry and toxicological properties of the metabolites produced by these 13 species are discussed.*

Molds are ubiquitous in nature; in fact it is hard to specify an area or place where a mold will not grow and proliferate. This fact engendered a tremendous impetus to study molds and the metabolites produced by molds. These studies progressed to the point where one may confidently say that molds can produce many secondary metabolites—some of which are acutely toxic and some of which have other toxic manifestations (*i.e.*, mutagenicity, teratogenicity, or carcinogenicity). However it was not until 1960 (when the problem of aflatoxin, elaborated by the mold *Aspergillus flavus,* became apparent) that concern arose over these metabolites in foods and feeds. Since that time mold species of many genera besides *Aspergillus* have been implicated as being capable of producing mycotoxins in foods and feeds; many of these toxins have been identified as the causative agents in various animal illnesses and deaths.

Since the number of species in the genus *Penicillium* known to produce toxic metabolites is extensive, it is necessary to exert some caution in assessing the significance of these findings. The studies of the toxins produced by the various *Penicillium* species over the past decade have implicated the molds in illnesses and deaths of animals. It is therefore essential to evaluate carefully the hazardous potential to humans resulting from exposure to these toxins.

To evaluate properly its hazardous potential, one must determine the species of *Penicillium* that produce mycotoxin in foods and feeds. For each species one must consider the following points: (a) how frequently is the species encountered and on what foods; (b) what quantity of such food is consumed by humans and at what age group; (c) what environmental conditions are required by the species for growth; (d) which mycotoxins the species produces; (e) what proportion of the isolates of a given species produces the toxin; (f) how much of the toxin the toxigenic isolate produces; (g) how toxic the toxin is in terms of both amount and effects; (h) does the toxin occur in foods and feeds, at what concentration, and is the toxin stable to food processing; (i) are species that occur frequently but with no history of toxigenicity actually toxic (*P. funiculosum* in field corn, for example).

To answer these questions we must consider the following facts: (a) the type of food will often determine the mold flora, *e.g., P. urticae* is commonly found in wheat flour products but rarely found in corn or beans; (b) the source and processing stage of the food also determines the flora, *e.g., P. oxalicum* and *P. funiculosum* are commonly found on corn in the field whereas in storage *P. cyclopium* and *P. viridicatum* predominate; (c) conditions of temperature and moisture prior to and during food storage greatly influence the mold flora; (d) detection and identification of the mold species is not always straightforward. This is particularly true for species of *Penicillium;* most species of *Penicillium* are difficult to identify and are frequently referred to in the literature as a *Penicillium* sp. Others are slow growers (*e.g., P. islandicum* and *P. purpurogenum*) and may go undetected because of the overgrowth of fast growing species of *Penicillium* or some other genus (*e.g., Rhizopus*). From our own studies it is apparent that the manner in which the molds are isolated from the food is important. For example, to determine the mold flora of peppercorns, the isolation medium used was potato-dextrose agar, and much *P. islandicum* was detected; with dried beans, however, malt agar with 7.5% NaCl had to be used to prevent bean germination on the plate, and no *P. islandicum* was observed. It is possible that this species was not able to establish growth on the latter medium.

Considering these facts we proposed that the *Penicillium* species listed in Table I should be carefully investigated and evaluated for their

Table I.   *Penicillium* Species Encountered on Foods and Feeds

I	II	III
P. cyclopium	P. oxalicum	P. urticae
P. viridicatum	P. expansum	P. islandicum
	P. chrysogenum	P. citrinum
	P. brevi-compactum	P. variable
	P. funiculosum	P. frequentans
		P. purpurogenum

hazardous potential arising from their occurrence on foods and feeds (*1*). This list is based on the extensive experience of mycologists relative to the presence and rate of occurrence of these *Penicillium* species on foods and feeds. The occurrence of *Penicillium* species is listed in Table I in three groups: group I—very frequently encountered, group II—frequently encountered, and group III—occasionally encountered. The metabolites elaborated by each of these species will be discussed later. Some of the FDA-generated data concerning natural occurrence on which Table I is based are found in Tables II and III (*2, 3*).

Table II. Toxicogenic Penicillia Isolated from Commodities During FDA Surveys

Commodity	Species	% Incidence[a] NSD	SD	Myco- toxin	No. Isolates Positive
Dried Beans	P. brevi-compactum	1.7	0.1	—	—
(114 Samples)	P. citrinum	3.5	0.4	Citrinin	10 of 10
	P. cyclopium	17.3	3.3	Penicillic Acid	38 of 51
	P. viridicatum	18.0	2.4	Citrinin	3 of 15
	P. viridicatum	18.0	2.4	Ochratoxin	0 of 15
	P. urticae	0.4	0.1	Patulin	9 of 9
	P. urticae	0.4	0.1	Griseo- fulvin	9 of 9
White Pepper-	P. islandicum	98.0	2.8	—	—
corns	P. citrinum	2.9	23.0	Citrinin	10 of 10
(24 Samples)					
Black Pepper-	P. islandicum	0.1	0.0	—	—
corns	P. citrinum	1.4	0.0	Citrinin	1 of 1
(108 Samples)					

[a] NSD = not surface disinfected; SD = surface disinfected.

Several other studies support the importance of the species of *Penicillium* listed in Table I as invaders of foods and feeds. In a study of the species of *Penicillium* capable of rotting pomaceous fruits (in addition to *P. expansum* which is notorious in this respect) Mislivec found that *P. cyclopium, P. funiculosum,* and *P. purpurogenum* were highly effective rotters of apple and apple products (*4*).

Mislivec and Tuite (*5*) also studied dent corn kernels obtained from fields at harvest, from cribs and bins, and from experimental storage tests during 1964–1968. *Penicillium* species were found consistently in unstored corn (6.4% of kernels infected), in crib samples (13.4%), and in commercial samples of poor quality. The chief species isolated from unstored kernels were *P. oxalicum, P. funiculosum,* and to a limited extent *P. cyclopium.* The chief species isolated from stored kernels were *P.*

Table III.   Incidence of Penicillia in
11 Wheat Paste Product Samples

Species	No. Samples with Each Species
P. cyclopium	11 of 11
P. frequentans	2 of 11
P. funiculosum	2 of 11
P. islandicum	4 of 11
P. luteum	1 of 11
P. purpurogenum	5 of 11
P. urticae	11 of 11
P. viridicatum	5 of 11

cyclopium, P. brevi-compactum, and *P. viridicatum.* Hesseltine and Graves (6) found in an exhaustive study that *P. cyclopium, P. urticae,* and *P. citrinum* occurred most frequently in flour and refrigerated dough products.

Finally Ciegler, Mintzlaff, and Leistner (7) reported the isolation of 422 *Penicillium* strains from 44 mold-ripened sausages collected in 11 countries; *P. viridicatum* and *P. expansum* were most frequently encountered. Earlier studies by Leistner and Ayres (8) of molds occurring on cured meats (sausages and hams) showed *Penicillium* species present on 89% of the sausages and on 83% of the hams. The most frequently observed molds belonged to *P. expansum, P. janthinellum, P. chrysogenum, P. commune,* and *P. viridicatum.*

Table IV is an attempt to summarize the various literature reports of observed illnesses and deaths of experimental animals when exposed to a substrate molded with the *Penicillium* species listed in Table I. Also included are natural outbreaks of mycotoxicoses. Several review articles also appeared in which various species of *Penicillium* have been implicated in mycotoxicoses; thus Borker and co-workers (9) cited 22 species of *Penicillium* as being mycotoxigenic including *P. citrinum, P. cyclopium, P. islandicum, P. expansum, P. purpurogenum,* and *P. urticae.* Brook and White (10) have listed 26 species including *P. brevi-compactum, P. chrysogenum, P. citrinum, P. cyclopium, P. islandicum, P. oxalicum, P. urticae,* and *P. viridicatum.*

Once studies such as those outlined above have identified molds frequently found on foods and feeds, we can determine what metabolites are produced by a particular species and whether these metabolites are toxic. These questions are particularly relevant if the food or feed associated with the fungal species has been implicated in animal illnesses or deaths. With this in mind let us examine the known information relative to each of the molds listed in Table I.

Table IV. *Penicillium—*

Mold	Substrate	Subject
P. cyclopium	—	rat
	corn	mouse
	corn [a]	sheep
	corn [a]	cattle
	corn, beans, flour, pickles	mouse
P. viridicatum	maize [a]	swine, horses
	barley [a]	pigs, rats
	corn	mice, rats, guinea pigs
	rice	mice
	rice	rats
	rice, wheat, flour, beans, seaweeds	mouse
P. oxalicum	maize meal	ducks, mice, rats
	corn	mouse
	rice, miso, beans	mouse
P. expansum	culture filtrate	Japanese quail
	corn	mouse
P. chrysogenum	cereal	rabbit
	corn	mouse
P. brevi-compactum	cereal	rabbit
	miso	mouse
P. funiculosum	corn	mouse
P. urticae	maize meal	mouse
	malt [a]	cattle
	flour	mouse
P. islandicum	flour	mouse
	rice	mouse
	rice	human
	rice	chick
P. citrinum	wheat, flour, beans	mouse
P. variable	corn	
P. frequentans	corn	mouse
P. purpurogenum	rice, wheat, flour	mouse
	grain	chicks
	corn	mouse

[a] Natural outbreaks of mycotoxicoses.

Group I

In terms of frequency of occurrence in foods and feeds *P. cyclopium* and *P. viridicatum* appear to be most important. Both of these species have been studied extensively, and they apparently produce a host of secondary metabolites, some of which are extremely toxic and some of

Mycotoxicoses Associations

Effects (Oral)	Ref.
focal necrosis of most organs, death	*11, 10*
liver and kidney lesions	*12*
death	*13*
death	*14*
hepatotoxic, nephrotoxic	*26*
poisoning	*15*
chronic kidney degeneration	*16*
liver lesions, death	*17, 18*
pulmonary tumors	*19*
hepatic, renal, gastric and scrotal lesions	*20*
neurotoxic, hepatotoxic, nephrotoxic	*26*
death	*21, 10*
reduction in weight gain, death	*22*
hepatotoxic, nephrotoxic	*26*
liver lesions	*23*
reduction in weight gain	*22*
skin reaction	*24, 10*
death	*22*
skin reaction	*24, 10*
nephrotoxic, death	*26*
reduction in weight gain	*22*
death	*21*
death	*25*
nephrotoxic	*26*
hepatotoxic, nephrotoxic	*26*
hepatoma	
hepatotoxic, death	*27, 28, 29*
edema of leg	
death	
nephrotoxic	*26*
reduction in weight gain, death	*22*
reduction in weight gain, death	*22*
hepatotoxic, nephrotoxic	*26*
congestion, hemorrhage, liver and kidney damage	*30*
liver lesions	*22*

which are known to exhibit other toxic manifestations. In each instance the mold has been implicated as the causative organism in many cases of animal illness and death (*see* Table IV).

P. cyclopium. Extensive studies of this organism resulted in the identification of a variety of mycotoxins, some of which have been commonly associated with other mold species. For example, ochratoxin A

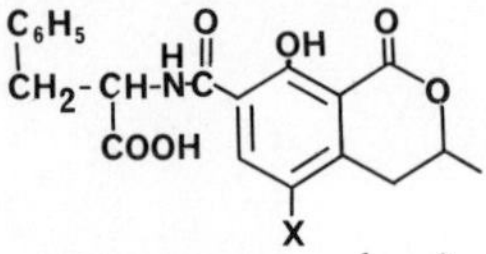

OCHRATOXIN A (X=Cl)
          B (X=H)   PENICILLIC ACID   CYCLOPIAZONIC ACID

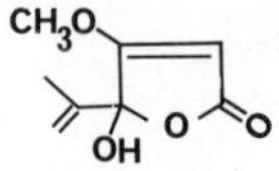

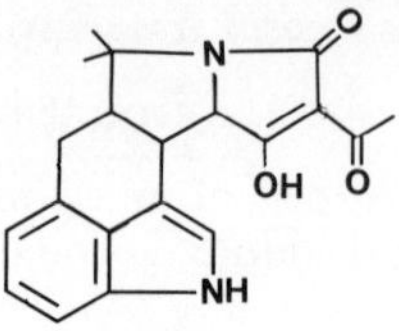

I   II   III

(Structure I), a mycotoxin more commonly associated with *Aspergillus ochraceus,* has been found to be produced by *P. cyclopium* (*31*). Ochratoxin A is acutely toxic (LD_{50} = 20–22 mg/kg, rat, oral) (*32*) and has been implicated as a potent teratogen (*33*). *P. cylopium* also produces penicillic acid (Structure II) (*34*), a mycotoxin (LD_{50} = 12 mg/20 g, mouse, oral) (*35*) that has been implicated as a possible carcinogen (*36*) and that is produced by at least 12 other species of *Penicillium.* Later a series of extremely toxic tremorgenic toxins were isolated from *P. cyclopium* (*37*); these include penitrem A (LD_{50} = 1.05 mg/kg, mouse, IP), penitrem B (LD_{50} = 5.84 mg/kg, mouse, IP), and penitrem C. These materials will be described in Chapter 10.

Table V.   *P. cyclopium*

Compound	Formula	MW	M.P., °C
Ochratoxin A	$C_{20}H_{18}ClNO_6$	404	169–72
Penicillic acid	$C_8H_{10}O_4$	170	86
Penitrem A (Tremortin A)	$C_{37}H_{44}O_6NCl$	633	237–9d
Penitrem B (Tremortin B)	$C_{37}H_{45}O_5N$	583	185–95d
Cyclopiazonic acid	$C_{20}H_{20}N_2O_3$	336	245–6
Cyclopiazonic acid imine	$C_{20}H_{21}N_3O_2$	335	277–8
Bissecodehydro-cyclopiazonic acid	$C_{20}H_{22}N_2O_3$	338	168–9
Cyclopiamine	$C_{26}H_{33}N_3O_5$	468	
Cyclopeptin	$C_{17}H_{16}N_2O_2$	280	95
Dehydrocyclopeptin	$C_{17}H_{14}N_2O_2$	278	202
Cyclopenin	$C_{17}H_{14}O_3N_2$	294	184
Cyclopenol	$C_{17}H_{14}O_4N_2$	310	210–11 215d
Viridicatin	$C_{15}H_{11}O_2N$	237	268
Viridicatol	$C_{15}H_{11}O_3N$	253	280
Palitantin	$C_{14}H_{22}O_4$	254	164–5
Puberulic acid	$C_8H_6O_6$	198	318
Puberulonic acid	$C_9H_4O_7$	224	298d
Cyclopolic acid	$C_{11}H_{12}O_6$	240	147d
Cyclopaldic acid	$C_{11}H_{10}O_6$	238	224–5
Isoerythritol	$C_4H_{10}O_4$	122	116–20
Mannitol	$C_6H_{14}O_6$	182	166–8
Emodic acid	$C_{15}H_8O_7$	300	363–5
ω-Hydroxyemodin	$C_{15}H_{10}O_6$	286	288

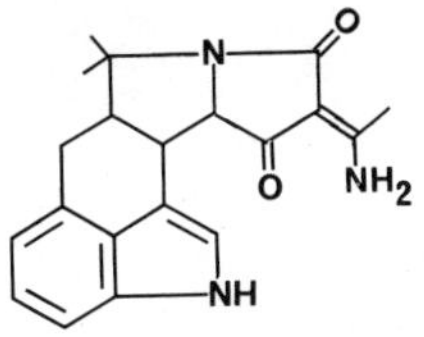

CYCLOPIAZONIC ACID IMINE
IV

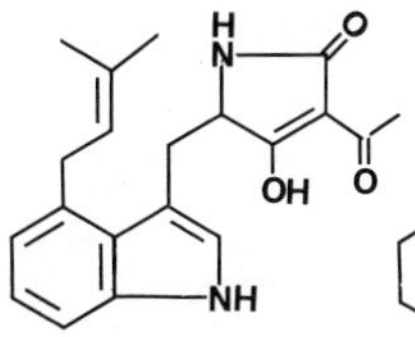

BISSECODEHYDRO CYCLOPIAZONIC ACID
V

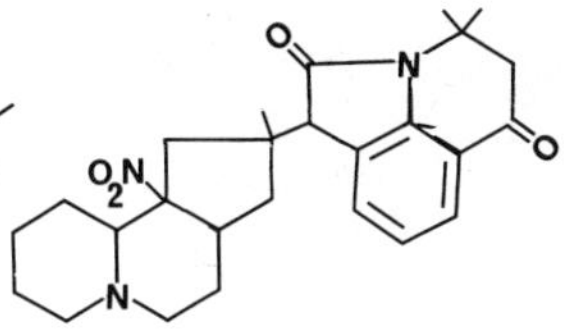

CYCLOPIAMINE
VI

P. cyclopium produces many other metabolites (*see* Table V); among these are a group of complex alkaloids: cyclopiazonic acid (Structure III), cyclopiazonic acid imine (Structure IV), bissecodehydrocyclopiazonic acid (Structure V), and cyclopiamine (Structure VI). Cyclopiazonic acid has been studied toxicologically (*51*) and is apparently the major toxic component in certain *P. cyclopium* isolates; 2.3 mg/kg (male rat, IP) caused convulsions followed by death suggesting that it may act as a neurotoxin. Oral administration did not cause convulsions. The major site of action of the toxin on oral administration appeared to be the spleen and the kidney (LD_{50} = 36 mg/kg, male rat, oral).

Metabolites

UV, nm (solvent)	Ref.
215, 333 (EtOH)	*32*
226 (H₂O)	*38*
295, 333 (MeOH)	*39*
227, 286, 297sh (MeOH)	*39*
225, 253, 384 (MeOH)	*40*
224, 293 (MeOH)	*41*
225, 276, 296sh (MeOH)	*41*
	42
293 (MeOH)	*43*
286 (MeOH)	*43*
211, 290	*44*
285 (EtOH)	*44*
230, 320 (EtOH)	*45*
226, 284, 304sh, 316, 329sh (MeOH)	*45*
232	*46*
	47
	47
	48
245, 278, 322	*48*
	49
	49
	50
	50

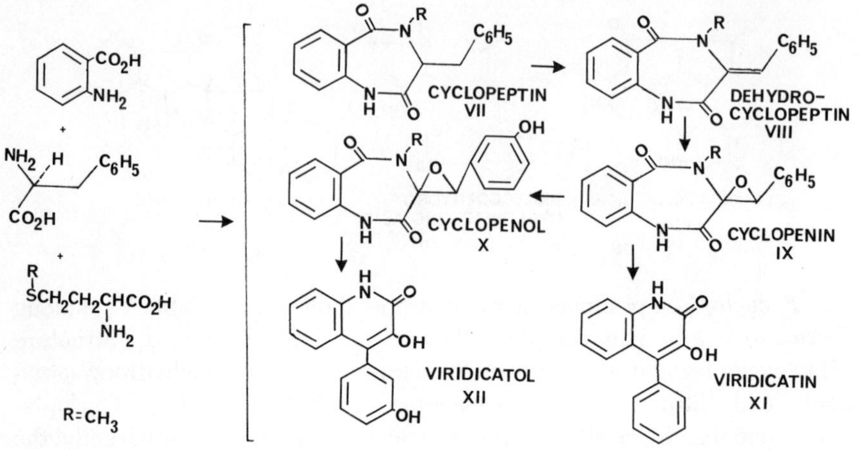

Figure 1. P. cyclopium *metabolites*

The structural elucidation of these complex materials is described in a review article by Holzapfel (*42*) as well as in many previous publications by the same author; for Structure III this involved basically recognition and combination of the indole nucleus and the tenuazonic acid systems. Treatment of cyclopiazonic acid with 25% aqueous ammonia generated Structure IV which accumulated during later stages of the fermentation process. Structure V is probably a precursor of Structure III since it accumulates during early stages of fermentation and is converted into Structure III by β-cyclopiazonate oxidocyclase (*52*). Structure VI and its stereoisomer isocyclopiamine were produced by a *P. cyclopium* isolate from moldy peanuts (*42*).

Another group of interrelated alkaloids produced by *P. cyclopium* is presumably derived from anthranilic acid, S-phenylalanine, and methionine (*43*) (*see* Figure 1). These include cyclopeptin (Structure VII), dehydrocyclopeptin (Structure VIII), cyclopenin (Structure IX), cyclopenol (Structure X), viridicatin (Structure XI), and viridicatol (Structure XII). Structures XI and XII were isolated and identified first. Thus oxidative degradation of Structure XI readily yields oxalic acid and 2-aminobenzophenone, while Structure XII yields 2-amino-3'-hydroxy-benzophenone (*45, 53*). These structures were later confirmed through total synthesis (*53, 54*). The structures of the benzodiazepin alkaloids (Structures IX and X) were more difficult to obtain; however, degradation studies leading to anthranilic acid and the appropriate benzoic acid, as well as physical data, indicated the nature of the ring system involved (*44*). At that time it was known that treatment with acid converted Structures IX and X to carbon dioxide, methyl amine, and viridicatin and

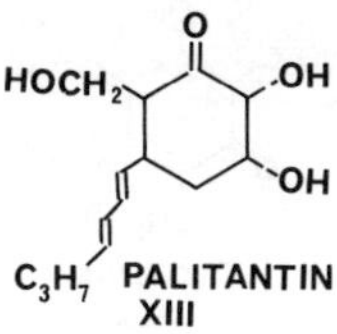

HOCH₂ ... PALITANTIN XIII   C₃H₇

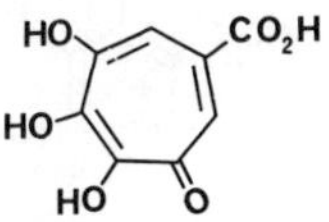

PUBERULIC ACID XIV

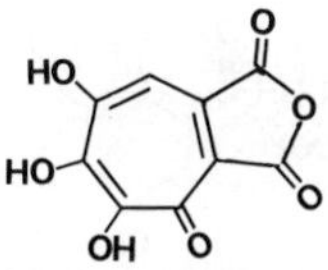

PUBERULONIC ACID XV

viridicatol. Structures IX and X were later confirmed by total synthesis (55). Furthermore an enzyme (cyclopenase) obtained from the mycelium of *P. viridicatum* accomplished the same conversion (57). Based on the formula of Structure IX it was relatively simple to formulate Structures XI and XII. No studies have been reported relative to the toxicity of any of these metabolites.

Finally *P. cyclopium* has been reported to produce a number of other metabolites including palitantin (Structure XIII), puberulic (Structure XIV) and puberulonic (Structure XV) acids, cyclopolic (Structure XVI) and cylopaldic (Structure XVII) acids, isoerythritol, mannitol, and a pair of anthraquinones, emodic acid (Structure XVIII) and ω-hydroxyemodin (Structure XIX) (*see* Table V). No toxicological studies have been reported for any of these materials.

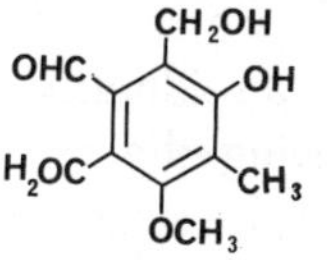

CYCLOPOLIC ACID

XVI

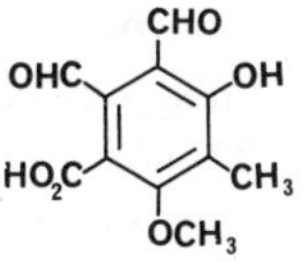

CYCLOPALDIC ACID

XVII

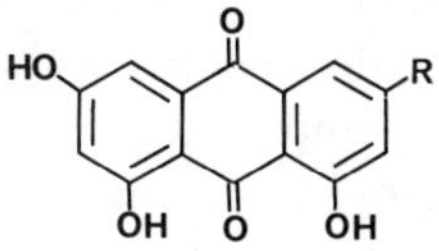

EMODIC ACID (R=CO₂H)
w-HYDROXYEMODIN (R=CH₂OH)

XVIII
XIX

P. viridicatum. This mold is frequently encountered in stored grains and on decaying vegetation of the soil; it has been implicated as the causative agent in many instances of animal illnesses and deaths (*see* Table IV). These facts, along with the report (19) of carcinogenicity in mice attributed to administration of rice cultures of *P. viridicatum* engendered extensive research into the metabolites produced by this mold. These studies appear to indicate that the reported toxicity associated with this mold must arise from a variety of mycotoxins, only some of which have been identified.

P. viridicatum has been observed to produce many of the same metabolites that are produced by *P. cyclopium* including ochratoxin A (56), viridicatin (15), viridicatol (57), cyclopenin and cyclopenol (45), cyclopolic and cyclopaldic acid (48), mannitol, and isoerythritol (*see* Table V). In addition recent findings show that ochratoxin B (Structure

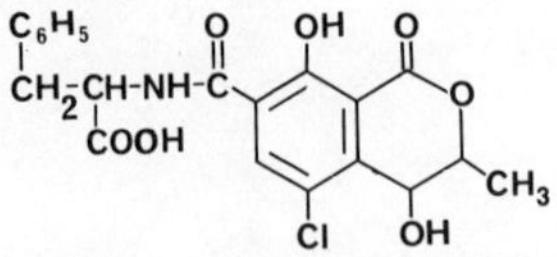

4-HYDROXYOCHRATOXIN A
XX

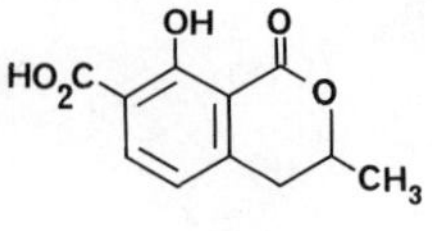

XXI

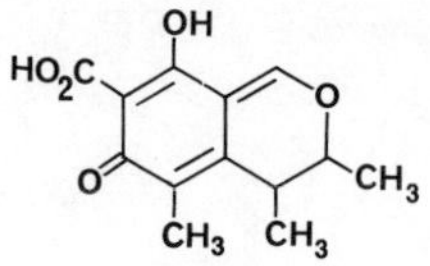

CITRININ
°XXII

I), 4-hydroxyochratoxin A (Structure XX), and 7-carboxy-3,4-dihydro-8-hydroxy-3-methyl isocoumarin (Structure XXI) are elaborated by *P. viridicatum* (*58*). These structures were elucidated by carefully evaluating spectral data; toxicological studies indicate that these derivatives of ochratoxin A are relatively nontoxic (*32*).

Krogh and co-workers (*16, 17*) in their studies of fungal nephrotoxicity isolated and identified oxalic acid and citrinin (Structure XXII) from corn-steep liquor cultures of *P. viridicatum*. Citrinin was isolated originally from *P. citrinum* cultures (*59*). Friis, Hasselager, and Krogh (*16*) observed that feeding Structure XXII to swine resulted in a nephropathy similar to the naturally occurring porcine nephropathy; also citrinin was acutely toxic to mice ($LD_{50} = 35$ mg/kg, S C) (*60*). Much effort was expended to assign the structure of citrinin; it was known (*59*) that dilute acid converted citrinin into two phenols (A_1, optically active and B_1, optically inactive) that when fused with a base yielded a material with the empirical formula $C_9H_{12}O_2$. This material was later identified as 4-methyl-5-ethyl-resorcinol (Figure 2) (*61*). Reconverting the optically actively phenol ($C_{11}H_{16}O_3$) to citrinin then established the structure for citrinin (*61, 62*).

Mycophenolic acid (Structure XXIII) has also been isolated from *P. viridicatum* (*64*). This material was originally isolated from *P. brevicompactum* and is often referred to as the first antibiotic substance isolated and purified from molds ($LD_{50} = 2500$ mg/kg, mouse, oral). A

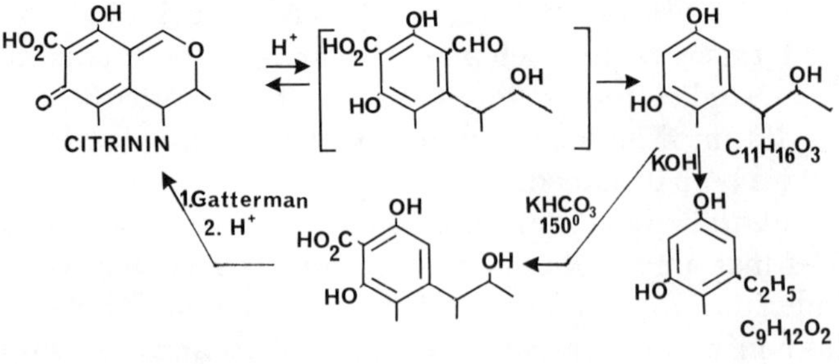

Figure 2.   The structure of citrinin

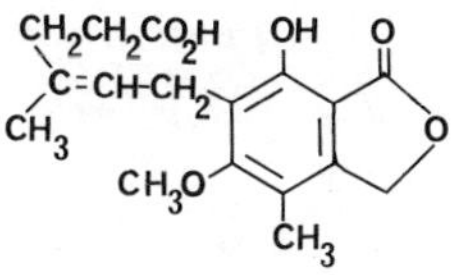

MYCOPHENOLIC ACID
XXIII

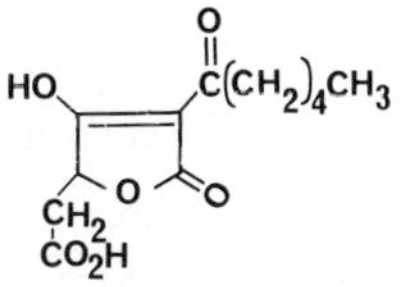

VIRIDICATIC ACID
XXIV

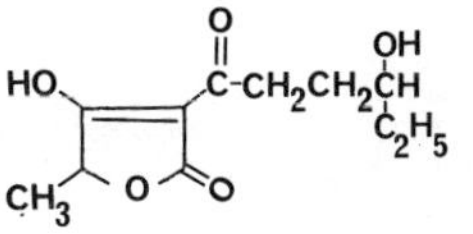

TERRESTRIC ACID
XXV

good review by B. J. Wilson covering the structural identification and biological activity of this material has been published (*65*). In addition to mycophenolic acid culture filtrates of *P. viridicatum* also produce the tetronic acids viridicatic acid (Structure XXIV) and terrestric acid (Structure XXV); from the mycelium mannitol, isoerythritol, and ergosteryl palmitate were obtained (*66*). Structure XXIV was determined by relating its physical properties to those of carlosic acid which has a butyryl group in the α-position, and by hydrolysis to *n*-hexanoic acid and β-hydroxylaevulic acid.

Two further metabolites of *P. viridicatum* have been isolated and identified: brevianamide A (Structure XXVI) (*67*), a compound originally isolated from *P. brevi-compactum* (*68*), and xanthomegnin (Structure XXVII) (*69*), a compound originally isolated from *Trichophyton*

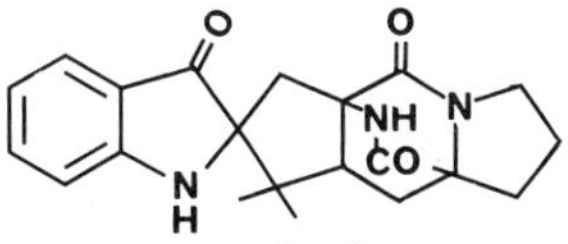

(A, B)
XXVI

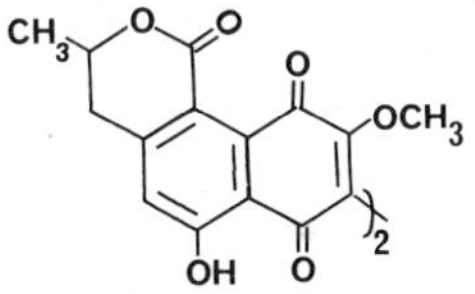

XANTHOMEGNIN
XXVII

magnini (*70*). Neither of these materials appears appreciably orally toxic to mice. Finally a report (*71*) recently appeared describing a new mycotoxin, viridicumtoxin ($C_{30}H_{31}NO_{10}$) (LD_{50} = 122.4 mg/kg, rat, oral), of unknown structure (Table VI).

Group II

The molds in this group are encountered frequently on foods and feeds (Table I) and have the potential to produce toxin (Table IV). However these molds have not yielded the large numbers of toxins noted for Group I molds, nor have they been studied as extensively (with the possible exception of *P. chrysogenum*).

P. oxalicum. Very few metabolites have been isolated and identified from this mold. It produces oxalic acid (*71*) which apparently is toxic

		Table VI.	*Penicillium*
Compound	*Formula*	*MW*	*M.P., °C*
Ochratoxin B	$C_{20}H_{19}NO_6$	369	220–1
4-Hydroxyochratoxin A	$C_{20}H_{18}ClNO_7$	419	216–8
7-Carboxy-3,4-dihydro-8-hydroxy-3-methyl isocoumarin	$C_{11}H_{10}O_5$	222	223
Oxalic acid	$C_2H_2O_4$	90	101
Citrinin	$C_{13}H_{14}O_5$	250	175d
Mycophenolic acid	$C_{17}H_{20}O_6$	320	141
Viridicatic acid	$C_{12}H_{16}O_6$	256	174.5
Terrestric acid	$C_{11}H_{14}O_4$	211	89
Brevianamide A	$C_{21}H_{23}N_3O_3$	365	215–230
Xanthomegnin	$C_{30}H_{22}O_{12}$	574	285–300d
Viridicumtoxin	$C_{30}H_{31}NO_{10}$	565	211

only in extremely high dosage. Recently, however, *P. oxalicum* has also been shown to produce secalonic acid D (Structure XXVIII) and two new alkaloids of unknown structure, one of which was called oxaline (*see* Table VII). The structure of secalonic acid D was determined spectroscopically by relating its properties to those of its optical antipode (secalonic acid A), one of the toxic pigments elaborated by *Claviceps purpurea*.

P. expansum. Again little is known of the metabolites produced by this mold species. The major toxin isolated and identified appears to be patulin (73) (Structure XXIX) which is more commonly associated with the mold *P. urticae* (*see* discussion of *P. urticae*). The fact that *P. expansum* is the major contributor to apple rot has engendered much interest in the possible occurrence of patulin in apple products. *P. expansum* is also known to produce curvularin (Structure XXX), a material closely related to the estrogenic material zearalenone (106).

P. chrysogenum. This mold has been extensively studied from the standpoint of penicillin production. Toxic metabolites have not been reported for this species although a wide diversity of metabolites have

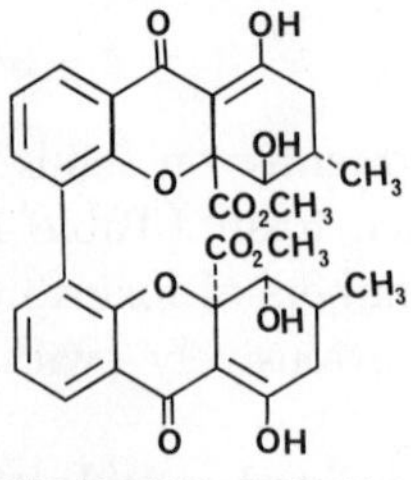

SECALONIC ACID D
XXVIII

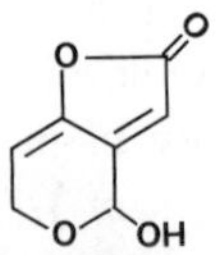

PATULIN
XXIX

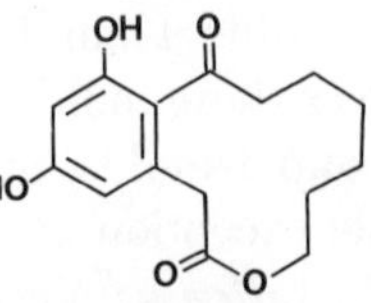

CURVULARIN
XXX

viridicatum **Metabolites**

UV, nm (solvent)	Ref.
218, 318 (EtOH)	58
213, 334 (EtOH)	58
218, 322 (EtOH)	58
	16, 17
222, 253, 319 (EtOH)	63
	64
230, 268 (EtOH)	66
	66
234, 256sh, 405 (MeOH)	67
227, 290sh, 395 (CHCl₃)	69
237, 285, 317, 331, 347, 424 (EtOH)	71

been reported (*see* Table VII). These include penicillin F (Structure XXXI), dethiobiotin (Structure XXXII), adenosine-5-phosphate, inosine-5-phosphate, adenylosuccinic acid, chrysogine (Structure XXXIII), and tetracosanoic acid. Ballio and co-workers detected at least 16 derivatives of adenosine, guanosine, inosine, cytidine, and uridine in the mycelium of *P. chrysogenum* (77). In addition Suter and Turner (82) reported

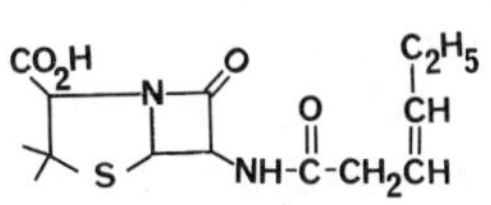

PENICILLIN F
XXXI

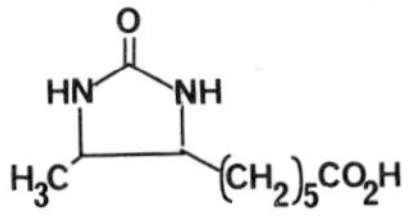

DETHIOBIOTIN
XXXII

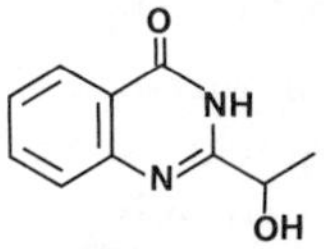

CHRYSOGINE
XXXIII

the presence of 2-pyruvoylaminobenzamide (Structure XXXIV; not shown) in the culture filtrate of *P. chrysogenum*. No toxicity has been associated with any of these compounds.

   P. brevi-compactum. This mold is of particular interest since it was involved in one of the earliest attempts (1896) to relate a toxin produced by a mold to the incidence of a human illness—pellagra in this case (83). Although no relationship could be established, work in this area did result in the first chemical detection system devised to detect spoilage of maize based on the color reaction between ferric chloride and phenolic metabolites. Raistrick and co-workers isolated and identified (83) a series of phenolic materials including mycophenolic acid (Structure XXIII) (Table VI), 3,5-dihydroxy-2-carboxybenzyl methyl ketone (Structure XXXV), 3,5-dihydroxy-2-carboxyphenylacetyl carbinol (Structure XXXVI), 3,5-dihydroxy-2-carboxylbenzoyl methyl ketone (Structure XXXVII), and 3,5-dihydroxyphthalic acid (Structure XXXVIII). Later

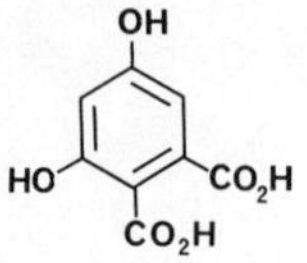

XXXV 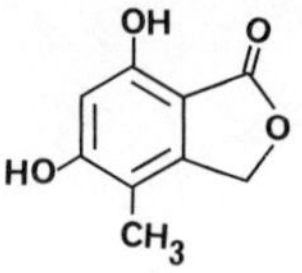   XXXVI 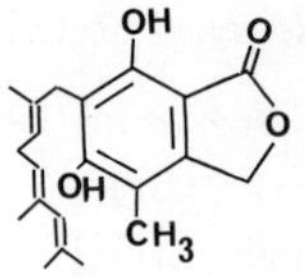   XXXVII

workers investigating the biosynthesis of mycophenolic acid isolated two additional metabolites: 5,7-dihydroxy-4-methylphthalide (Structure XXXIX) and 6-farnesyl-5,7-dihydroxy-4-methylphthalide (Structure XL). Finally several other mycophenolic acid derivatives (Structures XLI–XLIII) have been reported (Table VIII).

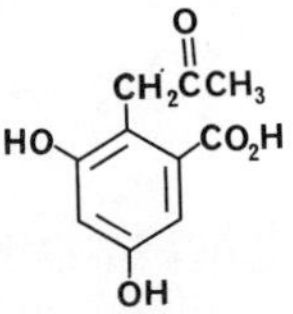

XXXVIII 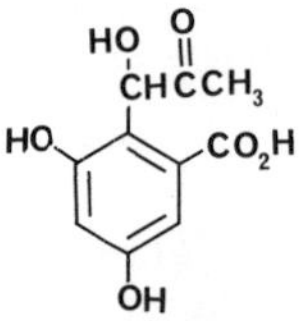   XXXIX 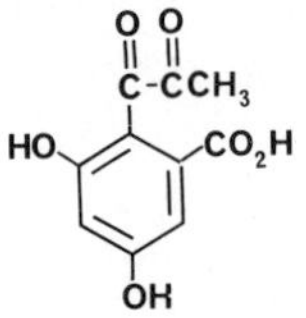   XL

In attempting to isolate the hepatotoxic substances produced by *P. brevi-compactum* Birch and co-workers isolated a series of neutral compounds, mostly pigments: brevianamides A–F (Table VIII). Structure XXVI (brevianamide A) was determined first, based on a combination of physical methods with biogenetic hypotheses. Brevianamide B was quickly shown to be a stereoisomer of Structure XXVI. Irradiation of Structure XXVI (A and B) yields brevianamides C (Structure XLIV) and D (Structure XLV) which are simply cis–trans isomers; reduction of these isomers with NaBH$_4$ yields a single indole (Structure XLVI).

Table VII.   Metabolites of *P. oxalicum*,

Compound	*Formula*	*MW*	*M.P., °C*
Oxalic acid	$C_2H_2O_4$	90	101
Secalonic acid D	$C_{32}H_{30}O_{14}$	638	253–254
Oxaline	$C_{24}H_{25}N_5O_4$		
Patulin	$C_7H_6O_4$	154	111
Curvularin	$C_{16}H_{20}O_5$	292	206–7
Penicillin F	$C_{14}H_{20}O_4N_2S$	312	204d
Dethiobiotin	$C_{10}H_{18}O_3N_2$	214	156–8
Adenosine-5′-phosphate	$C_{10}H_{14}O_7N_5P$	347	178
Inosine-5′-phosphate	$C_{10}H_{13}O_8N_4P$	347	191–5d
Adenylosuccinic acid	$C_{14}H_{18}O_{11}N_5P$	468	
Choline sulfate	$C_5H_{13}O_4N_5$	183	
Chrysogine	$C_{10}H_{10}O_2N_2$	190	189–90
Tetracosanoic acid	$C_{24}H_{48}O_2$	369	87.5
2-Pyruvoylaminobenzamide	$C_{10}H_{10}N_2O_3$	206	181–4

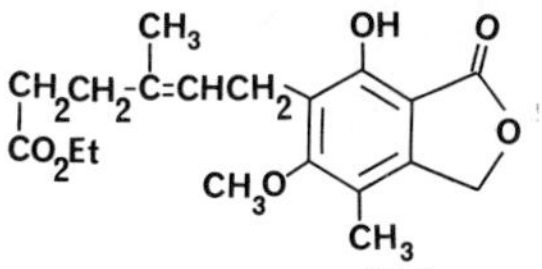

XLI 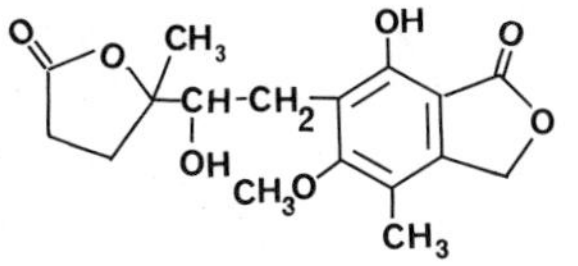   XLII 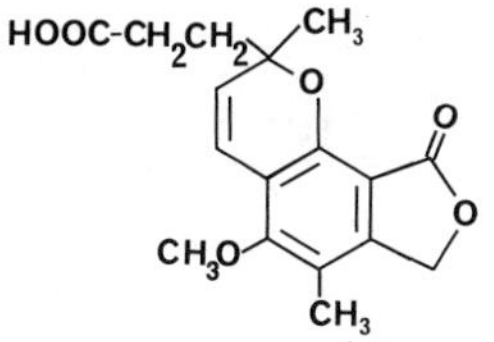   XLIII

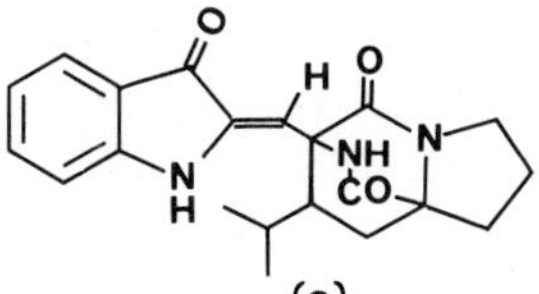

(c)   (D)
XLIV   XLV

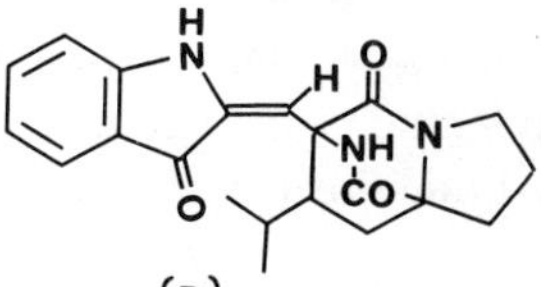

Brevianamide E and F were assigned Structures XLVII and XLVIII based on physical data. The biogenetic precursor Structure XLIX postulated by Birch (*90*) has recently been isolated from *Aspergillus ustus* (*91*). Details of the biosynthesis of the brevianamides as well as their toxicological effects are under study.

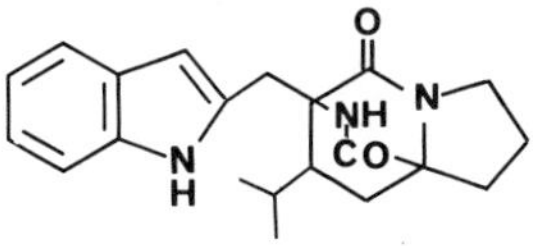

XLVI 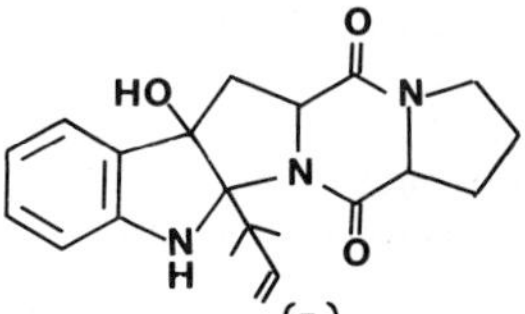   (E)
                       XLVII

P. expansum, and P. chrysogenum

UV, nm (*solvent*)   *Ref.*

	71
248, 337 (EtOH)	*72*
	72
277 (MeOH)	*73*
223, 271.5, 304 (EtOH)	*74*
	75
	76
	77
	77
	78
	79
226, 230, 238, 265, 273, 292, 305, 316 (EtOH)	*80*
	81
211, 247, 302 (MeOH)	*83*

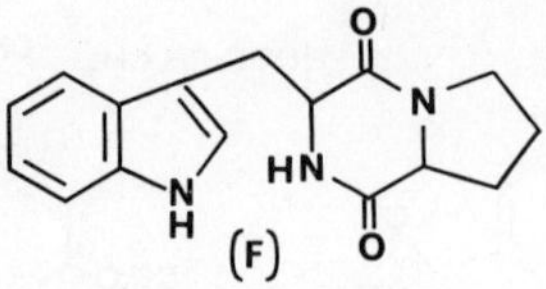

XLVIII   XLIX

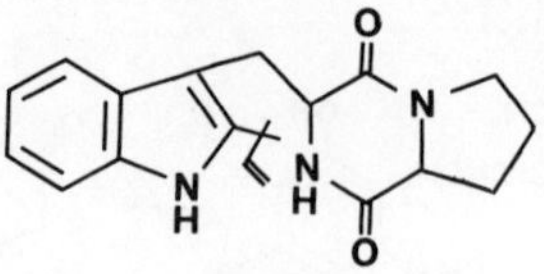

P. funiculosum. Metabolites produced by this mold species include malonic acid, orsellinic acid (Structure L), an uncharacterized antiviral agent, helenine, which is thought to be a nucleoprotein, and the anthraquinone funiculosin which is identical to islandicin (Structure LI) (*see*

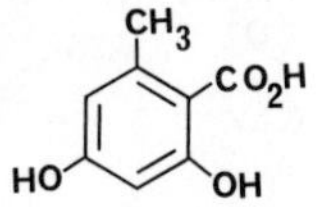

ORSELLINIC ACID   ISLANDICIN
L   LI

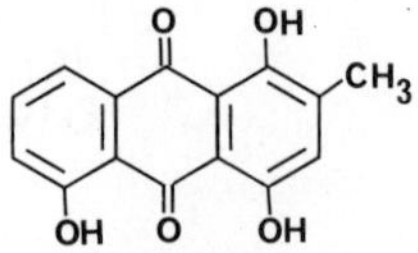

		Table VIII.	Metabolites of
Compound	*Formula*	*MW*	*M.P., °C*
3,5-Dihydroxy-2-carboxy-benzyl-methyl ketone	$C_{10}H_{10}O_5$	210	152–6d
3,5-Dihydroxy-2-carboxy-phenyl-acetyl carbinol	$C_{10}H_{10}O_6$	226	200d
3,5-Dihydroxy-2-carboxy-benzoyl methyl ketone	$C_{10}H_{10}O_7$	224	125–35
3,5-Dihydroxyphthalic acid	$C_8H_6O_6$	198	188 (206)
6-Farnesyl-5,7-dihydroxy-4-methylphthalide	$C_{24}H_{32}O_4$	384	98–100
Ethyl mycophenate	$C_{19}H_{24}O_6$	348	88–90
Structure XLII	$C_{17}H_{20}O_7$	336	218–20
Mycochromenic acid	$C_{17}H_{18}O_6$	318	163–165
Brevianamide A	$C_{21}H_{23}N_3O_3$	365	190–220
B	$C_{21}H_{23}N_3O_3$	365	324–8d
C	$C_{21}H_{23}N_3O_3$	365	Glass
D	$C_{21}H_{23}N_3O_3$	365	Glass
E	$C_{21}H_{25}N_3O_3$	367	Glass
F	$C_{16}H_{17}N_3O_2$	283	173–5
Isoerythritol	$C_4H_{10}O_4$	122	116–20
Dihydroxyacetone	$C_3H_6O_3$	90	75–80
Malonic acid	$C_3H_4O_4$	104	135
Orsellinic acid	$C_8H_8O_4$	168	176
Funiculosin	$C_{15}H_{10}O_5$	270	218
Mitorubrin	$C_{21}H_{18}O_7$	382	218
Mitorubrinol	$C_{21}H_{18}O_8$	398	219–21
Mitorubrinic acid	$C_{21}H_{16}O_9$	412	
Funicone	$C_{19}H_{18}O_8$	374	176–8

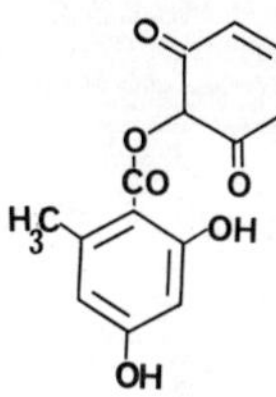

MITORUBRIN   R=CH₃   LII
MITORUBRINOL   R=CH₂OH   LIII
MITORUBRINIC ACID R=CO₂H   LIV

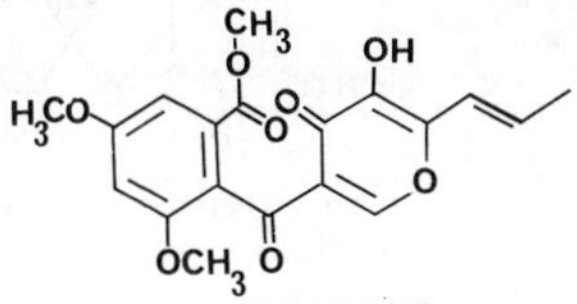

FUNICONE
LV

Table VIII). In addition a series of metabolites have been isolated which are structurally similar to the sclerotiorin (azaphilone) group of metabolites (93); these include mitorubrin (Structure LII), a compound originally isolated from *P. rubrum*, mitorubrinol (Structure LIII), mitorubrinic acid (Structure LIV), and funicone (Structure LV) (*see* Table VIII).

P. brevi-compactum and *P. funiculosum*

UV, nm (solvent)	*Ref.*
	83
	83
	83
	84
	85, 86
303	*87*
	87
245, 280, 321.5, 332.5	*87*
235, 256, 404 (MeOH)	*88*
236, 254, 400 (EtOH)	*89*
234, 259, 450 (EtOH)	*89*
235, 264, 306, 470 (EtOH)	*89*
239, 296 (EtOH)	*89*
277, 283, 292 (EtOH)	*89*
	49
	92
	94
	95
	96
216, 266, 292, 346 (EtOH)	*97*
216, 266, 292, 346 (EtOH)	*97*
	98
245, 310 (95% EtOH)	*98*

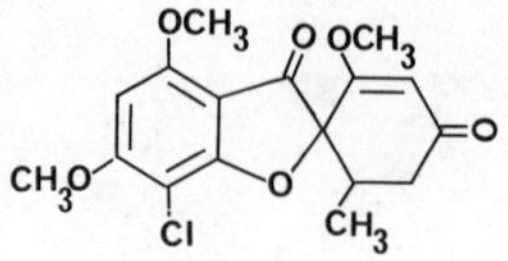

GRISEOFULVIN
LVI

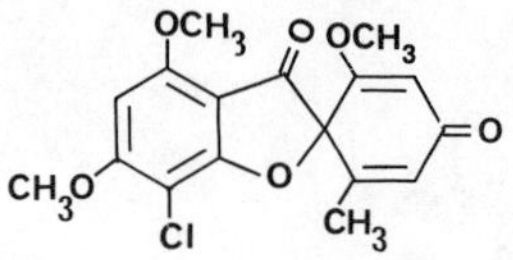

DEHYDROGRISEOFULVIN
LVII

Group III

Molds in this group are only occasionally found on foods and feeds. However, they are important with respect to certain types of foods and do produce some very toxic, and in some cases carcinogenic, metabolites.

P. urticae (*P. patulum*). This mold species has been implicated as the causative agent in an outbreak of fatal poisoning of dairy cows in Japan (99). It was concluded that the toxin involved was patulin (Structure XXIV). Patulin is produced in high yields by *P. urticae* and is extremely toxic ($LD_{50} = 0.7$ mg/20 g, mouse, oral); patulin has also been implicated as a carcinogen (36). Its chemistry and toxicology have been reviewed by Ciegler, Detroy, and Lillehoj (106).

P. patulum also produces the extremely useful antimicrobial agent griseofulvin (Structure LVI). It is still prescribed as a systemic therapeutic agent for cutaneous fungal infections, although it apparently has some carcinogenic properties (107). The chemical and toxicological properties of griseofulvin are carefully reviewed in B. J. Wilson's article

Table IX.   Metabolites of

Compound	Formula	MW	M.P., °C
Griseofulvin	$C_{17}H_{17}O_6Cl$	353	220
Dehydrogriseofulvin	$C_{17}H_{15}O_6Cl$	351	270–275
2,6-Dihydroxy-4-methyl-8-methoxyxanthone	$C_{15}H_{12}O_5$	272	253–5
4,6-Dimethoxy-2'-methyl-grisan-3,4',6'-trione	$C_{16}H_{16}O_6$	304	245–8d
Structure LX	$C_{17}H_{17}O_5Cl$	337	181–2
Structure LXI	$C_{17}H_{17}O_6Cl$	353	212–4
Gentisic acid	$C_7H_6O_4$	154	199
Gentisaldehyde	$C_7H_6O_3$	138	
Gentisyl alcohol	$C_7H_8O_3$	140	100
6-Methysalicylic acid	$C_8H_8O_3$	152	170
6-Formylsalicylic acid	$C_8H_6O_4$	166	134
3-Hydroxyphthalic acid	$C_8H_6O_5$	182	154
Pyrogallol	$C_6H_6O_3$	126	134
p-Hydroxybenzoic acid	$C_7H_6O_3$	138	213
Anthranilic acid	$C_7H_7O_2N$	137	144
Gentisylquinone	$C_7H_6O_3$	138	76

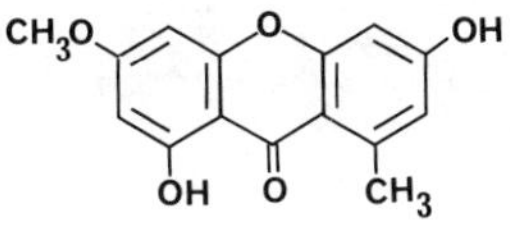

LVIII

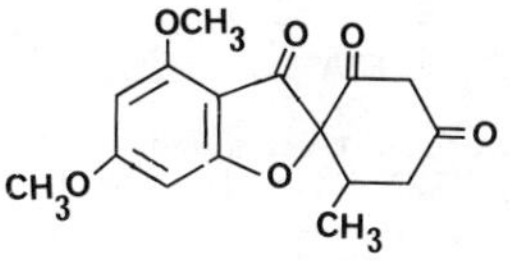

LIX

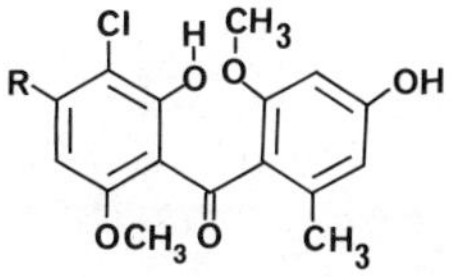

LX R=OCH₃

LXI R=CH₃

on miscellaneous *Penicillium* toxins (*108*). In addition, *P. patulum* produces five additional materials related to dehydrogriseofulvin (Structure LVII), 2,6-dihydroxy-4-methyl-8-methoxyxanthone (Structure LVIII), 4,6-dimethoxy-2′-methylgrisan-3,4′,6′-trione (Structure LIX), and a pair of susbtituted benzophenones (Structures LX and LXI) (Table IX). The toxicological properties of these materials are apparently not known. Finally *P. patulum* produces many phenolic compounds (*see* Table IX) which apparently are interrelated biosynthetically (*see* Figure 3) (*104*). No toxicity has been associated with these materials.

   P. islandicum. Few molds have been studied more extensively or systematically than *P. islandicum.* Interest in the metabolites of *P. islandi-*

P. urticae (P. patulum)

UV, nm (solvent)	Ref.
236, 252, 241, 324 (MeOH)	100
242, 289, 330 (EtOH)	109
242, 269, 309, 340 (EtOH)	109
	109
296 (EtOH)	109
298 (EtOH)	109
	101
	101
	102
	103
	104
323	104
	104
	104
	104
	105

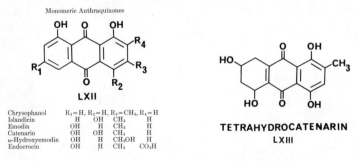

Figure 3.   Metabolites of P. patulum

cum arises mainly from early findings that rice naturally molded by *P. islandicum* (yellowed rice) could cause acute and chronic liver damage when fed to mice (*110*). This finding coupled with the fact that Asiatic populations in which rice forms a major portion of the diet also suffer from a high incidence of liver diseases including primary hepatic carcinoma (*99*) gave impetus to a great deal of research into the metabolites produced by *P. islandicum* and their toxicological properties. These studies led eventually to the isolation of two extremely potent hepatotoxins, luteoskyrin ($LD_{50} = 2.21$ mg/kg, mouse, oral) and cyclochlorotine ($LD_{50} = 6.55$ mg/kg, mouse, oral), both of which are believed carcinogenic (*28*). In addition a second extremely toxic peptide, islanditoxin (minimum lethal dose 3.6 mg/kg, SC, mouse) has been isolated and identified (*111, 112*). An excellent review of these materials as well as other toxins related to yellowed rice has appeared (*113*).

P. islandicum produces at least 27 quinoidal pigments (*see* Table X) which may be conveniently arranged in three groups. The first group

Monomeric Anthraquinones

LXII

Chrysophanol	$R_1=H$, $R_2=H$, $R_3=CH_3$, $R_4=H$			
Islandicin	H	OH	CH₃	H
Emodin	OH	H	CH₃	H
Catenarin	OH	OH	CH₃	H
ω-Hydroxyemodin	OH	H	CH₂OH	H
Endocrocin	OH	H	CH₃	CO₂H

TETRAHYDROCATENARIN
LXIII

contains the monomeric anthraquinones, all of which are derivatives of chrysophanol (Structure LXII): islandicin, emodin, catenarin, ω-hydroxy-emodin, endocrocin, tetrahydrocatenarin (Structure LXIII), and dihydro-catenarin. The structures of these quinones are readily derived by comparing their physical properties, including color tests (magnesium acetate), uv, ir, NMR spectra, and x-ray diffraction data, with those of equivalent materials obtained through total synthesis. These synthetic procedures generally involve the Friedel–Crafts condensation of a phthalic anhydride with a suitable phenol. Recently Kende et al. (*119*) reported a new approach to the total synthesis of islandicin involving regiospecific photo-Fries rearrangement (*see* Figure 4).

Dimeric Anthraquinones

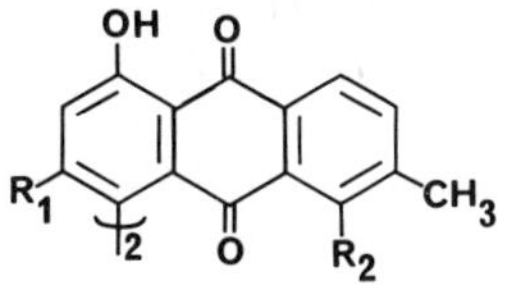

LXV

Dianhydrorugulosin	$R_1 = R_2 = H$
Iridoskyrin	$R_1 = H, R_2 = OH$
Skyrin	$R_1 = OH, R_2 = h$
Dicatenarin	$R_1 = R_2 = OH$
Oxyskyrin	One methyl of skyrin = CH_2OH
Skyrinol	Both methyls of skyrin = CH_2OH
Roseoskyrin	(chrysophanol + islandicin)
Auroskyrin	(chrysophanol + emodin)
Rhodoislandin A	(chrysophanol + catenarin)
Rhodoislandin B	(emodin + islandicin)
Punicoskyrin	(catenarin + islandicin)
Aurantioskyrin	(catenarin + emodin)

The second group contains the dimeric anthraquinones (Structure LXV): dianhydrorugulosin, iridoskyrin, skyrin, dicatenarin, oxyskyrin, skyrinol, roseoskyrin, auroskyrin, rhodoislandin A, rhodoislandin B, puni-coskyrin, and aurantioskyrin (Table X). The structures of these materials were established primarily through reductive cleavage with alkaline

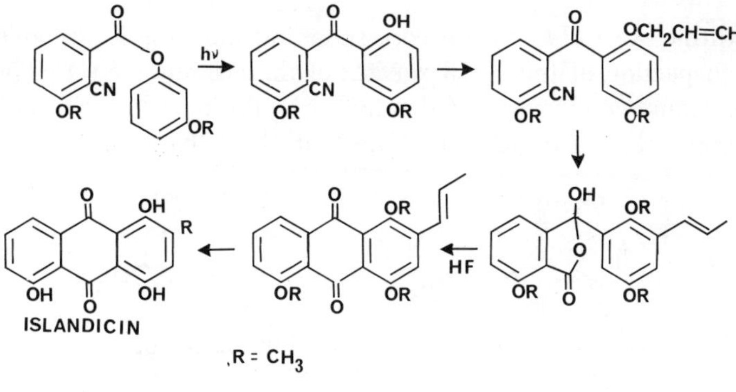

Figure 4.   Total synthesis of islandicin

Table X.   Metabolites

Compound	Formula	MW	M.P., °C
Chrysophanol	$C_{15}H_{10}O_4$	254	195–6
Islandicin	$C_{15}H_{10}O_5$	270	218
Emodin	$C_{15}H_{10}O_5$	270	256–7
Catenarin	$C_{15}H_{10}O_6$	286	244–6
ω-Hydroxyemodin (citreorosein)	$C_{15}H_{10}O_6$	286	288
Endocrocin (clavoxanthin)	$C_{16}H_{10}O_7$	314	290–320d
Tetrahydrocatenarin	$C_{15}H_{14}O_6$	290	∼130d
Dihydrocatenarin	$C_{15}H_{12}O_6$	288	95–105d
(+) Dianhydrorugulosin	$C_{30}H_{18}O_{10}$	538	321
(+) Iridoskyrin	$C_{30}H_{18}O_{10}$	538	358–60d
(+) Skyrin	$C_{30}H_{18}O_{10}$	538	>360d
(+) Dicatenarin	$C_{30}H_{18}O_{12}$	570	>300d
(+) Oxyskyrin	$C_{30}H_{18}O_{11}$	554	>360d
(+) Skyrinol	$C_{30}H_{18}O_{12}$	570	>360
(+) Roseoskyrin	$C_{30}H_{18}O_9$	522	275–380d
(+) Auroskyrin	$C_{30}H_{18}O_9$	522	>300
(+) Rhodoislandin A	$C_{30}H_{18}O_{10}$	538	>300
(+) Rhodoislandin B	$C_{30}H_{18}O_{10}$	538	>300
(+) Punicoskyrin	$C_{30}H_{18}O_{11}$	554	>300
(+) Aurantioskyrin	$C_{30}H_{18}O_{11}$	554	>300
(−) Luteoskyrin	$C_{30}H_{22}O_{12}$	574	281d
(−) Rubroskyrin	$C_{30}H_{22}O_{12}$	574	289d
(−) Flavoskyrin	$C_{30}H_{24}O_{10}$	544	215d
(−) Rugulosin	$C_{30}H_{22}O_{10}$	542	290d
(−) Deoxyluteoskyrin	$C_{30}H_{22}O_{11}$	558	293
(−) Deoxyrubroskyrin	$C_{30}H_{22}O_{11}$	558	255
(−) 4-α-Oxyluteoskyrin	$C_{30}H_{22}O_{13}$	590	>250d
Erythroskyrine	$C_{26}H_{33}O_6N$	455	130–3
Islanditoxin	$C_{24}H_{31}O_7N_5Cl_2$	572	258
Cyclochlorotine	$C_{25}H_{36}O_8N_5Cl_2$	605	251d
3-Hydroxyphthalic acid	$C_8H_6O_5$	182	166
Malonic acid	$C_3H_4O_4$	104	135

sodium dithionite (*114*) to the corresponding monomeric quinones and through inspection of the NMR spectra of the acetates (*120*). Thus, for example, reductive cleavage of dianhydrorugulosin yields two molecules of chrysophanol (*see* Figure 5). Note that all of these materials exhibit

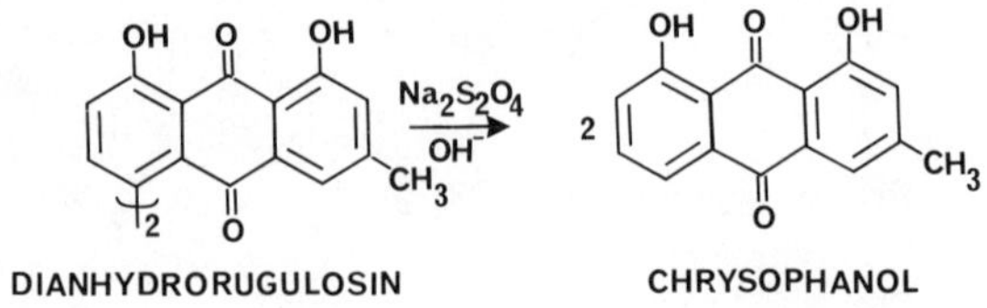

DIANHYDRORUGULOSIN   CHRYSOPHANOL

Figure 5.   Reduction of dimeric anthraquinones

of *P. islandicum*

UV, nm (solvent)	Ref.
228, 257, 277, 287, 429 (EtOH)	*114*
231.5, 252, 288, 490, 512 (EtOH)	*115*
253, 266, 289, 436 (EtOH)	*116*
231, 257, 282, 492, 525 (EtOH)	*116*
221, 252, 290, 438, 458 sh (EtOH)	*117*
274, 442 (MeOH)	*118*
485, 514, 554 (EtOH)	*117*
495 (530i, 570i) (EtOH)	*117*
282 sh, 439 (Dioxin)	*128*
286, 502 (Dioxin)	*121*
257, 300, 462 (EtOH)	*114*
	120
257, 300, 462 (EtOH)	*122*
258, 290, 448 (Dioxan)	*120*
	120
	120
	120
	120
	120
	120
280, 350, 440 (EtOH)	*124*
275, 415, 435, 530, 540 (CHCl₃)	*124*
267, 303, 312, 328, 368, 414 (Dioxane)	*125*
253, 396.5 (CHCl₃)	*124*
	124
280, 369, 380, 510, 531, 570 (Dioxane)	*124*
	124
392, 409 (EtOH)	*126*
	112
253, 259, 265 (MeOH)	*127*
	128
	129

optical activity attributable to restricted rotation around the bond connecting the two monomeric halves. Currently no information is available concerning the toxicity of these dianthraquinones.

The third group contains the modified bianthraquinones (Table X): luteoskyrin (Structure LXVI, R=OH), rubroskyrin (Structure LXVII, R=OH), flavoskyrin (Structure LXVIII), rugulosin (Structure LXIX), deoxyluteoskyrin (Structure LXVI, R=H), deoxyrubroskyrin (Structure LXVII, R=H), and 4-α-oxyluteoskyrin (Structure LXX). The structures of these compounds were very difficult to determine; they were finally resolved by careful interpretation of the NMR spectra and were confirmed, at least for rugulosin, by x-ray diffraction studies (*123*). Figure 6

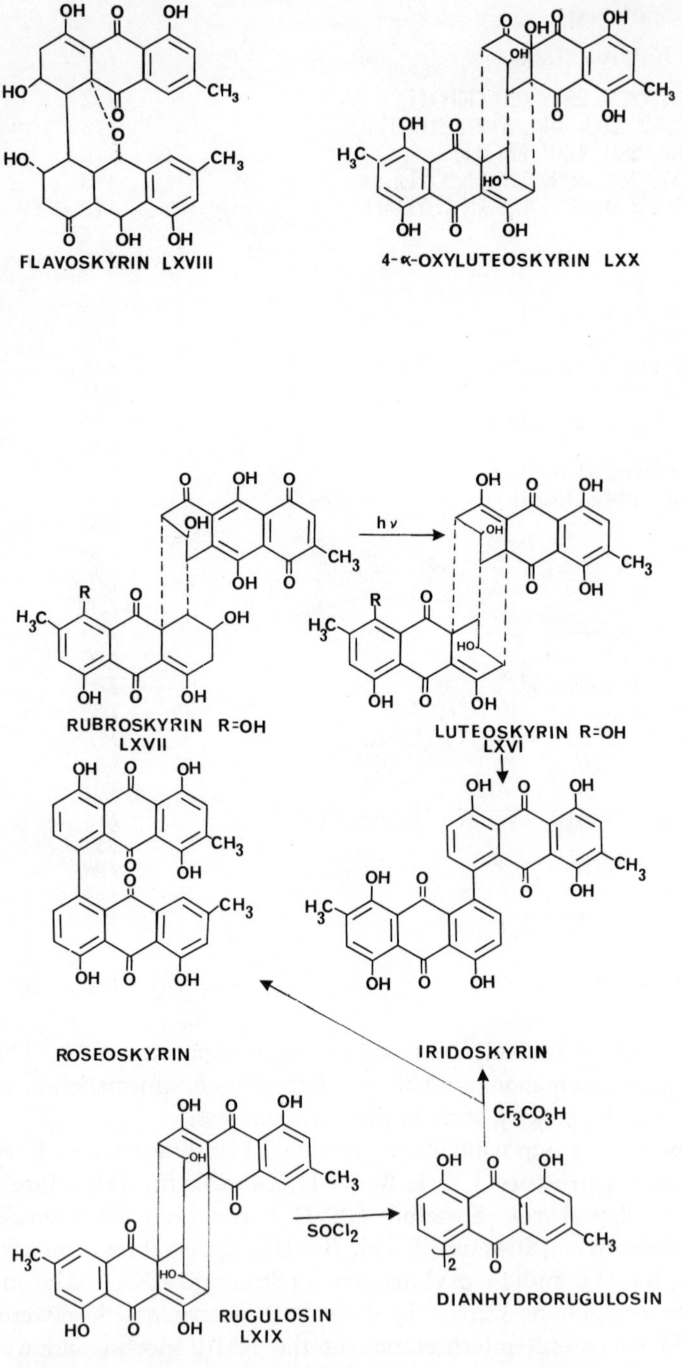
FLAVOSKYRIN LXVIII
4-α-OXYLUTEOSKYRIN LXX
hν
RUBROSKYRIN R=OH
LXVII
LUTEOSKYRIN R=OH
LXVI
ROSEOSKYRIN
IRIDOSKYRIN
CF3CO3H
SOCl2
RUGULOSIN
LXIX
DIANHYDRORUGULOSIN

Figure 6. Modified bianthraquinones from P. islandicum

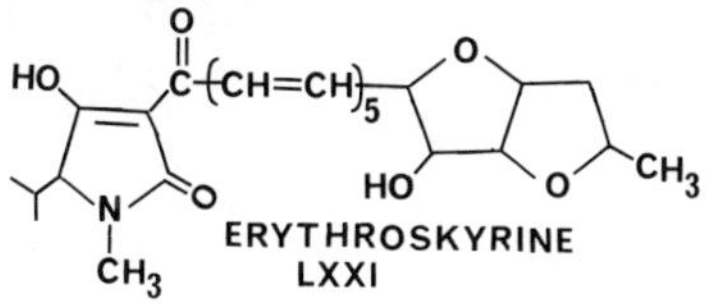

ERYTHROSKYRINE
LXXI

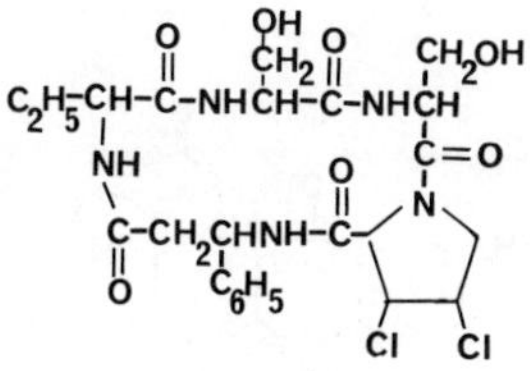

ISLANDITOXIN
LXXII

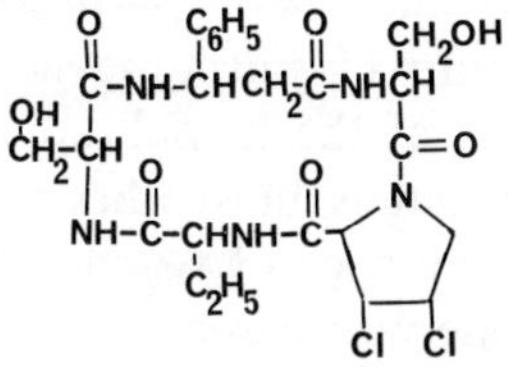

CYCLOCHLOROTINE
LXXIII

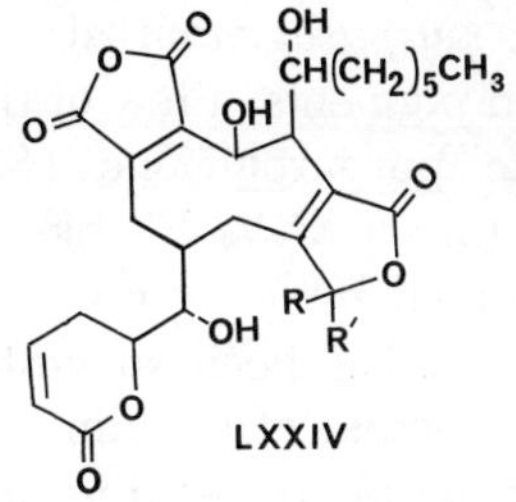

LXXIV

RUBRATOXIN A (R=H, R'=OH)
         B (R,R'= =O)

shows some of the observed interrelationships between these materials.

P. *islandicum* also produces the extremely toxic (LD_{50} = 60 mg/kg, mouse, ip) metabolite erythroskyrine (Structure LXXI) (*113, 126*). The structure of this pigment was determined by chemical degradation experiments which indicated the presence of the polyene system (—CH= CH—)$_5$, the tenuazonic acid moiety, and the dianhydrosorbitol structure. The role of this compound in intoxication by P. *islandicum*-infested rice has not yet been determined.

Finally P. *islandicum* produces two water-soluble, hexatotoxic, cyclic peptides—islanditoxin (Structure LXXII) and cyclochlorotine (Structure LXXIII) (*see* Table X). The tentative structures of these extremely toxic materials have been deduced by hydrolysis experiments (*112, 127*); however some of the investigators in this field feel that these two toxins may be identical (*129*).

P. *variable*. Little is known of the metabolites produced by this mold. However it produces (+)-rugulosin (Structure LXIX), ergosterol, and its peroxide (*130*).

P. *purpurogenum*. This mold is frequently found on foods and feeds and has been implicated in many cases of animal illnesses and deaths (Table IV). It has recently been shown (*131*) capable of producing high yields of the extremely toxic materials rubratoxins **A and B** (Structure LXXIV) (LD_{50} = 100–200 mg/kg, oral, rat). These mycotoxins have been commonly associated with P. *rubrum;* an excellent review of the subject by M. O. Moss has been published (*132*).

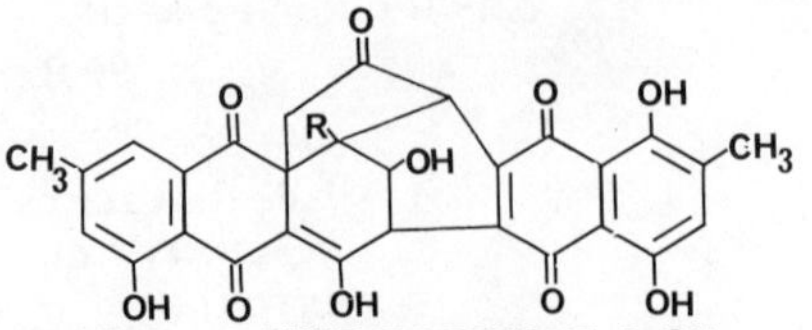

LXXV   PURPUROGENONE R=OH
LXXVI   DEOXYPUPUROGENONE R=H

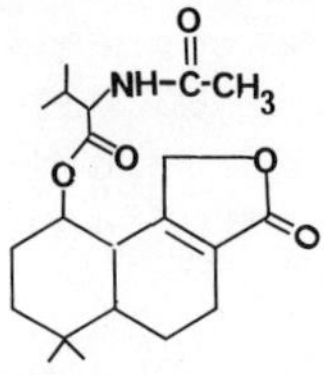

PURPURIDE
LXXVII

P. *purpurogenum* also produces copious amounts of some highly colored pigments; a few of these have been isolated and identified. These include purpurogenone (Structure LXXV) and deoxypurpurogenone (Structure LXXVI, Table XI). The structure of purpurogenone was determined by x-ray crystallographic analysis of the monobromoacetate (145). It has been suggested that the pigment is biosynthesized from two molecules of emodin *via* an undefined sequence of reactions (134). The structure assigned to deoxypurpurogenone was based on a comparison of its spectral data with those obtained from purpurogenone, the formation of a pentaacetate instead of a hexaacetate and oxidative degradation to 3-hydroxy-5-methylphthalic acid and 1,4-dihydroxy-2-methylanthraquinone (135). In addition to Structures LXXV and LXXVI a third, colorless material was isolated and given the trivial name purpuride (Structure LXXVII) which was determined by direct x-ray analysis. The toxicological properties of these compounds have not been investigated.

Table XI.   Metabolites Produced by

Compound	Formula	MW	M.P., °C
Purpurogenone	$C_{29}H_{20}O_{11}$	544	310d
Deoxypurpurogenone	$C_{29}H_{20}O_{10}$	528	>300d
Purpuride	$C_{22}H_{33}NO_5$	391	200–201
Glauconic acid	$C_{18}H_{20}O_7$	348	202
Glaucanic acid	$C_{18}H_{20}O_6$	332	186
Antibiotic SL 3238	$C_{27}H_{41}NO_7$	492	160–1
D-Mannonic acid	$C_6H_{12}O_7$	196	
Alloisocitric acid	$C_6H_6O_6$	174	140–1
Citromycetin	$C_{14}H_{10}O_7$	290	283–5d
Frequentin	$C_{14}H_{20}O_4$	252	134
Sulochrin	$C_{17}H_{16}O_7$	332	226–7
Asterric acid	$C_{17}H_{16}O_8$	348	213–5
(+) Bisdechlorogeodin	$C_{17}H_{14}O_7$	330	170–3
Questin	$C_{16}H_{12}O_5$	284	301–3
Questinol	$C_{16}H_{12}O_6$	300	280–2
Hadacidin	$C_3H_5NO_4$	119	119–20
Rubratoxin A	$C_{26}H_{32}O_{11}$	520	213–5
Rubratoxin B	$C_{26}H_{30}O_{11}$	518	170–1d
Mannitol	$C_6H_{14}O_6$	182	163

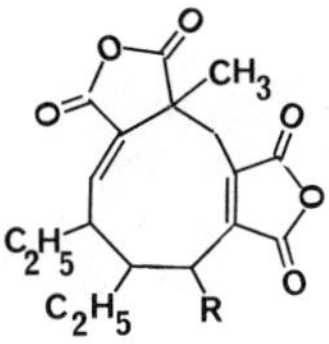

GLAUCONIC ACID R=OH LXXVIII
GLAUCANIC ACID R=H   LXXIX

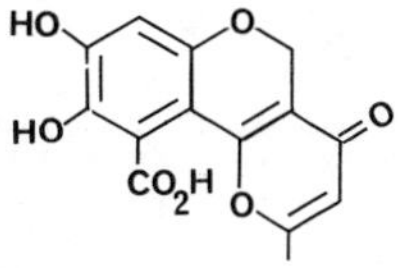

CITROMYCETIN LXXX

P. purpurogenum also produces a pair of nonadrides, glauconic (Structure LXXVIII) and glaucanic (Structure LXXIX) acids, so named because they are constructed from two identical C_9 fragments. Like the rubratoxins these acids contain the relatively stable bisanhydride structure. The structures of these compounds were established primarily by degradation experiments coupled with x-ray crystallographic data (*146*). The key pyrolytic degradation product, glauconin, was identified as a Cope rearrangement product, and its structure was proved by synthesis (*see* Figure 7). Finally an antibiotic (SL 3238-$C_{27}H_{41}NO_2$) of unknown structure is reported to be produced by *P. purpurogenum* (*see* Table XI). No toxicological information is available about this material.

P. frequentans. As its name implies, this mold is commonly found in all types of materials. None of the commonly known mycotoxins, however, have been isolated from this mold although several metabolites are known (*see* Table XI). These include citromycetin (Structure LXXX),

P. purpurogenum and P. frequentans

UV, nm (solvent)	Ref.
253, 308, 388, 499, 530, 570 (CHCl₃)	*134*
251, 275, 309, 389, 490, 529 (CHCl₃)	*135*
216.5 (EtOH)	*136*
223	*137*
220	*137*
	138
	139
	140
	141
232, 290 (Dioxane)	*142*
	143
250, 317 (EtOH)	*143*
215, 285 (EtOH)	*143*
224, 248, 285, 425 (EtOH)	*143*
224, 247, 286, 432 (EtOH)	*143*
	144
250 (CH₃CN)	*133*
250 (CH₃CN)	*133*
	131

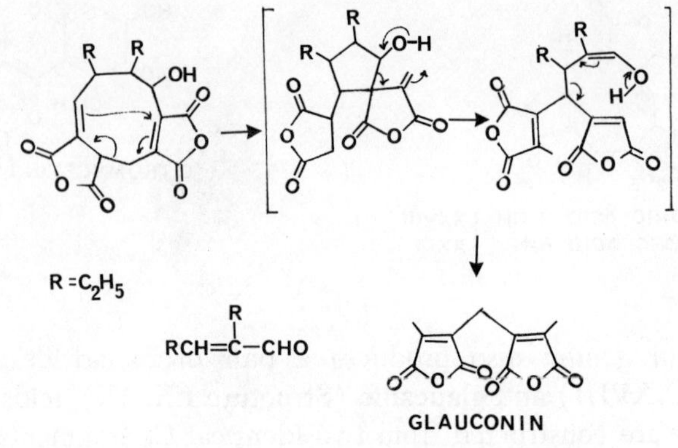

R = C_2H_5

$RCH=\overset{R}{\underset{}{C}}-CHO$

GLAUCONIN

Figure 7. Formation of glauconin from glauconic
acid

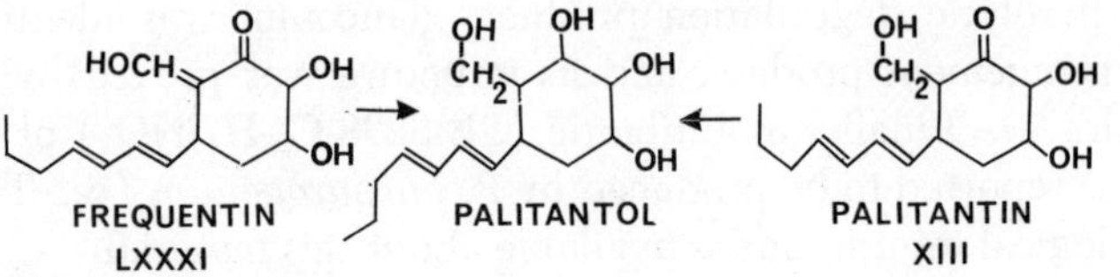

FREQUENTIN
LXXXI

PALITANTOL

PALITANTIN
XIII

Figure 8. Relationship between frequentin and palitantin

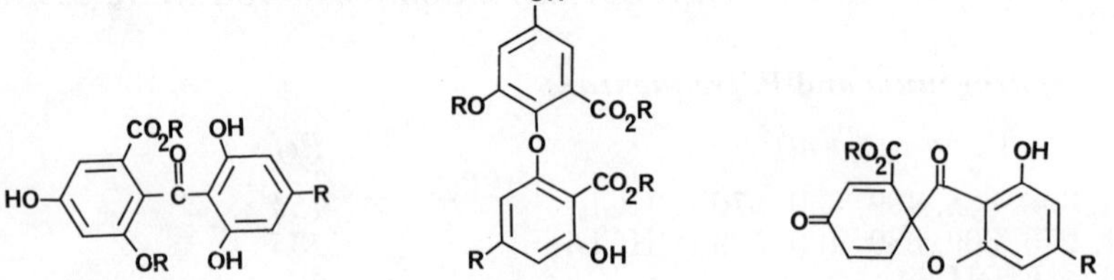

SULOCHRIN
LXXXII

ASTERRIC ACID
LXXXIII

BISDECHLOROGEODIN
LXXXIV

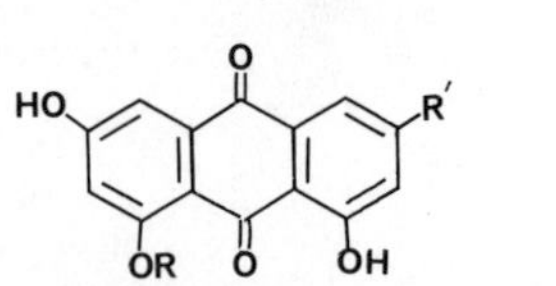

QUESTIN R=CH_3 LXXXV
QUESTINOL R'=CH_2OH LXXXVI

frequentin (Structure LXXXI; Figure 8), palitantin (Structure XIII; see
P. cyclopium), sulochrin (Structure LXXXII), asterric acid (Structure
LXXXIII), bisdechlorogeodin (Structure LXXXIV), and a pair of anthraquinone pigments, questin (Structure LXXXV) and questinol (Structure LXXXVI). The structure of citromycetin was based primarily on

degradation results in which methyl-*O*-dimethylcitromycetin was cleaved with permanganate to yield 2-carboxy-3-hydroxy-5,6-dimethoxybenzoate (*137*). Frequentin (Structure LXXXI) was quickly deduced by its ready conversion into palitantol, a product readily obtained from palitantin (Structure XIII) by NaBH₄ reduction (Figure 8). *P. frequentans* also produces sulochrin (Structure LXXXII), asterric acid (Structure LXXXIII), and bisdechlorogeodin (Structure LXXXIV); the latter two compounds are interrelated in that bisdechlorogeodin is easily converted into asterric acid simply by heating in water. All three compounds had been previously isolated from *Oospora sulphurea-ochracea,* and the structure of bisdechlorogeodin has been confirmed by total synthesis (*143*). The structures of questin (Structure LXXXV) and questinol (Structure LXXXVI) were established through degradation experiments and comparison with derivatives of emodin and ω-hydroxyemodin. No toxicity has been associated with any of these materials.

Conclusion

The 13 *Penicillium* species identified as commonly found on foods produce a large number of metabolites; some of these may be classified as true mycotoxins. However, little is known about the toxicological properties of many of the metabolites, and this needs to be studied. Finally very little is known about the occurrence of these metabolites in foods and feeds.

Literature Cited

1. Mislivec, P., private communication.
2. Mislivec, P., Bruce, V., Dieter, C., unpublished data.
3. Mislivec, P., unpublished data.
4. Mislivec, P., Ph.D. Thesis, Purdue University, 1968.
5. Mislivec, P. B., Tuite, J., *Mycologia* (1970) **62** (1), 67.
6. Hesseltine, C. W., Graves, R. R., *Econ. Bot.* (1966) **20,** 156.
7. Ciegler, A., Mintzlaff, H. J., Leistner, L., *Fleischwirtschaft* (1972) **52** (10), 1311.
8. Leistner, L., Ayres, J. C., *Fleischwirtschaft* (1968) **48** (1), 62.
9. Borker, E., Insalata, N. F., Levi, C. P., Witzman, J. S., *Advan. Appl. Microbiol.* (1966) **8,** 315.
10. Brook, P. J., White, E. P., *Annu. Rev. Phytopathol.* (1966) **4,** 171.
11. Purchase, I. F. H., *Toxicol. Appl. Pharmacol.* (1971) **18,** 114.
12. Carlton, W. W., Tuite, J., *Toxicol. Appl. Pharmacol.* (1970) **17,** 289.
13. Wilson, B. J., Wilson, C. H., Hayes, A. W., *Nature* (1968) **220,** 77-78.
14. Albright, J. L., Aust, S. D., Byers, J. M., Fritz, T. E., Brodie, B. O., Olsen, R. E., Link, R. P., Simon, J., Rhoades, H. E., Brewer, R. L., *J. Amer. Vet. Med. Assoc.* (1964) **144,** 1013.
15. Cunningham, K. G., Freeman, G. G., *Biochem. J.* (1953) **53,** 328.
16. Friis, P., Hasselager, E., Krogh, P., *Acta Pathol. Microbiol. Scand.* (1969) **77,** 559.

17. Krogh, P., Hasselager, E., Friis, P., *Acta Pathol. Microbiol. Scand.* (1970) **78**, 401.
18. Carlton, W. W., Tuite, J., *Pathol. Vet.* (1970) **7**, 68.
19. Zwicker, G. M., Carlton, W. W., Tuite, J., *Food Cosmet. Toxicol.* (1973) **11**, 989.
20. McCracken, M. D., Carlton, W. W., Tuite, J., *Food Cosmet. Toxicol.* (1974) **12**, 79.
21. Scott, D. B., *Mycopathol. Mycol. Appl.* (1965) **25**, 213.
22. Carlton, W. W., Tuite, J., Mislivec, P., *Toxicol. Appl. Pharmacol.* (1968) **13**, 372.
23. Mintzlaff, H. J., *Fleischwirtschaft* (1971) **51**, 344.
24. Joffe, A. Z., *Mycopathol. Mycol. Appl.* (1962) **16**, 201.
25. Yamamoto, T., *J. Pharm. Soc. Jap.* (1954) **74**, 797.
26. Enomoto, M., Saito, M., *Ann. Rev. Microbiol.* (1972) **26**, 279.
27. Kobayashi, M. *et al.*, *Proc. Jap. Acad.* (1959) **35**, 501.
28. Uraguchi, K. *et al.*, *Food Cosmet. Toxicol.* (1972) **10**, 193.
29. Tsunoda, H., *Proc. U.S.–Jap. Conf. Toxic Microorganisms, 1st, Honolulu, 1968,* "U.S. Dept. of Interior and U.J.N.R. Panels on Toxic Microorganisms," Washington, D.C., p. 143.
30. Forgacs, J., Koch, H., Carll, W. T., White–Stevens, R. H., *Amer. J. Vet. Res.* (1958) **19**, 744.
31. Ciegler, A., Fennell, D. I., Mintzlaff, H. J., Leistner, L., *Naturwissenschaften* (1972) **59**, 365.
32. Chu, F. S., *Crit. Rev. Toxicol.* (1974) **2** (4), 499.
33. Hayes, A. W., Hood, R. D., Lee, H. L., *Teratology* (1974) **9**, 93.
34. Birkinshaw, J. H., Oxford, A. E., Raistrick, H., *Biochem. J.* (1936) **30**, 394.
35. Murnagham, M. F., *J. Pharmacol. Exp. Ther.* (1946) **88**, 119.
36. Dickens, F., Jones, H. E. H., *Brit. J. Cancer* (1965) **19**, 392.
37. Hou, C. T., Ciegler, A., Hesseltine, C. W., *Appl. Microbiol.* (1971) **21** (6), 1101.
38. Ciegler, A., Kurtzman, C. P., *Appl. Microbiol.* (1970) **20** (5), 761.
39. Hou, C. T., Ciegler, A., Hesseltine, C. W., *Can. J. Microbiol.* (1971) **17** (5), 599.
40. Holzapfel, C. W., *Tetrahedron* (1968) **24**, 2101.
41. Holzapfel, C. W., Hutchison, R. D., Wilkins, D. C., *Tetrahedron* (1970) **26**, 5239.
42. Holzapfel, C. W., in "Microbial Toxins," A. Ciegler, S. Kadis, J. Ajl, Eds., p. 435, Academic, New York, 1971.
43. Framm, J., Nover, L., Azzouny, A. E., Richter, H., Winter, K., Werner, S., Luckner, M., *Eur. J. Biochem.* (1973) **37**, 78.
44. Mohammed, Y. S., *Tetrahedron Lett.* (1963) **28**, 1953.
45. Birkinshaw, J. H., Luckner, M., Mohammed, Y. S., Mothes, K., Stickings, C. E., *Biochem. J.* (1963) **89**, 196.
46. Birch, A. J., Kocor, M., *J. Chem. Soc.* (1960) 866.
47. Aulin-Erdtman, G., Theorell, H., *Acta Chem. Scand.* (1950) **4**, 1490.
48. Birkinshaw, J. H., Raistrick, H., Ross, D. J., Stickings, C. E., *Biochem. J.* (1952) **50**, 610.
49. Oxford, A. E., Raistrick, H., *Biochem. J.* (1935) **29**, 1599.
50. Anslow, W. K., Breen, J., Raistrick, H., *Biochem. J.* (1940) **33**, 159.
51. Purchase, I. F. H., *Toxicol. Appl. Pharmacol.* (1971) **18**, 114.
52. Schabort, J. C., Wilkins, D. C., *J. S. Afr. Chem. Inst.* (1969) **22**, S9.
53. Bracken, A., Pocker, A., Raistrick, H., *Biochem. J.* (1954) **57**, 587.
54. White, J. D., Haefliger, W. E., Dimsdale, M. J., *Tetrahedron* (1970) **26**, 233.
55. Martin, P. K., Rapoport, H., Smith, H. W., Wong, T. L., *J. Org. Chem.* (1969) **34** (5), 1359.

56. van Walbeek, W., Scott, P. M., Harwig, J., Lawrence, J. W., Can. J. Microbiol. (1969) **15**, 1281.
57. Luckner, M., Mohammed, Y. S., Tetrahedron Lett. (1964) **29**, 1987.
58. Hutchison, R. D., Steyn, P. S., Thompson, D. L., Tetrahedron Lett. (1971) **43**, 4033.
59. Hetherington, A. C., Raistrick, H., Trans. Roy. Soc. (London) (1931) **B 220**, 269.
60. Cartwright, N. J., Robertson, A., Whalley, W. B., Nature (1949) **163**, 94.
61. Brown, J. P., Cartwright, N. J., Robertson, A., Whalley, W. B., Nature (1948) **162**, 72.
62. Johnson, D. H., Robertson, A., Whalley, W. B., J. Chem. Soc. (1950) 2971.
63. Cartwright, N. J., Robertson, A., Whalley, W. B., J. Chem. Soc. (1949) 1563.
64. Burton, H. S., Brit. J. Exp. Pathol. (1949) **30**, 151.
65. Wilson, B. J., in "Microbial Toxins," Vol. VI, A. Ciegler, S. Kadis, S. J. Ajl, Eds., p. 459, Academic, New York, 1971.
66. Birkinshaw, J. H., Samant, M. S., Biochem. J. (1960) **74**, 369.
67. Wilson, B. J., Yang, D. T., Harris, T. M., Appl. Microbiol. (1973) **26** (4), 633.
68. Birch, A. J., Wright, J. J., Chem. Commun. (1969) 644.
69. Pohland, A. E., Stack, M. E., unpublished data.
70. Just, G., Day, W., Blank, F., Can. J. Chem. (1963) **41**, 74.
71. Hutchinson, R. D., Steyn, P. S., van Rensburg, S. J., Toxicol. Appl. Pharmacol. (1973) **24**, 507.
72. Steyn, P. S., Tetrahedron (1970) **26**, 51.
73. Scott, P. M., Miles, W. F., Taft, P., Dube, J. G., J. Agric. Food Chem. (1972) **20** (2), 450.
74. Birch, A. J., Musgrave, O. C., Richards, R. W., Smith, H., J. Chem. Soc. (1959) 3146.
75. Clarke, H. J., Johnson, J., Robinson, R., "The Chemistry of Penicillin," Princeton University, Princeton, 1949.
76. Tatum, E. L., J. Biol. Chem. (1945) **160**, 455.
77. Ballio, A., Casinovi, C., Serlupi–Crescenzi, G., Biochim. Biophys. Acta (1956) **20**, 414.
78. Ballio, A., Serlupi–Crescenzi, G., Nature (1957) **179**, 154.
79. deFlines, J., J. Amer. Chem. Soc. (1955) **77**, 1676.
80. Hikino, H., Nabetani, S., Takemoto, T., J. Pharm. Soc. Jap. (1973) **93** (5), 619.
81. Peck, R. L., Anderson, R. J., J. Biol. Chem. (1941) **140**, 89.
82. Suter, P. J., Turner, W. B., J. Chem. Soc. (1967) 2240.
83. Clutterbuck, P. W., Oxford, A. E., Raistrick, H., Smith, G., Biochem. J. (1932) **26**, 1441.
84. Oxford, A. E., Raistrick, H., Biochem. J. (1932) **26**, 1902.
85. Canonica, L., Kroszcynski, W., Ranzi, B. M., Rindone, B., Scolastico, C., Chem. Commun. (1971) 257.
86. Ibid. (1970) 1357.
87. Campbell, I. M., Calzadilla, C. H., McCorkindale, N. J., Tetrahedron Lett. (1966) **42**, 5107.
88. Birch, A. J., Wright, J. J., Tetrahedron (1970) **26**, 2329.
89. Birch, A. J., Russel, R. A., Tetrahedron (1972) **28**, 2999.
90. Birch, A. J., J. Agric. Food Chem. (1971) **19** (6), 1088.
91. Steyn, P. S., Tetrahedron (1973) **29**, 107.
92. Godin, P., Biochim. Biophys. Acta (1953) **11**, 114.
93. Whalley, W. B., Pure Appl. Chem. (1963) **7**, 565.
94. Yamamoto, T., J. Pharm. Sci. Jap. (1955) **75**, 761.
95. Mosbach, K., Z. Naturforsch. (1959) **14b**, 69.

96. Igarasi, H., *J. Agric. Chem. Soc. Jap.* (1939) **15**, 225.
97. Buchi, G., White, J. D., Wogan, G. N., *J. Amer. Chem. Soc.* (1965) **87** (15), 3484.
98. Merlini, L., Nasini, G., Selva, A., *Tetrahedron* (1970) **26**, 2739.
99. Uraguchi, K., Tatsuno, T., Tsukioka, M., Sakai, Y., Sakai, F., Koboyashi, Y., Saito, M., Enomoto, M., Miyaki, M., *Jap. J. Exp. Med.* (1961) **31**, 1.
100. Grove, J. F., MacMillan, J. T., Mulholland, T. P. C., Rogers, M. A. T., *J. Chem. Soc.* (1952) 3949.
101. Birkinshaw, J. H., Bracken, A., Michael, S. A., Raistrick, H., *Lancet* (1943) **245**, 625.
102. Birkinshaw, J. H., Bracken, A., Raistrick, H., *Biochem. J.* (1943) **37**, 726.
103. Anslow, W. K., Raistrick, H., *Biochem. J.* (1931) **25**, 39.
104. Bassett, E. W., Tanenbaum, S. W., *Experientia* (1958) **14**, 38.
105. Engel, B. G., Brzesk, W., *Helv. Chim. Acta* (1947) **30**, 1472.
106. Ciegler, A., Detroy, R. W., Lillehoj, E. B., in "Microbial Toxins," Vol. VI, A. Ciegler, S. Kadis, S. J. Ajl, Eds., p. 409, Academic, New York, 1971.
107. Paget, G. E., Walpole, A. L., *Nature* (1958) **182**, 1320.
108. Wilson, B. J., in "Microbial Toxins," Vol. VI, A. Ciegler, S. Kadis, S. J. Ajl, Eds., Academic, New York, 1971.
109. McMaster, W. J., Scott, A. I., Trippett, S., *J. Chem. Soc.* (1960) 4628.
110. Miyake, M., Saito, M., Enomoto, M., Shikata, T., Ishiko, T., Uraguchi, K., Sakai, F., Tatsuno, T., Tsukioka, M., Sakai, Y., Sato, T., *Acta Pathol. Jap.* (1960) **10**, 75.
111. Marumo, S., Sumiki, Y., *J. Agric. Chem. Soc.* (1955) **29**, 305.
112. Marumo, S., *Bull. Agric. Chem. Soc. Jap.* (1959) **23** (5), 428.
113. Saito, M., Enomoto, M., Tatsuno, T., in "Microbial Toxins," Vol. VI, A. Ciegler, S. Kadis, S. J. Ajl, Eds., p. 299, Academic, New York, 1971.
114. Howard, B. H., Raistrick, H., *Biochem. J.* (1954) **56**, 56.
115. Howard, B. H., Raistrick, H., *Biochem. J.* (1949) **44**, 227.
116. Gatenbeck, S., *Acta Chem. Scand.* (1958) **12**, 1985.
117. Bu'Lock, J. D., Smith, J. R., *J. Chem. Soc.* (1968) 1941.
118. Gatenbeck, S., *Acta Chem. Scand.* (1959) **13** (2), 386.
119. Kende, A. S., Belletire, J. L., Hume, E. L., *Tetrahedron Lett.* (1973) **31**, 2935.
120. Ogihara, Y., Kobayashi, N., Shibata, S., *Tetrahedron Lett.* (1968) **15**, 1881.
121. Howard, B. H., Raistrick, A., *Biochem. J.* (1954) **57**, 212.
122. Shibata, S., Takido, M., Ohta, A., Kurosu, T., *Chem. Pharm. Bull.* (1957) **6**, 573.
123. Kobayashi, N., Iitaka, Y., Sankawa, U., Ogihera, Y., Shibata, S., *Tetrahedron Lett.* (1968) **58**, 6135.
124. Takeda, N., Seo, S., Ogihara, Y., Sankawa, U., Iitaka, I., Kitagawa, I., *Tetrahedron Lett.* (1973) **29**, 3703.
125. Seo, S., Sankawa, U., Ogihara, Y., Iitaka, Y., Shibata, S., *Tetrahedron* (1973) **29**, 3721.
126. Shojii, J., Shibata, S., *Chem. Ind.* (1964) 419.
127. Ishikawa, I., Ueno, Y., Tsunoda, H., *J. Biochem.* (1970) **67** (6), 753.
128. Gatenbeck, S., *Acta Chem. Scand.* (1957) **11** (3), 555.
129. Shibata, S., private communication.
130. Yamazaki, M., Fujimoto, H., Miyaki, K., *Yakugaku Zasshi* (1972) **92** (1), 101.
131. Natori, S., Sakaki, S., Kurata, H., Udagawa, S., Ichinoe, M., Saito, M., Umeda, M., Ohtsubo, K., *Appl. Microbiol.* (1970) **19** (4), 613.
132. Moss, M. O., in "Microbial Toxins," Vol. VI, A. Ciegler, S. Kadis, S. J. Ajl, Eds., p. 381, Academic, New York, 1971.
133. Buchi, G., Snader, K. M., White, J. D., Gougoutas, J. Z., Singh, S., *J. Amer. Chem. Soc.* (1970) **92**, 6638.

134. Roberts, J. C., Thompson, D. J., *J. Chem. Soc.* (1971) 3488.
135. Roberts, J. D., Thompson, D. J., *J. Chem. Soc.* (1971) 3493.
136. King, T. J., Roberts, J. C., Thompson, D. J., *J. Chem. Soc.* (1973) 78.
137. Barton, D. H. R., Sutherland, J. K., *J. Chem. Soc.* (1965) 1769.
138. Bollinger, P., Sigg, H. P., Haerri, E., Ger. Patent **2,005,976** (1970); *Chem. Abstr.* (1970) **73,** 108.
139. Angeletti, A., Cerruti, C. F., *Ann. Chim. Appl.* (1930) **20,** 424.
140. Beppu, T., Abe, S., Sakaguchi, R., *Bull. Agric. Chem. Soc.* (1957) **21,** 263.
141. Cavill, G. W., Robertson, A., Whalley, W. B., *J. Chem. Soc.* (1950) 1031.
142. Sigg, H. P., *Helv. Chim. Acta* (1963) **46,** 1061.
143. Mahmoodian, A., Stickings, C. E., *Biochem. J.* (1964) **92,** 369-378.
144. Kaczka, E. A., Citterman, C. O., Dulaney, E. L., Folkers, K., *Biochem. J.* (1962) **1,** 340-43.
145. King, T. J., Roberts, J. C., Thompson, D. J., *Chem. Commun.* (1970) 1499.
146. Baldwin, J. E., Barton, D. H. R., Bloomer, J. L., Jackman, L. M., Rodriguez–Hahn, L., Sutherland, J. K., *Experientia* (1962) **18,** 345.

RECEIVED November 8, 1974.

8

Chemical and Biochemical Studies of the Trichothecene Mycotoxins

JAMES R. BAMBURG

Department of Biochemistry, Colorado State University, Ft. Collins, Colo. 80521

Several naturally occurring sesquiterpene compounds in the trichothecene family have been implicated in economically important mycotoxicoses such as moldy corn toxicosis of cattle and poultry, and stachybotryotoxicosis. The trichothecenes in general are stable compounds but under appropriate conditions undergo several types of intramolecular rearrangements. These reactions as well as the complete chemical synthesis of the trichothcene, trichodermin, are reviewed. Assignments have been made for the signals in the ^{13}C-NMR spectra of several trichothecenes, and this technique along with ^{14}C-labeling studies has proved useful in investigations of the biosynthetic origin of the trichothecene ring system. The mechanism of action of the trichothecenes in their inhibition of eukaryotic ribosomal protein synthesis is reviewed, and structure–function relationships are discussed.

More than 20 naturally occurring members of the trichothecene family of sesquiterpene compounds had been characterized by 1970. The structures and chemical and biological properties of these compounds have been reviewed extensively (1). The purpose of this paper is to summarize current research on the chemistry and mechanism of action of this important group of mold metabolites. The total number of naturally occurring trichothecenes known today approaches 30 (Figures 2, 3, and 4) with the identification of calonectrin (Figure 1l) and 15-desacetylcalonectrin (Figure 1m) isolated from a fungus identified as *Calonectria nivalis* (16) but recently revised to *Fusarium culmorum* (25), trichothecene (Figure 1n) and 4β, 8α-dihydroxytrichothecene (Figure 1o) from *Trichothecium roseum* (17), and monoacetoxyscirpendiol and trihydroxyscirpene from *Fusarium roseum* (7). In addition, several compounds which appear to be derivatives of verrucarol (Figure 1b) have been isolated from *Stachybotrys atra* cultures (33). Although not yet identified they appear to be different from the known verrucarins and roridins (33).

The chemical structures of all the trichothecenes known have been proved by interconversion to one of the known trichothecene derivatives which was itself related to the structure of trichodermol determined by x-ray crystallography of its *p*-bromobenzoate ester (34, 35). Increasing awareness of the potential dangers of mycotoxicoses and increasing knowledge of the physiological effects of mycotoxins have led to the discovery and probable involvement of several trichothecenes in actual field cases of mycotoxin diseases. The trichothecene T-2 toxin (Figure 1h) which was originally implicated in moldy corn toxicosis of cattle has been isolated from the feed of a herd of cows suffering from moldy corn toxicosis (36). In addition, outbreaks of mycotoxicoses in commercial flocks of chickens led to symptoms in the birds which could be produced by T-2 toxin alone (37). Stachybotryotoxicosis, a disease mainly of horses but which affects poultry and swine as well is at least partially caused by trichothecenes, specifically trichodermol (Figure 1a) (roridin C), and two derivatives of verrucarol which are as yet uncharacterized (33).

Little progress has been made over the past few years to determine the metabolites of the trichothecene ring system when toxins are admin-

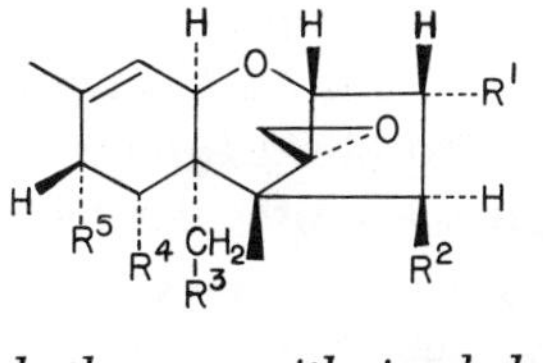

Figure 1.   Structures of trichothecenes with simple hydroxyl or acyl substituents

		Ref.	R^1	R^2	R^3	R^4	R^5
a.	Trichodermol	2, 3, 4, 5	H	OH	H	H	H
b.	Verrucarol	5	H	OH	OH	H	H
c.	Scirpenetriol	6, 7	OH	OH	OH	H	H
d.	T-2 Tetraol	8	OH	OH	OH	H	OH
e.	Diacetoxyscirpenol	6, 9, 10, 11	OH	OAc	OAc	H	H
f.	Trichodermin	3, 4	H	OAc	H	H	H
g.	Diacetylverrucarol	12	H	OAc	OAc	H	H
h.	T-2 Toxin	8	OH	OAc	OAc	H	OOCCH₂CHMe₂
i.	HT-2 Toxin	13	OH	OH	OAc	H	OOCCH₂CHMe₂
j.	(C₂₁H₂₈O₁₀ Triacetate from F. Scirpi)	14	OH	OAc	OAc	OH	OAc
k.	Neosolaniol	15	OH	OAc	OAc	H	OH
l.	Calonectrin	16	OAc	H	OAc	H	H
m.	15-Desacetylcalonectrin	16	OAc	H	OH	H	H
n.	Trichothecene	17	H	H	H	H	H
o.	4,8-Dihydroxytrichothecene	17	H	OH	H	H	OH
p.	Triacetoxyscirpene	6	OAc	OAc	OAc	H	H
q.	Acetoxyscirpendiol	7, 18	OH	OH	OAc	H	H

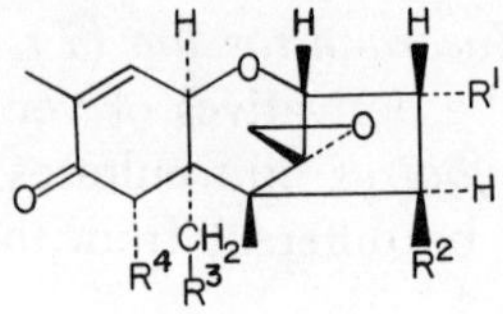

Figure 2.   Structures of 8-keto trichothecenes

	Ref.	R¹	R²	R³	R⁴
a. Trichothecolone	19, 20	H	OH	H	H
b. Nivalenol	21	OH	OH	OH	OH
c. Trichothecin	3, 22	H	OOCCHCHMe	H	H
d. Diacetylnivalenol	15, 23, 24	OH	OAc	OAc	OH
e. Fusarenon-X	25	OH	OAc	OH	OH
f. C₁₇H₂₂O₇ from F. culmorum	25	OAc	H	OH	OH

istered in low doses over long periods. *In vitro* metabolic studies indicate that T-2 toxin is converted to HT-2 toxin (Figure 1i) by the liver (*38*); this is hardly a detoxification mechanism since the toxicities of both compounds are nearly identical. Research in this area has been slow because of the lack of a specific radiolabelled trichothecene compound to identify nontoxic metabolites, but rapid progress should be made when sufficient labelled material is available.

Chemistry of Trichothecenes

Rearrangements and Modification Reactions. A variety of modification reactions to trichothecene compounds have been reported. The most important of these reactions are those involving intramolecular rearrangements because the 12,13-spiroepoxide group is extremely stable to extramolecular, nucleophilic attack. Although these reactions have been reviewed (*1*), they are important to understand because any attempts to modify these compounds must avoid conditions that lead to the rearrangements. For example diacetyl verrucarol (Figure 1g) (*5, 6*), triacetoxyscirpene (Figure 1p) (*6*), and calonectrin (Figure 1l) (*16*) all undergo a hydration upon prolonged boiling in water to give the rearranged diol (Figure 5). Acid treatment of many of the trichothecenes

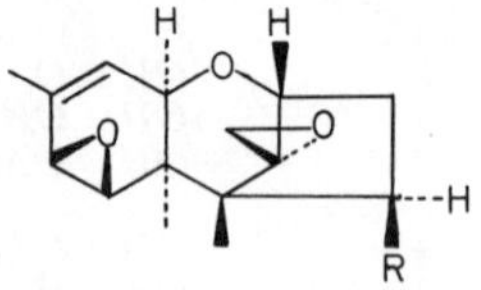

Figure 3.   Structures of 7,8-epoxytrichothecenes

	Ref.	R
a. Crotocol	26	OH
b. Crotocin	26	OOCCHCHMe

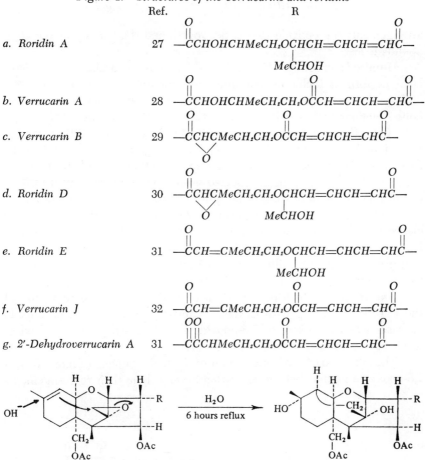

Figure 4.   Structures of the verrucarins and roridins

		Ref.	R
a.	Roridin A	27	—CCHOHCHMeCH₂OCHCH=CHCH=CHC—

$$\text{a. Roridin A} \quad 27 \quad -\overset{O}{\overset{\|}{C}}CHOHCHMeCH_2OCHCH{=}CHCH{=}CH\overset{O}{\overset{\|}{C}}-$$
$$\underset{Me\overset{|}{C}HOH}{}$$

$$\text{b. Verrucarin A} \quad 28 \quad -\overset{O}{\overset{\|}{C}}CHOHCHMeCH_2CH_2O\overset{O}{\overset{\|}{C}}CH{=}CHCH{=}CH\overset{O}{\overset{\|}{C}}-$$

$$\text{c. Verrucarin B} \quad 29 \quad -\overset{O}{\overset{\|}{C}}CHCMeCH_2CH_2O\overset{O}{\overset{\|}{C}}CH{=}CHCH{=}CH\overset{O}{\overset{\|}{C}}-$$
$$\underset{O}{\overset{\diagdown\diagup}{}}$$

$$\text{d. Roridin D} \quad 30 \quad -\overset{O}{\overset{\|}{C}}CHCMeCH_2CH_2OCHCH{=}CHCH{=}CH\overset{O}{\overset{\|}{C}}-$$
$$\underset{O \qquad\quad Me\overset{|}{C}HOH}{\overset{\diagdown\diagup}{}}$$

$$\text{e. Roridin E} \quad 31 \quad -\overset{O}{\overset{\|}{C}}CH{=}CMeCH_2CH_2OCHCH{=}CHCH{=}CH\overset{O}{\overset{\|}{C}}-$$
$$\underset{Me\overset{|}{C}HOH}{}$$

$$\text{f. Verrucarin J} \quad 32 \quad -\overset{O}{\overset{\|}{C}}CH{=}CMeCH_2CH_2O\overset{O}{\overset{\|}{C}}CH{=}CHCH{=}CH\overset{O}{\overset{\|}{C}}-$$

$$\text{g. 2'-Dehydroverrucarin A} \quad 31 \quad -\overset{OO}{\overset{\|\|}{CC}}CHMeCH_2CH_2O\overset{O}{\overset{\|}{C}}CH{=}CHCH{=}CH\overset{O}{\overset{\|}{C}}-$$

Figure 5.   Hydration of diacetylverrucarol (R=H) and triacetoxyscirpene (R=OAc). Data from Refs. 5 and 6.

also yields a product in which ring rearrangement has occurred such as with verrucarol (Figure 1b) (5) and trichodermol (Figure 1a) (4) (Figure 6). Concentrated mineral acids such as HCl will cause similar rearrangements to give the chlorohydrin derivative. In all of these re-

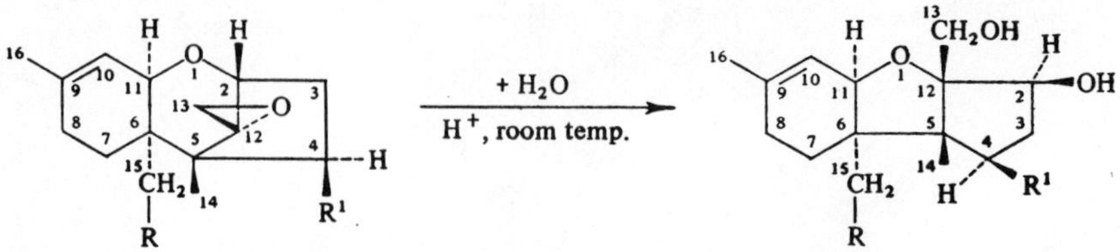

Figure 6. Acid catalyzed rearrangement of trichodermol (R=H,R¹=OH) and
verrucarol (R=R¹=OH). Data from Refs. 4 and 5.

arrangements the epoxide ring is destroyed, and the toxicity of the compounds is lost.

Hundreds of other chemical modifications of trichothecenes have
been performed including chromic acid oxidation of primary and secondary alcohols (epoxide is stable to this treatment), acylation of alcoholic functions with acetate, propionate, butyrate, and other acyl groups,
reduction of ketones and epoxides with LiAlH₄, etc. Very little work has
been done however to modify the type of linkage from the trichothecene
ring system to the acyl functional group. No ether, thioether, amine, or
amide derivatives have been reported even though the biological properties of these compounds might be quite interesting for future studies.

Tratment of diacetoxyscirpenol (Figure 1e) with CrO₃ gives rise to
cleavage of ring C between C3 and C4 (Figure 7) (9). This reaction
leaves the epoxide group intact but destroys the rigidity of the structure
that prevented nucleophilic attack. The acid aldehyde product is therefore very susceptible to nucleophilic attack at C12.

One reaction which occurs in all trichothecenes is the reduction of
the 12,13-epoxy group with LiAlH₄. A tertiary alcohol is the product in
all cases when no 8-keto or 7,8-epoxide functions are present and when
no ring system rearrangement occurs (Figure 8).

The 8-keto trichothecenes (Figure 2) and crotocin (Figure 3b), a
7,8-epoxy derivative, behave somewhat differently in their rearrangements

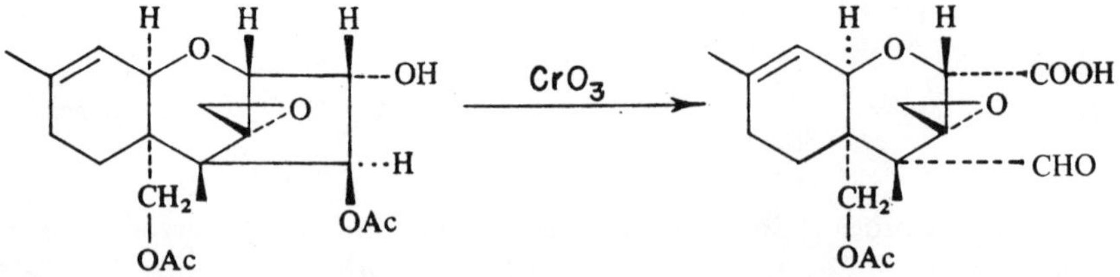

Figure 7. Chromium trioxide oxidation of diacetoxyscirpenol. Data from
Ref. 9.

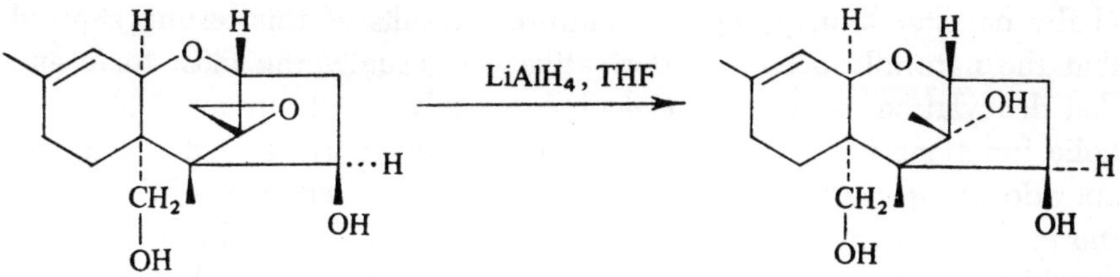

Figure 8.   Reduction of 12,13-spiroepoxide of verrucarol with LiAlH₄. Data from Refs. 5 and 6.

than do the trichothecenes not substituted in these positions. Alkali treatment of either trichthecolone (Figure 2a) (*39*) or crotocol (Figure 3a) (*26*) gave the corresponding iso compound (Figure 9). Crotocin (Figure 3b) and crotocol undergo several other rearrangements as well, generally under fairly mild conditions. Virtually all of the trichothecenes can be reduced with H_2 gas and Pt or Pd catalysts to the corresponding dihydro derivative. Crotocol (Figure 3a), however, undergoes intramolecular rearrangement under these conditions to give a mixture of dihydroisocrotocol derivatives (*26*).

Using these and other modification reactions several workers prepared various derivatives of trichothecenes for toxicity testing. Grove and Mortimer (*40*) prepared several derivatives of verrucarin A (Figure 4b), diacetoxyscryrpenol (Figure 1e), and trichothecin (Figure 2c) which were tested for toxicity against HEp2 cells (human) and BHK

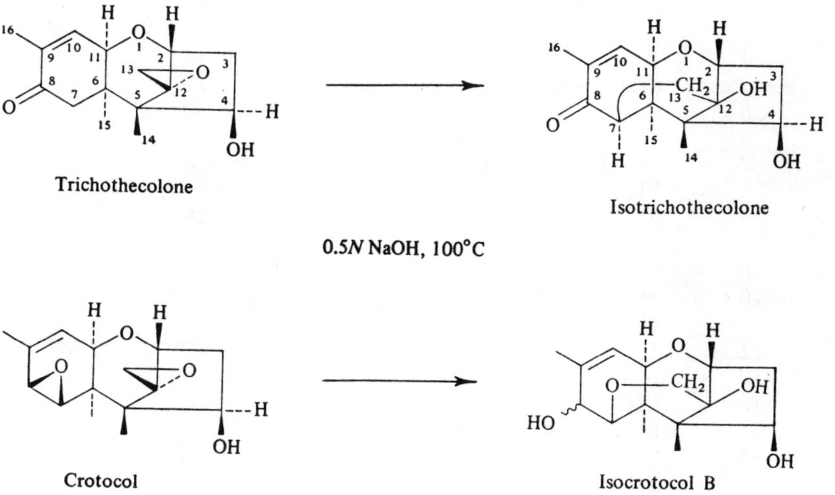

Trichothecolone

Isotrichothecolone

0.5*N* NaOH, 100°C

Crotocol

Isocrotocol B

Figure 9.   Base catalyzed rearrangement of trichothecolone and crotocol. Data from Refs. 26 and 39.

(baby hamster kidney) cells in culture. Results of this testing showed that the naturally occurring derivative was usually the most toxic and that deacylation to the parent alcohol or acylation of any available alcoholic functions usually lower the toxicity. Any derivative that had the epoxide group destroyed was nontoxic as were derivatives which had the epoxide but where ring C was cleaved (*i.e.* Figure 7) so that the epoxide became available for rearside nucleophilic attack. Reduction of the 9–10 double bond also decreased the toxicity of the compound but did not destroy it completely. It was concluded that both water and lipid solubility were important characteristics of the compound for toxicity and that the presence of the stable epoxide group was an absolute necessity for toxicity.

   ^{13}C-NMR. The assignments of the ^{13}C-NMR signals for a wide variety of trichothecenes has recently been reported (*41*). Assignments were made on the basis of comparative chemical shifts of signals in substituted *vs.* unsubstituted derivatives for the carbon atom in question and

Table I.   ^{13}C-NMR Chemical Shifts and Splitting for Signals from Substituted Trichothecenes[a]

Carbon Atom	Substituent	Chemical Shift	Splitting
2	H	68–71	d
3	2H	36–42	t
	α-OH or OAc, β-H (C4, R = 2H)	68–71	d
	α-OH or OAc, β-H (C4, R = OAc)	78–84	d
4	2H	39–42	t
	α-H, β-OH or OAc	73–78	d
5	—	45–50	s
6	—	40–44	s
7	2H (C8, R = 2H)	21–25	t
	2H (C8, R = O)	42	t
8	2H	27–28	t
	O	198–199	s
9	—	138–140	s
10	H (C8, R = 2H)	118–120	d
	H (C8, R = O)	137	d
11	H	76–80	d
12	—	64–66	s
13	2H	47–50	t
14	3H (C4, R = β–OH or OAc)	5–7	q
15	3H	15–16	q
	2H, OAc	63–64	t
16	3H (C8, R = 2H)	23–24	q
	3H (C8, R = O)	18–19	q

[a] Data from Ref. *41*.

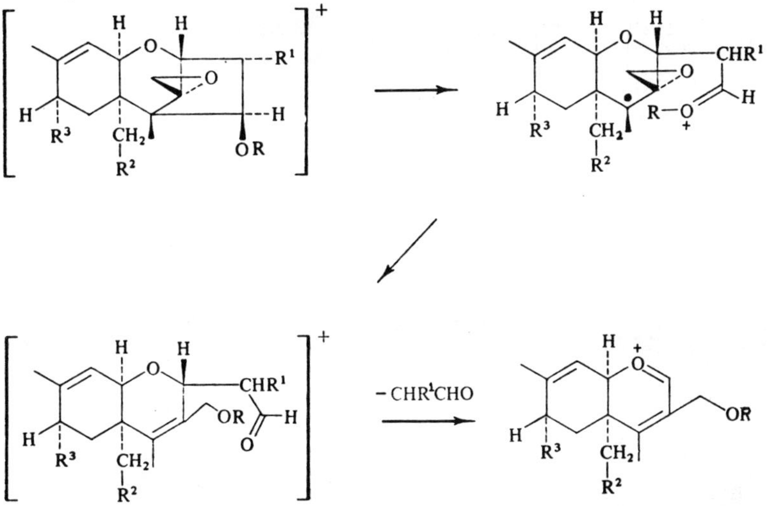

Figure 10. Proton or acyl transfer from C4 to epoxide oxygen for several trichothecenes in the mass spectrometer. Data from Ref. 1.

on peak splittings which would be expected for the substitutions reported. Table I lists the approximate expected chemical shifts and the peak splitting for signals from trichothecenes with various substituents.

Mass Spectrometry. The mass spectra of the trichothecenes are quite complex, and no single characteristic cleavage pattern emerges for the family as a whole which would allow ready identification of the trichothecene ring system. The fragmentation pattern varies between compounds and depends on the nature and position of the ring substituents. One unusual rearrangement which seems to occur on trichothecenes substituted at C4 with either hydroxyl, acyl, or trimethylsilyl function is a transfer of the oxygen bearing substituent to the epoxide oxygen with a subsequent loss of the C3–C4 bridge as shown in Figure 10. This fragmentation scheme has been supported by deuterium labelling of the C4 position. When the deuterium is on the C4 carbon, a fragment of mass 44 (CH_2CDO) is lost. When the deuterium is on the oxygen at C4 (Figure 1a), a fragment of mass 43 is lost (CH_2CHO); the deuterium is transferred to the epoxy group. Trichodermol-d_3-acetate and TMS–trichodermol also show a loss of mass 43 which again probably comes from the C3–C4 bridge. This same fragmentation pattern also occurs in trichothecenes substituted at C3; a loss of a fragment with mass 59 was observed for scirpenetriol (Figure 1c) and T-2 tetraol (Figure 1d) (*1*).

Chemical Synthesis of Trichodermin

Several approaches to the synthesis of trichothecenes have been taken (*42, 43, 44*), but to date only one method has yielded a successful

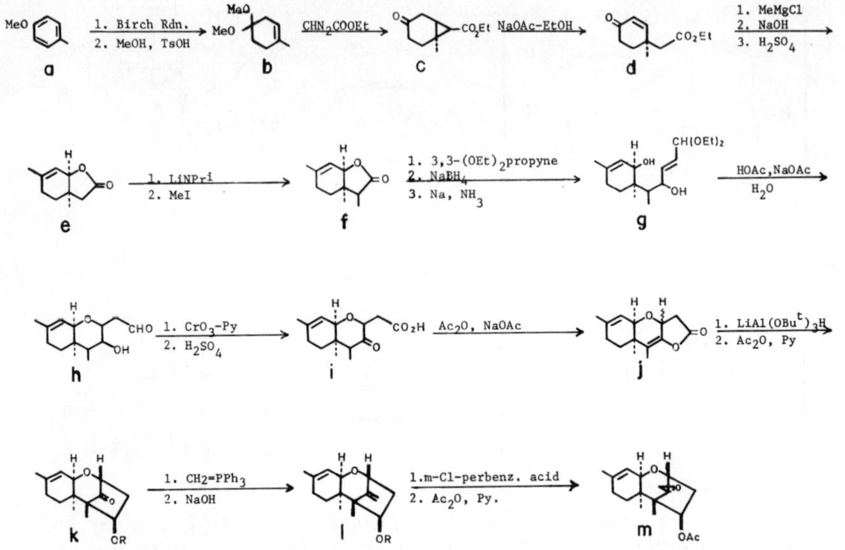

Figure 11.   Chemical synthesis of (±) trichodermin.   Data from Refs. 43 and 44.

synthesis of the trichothecene ring system (*43, 44*). The complete chemical synthesis of the racemic mixture (±)-trichodermin (Figure 1f) has been reported by Colvin et al. (*44*). To achieve the synthesis, the first goal was the production of cis-fused bicyclic rings which was accomplished by the Birch reduction of *p*-methoxytoluene (Figure 11a) and transformation of the resulting dihydrocompound into a 4,4-disubstituted cyclohexanone (Figure 11d) by reaction with ethyl diazoacetate followed by transacetalation with acetone (Figure 11). Reaction of this substituted cyclohexenone with CH_3MgCl followed by base hydrolysis and acidification gave the cis-fused α-lactone (Figure 11e).

The α-methyl homolog of the lactone (Figure 11f) was prepared by a reaction with lithium diisopropylamide followed by direct methylation with iodomethane. Reaction of this lactone with the lithium salt of 3,3-diethoxypropyne gave a hemiacetal which was reduced with sodium borohydride to the corresponding diol. Reduction of the diol in liquid ammonia by sodium gave the transacetal which upon mild acid hydrolysis gave the cis-fused bicyclic hydroxyaldehyde (Figure 11h). The hydroxyaldehyde was oxidized with chromium trioxidepyridine and chromic acid to the corresponding keto acid (Figure 11i). Acetic anhydride treatment of this compound gave the two racemates of the enol lactone (Figure 11j).

The final step in the conversion of the enol lactone to the trichothecene ring system made use of the highly stereoselective, hydride reduction of lactones by the configuration-holding, coordination, metal complex.

Treatment of the enol lactone with lithium hydridotri-*tert*-butoxyalumi-
nate gave two products: a ketoaldehyde and keto alcohol (Figure 11k)
which proved to have a trichothecene-like structure. The ketone was
converted to the corresponding methylene compound (Figure 11l) by
a Wittig reaction with methylenetriphenylphosphorane. Following hydrolysis of the ester to the parent alcohol, stereoselective epoxidation of
the desired double bond was achieved with *m*-chloroperbenzoic acid used
in stoichiometric amounts to prevent epoxidation of the 9,10 double bond.
The final product was acetylated and was identical in all respects (NMR,
IR, mass spectrum, TLC and GLC behavior) except optical rotation with
authentic (−)-trichodermin. During the course of this synthesis several
interesting compounds were produced; perhaps the most fascinating was
12-epitrichodermin (Figure 12). No reports of its biological activity have
as yet appeared in the literature.

Biosynthesis of Trichothecenes

Investigations into the biosynthesis of the trichothecenes occurred
before the correct structure of the trichothecene ring system was known.
Jones and Lowe (*45*) degraded the trichothecene (Figure 2c) which
was derived from 2-^{14}C-mevalonic acid to show that labelling occurred
in C4, C10, and C14. On the basis of this information, these workers
proposed a model for trichothecene biosynthesis from farnesyl pyrophosphate which, based on the correct structure of the trichothecene ring
system, would imply an α-bisabolene intermediate.

More recent studies have shown that farnesyl pyrophosphate is a
precursor to trichothecene biosynthesis (*46, 47*). However α-bisabolene
(as well as α-bisabolol and β-bisobolene) have been excluded as precursors for the trichothecenes (*48*). A reinvestigation of the labelling
pattern of the trichothecene ring both from 2-^{14}C-mevalonate followed
by chemical degradationand from 2-^{13}C-mevalonate incorporation and
position of the label measured by ^{13}C-NMR have shown that the labelled
carbon atoms in the trichothecene structure are C4, C8, and C14 (*41*)
and not C10 as originally reported. These studies coupled with the
recent isolation of trichodiol, trichodiene, and trichothecene (Figure 1n)

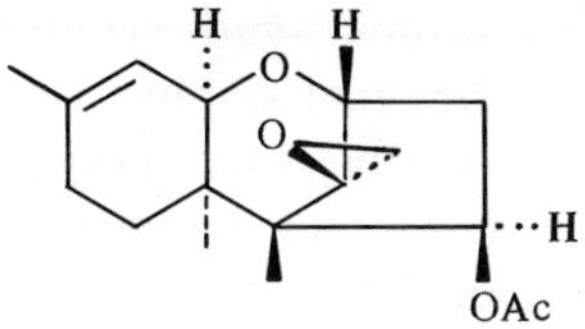

*Figure 12.   The structure of 12-
epitrichodermin. Data from Ref.
43.*

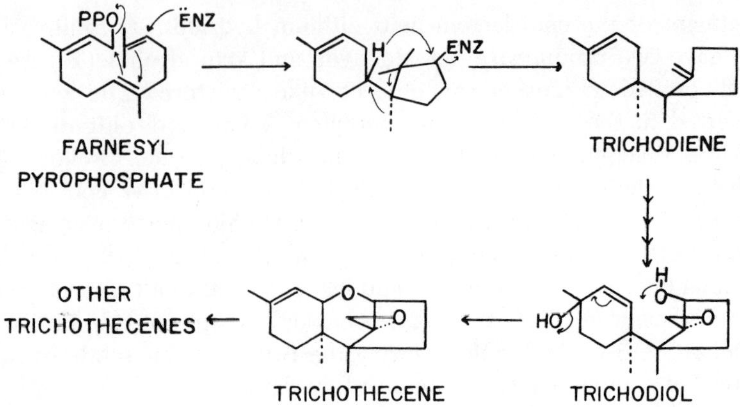

Figure 13.   Proposed pathway for the biosynthesis of the trichothecene ring system. Data from Refs. 17 and 47.

from cultures of *Trichothecium roseum* (49) led to the postulated scheme of biosynthesis and folding of the farnesyl pyrophosphate shown in Figure 13 (47, 49). The compound originally referred to as trichodiol (49) has been shown to be an artifact derived from trichodiol by alkali treatment and is now referred to as trichodiol A (49). In the case of the biosynthesis of trichothecin, the diepoxide crotocin has been postulated as an intermediate since it co-occurs with trichothecin in cultures of *T. roseum* (46).

The dihydroxytrichothecene shown in Figure 13 has also been found in cultures of *T. roseum* and may be an intermediate in the synthesis of trichothecin either through a crotocin intermediate or by direct oxidation. In the synthesis of other trichothecenes we should see when and how the oxidation of other positions on the ring occurs.

Mechanism of Action of Trichothecenes

More progress has been made on the mechanism of action of the trichothecenes in the past few years than for any other mycotoxin. In 1968 Ueno et al. (50) reported that the newly isolated and characterized trichothecene, nivalenol (Figure 2b), inhibited protein synthesis in cultured cells and in cell free protein synthesizing systems. Both the rabbit reticulocyte and rat liver ribosomal systems were used, and both poly U directed polyphenylalanine synthesis and poly A directed polylysine synthesis were inhibited. The site of inhibition was determined at the ribosomal level since nivalenol had no effect on the activation reaction for amino acids catalyzed by aminoacyl-tRNA synthetases (50). In addition the trichothecenes are virtually nontoxic to bacterial systems; this means that either bacterial ribosomes are resistant to these compounds or that trichothecenes do not get into bacteria. In vitro experiments with *E. coli* extracts revealed that trichothecenes did not inhibit bacterial ribosomal protein synthesis (50).

Further studies on the mechanism of action of the trichothecenes were reported in 1972. Ohtsubo et al. (51) reported that the trichthecene, fusarenon-X (Figure 2e), caused a rapid breakdown in the polysomes from cultured mouse fibroblasts. A similar effect was also seen for T-2 toxin (Figure 1h), diacetoxyscirpenol (Figure 1e), and neosolaniol (Figure 1k) on the polysomal profile of rabbit reticulocytes (52). The effects of these toxins on polysome degradation was rapidly reversible when the toxins were washed from the cell culture (52). These effects on polysome profiles could be interpreted in one of two ways: either the toxins inhibited the initiation of translation on the ribosomes, or they stimulated premature release or degradation of the message. In 1973 several reports appeared which seemed to contradict these findings if all trichothecenes were assumed to have the same mechanism of action. Trichodermin (Figure 1f) was reported to inhibit the peptidyl transferase center on the ribosome (53, 54) and to effect the termination step which also involves the peptidyl transferase (54, 55). However fusarenon-X (Figure 2e) and verrucarin A (Figure 3b) were potent inhibitors of peptidyl transferase (53), yet fusarenon-X (Figure 2e) had already been shown to degradete polysomes (51).

The confusion on the mechanism of action of these compounds did not lessen during 1973 although other reports substantiated the effects of trichodermin as an inhibitor of the chain termination reaction (56, 57) and showed T-2 toxin had similar effects on the peptidyl transferase reaction on reticulocyte ribosomes and as an inhibitor of chain termination with reticulocyte releasing factor (55). Other intermediate steps of chain elongation were not affected by these trichothecenes (51). Further studies specifically with trichodermin have shown that this compound has no effect on polysome profiles even though protein synthesis is inhibited. The use of a new in vitro test to distinguish elongation inhibitors from termination inhibitors showed that trichodermin inhibited protein synthesis by blocking the activity of peptidyl transferase required for termination (54, 58).

Reports published during 1974 tended to clear up the confusion on the mechanism of action of the trichothecenes. Cundliffe et al. (59) found that nivalenol (Figure 2b), T-2 toxin (Figure 1h), and verrucarin A (Figure 4b) all caused a breakdown of polysomes to monoribosomes; however the breakdown was inhibited by anisomycin, cycloheximide, and trichodermin (Figure 1f). These authors conclude that trichodermin inhibits chain termination (or elongation) but that nivalenol, T-2 toxin, and verrucarin A inhibit the polypeptide chain initiation steps of eukaryo-

tic protein synthesis (59). The results of earlier reports of verrucarin A
and fusarenon-X being inhibitors of peptidyl transferase can be explained
in light of the new results. These compounds were tested for activity in
systems containing monoribosomes, and their effects on peptidyl transferase under those conditions are real. However if the *in vivo* effects of
these antibiotics inhibit initiation of protein synthesis, their secondary
effects on elongation or termination, although real, are not as important
in their toxic effects to cells. Knowing that these initiation inhibitors
bind at or near the same site on the ribosome however can give important
clues to how they function.

The structure–function relationships of several trichothecenes have
been explored to understand what structural features inhibit initiation
while others inhibit the termination reaction. An initial postulate by
Cundliffe et al. stated that substitution on the C15 position of the trichothecene was critical to inhibit initiation. Of the eight trichothecenes
tested by Schindler (60) the four that had oxygen containing substituents
on C15 had inhibitory activity against initiation, whereas the four not

Table II.   Trichothecene Substituents and Mode of Action in
             Inhibition of Protein Synthesis[a]

Compound	Type of Inhibition[b]	C3	C4	C7	C8	C15
T-2 Toxin	I	OH	OAc	H	iVal	OAc
Diacetoxyscirpenol	I	OH	OAc	H	H	OAc
Fusarenon-X	I	OH	OAc	OH	O	OH
Calonectrin	I	OAc	H	H	H	OAc
Verrucarin A	I	H	ester	H	H	ester
HT-2 Toxin	I	OH	OH	H	iVal	OAc
Nivalenol	I	OH	OH	OH	O	OH
Scirpentriol	I	OH	OH	H	H	OH
15-Acetoxyscirpendiol	I	OH	OH	H	H	OAc
Verrucarin E	I	H	ester	H	H	ester
Verrucarin J	I	H	ester	H	H	ester
Verrucarin H	I	H	ester	H	H	ester
Trichothecin	ET	H	i-crot.	H	O	H
Trichodermol	ET	H	OH	H	H	H
Trichodermin	ET	H	OAc	H	H	H
Verrucarol	ET	H	OH	H	H	OH
15-Desacetylcalonectrin	ET	OAc	H	H	H	OH
Trichothecolone	ET	H	OH	H	O	H
Crotocin	ET	H	i-crot.	epoxide		H
Crotocol	ET	H	OH	epoxide		H

[a] Data from Refs. *60* and *61*.
[b] I = initiation inhibitor; ET = elongation-termination inhibitor. Data from *Nature*
and from *Biochemical and Biophysical Research Communications*.

substituted at C15 all allowed initiation and inhibited at the termination step in protein synthesis. Further studies by Wei and McLaughlin (*61*) however have shown that verrucarol (Figure 1b) a C4, C15, dihydroxy-trichothecene does not inhibit initiation whereas the cyclic diester deriva-tives, verrucarins A (Figure 4b), E (Figure 3c), J (Figure 4f), and H all inhibit initiation (*61*). Therefore simple substitution on C15 is not enough to inhibit initiation. On the other hand all compounds tested that did not have substitution on C3 (except the verrucarins) did not inhibit initiation (Table II). Only one compound which was substituted at C3, 15-desacetylcalonectrin, had no observed effect on initiation, and this compound was also the only one in the group not to have substitution on C4.

Results in Table II are best interpreted using a model for the tri-chothecene nucleus. C15 and C3 substituents, both α to ring C, lie close to one another whereas C4 is β to ring C. A bulky C4 substituent how-ever restricts the repulsion between C3 and C15 substituents. To inhibit termination, a bulky substituent is needed on the α side of the C ring. When there is a substituent on C4, hydroxyl groups on C3 and C15 are enough to inhibit initiation as in the case of nivalenol (Figure 2b), scir-pentriol (Figure 1c), and fusarenon-X (Figure 2e). With no substituent on C4 or when only one of the two α groups is substituted (*i.e.* C3 or C15), larger substituents than hydroxyl groups are needed. Therefore verrucarol (Figure 1b) with only a C15 hydroxyl on the α side does not inhibit initiation whereas the verrucarins with long chain diesters on C15 (to C4) do. Calonectrin (Figure 1l), which has C3 and C15 acetoxy functions, also inhibits initiation whereas the monoacetate, 15-desacetyl-calonectrin (Figure 1m), does not.

A substituent on C4 is also necessary to inhibit the peptidyl transfer-ase reaction (*61*). Calonectrin (Figure 1l) and 15-desacetylcalonectrin (Figure 1m) are both inhibitors of the elongation–termination reaction, but they do not inhibit peptidyl transferase (*61*). It is probably just coincidence that most of the trichothecenes inhibit the peptidyl transfer-ase reaction since their site of inhibition may be on what is as yet an unknown reaction in the process of elongation–termination.

In further studies to characterize the ribosomal binding site of a large series of trichothecenes, a radio labelled trichodermin (^{3}H-acetyl) was prepared (*62*). Of the 17 compounds tested, all trichothecenes known to inhibit ribosomal functions required for either elongation–termination or initiation processes showed significant interference with trichodermin binding. Trichodermin bound to reticulocyte ribosomes with a K_a of 9.2×10^5 at 30°C (*62*). Extrapolation of the binding curve to infinite trichodermin concentration revealed a maximum binding ratio of 0.44 molecules trichodermin/ribosome (Figure 14). The binding property of

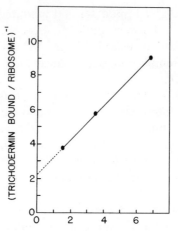

Figure 14. Ribosomal binding of trichodermin (^{3}H-acetyl). Intercept at infinite trichodermin concentration corresponds to 0.44 molecules/ribosome. Data from Ref. 62.

the ribosomes appears to be a function of the 80S ribosome since the 40S subunit had no binding affinity and since the 60S subunit had a much reduced affinity. The 60S subunit has the major role in the binding site since isolated yeast mutants which are resistant to trichodermin have an altered 60S subunit (63). This subunit is also the site of peptidyl transferase activity (64). A high correlation exists between the ability of a trichothecene to inhibit poly U directed polyphenylalanine synthesis *in vitro* and competition for the ^{3}H-trichodermin binding site (62). Verrucarin A (Figure 4b) and diacetoxyscirpenol (Figure 1e) and its derivatives, all of which inhibit initiation, show a good ability to compete with trichodermin binding indicating that the binding sites on the ribosomes are the same or overlap one another. The fact that only 0.44 trichodermin molecules are bound per ribosome even at infinite trichodermin concentration suggests that perhaps the stage of the ribosome function cycle is important in determining the exposure of this site. Since most trichothecenes appear to inhibit the peptidyl transferase reaction, the binding site probably involves this important part of the ribosome. In eukaryotic ribsomes it appears that the binding of initiation and elongation factors occurs at different sites because two sites of GTPase activity have recently been identified, one associated with each of these functions (65). However the sites where these factors bind may be very close together, and trichothecenes may bind in a way that large, bulky side chains on the α side of the C ring may interfere with binding of an initiation factor.

Trichothecene Toxicity as Compared to Their Inhibition of Protein Synthesis

Although the trichothecenes appear to be an exceedingly useful series of compounds to study events in eukaryotic protein synthesis, the original reason for developing a cytotoxicity assay and eventually an *in vitro* protein synthesis inhibition assay was to be able to screen many samples rapidly for compounds toxic to man or animals. From the results discussed above and the relative toxicities of some of the compounds in mice (Table III) it is easily seen that the most toxic of the trichothecenes are those that inhibit the initiation and not the elongation or termination of protein synthesis on polyribosomes (Table III). In the rabbit reticulocyte–poly-U system, however, compounds like trichothecin (Figure 2c) which have very low *in vivo* toxicity are better inhibitors than compounds like diacetoxyscirpenol (Figure 1e) which has an LD_{50} two orders of magnitude lower than trichothecin. Obviously other functional groups on the molecule such as the 8-keto function play a large role in the stability and metabolism of the compound in the animal. The proper degree of lipid and water solubility is also important since scirpenetriol (Figure 1c) and triacetoxyscirpenol (Figure 1p) are less toxic to whole cells than is diacetoxyscirpenol (Figure 1e) (*40*). Therefore although one can learn a great deal about the mechanism of action of trichothecenes through *in vitro* studies, more will have to be known about the metabolites of these compounds *in vivo,* and emphasis should be placed on those compounds which demonstrate high *in vivo* toxicity for these studies.

Table III. Animal, Cellular, and Subcellular Toxicities of Several Trichothecenes[a]

Compound	LD_{50} In Mice (mg/kg)	ID_{50} In Reticulocytes (μg/ml)	ID_{50} In Vitro (μg/ml)	Type of Inhibition
Verrucarin A	0.5–0.75	10	0.5	I
Fusarenon-X	3.3	0.25	0.2	I
Nivalenol	4.1	3.0	0.5	I
T-2 Toxin	5.2	0.03	0.15	I
HT-2 Toxin	9.0	0.03	0.08	I
Neosolaniol	14.5	0.25	—	—
Diacetoxyscirpenol	23	0.03	5.0	I
Trichothecin	<250	0.15	<5	ET
Crotocin	<500	<1.0	<5	ET
Trichodermin	500–1000	1.0	<5	ET

[a] Data from Refs. *52, 61, 60,* and *1.*

Directions for Future Research

Several useful and productive areas for research in the chemistry, pharmacology, and toxicology of trichothecenes remain. In considering trichothecenes as mycotoxins, one useful contribution that should be made soon is the preparation of antisera to the trichothecene ring system and the preparation of high specific activity ^{3}H-trichothecenes for use in a radioimmunoassay. A compound like trichodermol (Figure 1a) could be covalently linked to rabbit albumin and injected back into rabbits for antibody production against the trichothecene hapten. A radioimmunoassay would greatly help analytical laboratories concerned with the possible contamination of human and animal food with trichothecenes.

The evaluation of trichothecenes as useful pharmaceuticals is also worthy of consideration. In the areas of research associated with eukaryotic protein synthesis the trichothecenes could play a major role to understand ribosomal structure and function, particularly if suitable affinity labelled compounds become available. It would be particularly interesting to explore the binding properties of trichodermol (Figure 1a), carrying an affinity label in the 4β position, to verrucarol (Figure 1b) or desacetylcalonectrin (Figure 1m), carrying an affinity label at the 3α or C15 position (α to the C ring). It might be possible in this manner to identify ribosomal components involved in elognation–termination reactions as distinct from components needed for the initiation reaction. One possible type of affinity label which has recently been used with puromycin (66) to bind to peptidyl transferase is shown attached to trichodermol (see Figure 15).

For clinically useful pharmaceuticals in the treatment of solid tumors advantage could be taken of the fact that relatively non-toxic compounds such as trichothecin have a high cytostatic activity in both cultured cells and in vitro protein synthesizing system. Local application of compounds of this type may not pose a great hazard to the organism as a whole but in high local concentration should be very effective against rapidly grow-

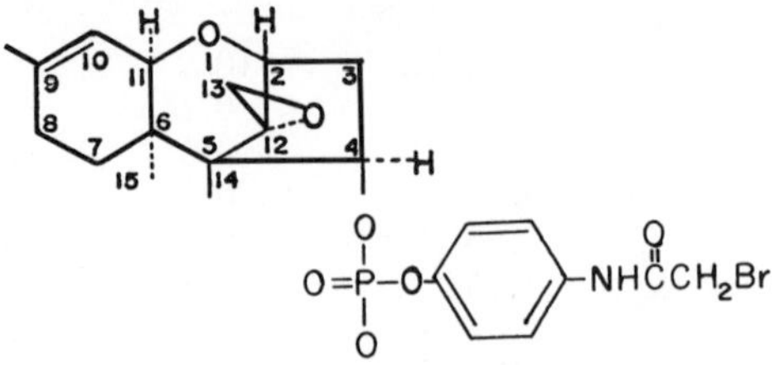

Figure 15. Trichodermol bearing an affinity label. The structure of 4β-O-(N-bromacetyl-p-aminophenylphosphoryl-12,13-epoxu-Δ⁹-trichothecene).

ing tumor cells. The high lipid solubility and penetrating power of many of the trichothecenes could make them ideal pharmaceuticals to treat papillomas and perhaps even viral and fungal skin diseases.

As a final point, further understanding of the structure–function relationships among the trichothecenes should allow a much more rational approach to drug design. The use of ionic functional groups that are chosen with regard to the transport systems in the cells that the drugs are to be directed against could give rise to compounds of much lower general toxicity (more rapid excretion) combined with a greater selectivity for the target tissue. An understanding of the chemical stability of the trichothecenes and their structure–function relationships will be necessary to achieve the chemical modifications desired.

Literature Cited

1. Bamburg, J. R., Strong, F. M., in "Microbial Toxins," Vol. VII, S. Kadis, A. Ciegler, S. J. Ajl, Eds., pp. 207-292, Academic, New York, 1971.
2. Härri, E., Loeffler, W., Sigg, H. P., Stahelin, H., Stoll, Ch., Tamm, Ch., Wiesinger, D., *Helv. Chim. Acta* (1962) **45**, 839.
3. Godtfredsen, W. O., Vangedal, S., *Proc. Chem. Soc.* (1964) 188.
4. Godtfredsen, W. O., Vangedal, S., *Acta Chem. Scand.* (1965) **19**, 1088.
5. Gutzwiller, J., Mauli, R., Sigg, H. P., Tamm, Ch., *Helv. Chim. Acta* (1964) **47**, 2234.
6. Sigg, H. P., Mauli, R., Flury, E., Hauser, D., *Helv. Chim. Acta* (1965) **48**, 962.
7. Pathre, S. V., Behrens, J., Mirocha, C. J., "Abstracts of Papers," 168th Natl. Meetg., ACS, Atlantic City, N. J., 1974, AGFD 56.
8. Bamburg, J. R., Riggs, N. V., Strong, F. M., *Tetrahedron* (1968) **24**, 3329.
9. Flury, E., Mauli, R., Sigg, H. P., *Chem. Commun.* (1965) 27.
10. Dawkins, A. W., Grove, J. F., Tidd, B. K., *Chem. Commun.* (1965) 27.
11. Dawkins, A. W., *J. Chem. Soc.* (1966) 116.
12. Okuchi, M., Itoh, M., Kaneko, Y., Doi, S., *Agric. Biol. Chem.* (1968) **32**, 394.
13. Bamburg, J. R., Strong, F. M., *Phytochemistry* (1969) 8, 2405.
14. Grove, J. R., *J. Chem. Soc.* (1970) 379.
15. Ueno, Y., Ishii, K., Sakai, K., Kanaeda, S., Tsunoda, H., Tanaka, T., Enomoto, M., *Jap. J. Exp. Med.* (1972) **42**, 187.
16. Gardner, D., Glen, A. T., Turner, W. B., *J. Chem. Soc., Perkin Trans. 1* (1972) 2576.
17. Machida, Y., Nozoe, S., *Tetrahedron* (1972) **28**, 5113.
18. Loeffler, W., Mauli, R., Rüsch, M. E., Stähelin, H., Ger. Patent 1,233,098; *Chem. Abstr.* **66**, 84744u (1967).
19. Freeman, G. G., Gill, J. E., *Nature* (1950) **166**, 698.
20. Achilladelis, B., Hanson, J. R., *Phytochemistry* (1969) 8, 765.
21. Tatsuno, T., Saito, M., Enomoto, M., Tsunoda, H., *Chem. Pharm. Bull.* (1968) **16**, 2519.
22. Freeman, G. G., Morrison R. I., *Nature* (1948) **162**, 30.
23. Tidd, B. K., *J. Chem. Soc.* (1967) 218.
24. Grove, J. F., *J. Chem. Soc.* (1970) 375.
25. Ueno, Y., Ueno, I., Tatsuno, T., Ohokubo, K., Tsunoda, H., *Experientia* (1969) **25**, 1062.
26. Gyimesi, J., Melera, A., *Tetrahedron Lett.* (1967) 1655.
27. Böhner, B., Tamm, Ch., *Helv. Chim. Acta* (1966) **49**, 2527.

162   MYCOTOXINS

28. Gutzwiller, J., Tamm, Ch., *Helv. Chim. Acta* (1965) **48**, 157.
29. Gutzwiller, J., Tamm, Ch., *Helv. Chim. Acta* (1965) **48**, 177.
30. Böhner, B., Tamm, Ch., *Helv. Chim. Acta* (1966) **49**, 2547.
31. Zuercher, W., Tamm, Ch., *Helv. Chim. Acta* (1966) **49**, 2594.
32. Fetz, E., Böhner, B., Tamm, Ch., *Helv. Chim. Acta* (1965) **48**, 1669.
33. Eppley, R. M., Bailey, W. J., *Science* (1973) **181**, 758.
34. Abrahamsson, S., Nilsson, B., *Proc. Chem. Soc.* (1964) 188.
35. Abrahamsson, S., Nilsson, B., *Acta Chem. Scand.* (1966) **20**, 1044.
36. Hsu, I., Smalley, E. B., Strong, F. M., Ribelin, W. E., *Appl. Microbiol.* (1972) **24**, 684.
37. Wyatt, R. D., Harris, J. R., Hamilton, P. B., Burmeister, H. R., *Avian Dis.* (1972) **16**, 1123.
38. Ellison, R. A., Kotsonis, F. N., *Appl. Microbiol.* (1974) **27**, 423.
39. Gutzwiller, J., Tamm, Ch., *Tetrahedron Lett.* (1965) **50**, 4495.
40. Grove, J. F., Mortimer, P. H., *Biochem. Pharmacol.* (1969) **18**, 1473.
41. Hanson, J. R., Martin, T., Siverns, M., *J. Chem. Soc., Perkin Trans. 1* (1974) 1033.
42. Goldsmith, D. J., Helms, C. T., Jr., *Synth. Commun.* (1973) **3**, 231.
43. Colvin, E. W., Malchenko, S., Raphael, R. A., Roberts, J. S., *J. Chem. Soc., Perkin Trans. 1* (1973) 1989.
44. Colvin, E. W., Raphael, R. A., Roberts, J. S., *Chem. Commun.* (1971) 858.
45. Jones, E. R. H., Lowe, G., *J. Chem. Soc.* (1960) 3959.
46. Adams, P. M., Hanson, J. R., *Chem. Commun.* (1970) 1569.
47. Achilladelis, B. A., Adams, P. M., Hanson, J. R., *J. Chem. Soc., Perkin Trans. 1* (1972) 1425.
48. Forrester, J. M., Money, T., *Can. J. Chem.* (1972) **50**, 3310.
49. Nozoe, S., Machida, Y., *Tetrahedron* (1972) **28**, 5105.
50. Ueno, Y., Hosoya, M., Morita, Y., Ueno, I., Tatsuno, T., *J. Biochem. (Tokyo)* (1968) **64**, 479.
51. Ohtsubo, K., Kaden, P., Mittermayer, C., *Biochim. Biophys. Acta* (1972) **287**, 520.
52. Ueno, Y., Nakajima, M., Sakai, K., Ishii, K., Sato, N., Shimoda, N., *J. Biochem. (Tokyo)* (1973) **74**, 285.
53. Carrasco, L., Barbacid, M., Vazquez, D., *Biochim. Biophys. Acta* (1973) **312**, 368.
54. Stafford, M. E., McLaughlin, C. S., *J. Cell Physiol.* (1973) **82**, 121.
55. Tate, W. P., Caskey, C. T., *J. Biol. Chem.* (1973) **248**, 7970.
56. Hansen, B. S., Vaughan, M. H., Jr., *Fed. Proc., Fed. Amer. Soc. Exp. Biol.* (1973) **32**, 494 abs.
57. Wei, C., McLaughlin, C. S., *Fed. Proc., Fed. Amer. Soc. Exp. Biol.* (1973) **32**, 494 abs.
58. Wei, C., Hansen, B. S., Vaughan, M. H., Jr., McLaughlin C. S., *Proc. Nat. Acad. Sci. U.S.A.* (1974) **71**, 713.
59. Cundliffe, E., Cannon, M., Davies, J., *Proc. Nat. Acad. Sci. U.S.A.* (1974) **71**, 30.
60. Schindler, D., *Nature* (1974) **249**, 38.
61. Wei, C., McLaughlin, C. S., *Biochem. Biophys. Res. Commun.* (1974) **57**, 838.
62. Wei, C., Campbell, I. M., McLaughlin, C. S., Vaughan, M. H., *Mol. Cell Biochem.* (1974) **3**, 215.
63. Schindler, D., Grant, P., Davies, J., *Nature* (1974) **248**, 535.
64. Traut, R. R., Monro, R. E., *J. Mol. Biol.* (1964) **10**, 63.
65. Lockwood, A. H., Maitra, U., *J. Biol. Chem.* (1974) **249**, 346.
66. Harris, R. J., Greenwell, P., Symons, R. H., *Biochem. Biophys. Res. Commun.* (1973) **55**, 117.

RECEIVED November 8, 1974.

Tremorgenic Mycotoxins

ALEX CIEGLER and RONALD F. VESONDER

Northern Regional Research Laboratory, Agricultural Research Service,
United States Department of Agriculture, Peoria, Ill. 61604

RICHARD J. COLE

National Peanut Research Laboratory, Dawson, Ga. 31742

*Ten tremorgenic mycotoxins have been reported in the
literature, but structures have been determined for only
five of these. The toxins can be separated into three groupings based on their nitrogen content: one, three, or four
atoms per molecule. Structural investigations are underway
on one of the major unidentified tremorgens, penitrem A;
current data indicate the presence of an indole nucleus and
an isoprene unit.*

Most described mycotoxins function as hepatotoxins, nephrotoxins, or dermal toxins, but two classes of substances have been isolated that appear to act at the level of the central nervous system. The first of these, citreoviridin, causes paralysis in the extremities of laboratory animals sometimes followed by convulsions and respiratory arrest (*1*); tremoring has not been ascribed to this substance. The second class encompasses several compounds which cause sustained trembling in host animals. This review covers only the second set of substances, the tremorgens.

It is unusual for secondary fungal metabolites to elicit a sustained tremoring response in animals. Only 10 tremorgenic compounds have been reported in the literature, and structures have been determined for five of these, verruculogens TR-1 and TR-2, fumitremorgen B, tryptoquivaline, and tryptoquivalone. The tremorgens can be divided into three groupings based on their nitrogen content: Group A composed of penitrems A, B, and C (PA, PB, and PC) contain only one nitrogen per molecule; Group B composed of fumitremorgens A and B (FTA and FTB) and verruculogens (TR-1 and TR-2) contain three nitrogen atoms per molecule (*2*); Group C composed of tryptoquivaline and tryptoquivalone contain four nitrogens per molecule. No elemental analysis is available on the tenth compound isolated from *Aspergillus flavus* by Wilson and Wilson (*3*) although a molecular weight of 501 has been published (*4*).

Group A

Penitrem A was originally extracted from two strains of *Penicillium cyclopium* (later identified as *P. crustosum*) that were the principal contaminants of feedstuffs causing disease outbreaks among sheep and horses (*4*). A third producing strain came from peanuts not involved in food intoxication. Subsequently the same toxin was isolated from *P. palitans* NRRL 3468, a culture found in almost monotypic growth on a sample of moldy commercial feed suspected of being implicated in deaths of dairy cows (*5*). The tremorgen found by Ciegler (*5*) was named tremortin A. This name is now withdrawn in deference to the trivial name penitrem A advanced by Wilson (*4*) who had initially discovered this class of tremorgenic substances.

Because the two known PA-producing Penicillia were closely related, Ciegler and Pitt (*6*) screened additional *Penicillium* species to determine if tremorgen production had taxonomic significance and to what extent the occurrence of various Penicillia in foods and feeds might represent a potential health hazard. Tremorgen production among the Penicillia was confined to several species in the subsection Fasiculata, section Asymetrica. Other subsections in Asymetrica or sections other than Asymetrica tested show no production of tremorgen.

Some of the species that produce PA are common contaminants of grains or specific foodstuffs. *P. crustosum*, a good tremorgen producer, is a contaminant of various refrigerated foods, grains, and cereal products and causes a soft brown rot in apples. Whether or not tremorgen is produced during the apple-rotting process is not known. Four cultures (*P. cyclopium, P. palitans, P. crustosum, P. puberulum*) isolated from moldy commercial feedstuffs were capable of producing PA on a variety of agricultural commodities with low temperatures favoring toxin accumulation (*7*). It was subsequently found that most of the PA producers also synthesized two additional closely related tremorgens, PB and PC (*8*).

PA caused perceptible tremors in mice at 250 μg/kg; PB required 1.3 mg/kg for a similar reaction. The single dose LD_{50} of PA for mice calculated according to Weil's formula (*9*) was 1.05 with a 95% confidence interval of 0.51–2.17 mg/kg; the PB dose was 5.84 mg/kg with a 95% confidence interval of 4.13–8.26 mg/kg (*8*). PC is far less toxic than PA or PB, but studies on its properties and toxicity were limited by low yields. Further toxicological effects of penitrem have been described

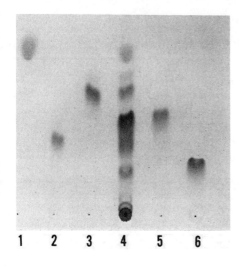

1 2 3 4 5 6

Applied Microbiology

Figure 1. Thin-layer chromatogram (silica gel G-HR, developed in chloroform:acetone, 93:7; sprayed with FeCl₃) of a crude solvent extract of Penicillium palitans. 1: erogsterol; 2: penitrum C; 3: penitrum B; 4: crude solution; 5: penitrum A; 6: viridicatin.

by Wilson et al. (*4, 10*) and Cysewski (*11*). Stern (*12*) speculated that PA produces tremor by inhibiting the interneurons which inhibit the α-motor cells of the anterior horn of the spinal column.

The penitrems can be readily extracted from mold mycelia or contaminated agricultural commodities by maceration in a blendor with chloroform–methanol; they can be detected using thin-layer chromatography (TLC) on silica gel G-HR (Merck) developed in chloroform–acetone (93:7, v/v) and sprayed with $FeCl_3$. The pattern of $FeCl_3$-positive compounds on the TLC plate appears to be the same for most penitrem producers and is illustrated in Figure 1.

A simple and specific colorimetric assay depends on the formation of a blue color via methanolysis (*13*); absorbance at 630 nm is a linear function of penitrem concentration between 2.5 and 30 μg/ml. Penitrems can be crystallized from ethanol–water in the form of fine needles: mp PA, 237°–239°C (decomposition, turning reddish brown); PB decomposes similarly between 185° and 195°C. The penitrems are soluble in diethyl ether, chloroform, acetone, and methanol; they have limited solubility in water and in both hydrochloric acid and sodium hydroxide (5% concentrations). Both penitrems are rapidly degraded to form a yellowish solution, progressing through green and then to blue, when dissolved in alcohols or acetone and treated with various dilute acids. These changes are concurrent with loss of toxicity. Purified penitrems are unstable in chloroform when exposed directly to light. This change is presumably a result of acid formation in the solvent.

The structures of the penitrems have not been determined. The elemental analysis and the heaviest detectable ion in the mass spectra of both toxins correspond to a formula of $C_{37}H_{44}NO_6Cl$ for PA and

Table I.   NMR[a] Data of PA in Pyridine-d_5

PPM, δ	Proton Count	Assignment
1.35 s	3	quarternary methyl
1.5 s	3	CH_3-C—O
1.7 s	3	olefinic methyl
1.8 s	3	olefinic methyl
2.15 s	3	aromatic methyl
3.6–2.0	12	
3.75 S	1	
3.85 d (J, Hz 20)	1	
4.3 d	1	
4.4 s	1	
4.7 t,s	3	
5.0 b,s	2	
5.15 b,s	1	
5.4 d	1	
5.45 s	1	
6.0 s	1	
6.1 d	1	
6.9 s	1	
11.7	1	acidic OH
Total	43	

[a] NMR = nuclear magnetic resonance; PA = penitrem A.

$C_{37}H_{45}NO_5$ for PB (8). Both tremorgens give a positive Lieberman–Burchard reaction, but neither is precipitated with digitonin. No amino acids or sugars can be detected in the acid hydrolyzate of either compound.

The ultraviolet (uv) spectrum of PA in methanol shows absorption at 295 ($\epsilon = 11,600$) and 233 nm ($\epsilon = 37,000$); PB has peaks at 286 ($\epsilon = 13,100$) and 227 nm ($\epsilon = 38,450$) and a shoulder at 297 nm ($\epsilon = 11,000$). In 0.1N HCl PA has new peaks at 272 ($\epsilon = 15,400$) and 254 nm ($\epsilon = 23,700$); the peak at 295 nm disappeared, and the peak at 233 nm shifted to 227 nm ($\epsilon = 25,500$). These spectra suggest an indole nucleus. The only change in spectrum for PB in acid solution is a new broad absorption between 230 and 245 nm ($\epsilon = 28,200$). Both tremorgens show no spectrum changes in alkaline solution (8).

In unpublished data we have shown some structural features by ir, NMR, and chemical transformations. The ir spectrum of PA in chloroform showed strong OH absorption at 3580 cm^{-1}; a band at 3475 cm^{-1} indicated either an N–H stretch as in pyrroles (indoles) or a hydrogen bonded OH; a medium band at 1650 cm^{-1} could result from C=C stretching attributed to alkyl CH_3, CH_2; methyl absorption at 1370 and 1360 cm^{-1}; hydroxyl at 1055 cm^{-1}.

The NMR spectrum of PA in deuterated pyridine (TMS as reference) exhibited signals which account for 43 of its 44 protons. Assignments were made only to the methyl signals (Table I). The H proton of the NH could not be seen as it occurs as a broad signal at δ 7.4 where pyridine also exhibits signals.

Acetylation of PA gave a product with a mp 203°–205°C (decomposes, turns dull red). High-resolution mass spectroscopy was in accord for a molecular formula $C_{39}H_{46}NO_7Cl$ incorporating one acetyl group. The ir of the acetylated material still showed OH (possibly a hindered OH which does not acetylate with pyridine–acetic anhydride at room temperature), and a peak at 657 (M, 18) in the mass spectrum was in agreement for a hydroxyl group. The band at 3480 cm^{-1}, strong evidence for an NH absorption, was still present in the ir. The NMR signals of acetylated PA are in Table II. The NMR spectrum is in agreement with the mass spectral analysis in that one hydroxyl group was actylated (one new methyl peak at δ 2.05). The peak at δ 6.9 in the NMR spectrum of PA disappears on acetylation, an indication that this peak could result from the proton of a hydroxyl group.

Table II.   NMR Data of Acetylated PA in Pyridine-d_5

PPM, δ	Proton Count	Assignment
1.39 s	3	methyl
1.42 s	3	methyl
1.5 s	2	isolated CH$_2$
1.7 s	3	methyl
1.72 s	3	methyl
1.85 s	2	isolated CH$_2$
2.05 s	3	acetate methyl
2.15 s	3	aromatic methyl
3.5–2.0	appearance of a new peak equivalent to one proton at δ 3.6 (b,s)	
5.6 d	this is apparently a shift of the 5.45 s peak in the PA spectrum	
6.1 d		
11.77	still present, could indicate an acidic OH	

NMR Decoupling Experiments. Irradiation of the proton for PA at δ 6.1 collapses the doublet at δ 4.3 to a smaller doublet, indicating allylic coupling to a methine proton of the following type:

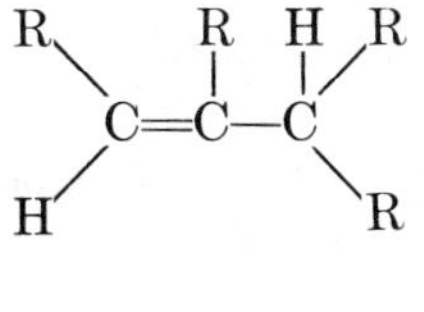

Geminal coupling of the type ——C——C——C——R is indi-

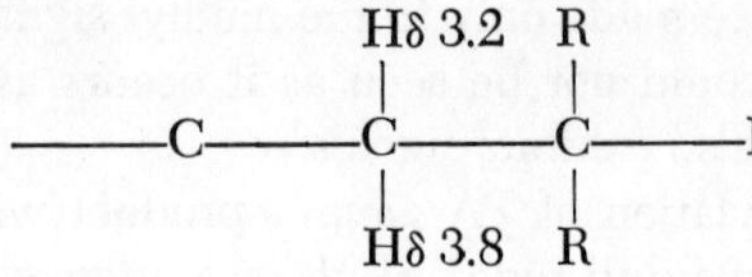

where the carbon chain shows: Hδ 3.2 and R on top of the second and third carbons, Hδ 3.8 and R on the bottom.

cated by irradiating the signal at δ 3.0 which causes the doublet at δ 3.85 to collapse to a broad singlet. Hydrogenation of acetylated PA using Adams catalyst appeared to cause decomposition. However the methyl protons at δ 2.15 remained; this is evidence of an aromatic methyl group.

Because limited material hindered further chemical analysis, only tentative speculation can be made on a structure for PA. Based on spectroscopic data the presence of an indole nucleus can be proposed with a fully substituted aromatic moiety, *e.g.*,

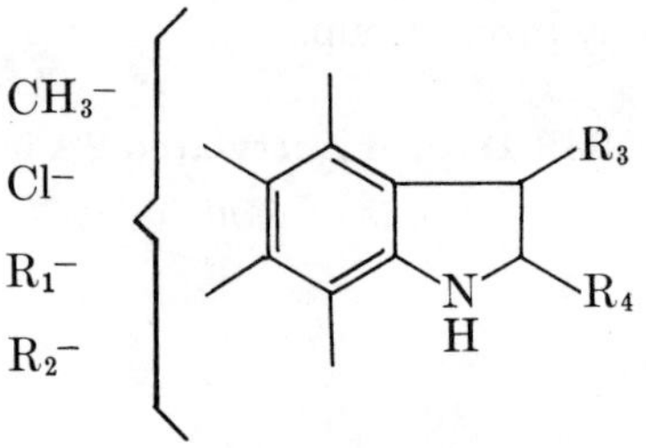

In addition one OH is readily acetylated, and apparently one is not acetylated. This would account for two of the oxygen functions. The proton at δ 11.77 in the NMR spectrum indicates an acidic OH or bonded OH (*e.g.*, hydroxyl group bonded to carbonyl function). If the latter is the case we could interpret the band at 1650 cm^{-1} in the IR to be a bonded carbonyl; this would account for two more oxygens. The remaining two oxygens could be accounted for by ether linkages. However the NMR does not exclude an epoxide linkage. More detailed structural analyses will depend on the availability of additional toxin.

Group B

Verruculogen. Verruculogen (TR-1), a tremorgenic mycotoxin, was produced by *Penicillium verruculosum* (ATCC #24640; NRRL 5881) isolated from peanuts that were molded as a result of improper storage conditions (*14*). In addition to causing severe tremors in mice and one-day old cockerels verruculogen has an LD$_{50}$ of 2.4 mg/kg in mice and 15.2 mg/kg in cockerels, i.p. When it was administered orally, the LD$_{50}$ was 126.7 mg/kg in mice and 365.5 mg/kg in cockerels.

Hotujac et al. (*15*) studied the mode of action of verruculogen using both mice and three- to seven-day old chickens. On the basis of their results using a substance which increased γ-aminobutyric acid levels in the central nervous system of mice and a γ-aminobutyric acid derivative which was capable of passing the blood-brain barrier, they concluded that verruculogen-induced tremors in mice were caused by a decrease of gamma-aminobutyric acid levels in the central nervous system.

In a subsequent study using three- to seven-day-old chickens in which γ-aminobutyric acid itself easily penetrated the blood–brain barrier, they found a direct antagonistic effect of γ-aminobutyric acid on verruculogen-induced tremors.

Although the biosynthesis of verruculogen has not been studied, it may be speculated on the basis of its chemical structure (Structure I)

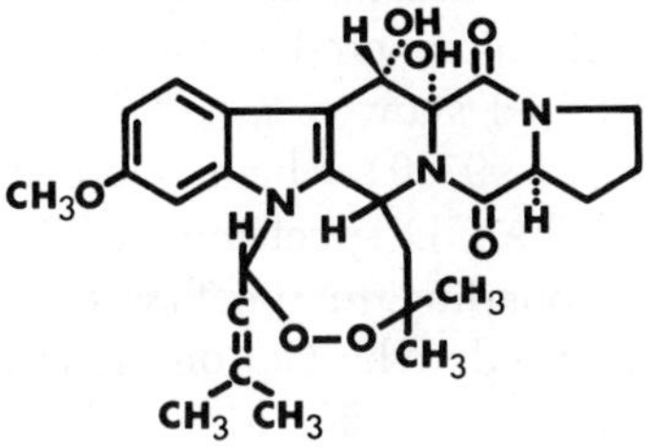

Structure I

that it is formed from the amino acids proline and tryptophan and two isoprene units.

The close structural and spectral similarities of TR-1 and a closely related substance TR-2 with those of fumitremorgen A and B (Structure II) (FTA and FTB) strongly suggest a common biosynthetic pathway. Perhaps TR-1 comes from FTB via hydroperoxide. FTA appears to contain an additional isoprene moiety. Although neither of the fumitremorgens was detected in extracts of the verruculogen-producing mold, a metabolite exhibting the same R_f on TLC and color reactions as those

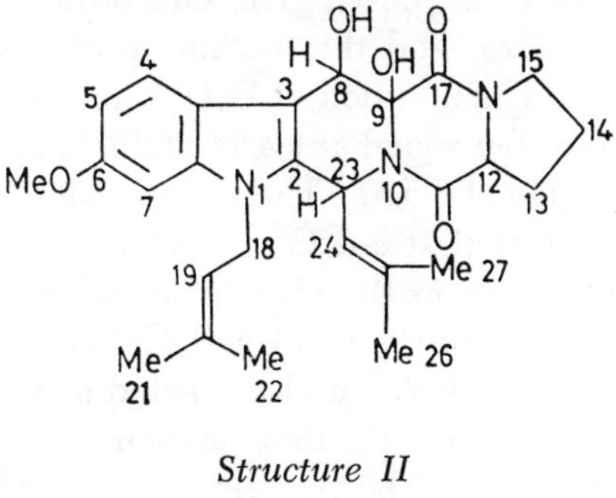

Structure II

observed for TR-2 was present. Since the conversion of TR-1 to TR-2 was observed only under the specific conditions reported (2) and since TR-2 was not a product from photodegradation, it is plausible that TR-2 is also of natural origin and may be a biosynthetic precursor to TR-1.

Verruculogen (mp 233°–235°C) was very soluble in chloroform, moderately soluble in benzene, ethyl acetate, acetone, and dimethylsulfoxide, sparingly soluble in ethanol, methanol, and toluene, and insoluble in hexane and water. The tremorgen rapidly degraded into several photo products when subjected to normal laboratory light conditions.

Because of its size and complexity, the chemical structure of verruculogen (Structure I) was elucidated by single crystal x-ray diffraction studies in lieu of chemical methods. The tremorgen was neutral and crystallized with one molecule of benzene ($C_{27}H_{32}O_7N_3 \cdot C_6H_6$). It was characterized by 6-O-methoxyindole, diketopiperazine, β-methylcrotonyl moieties, and a novel eight-membered peroxide ring system (2).

The uv spectrum of TR-1 showed λ_{max}^{EtOH} 226 ($\epsilon = 47{,}500$), 277 ($\epsilon = 11{,}000$), and 295 nm ($\epsilon = 9700$) which is typical of 2,3,6-substituted indole compounds (2). The CD spectrum of TR-1 in ethanol showed two Cotton effects corresponding to the first two uv bands; the third cotton effect was not observed. The Cotton effect at 290 nm was $\Delta\epsilon = +0.16$; at 265 nm it was $\Delta\epsilon = +0.56$. Major absorptions in the ir spectrum were 3520 and 3480 cm^{-1} (OH indole, or both), 1660 cm (diketopiperazine), and doublet at 1365–1355 cm^{-1} (gem-dimethyl).

The proton NMR spectrum of verruculogen (Figure 2) was characterized by extremely well-defined chemical shifts that were assigned as follows: The three aromatic protons had the typical pattern for an ortho doublet at δ 7.85 ($J = 9.0$ Hz) (C16), ortho–meta doublet of doublets at δ 6.74 ($J = 2.0$ and 9.0 Hz) (C17), and a meta doublet at δ 6.52 ($J = 2.0$ Hz) (C19). The latter signal was partially obscured by another proton signal (δ 6.57) assigned to the proton at (C21) (doublet; $J = 8.0$ Hz). A vinyl proton (C22) coupled to (C21) was observed as a doublet ($J = 8.0$ Hz) at δ 4.98. Vincinal coupling was observed between the OH and methine protons located on (C13). The OH proton appeared at δ 4.74 as a doublet ($J = 3.0$ Hz), and the methine proton was at δ 5.57 as a doublet ($J = 3.0$ Hz). The addition of D_2O to the NMR sample resulted in the disappearance of the signal at δ 4.74 and a concomitant collapse in the coupling of the signal at δ 5.57. The OH proton (D_2O exchangeable) located on (C12) resonated at δ 4.25 as a sharp singlet. The hydroxyls on (C12) and (C13) were in the cis configuration. The gem-dimethyl protons on the isovaleryl moiety (C24 and C25) were equivalent when analyzed in chloroform-d solution and resonated at δ 1.66 as a six proton singlet; in dimethyl sulfoxide-d_6 they appeared as two three-proton singlets at δ 1.58 and δ 1.70. The two geminal methyl groups (C29 and

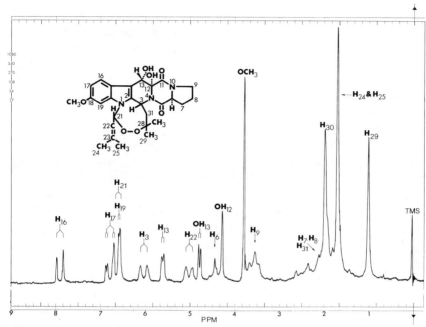

Figure 2. Proton magnetic resonance spectrum of verruculogen (Structure I) taken in chloroform-d solution

C30) attached to (C28) were observed at δ 1.95 and δ 0.97 as three-proton singlets. The two protons adjacent to the proline nitrogen at position 9 resonated as an ill-defined triplet at δ 3.50; the other four protons comprising the proline ring and the methylene protons at position 31 gave rise to an unstructured multiplet between δ 1.5 and 2.5. The proton at position 6 was assigned to the chemical shift at δ 4.40 (ill-defined triplet). The (C3) methine proton was strongly coupled to only one of the methylene protons on (C31) and appeared as a doublet at δ 5.98 ($J = 10.0$ Hz). The methoxy protons resonated as a three-proton singlet at δ 3.75. Doublet resonance experiments in both decoupling and INDOR modes verified the coupling between the protons on (C21) and (C22) and between (C13) and (OH13). The appearance of the C3) methine proton as a doublet was consistent with the geometry of the molecule as determined by x-ray crystallography.

Data from studies to determine the molecular formula were initially somewhat conflicting. However high resolution, mass spectral analysis effecting ionization via electron-impact at 70 eV provided the correct mass (m/e 511.2360) which analyzed for $C_{27}H_{33}N_3O_7$ (2). The mass spectrum showed, in addition to the molecular ion at m/e 511, prominent fragment ions at m/e 496 (loss of CH_3), m/e 493 (loss of H_2O), and m/e 427 (loss of C_5H_8O). The latter fragmentation also occurred chemically when verruculogen was hydrogenated using palladium on carbon (5%) in an ethanol solution (2). This chemical reaction yielded two products: one product was a small molecule identified as isovaleraldehyde ($C_5H_{10}O$) which originated via cleavage of the bonds between (C21) and the indole nitrogen and between the peroxide oxygens. Concomitantly the double bond between (C22) and (C23) was saturated to form isovaleraldehyde.

The product (TR-2) was assigned Structure II after comparing its spectral data with that of verruculogen (2). High resolution, mass spectral analysis of TR-2 showed the largest detectable mass at m/e 429.1898 with a computer-calculated formula of $C_{22}H_{27}N_3O_6$. Its UV spectrum showed λ_{max}^{EtOH} 224 ($\epsilon = 37{,}400$), 268 ($\epsilon = 6830$), and 294 nm ($\epsilon = 7540$) which is typical for 2,3,6-substituted indole compounds (2). The IR spectrum of TR-2 showed major absorptions at 3450 (OH and/or indole), 1660 (diketopiperazine), and 1380 cm^{-1} (CH$_3$).

Principal considerations were obtained from the proton and ^{13}C-NMR spectra (2). The proton NMR of TR-2 (Figure 3) had the typical chemical shifts for ortho doublet (δ 6.60, $J = 3.0$, and 9.0 Hz), and a meta doublet at δ 6.87 ($J = 3.0$ Hz) in accordance with the protons positioned at (C16), (C17), and (C19) of the indole ring. The proton assigned to position 3 was at δ 5.37 (multiplet). A chemical shift for one D$_2$O exchangeable proton appearing at δ 5.94 was assigned to the OH

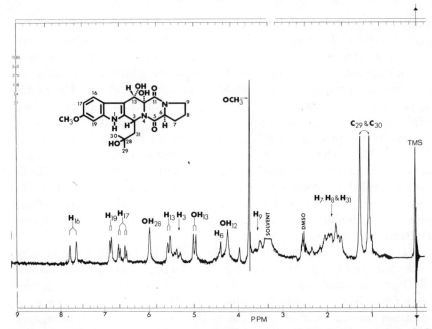

Figure 3.   The proton magnetic resonance spectrum of TR-2 taken in dimethyl sulfoxide-d$_6$

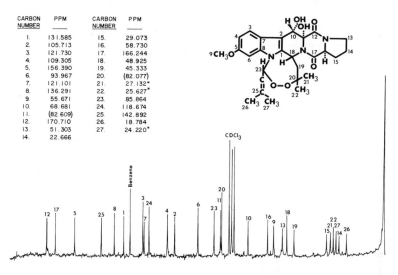

CARBON NUMBER	PPM	CARBON NUMBER	PPM
1.	131.585	15.	29.073
2.	105.713	16.	58.730
3.	121.730	17.	166.244
4.	109.305	18.	48.925
5.	156.390	19.	45.333
6.	93.967	20.	(82.077)
7.	121.101	21.	27.132*
8.	136.291	22.	25.627*
9.	55.671	23.	85.864
10.	68.681	24.	118.674
11.	(82.609)	25.	142.892
12.	170.710	26.	18.784
13.	51.303	27.	24.220*
14.	22.666		

*Figure 4. The ^{13}C-NMR spectrum of verruculogen (Structure I). ( )—Assignments may be reversed. *—Assignment uncertain. All values in ppm downfield from TMS; solvent CDCl$_3$.*

group formed on (C28). The six-proton signal in the spectrum of verruculogen resonating at δ 1.66 and assigned to the gem-dimethyl group attached to (C23) was absent in the spectrum of TR-2. Also absent were the two coupled methine protons resonating in the TR-1 spectrum at δ 6.57 (C21) and 4.98 (C22) (doublets; J = 8.0 Hz).

Further evidence supporting the (Structure II) proposed for TR-2 was provided when the ^{13}C-NMR spectra of TR-1 and TR-2 were compared (Figures 4 and 5). Those five carbons are present in the ^{13}C-NMR spectrum of TR-1 but are absent from the ^{13}C-NMR spectrum of TR-2 corresponded to (C23), (C24), (C25), (C26), and (C27). These data are consistent with that expected for the proposed conversion of verruculogen TR-1 to TR-2.

Fumitremorgens. Only two brief manuscripts have been published on fumitremorgens A and B (FTA and FTB), two closely related toxins produced by *A. fumigatus* (16, 17). The structure of FTB was established in the latter publication and was shown to contain proline and 6-methoxyindole groups (Structure III). FTB appears identical to

Structure III

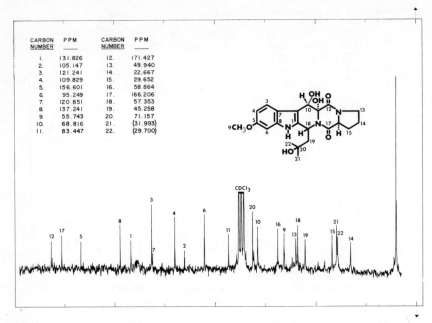

Figure 5. The ^{13}*C-NMR spectrum of TR-2 (Structure II). ( )—Assignments may be reversed. *—Assignment uncertain. All values in ppm downfield from TMS; solvent CDCl₃.*

lanosulin, the major metabolite of *Penicillium lanosum* (*18*). The structure of FTB appears almost identical to that of verruculogen (TR-1) except for the presence of the peroxide moiety linking the two isoprene fragments. Both FTA and FTB are soluble in chloroform and ethyl acetate, but only slightly soluble in methyl and ethyl alcohols.

In the uv spectra there are three maxima: λ_{max}^{EtOH} 225.5 ($\epsilon =$ 66,900), 275.5 ($\epsilon = 12,000$), and 295 nm ($\epsilon = 8500$). FTA has the following properties: Colorless prisms from methanol; mp 202.5°–203.5°C; elemental composition $C_{32}H_{41}N_3O_7$; m/e 579; ir spectra (KBr): 3420, 2940, 1670, 1565, 1440, 1370, 1300, 1160, 1070, and 1035 cm⁻¹. FTB crystallizes from methanol as colorless needles with the following characteristics: mp 211°–212°C; elemental composition $C_{27}H_{33}N_3O_5$; m/e 479; the IR spectra was similar to that of FTA.

Toxicity data indicated that 1 mg FTA/kg mice caused sustained trembling which was more severe when FTB was injected i.p. at a similar dose. The LD$_{50}$ was not determined, but 5 mg of either FTA or FTB (i.p.) caused 7% death within 96 hr. The fumitremorgens have not been indicated in any natural occurring mycotoxicosis.

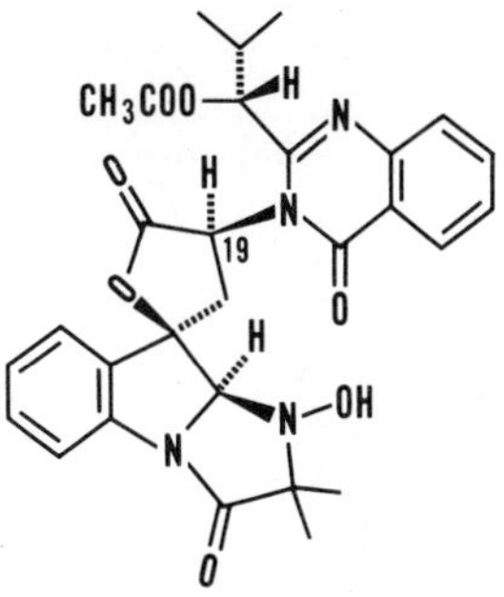

Structure IV 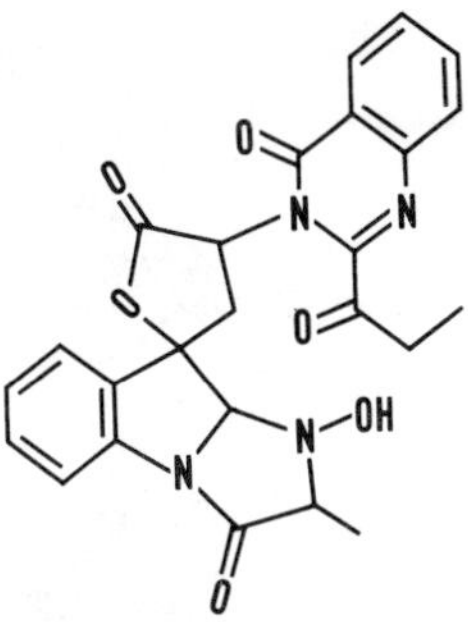   Structure V

Group C

In a privileged communication from G. Büchi, Massachusetts Institute of Technology (19), we learned that he and his colleagues had isolated two new tremorgenic toxins from *Aspergillus clavatus*—tryptoquivaline (Structure IV) and tryptoquivalone (Structure V). The producing fungus had been isolated originally from a sample of moldy rice collected in a Thai household where a young boy had died of an unidentified toxicosis. The isolated strain produced two new nontoxic metabolites, kotanin and desmethylkotanin (20), as well as small amounts of the highly toxic cytochalasin E (21).

The more polar of the two new tremorgens, tryptoquivaline, had the following properties: mp 153°–155°, $[\alpha]^{25}$ D 142°; m/e 546.2; elemental composition $C_{29}H_{30}N_4O_7$; IR (CHCl$_3$) 3520, 1790, 1735, 1680, and 1615 cm^{-1}; uv λ_{max}^{EtOH} 228 ($\epsilon = 37,000$), 275 ($\epsilon = 8550$), 305 ($\epsilon = 3800$), 317 nm ($\epsilon = 3040$); NMR (CDCl$_3$) δ 1.03 (d, 3, $J = 7$ Hz), 1.17 (d, 3, $J = 9$ Hz), 1.50 (s, 3), 1.52 (s, 3), 2.19 (s, 3), 2.63 (m, 1), 3.10 (d, 1, $J = 10$ Hz), 3.15 (d, 1, $J = 10$ Hz), 3.63 (b, 1), 4.04 (b, 1), 5.00 (s, 1), 5.61 (d, 1, $J = 9$ Hz), 5.70 (t, 1, $J = 10$ Hz), 7.12 ~ 7.90 (m, 7), 8.22 (d, 1, $J = 8$ Hz). Chemical and spectral data indicated that tryptoquivaline is a spiro-γ-lactone *rather than* a δ-lactone. Figure 6 shows a computer generated drawing of the x-ray model of the *p*-bromophenylurethane derivative of tryptoquivaline.

The less polar tremorgen, tryptoquivalone, had the following characteristics: mp 202°–204°; $[\alpha]^{25}$ D 254°; m/e 488.17; elemental composition $C_{26}H_{24}N_4O_4$; UV λ_{max}^{EtOH} 234 ($\epsilon = 34,950$), 292 ($\epsilon = 9550$), 320 nm ($\epsilon = 6300$); IR (CHCl$_3$) 2525, 1790, 1735, 1715, and 1680 cm^{-1}; NMR (CDCl$_3$) δ 1.24 (d, 3, $J = 7$ Hz), 1.31 (d, 3, $J = 7$ Hz), 1.59 (d, 3, $J = 7$ Hz), 3.09 (d of d, 1, $J = 10$, 14 Hz), 347 (d of d, 1, $J = 11$, 14 Hz), 5.12 (quintent, 1, $J = 7$ Hz), 4.36 (quartet, 1, $J = 7$ Hz), 5.24 (s, 1), 5.51 (t, 1, $J = 10$ Hz), 7.12 ~ 7.94 (m, 7), 8.28 (d, 1, $J = 8$ Hz).

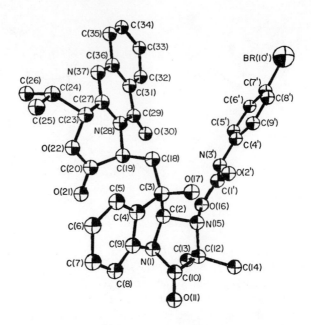

Figure 6. Computer generated drawing of the x-ray model of the p-bromophenyl–urethane derivative of tryptoquivaline. Data from Ref. 19.

Tryptoquivaline and tryptoquivalone appear to be tetrapeptides derived from tryptophane, anthranilic acid, valine and alanine, or methylalanine.

The two new tremorgens apparently are not as toxic as those tremorgenic substances previously reported. Glinsukon et al. (27) noted that the two compounds when injected into weanling rats at 500 mg/kg caused tremoring which persisted for five days; the animals died by eight days with no observable histopathologic changes.

Paspalum Staggers. A neurological disorder occurs in cattle and horses consuming Argentine Bahia grass (*Paspalum notatum*), Dallas grass (*P. dilatatum*), and brown-seed paspalum (*P. plicatulum*) whose seedheads have been infected by the ergot fungus *Claviceps paspali*. The symptoms in affected animals closely resemble those caused by the tremorgens isolated from other fungi except that severe structural damage was found in the brain, cerebellum, and spinal cord (*23, 24, 25, 26, 27*). No attempts have been reported to isolate the causative toxin; the problem has apparently been solved by discontinuing this family of grasses as fodder.

Acknowledgment

We thank Larry W. Tjarks for NMR analysis and William K. Rohwedder for mass spectral analyses of penitrem A. We also thank G. Büchi for supplying a preprint of his manuscript (*19*) on the two new tremorgens prior to publication.

Literature Cited

1. Ueno, Y., Ueno, I., *Jap. J. Exp. Med.* (1972) **42**, 91.
2. Cole, R. J., Kirksey, J. W., *J. Agric. Food Chem.* (1973) **21**, 927.
3. Wilson, B. J., Wilson, C. H., *Science* (1964) **144**, 177.
4. Wilson, B. J., Wilson, C. H., Hayes, A. W., *Nature* (1968) **220**, 77.
5. Ciegler, A., *Appl. Microbiol.* (1969) **18**, 128.
6. Ciegler, A., Pitt, J. I., *Mycopathol. Mycol. Appl.* (1970) **42**, 119.
7. Hou, C. T., Ciegler, A., Hesseltine, C. W., *Appl. Microbiol.* (1971a) **21**, 1101.
8. Hou, C. T., Ciegler, A., Hesseltine, C. W., *Can. J. Microbiol.* (1971b) **17**, 599.
9. Weil, C. S., *Biometrics* (1952) **8**, 249.
10. Wilson, B. J., Hockman, T., Dettbarn, W.-D., *Brain Res.* (1972) **40**, 540.
11. Cysewski, S. J., Jr., "A Tremorgénic Mycotoxin from *Penicillium puberulum*, Its Isolation and Neuropathic Effects," Ph.D. Thesis, Iowa State University, 1973.
12. Stern, P., *Yugoslav. Physiol. Pharmacol. Acta* (1971) **7**, 187.
13. Hou, C. T., Ciegler, A., Hesseltine, C. W., *Anal. Biochem.* (1970) **37**, 422.
14. Cole, R. J., Kirksey, J. W., Moore, J. H., Blankenship, B. R., Diener, U. L., Davis, N. D., *Appl. Microbiol.* (1972) **24**, 248.
15. Hotujac, L., Stern, P., Muftic, R. H., (abstract) VIII *Congr. Yogoslav. Physiol. Pharm. Soc.*, Opatia 25–28, September (1973).
16. Yamazaki, M., Suzuki, S., Miyaki, K., *Chem. Pharm. Bull.* (1971) **19**, 1739.
17. Yamazaki, M., Sasago, K., Mujaki, K., *Chem. Commun.* (1974) 408.
18. Dix, D. T., Martin, J., Moppett, C. E., *Chem. Commun.* (1972) 1168.
19. Clardy, J., Springer, J. P., Büchi, G., Matsuo, K., Wightman, R., private communication.
20. Büchi, G., Klaubert, D. H., Shank, R. C., Weinreb, S. M., Wogan, G. N., *J. Org. Chem.* (1971) **36**, 1143.
21. Büchi, G., Kitaura, Y., Yuan, S.-S., Wright, H. E., Clardy, J., Demain, A. L., Glinsukon, T., Hunt, N., Wogan, G. N., *J. Amer. Chem. Soc.* (1973) **95**, 5423.
22. Glinsukon, T., Yuan, S.-S., Wightman, R., Kitaura, Y., Büchi, G., Shank, R. C., Wogan, G. N., Christensen, C. M., *Plant Foods Man* (1974) **1**, 113.
23. Brown, H. B., *J. Agric. Res.* (1961) **7**, 401.
24. Hopkirk, C. S. M., *N.Z. J. Agric.* (1936) **53**, 105.
25. Grayson, A. R., *J. Dep. Agric. Victoria Aust.* (1941) **39**, 441.
26. Simms, B. T., *Auburn Vet.* (1945) **1**, 64.
27. Tatrishvili, P. S., *Tr. Vses. Inst. Eksp. Vet.* (1957) **20**, 226.

RECEIVED November 18, 1974. Mention of firm names or trade products does not imply that they are endorsed or recommended by the U.S. Department of Agriculture over other firms or similar products not mentioned.

10

Zearalenone and Related Compounds

S. V. PATHRE and C. J. MIROCHA

Department of Plant Pathology, University of Minnesota, St. Paul, Minn. 55101

Zearalenone [6-(10-hydroxy-6-oxo-trans-1-undecenyl)-β-re-sorcylic acid-μ-lactone] is a secondary metabolite of species of Fusarium *and is notable because of its estrogenic and anabolic activity in animals. Mass spectral, NMR, fluorescence, and x-ray diffraction properties are summarized with emphasis on fragmentation patterns resulting from analyses by mass spectrometry. Use of mass spectrometry in structure elucidation is illustrated. Zearalenone is biosynthesized via the acetate–malonyl–CoA pathway and can be metabolized to the two isomers of 8'-hydroxyzearalenone. Structure-activity relationships indicate that the most active derivative of the series is 7'-carboxyzearalane which is one-tenth as active as diethylstilbestrol and 100 times more active than the parent zearalenone. The naturally occurring macrolides related to zearalenone are radicicol, lasiodiplodin, and curvularin. The chemistry and total synthesis of this molecule are described and discussed.*

Zearalenone is a secondary metabolite produced by *Fusarium roseum, Fusarium tricinctum, Fusarium oxysporum, Fusarium culmorum,* and *Fusarium moniliforme.* It is usually produced on maize and barley in storage, and when fed to animals, particularly swine, it causes hyperestrogenism. A thorough treatment of this subject can be found in reviews by Mirocha et al. (*1*) and Mirocha and Christensen (*2*). Hyperestrogenism was first noted in swine by Buxton in 1927 (*3*) and Legenhausen in 1928 in herds in Iowa (*4*). Although they did not know its cause, they described symptoms in young gilts of the swelling and eversion of the vagina until, in some cases, the cervix was visible. Legenhausen also described a swelling of the prepuce in males. McNutt was the first to associate this disease with the consumption of moldy maize and to reproduce the estrogenic syndrome (*5*).

Stob et al. (*6*) isolated an active principle from cultures of *Gibberella zeae* (*Fusarium roseum,* Graminearum) in 1962 followed by Christensen et al. (*7*) in 1965. This metabolite had marked anabolic and uterotrophic activity when administered to mice, appeared to incite the estrogenic syndrome, and was called F-2 (*7*). Urry et al. (*8*) named the active principle zearalenone.

Zearalenone acts as a hormone in *Fusarium roseum* where it regulates the production of the sexual stage—*i.e.,* formation of perithecia (*9*). In the fungus system it acts in concert with cyclic 3′-5′-adenosine monophosphate to regulate perithecia production (*10*). Although it regulates the sexual stage in other genera of fungi as well, it has been found only within the genus *Fusarium* (*11*).

Zearalenone belongs to a group of natural products called resorcylates. In this paper the chemistry of zearalenone, its derivatives, and other related natural products are reviewed to summarize the more interesting and unusual features of macrocyclic resorcylates. An attempt is made to treat those aspects of zearalenone of special interest to the organic chemist and to the biologist as well.

Nomenclature. The estrogenic macrolide was designated zearalenone, an enone derivative of resorcylic acid lactone isolated from *Gibberella zeae* (*8*). Zearalane is a parent compound of zearalenone. The numbering system used throughout this paper for the zearalane system is shown in Figure 1. The chemical name commonly used for zearalane is 6-(10-hydroxy-1-undecyl)-β-resorcylic acid- μ-lactone. Accordingly, zearalenone is named 6-(10-hydroxy-6-oxo-*trans*-1-undecenyl)-β-resorcylic acid μ-lactone.

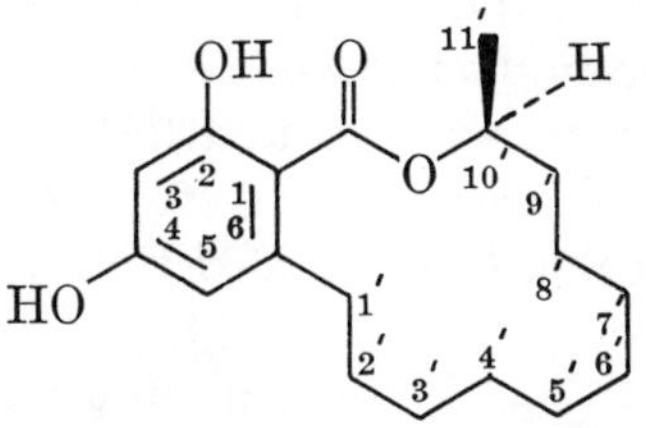

Figure 1.   Structure and numbering system for zearalane

Zearalenone

Structural Elucidation. Structure 1 of zearalenone ($C_{18}H_{22}O_5$) was elucidated in 1966 by Urry et al. (*8*) who found that it absorbed hydrogen in the presence of platinum to give a dihydro product 2 ($C_{18}H_{24}O_5$); however, hydrogenation over Raney nickel at 50 psi gave a mixture of two diastereomeric alcohols 3 ($C_{18}H_{26}O_5$). Chemical degradation of zearale-

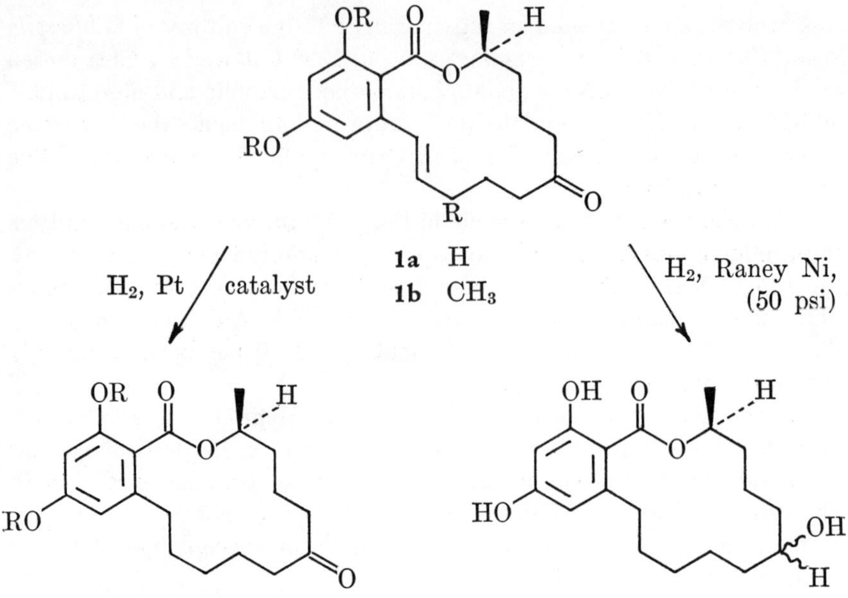

H$_2$, Pt / catalyst

1a H
1b CH$_3$

H$_2$, Raney Ni,
(50 psi)

2 C$_{18}$H$_{24}$O$_5$ R=H
4 R=CH$_3$

3 C$_{18}$H$_{26}$O$_5$

none (Scheme I) via Beckmann rearrangement yielded a product identified as 2(5-carboxy pentyl)-4,6-dimethoxybenzoic acid (5) determined
on the basis of NMR data. Ozonolysis of the dimethyl ether of zearalenone gave 2,4-dimethoxy-6-formylbenzoic acid. Zearalenone, when re-
fluxed 8 hr in 10% sodium bicarbonate solution, yields an alcohol 6
(C$_{17}$H$_{24}$O$_4$) after acidification. These studies established the positions
of the olefin and ketone in the alicyclic lactone ring. Also NMR spectral
data (see Spectral Properties) indicated the presence of trans olefinic
protons (J = 16 Hz) and a secondary methyl group. Thus the structure
of 1 is consistent with the data obtained from the studies listed above
(see Scheme I).

Absolute Configuration. Because of an asymmetric center at C10′,
naturally occurring zearalenone exhibits optical activity and purity
($[\alpha]^{25}_{546}$ = −170.5°, c = 1.0M MeOH). The absolute configuration of
this natural enantiomorph was determined by Kuo et al. (12) using a
method based on the kinetic resolution technique (13) of Horeou (14,
15, 16) to determine the configurations of secondary alcohols. They converted the natural zearalenone to the dihydroseco acid ketal 7, formed
the methyl ester 8, and then allowed it to react with (±)-α-phenylbutyric
anhydride in pyridine. The excess of α-phenylbutyric acid was recovered,
and its rotation was determined. The recovered acid exhibited a negative
rotation (corresponds to R(−)α-phenylbutyric acid) thereby denoting

SCHEME I

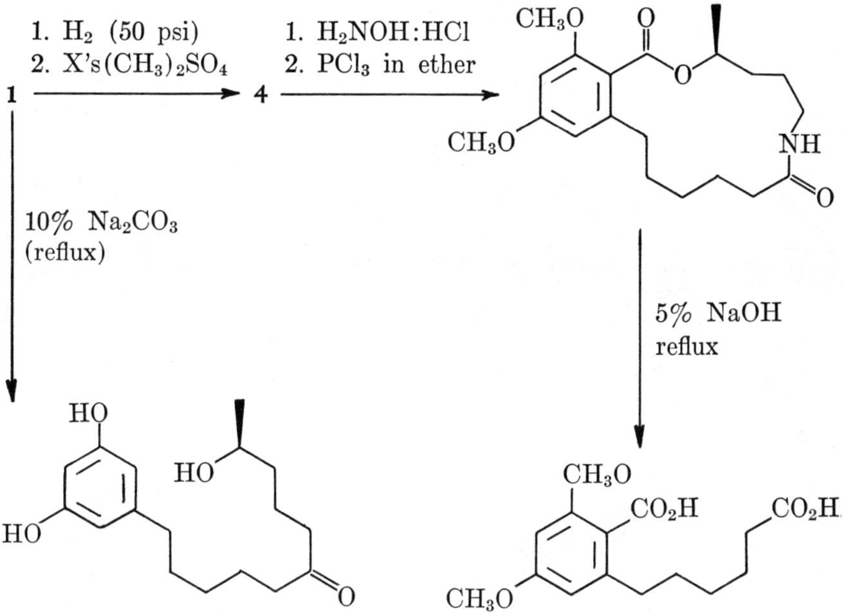

6 5

an S-configuration at the optically active 10′-center of zearalenone. Alternatively the lactone *9* derived from the exhaustive oxidation of zearalenone had an identical optical rotation to that of the S(−) enantiomer of 5-hydroxyhexanoic acid lactone.

Naturally Occurring Derivatives of Zearalenone

Mirocha et al. (*1*) reported the natural occurrence of at least seven derivatives of zearalenone from *Fusarium roseum* growing in culture on

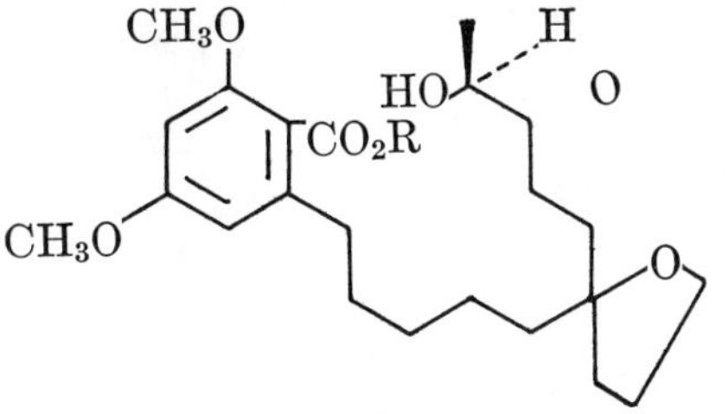

	R
7	H
8	CH_3

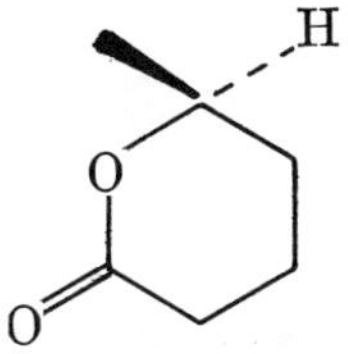

9

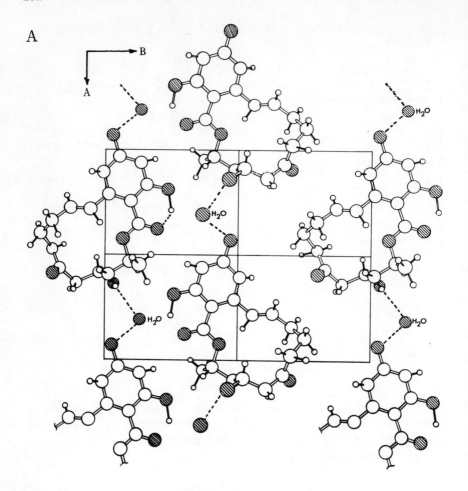

(8'R,10'S)-8'Hydroxyzearalenone

*Figure 2. (A) Packing of molecules in a crystal of 8'-dihydroxyzearalenone
(F-5-3) based on x-ray crystallography analysis. Note the intermolecular association arising from water of hydration. (Courtesy of I. F. Taylor.) (B) Stereochemistry of 8'-dihydroxyzearalenone.*

corn, and designated them as F-5-0 through F-5-7. The metabolites were partially characterized by their uv absorption spectra and separation by thin layer and gas–liquid chromatography. The most abundant of these derivatives were designated as F-5-3 (mp 198°–199°C) and F-5-4 (mp 168°–169°C), both of which have a mass of 334 and the empirical formula $C_{18}H_{23}O_6$. The structure was incorrectly reported as 3′-hydroxyzearalenone (alpha and beta isomers) by Mirocha et al. (*1*). Subsequent studies by Jackson et al. (*17*) revealed that the OH group of both isomers is in the 8′ position. Independently, Bolliger and Tamm (*18*) isolated two isomeric hydroxyzearalenones which when oxidized with Jones reagent (CrO_3–H_2SO_4 in acetone) yielded identical diketones ($[\alpha]_D^{24}$ = −93.2° and −92.8°) indicating the epimeric nature of the hydroxy group. Mass spectral data interpretation revealed that these isomeric hydroxyzearalenones were epimeric 8′-hydroxyzearalenones. By converting them into [S]-zearalanone, Jackson et al. (*17*) also showed that F-5-3 and F-5-4 are epimeric. Recently F-5-3 has been shown (*19*) to be (8′R,10′S)-hydroxyzearalenone, by x-ray crystallography (Figure 2).

Bolliger and Tamm (*18*) also reported the occurrence of 5-formylzearalenone **11** and 7′-dehydrozearalenone **12** in cultures of *Fusarium roseum* (Table I). Steele (*20*) isolated a compound from *Fusarium roseum* growing on a solid medium of shredded wheat which was identical with 6′,8′-dihydroxyzearalene **13**, $NaBH_4$-reduction product of F-5-3. He also isolated 7′-dehydrozearalenone **12** when the chloroform extract of the cultures was partitioned with $2N\ K_2CO_3$. However **12** was not detected when the base partition was eliminated.

Table I.   Naturally Occurring Derivatives of Zearalenone

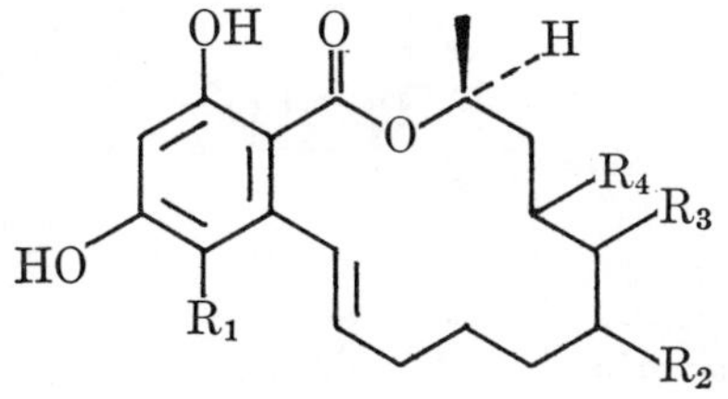

		R_1	R_2	R_3	R_4
10	8′-hydroxyzearalenone	—H	=O	=H_2	—OH
11	5-formylzearalenone	—CHO	=O	=H_2	=H_2
12	7′-dehydrozearalenone	—H	=O	—H	—H
13	6′,8′-dihydroxyzearalene	—H	—OH	=H_2	—OH

Reactions of Zearalenone

Ring Stability. Although zearalenone is a lactone, it is fairly stable in cold alkali; but prolonged exposure extensively hydrolyzes the lactone ring. The lactone function of 1 is easily hydrolyzed with sodium hydroxide in refluxing aqueous dimethyl sulfoxide (DMSO) and yields a racemized seco acid 14 in almost quantitative yield (21). The racemization of the seco acid is attributed to internal disproportionation arising from the presence of the 6' ketone (15 $\rightleftarrows$ 16) since the ethylene ketal 17 of zearalenone undergoes the opening of the lactone without racemization (21). Peters and Hurd (22) used this principle in opening the lactone ring of the naturally occurring (S)-zearalenone to prepare (R)-zearalanone, and they have inverted the configuration at C10' via the p-toluenesulfonic ester of the seco acid.

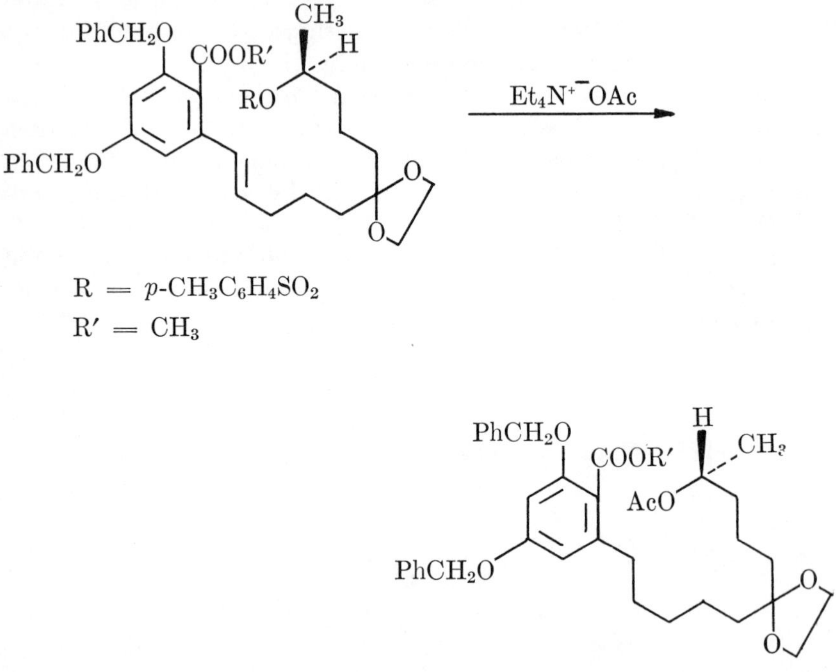

$PhCH_2O$ CH_3

$COOR'$ H

RO

$PhCH_2O$

$Et_4N^+\ ^-OAc$

O

O

$R = p\text{-}CH_3C_6H_4SO_2$

$R' = CH_3$

$PhCH_2O$ H $CH_?$

$COOR'$

AcO

$PhCH_2O$

O

O

Aromatic Substitution. Windholz and Brown (23) examined substitution of the carboxyl and formyl groups into the aromatic portion of zearalenone. When 1 is heated at 175° with anhydrous potassium carbonate at 800 psi CO_2 for 3 hr, it is carboxylated at the C3 position; however if the reaction time is increased to 5 hr, the carboxylation occurs at C-5 (24). These results are consistent with the conclusions (25) that such carboxylation is reversible and that, kinetically, substitution in the

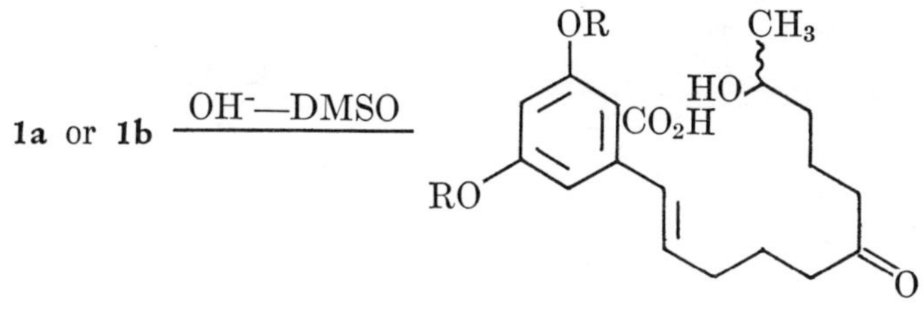

$$1a \text{ or } 1b \xrightarrow{\text{OH}^- \text{—DMSO}}$$

$\pm$ **14** R = H or CH$_3$

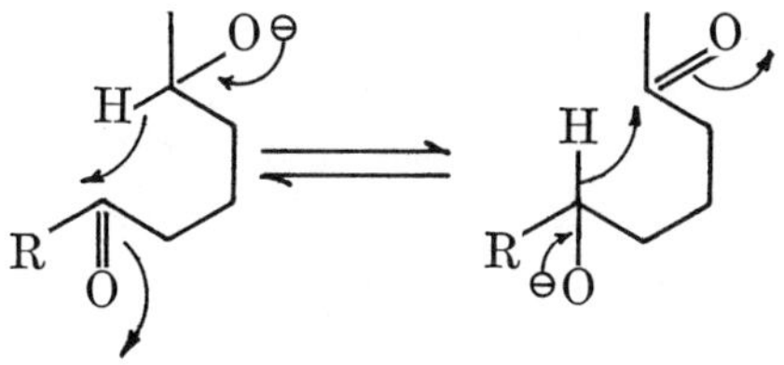

15   **16** 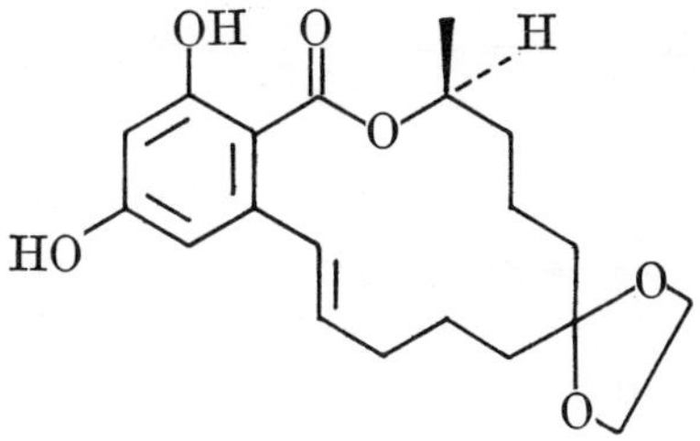   **17**

ortho position is favored, but, thermodynamically, the para position is favored. This is logical since the greater separation of the two negative charges (phenoxide and carboxylate) gives greater thermodynamic stability.

Zearalenone is formylated at the C3 position by allowing ethyl formate to react with aluminum chloride (Friedel–Craft formylation) (23) and by the Riemer–Tiemann and Gattermann reactions (18). (Reimer–Tiemann reaction is used to formylate sensitive aromatic rings; formylation occurs in chloroform in the presence of a strong base such as potassium hydroxide (see Ref. 26). The Gattermann reaction is used to formylate phenols (see Refs. 27 and 28). In these reactions formylation yielded a mixture of 3-formyl and 5-formyl zearalenone. The Gattermann reaction gave 89% of the formylated product in which the 3 and 5 formyl derivatives were in the ratio of 2:1, respectively.

Nitration of dimethyl ether zearalenone **1b** with a 50/50 mixture of concentrated sulfuric acid and nitric acid gives a mixture of 3,5-dinitro and 5-nitro derivatives (29). These nitro derivatives can be transformed into the corresponding amino derivatives by reduction with iron powder in a 50% methanolic solution containing hydrochloric acid (0.25 equiv). Johnston et al. (30) reported the conversion of 5-aminozearalenone **18** to 5-hydroxyzearalenone **20** by oxidizing the amino derivative with silver oxide–ammonium hydroxide to a 4-hydroxyquinone derivative **19** which yielded **20** when treated with aqueous sodium thiosulfate.

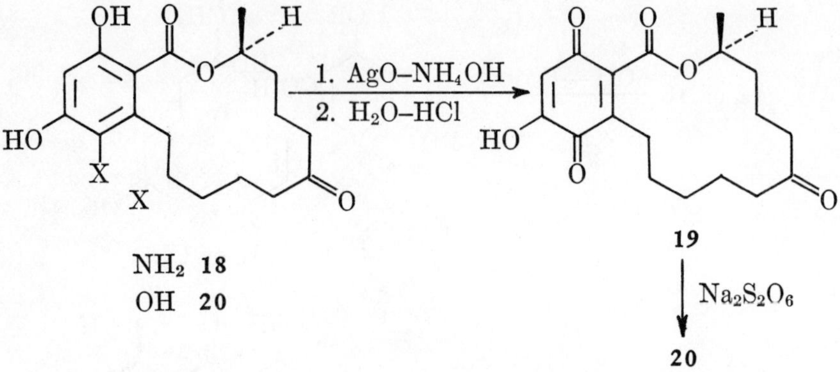

Halogen-substituted derivatives of zearalenone such as mono- and diiodozearalenone and monobromozearalenone have been reported (*31*). Halomercuric- and arsonic acid-substituted derivatives of zearalenone have also been prepared and show antibacterial and antifungal activity (*32*).

Diels–Alder Adducts. Several adducts of zearalenone have been prepared (Figure 3) to develop new growth-promoting agents (*33*). Maleic anhydride, sulfur dioxide, *p*-benzoquinone, 1,4-naphthoquinone, nitroethylene, and acrolein can easily form the 5-2′-adduct with zearalenone.

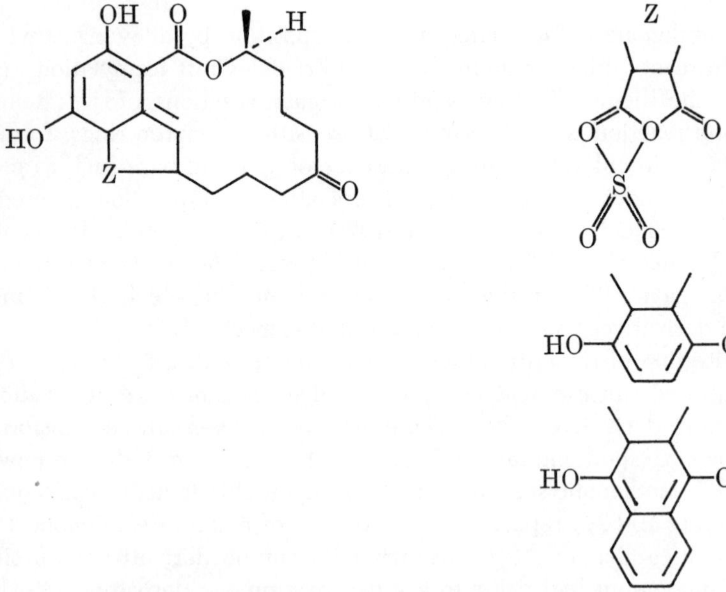

Figure 3.   Diels–Alder adduct of zearalenone

Birch Reduction. Birch reduction of zearalenone derivatives was studied by Windholz and Brown (*23*). The ethylene ketal of the dimethyl ether of zearalenone **21**, when treated with 4 equiv of sodium in liquid ammonia and *tert*-butyl alcohol yielded two rather unstable products (**22** and **23**), which on treatment with CrO_3 in pyridine aromatized to the deoxy derivatives **24** and **25**, respectively. The mechanistic interpretation of these reactions is shown in Scheme II (*23*). The deoxy product **26** was isomerized to **23** because of treatment with a base during isolation.

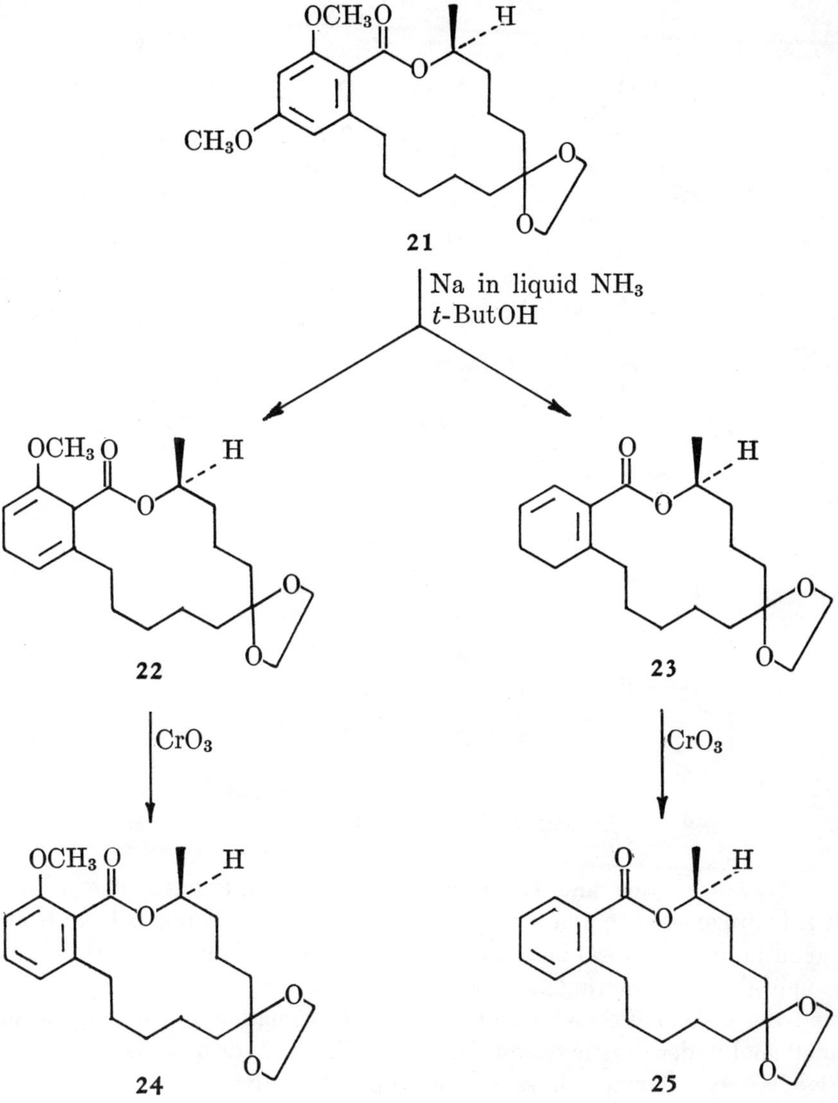

Scheme II

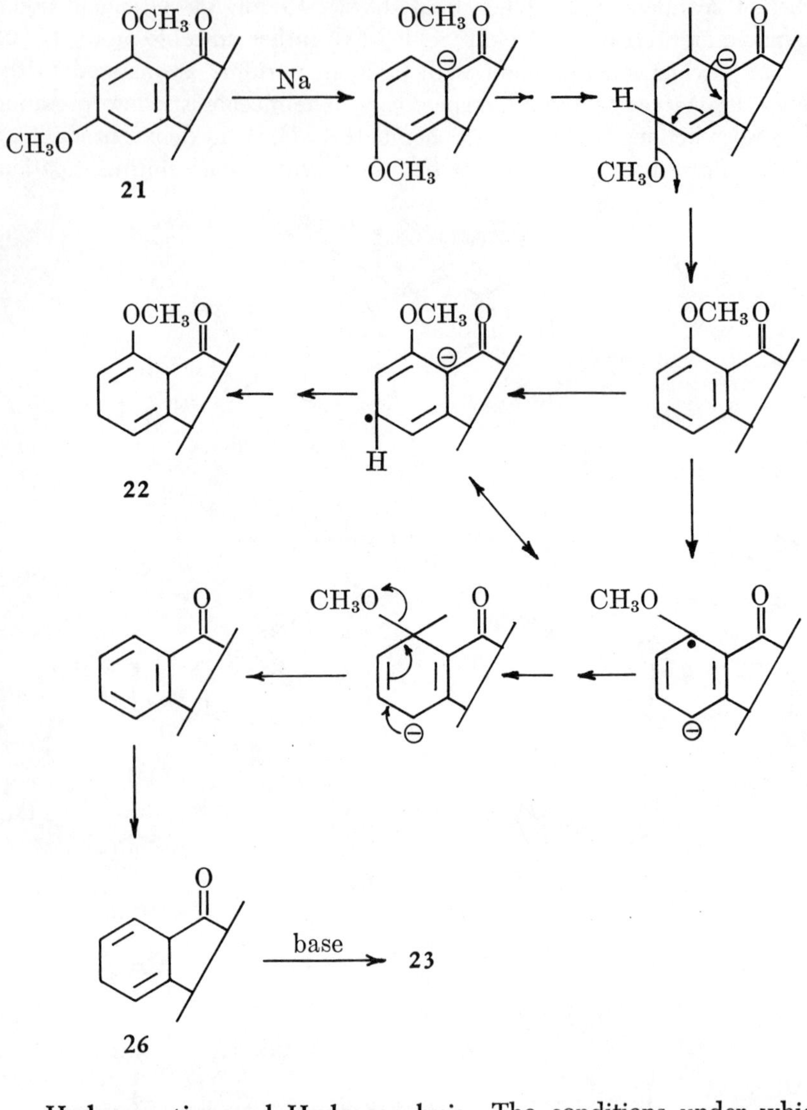

Hydrogenation and Hydrogenolysis. The conditions under which
1 is hydrogenated to 2 and to the diastereomeric zearalanols 3 have been
noted in our structural elucidation of zearalenone. The complete saturation of the aromatic ring 27 (concomitant with the reduction of the olefin
and the 6'-keto groups) occurs when hydrogenation is carried out in
methanol under drastic conditions (34). The perhydrozearalanol derivative has been shown to have anti-inflammatory activity (35).

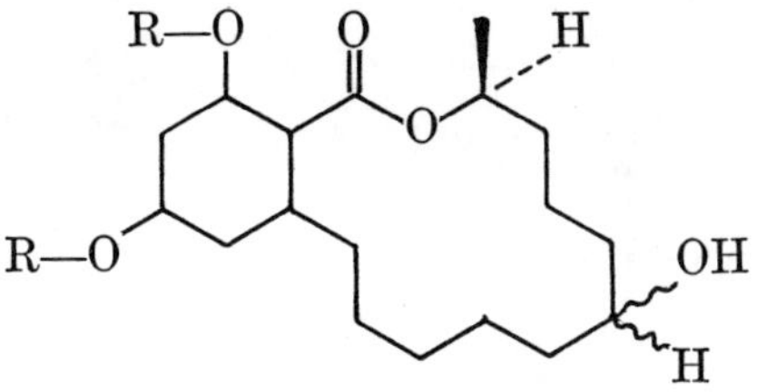

R—O   O   H

R—O   OH
                            H

R = H or CH₃

27

Hydrogenolysis of the phenolic hydroxyls in zearalenone has been reported by Johnston et al. (*30*) and Wehrmeister and Robertson (*36*). It involves preparation of the 1-phenyl-5-tetrazolyl **28** or benzyxazolyl **29** ethers and the subsequent hydrogenolysis with 5% Pd–C which also reduces the 1′-olefin.

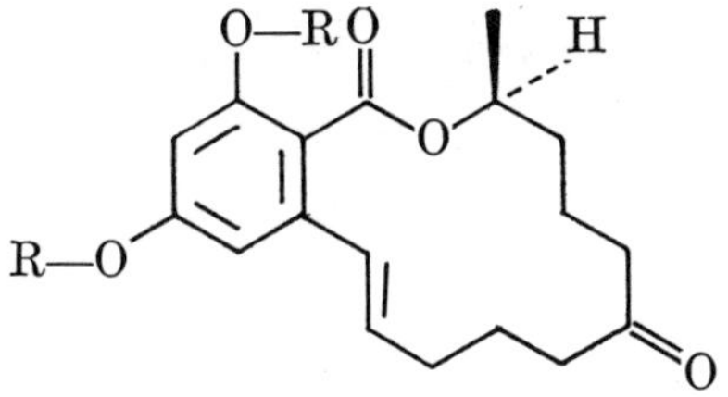

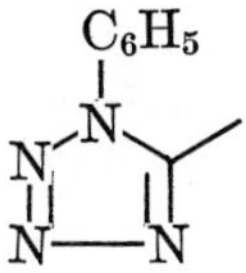

O—R O   H

R—O
                    O

C₆H₅

28

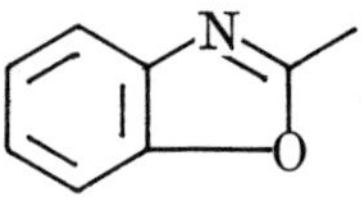

29

Oxidation. Zearalenone or its dimethyl ether, while refluxing in 14% nitric acid, oxidizes extensively to yield glutaric, succinic, and oxalic acids. The nitrated aromatic fragment can be isolated only by oxidizing the dimethyl ether derivative (*8, 37*). The advantage of such degradation was taken to determine the distribution of ¹⁴C in zearalenone (**Figure 4**) isolated from cultures of *Fusarium roseum* inoculated with [1-¹⁴C]-acetate (*37*).

The allylic oxidation of the ether of zearalenone **30** with Sarett reagent (CrO₃–pyridine complex) gives a 3-keto derivative **31** (*38*). The oxidation appears to be sensitive to the type of substituent at the 6′ position. The yield of the 3-keto derivative obtained from the other **30** was less than 15%; however the ethylene ketal **32** and the epimeric acetates **33** afforded the corresponding 3-keto derivatives in more than 70% yield. According to Jensen et al. (*38*) the change in hybridization of C6′ ($sp^2 \rightarrow sp^3$) allows a favorable ring conformation, and the presence of oxygen attached to sp^3 C6′ assists the attack at C3′.

Osmium tetroxide reacts smoothly with the double bond of the dibenzyl ether of zearalenone **34** to produce a mixture of epimeric 1′,2′-

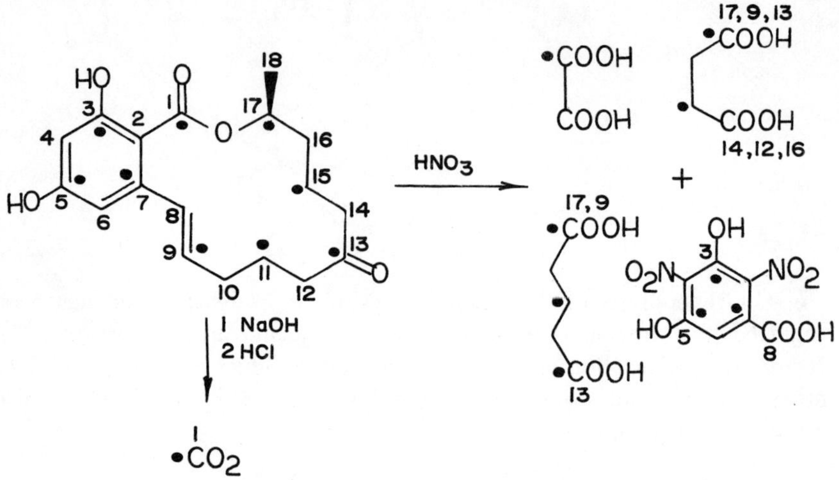

Figure 4.   Chemical degradation of ^{14}C-labelled zearalenone. The filled circles ($\bullet$) mark the location of ^{14}C atoms derived from 1-^{14}C-acetate.

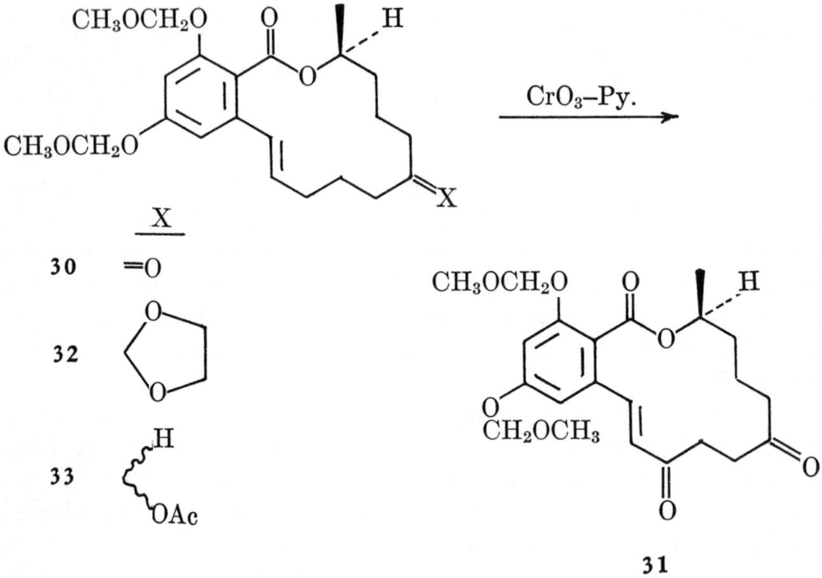

diol **35** which in the presence of an acid rearranges to give **36** (*38*), probably via acid-catalyzed openings of the lactone **35** to form **37**. The 2′,10′-diol **37** then undergoes an intramolecular ketal formation with the 6′-ketone.

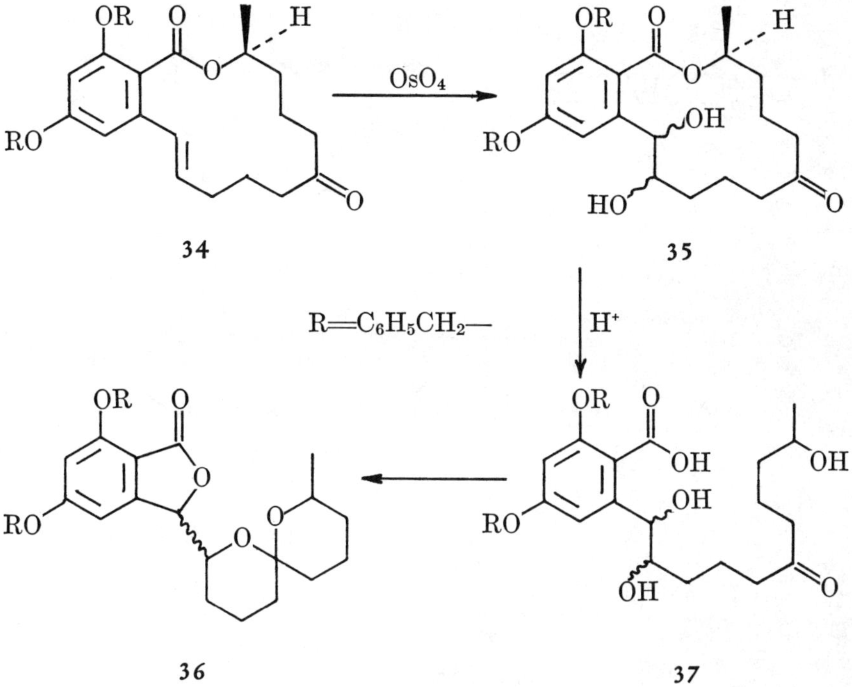

34   **35**

R=C₆H₅CH₂—   H⁺

36   **37**

Modification of the Lactone Ring. Reactions involving the aliphatic portion of zearalenone have been examined extensively either to modify the estrogenic acivity (*39*) or to synthesize naturally occurring derivatives of zearalenone; namely, 7'-dihydrozearalenone **12** and 8'-hydroxyzearalenone **10** (*40*).

Jensen et al. (*38*) reported that the reactions of activated methylenes (at 5' and 7') of zearalenone show considerable "regioselectivity" (*see* Ref. *41* for the definition). Formylation of zearalenone ethers in benzene under the conditions of sodium hydride and *tert*-butyl alcohol gave predominantly the C7' product **38** (< 70%). This preference for C7' formylation was also noticed in the zearalanone derivatives. Reaction of zearalenone-2-4-diacetate **39** with isopropenyl acetate in the presence of *p*-toluenesulfonic acid gave the enol acetate in which the major product isolated was **40** (enolization in C5' direction) in 61% yield. The other isomer (enolization in C7' direction) was isolated in *ca.* 4% yield. Whether such selectivity is kinetic or thermodynamic has not yet been determined. One postulation is that the acid-catalyzed enolization prior to enol acetate formation yields the isomer most favored thermodynamically while base-catalyzed alkylation favors that product resulting from reaction at the least sterically hindered position. Some preliminary observations on deuterium exchange experiments with zearalenone in sodium

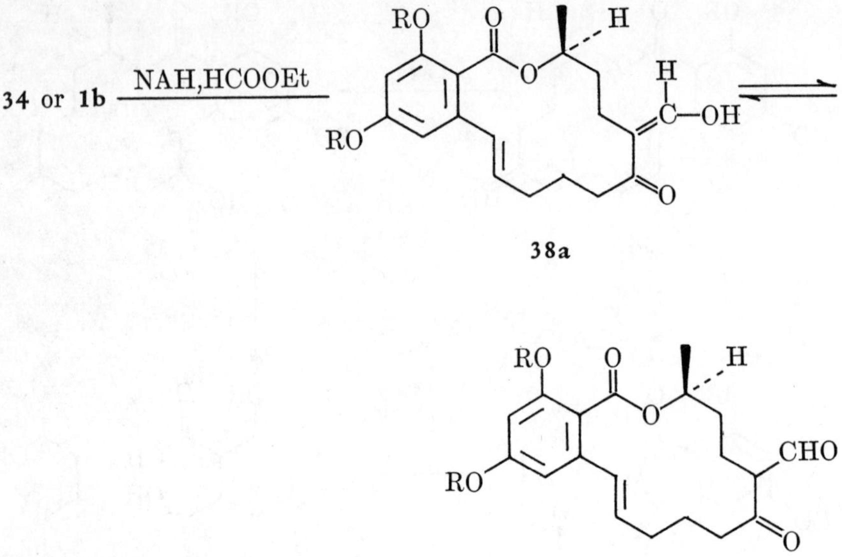

34 or 1b $\xrightarrow{\text{NAH,HCOOEt}}$

38a

38b

R = CH$_3$ or C$_6$H$_5$CH$_2$—

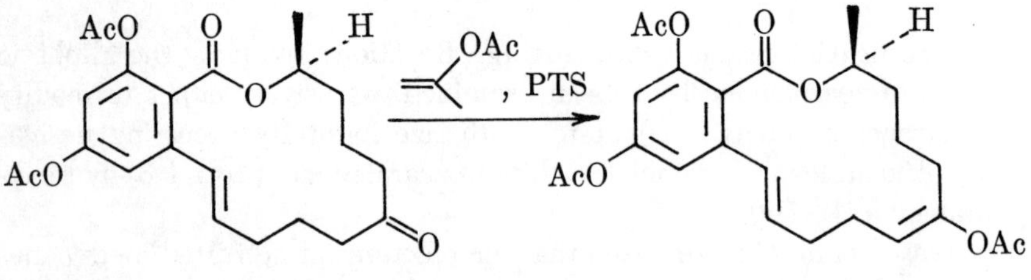

39   40

PTS = *p*-toluenesulfonic acid

methoxide–methanol indicated that exchange occurs rapidly at the C7′ position (42).

The selective introduction of formyl group at C7′ position is useful since it serves as a potential precursor in the synthesis of various zearalenone derivatives. Synthesis of isomeric zearalenone was reported by Jensen et al. (38) in which the hydroxymethylene derivative 38a was converted into zearalan-7′-one (Scheme III). Synthesis of 1′,7′-zearaldienone (7′-dehydrozearalenone) was attempted in which 7′-formylzearalenone-2,4-dimethyl ether 38b was used as an intermediate (40). Bromination of this ether was expected to yield the 7′-bromo derivative 41 which could be dehydrohalogenated to the dienone. However the crude bromi-

SCHEME III

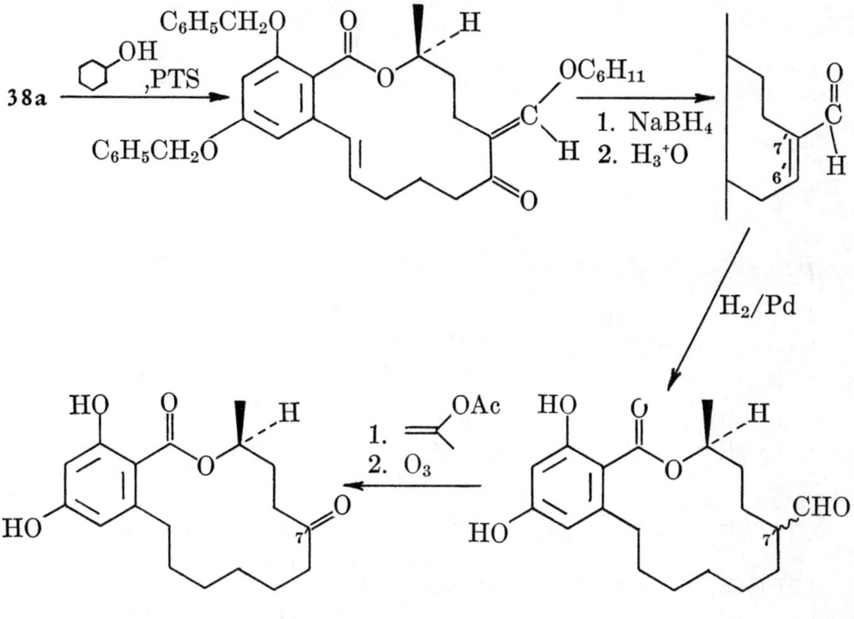

7'-Zearalanone

nation product was a mixture of monobromo **41** and dibromo derivatives **42** which on thin layer chromatography deformylated extensively without yielding a satisfactory separation. Dehydrobromination of this product with collidine gave 1',7'-zearaldienone in small yield as detected by combined gas chromatography–mass spectrometry (GC–MS).

The double bond in the macrocyclic lactone is quite resistant to bromination (*40*), epoxidation, and hydroboration (*38*). This is probably a result of the electron withdrawing effect of the ortho carboxyl group which makes the olefin electron defficient. Treating zearalenone with *N*-bromosuccinimide failed to produce the allylic bromide; instead the

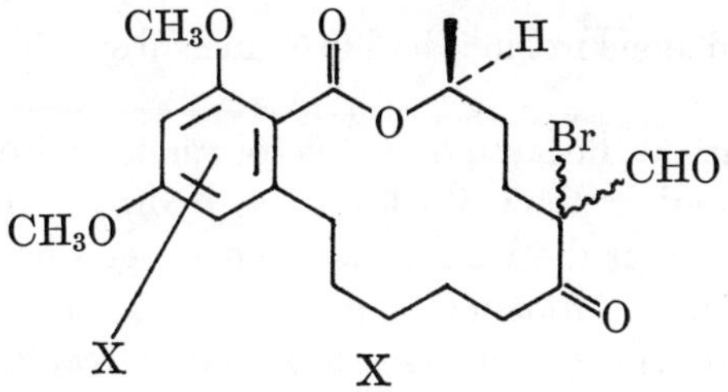

	X
41	H
42	Br

Table II.   Reaction Conditions for Forming Various Ethers of Zearalenone

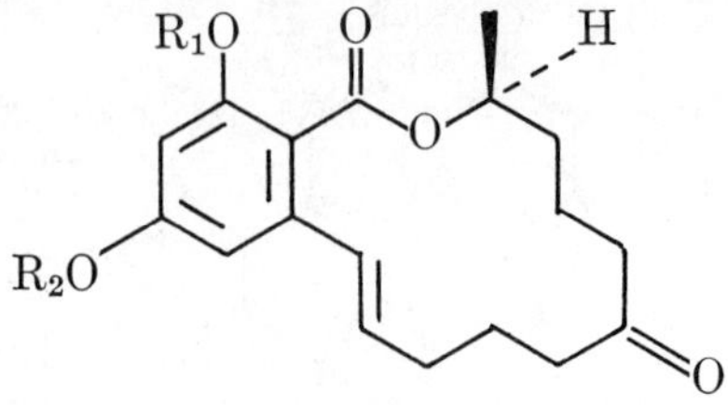

R_1	R_2	Conditions	Ref
H	CH_3	excess of CH_2N_2 in ether	8
CH_3	H	$(CH_3)_2SO_4$ in 10% NaOH	8
CH_3	CH_3	excess of $(CH_3)_2SO_4$ in 10% NaOH or CH_3I in acetone in the presence of K_2CO_3 at reflux	8 / 18
—$CH_2C_6H_5$	H	$C_6H_5CH_2Cl$ in anhydrous MeOH in the presence of K_2CO_3 at reflux (see Scheme IV)	30
—$CH_2C_6H_5$	—$CH_2C_6H_5$	$C_6H_5CH_2Cl$ in acetone in the presence of K_2CO_3 at reflux for 5 days	38
—CH_2OCH_3	—CH_2OCH_3	1) NaH in DMF at 0°; 2) CH_3OCH_2Cl in DMF at 0°	38
H	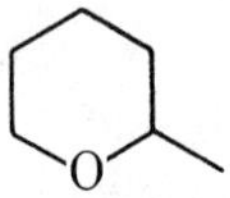	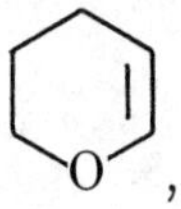	30
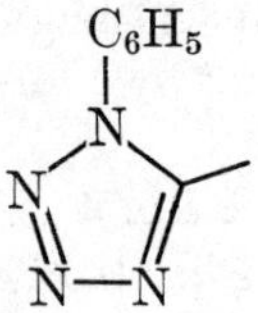	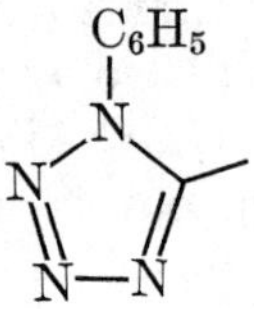	1-phenyl-5-chlorotetrazole in refluxing anhydrous acetone in the presence of K_2CO_3	30
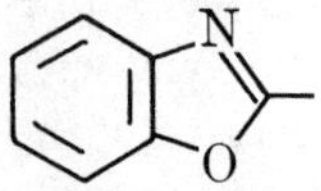	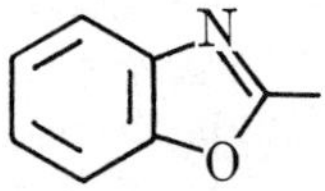	2-chlorobenzoxazole in acetone in the presence of K_2CO_3 at reflux for 24 hr	36

brominated zearalenone isolated had bromine substituted on the aromatic ring (40).

Ether Formation. Because of its two phenolic hydroxyls, zearalenone forms a variety of ethers; however these two hydroxyls differ in reactivity. The phenolic proton at the C2 position is hydrogen bonded to the peri-carbonyl of the lactone function. Therefore it is more acidic, and reactions of this hydroxyl demand high steric requirements. Table II shows the reaction conditions for preparing different ethers of zearalenone with corresponding references. Although the C2 OH proton is more acidic

SCHEME IV

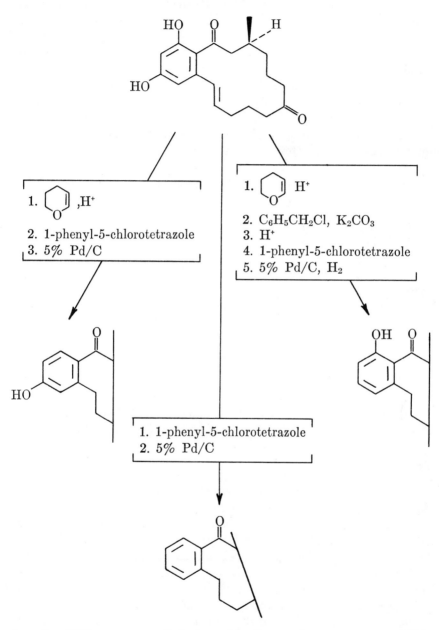

than the 4OH proton, methylation with diazomethane occurs at 4OH. This can be attributed to the strong intramolecular H bonding which precludes the transfer of the bonded proton (C2 OH) to diazomethane.

However, in the presence of alkali the C2 phenoxide can be selectively formed to effect the corresponding etherification by metathesis when steric requirements are not high. Such selective etherification has been used (30) to make the 2- or 4-deoxy derivative of zearalenone as shown in Scheme IV. The key reaction in this sequence is the selective mono-tetrahydropyranyl ether formation at C4 in good yield.

Cis-trans Isomerization. The geometrical isomerization of zearalene derivatives is accomplished photochemically. This can be brought about by light of a wavelength that is absorbed by the olefinic system (usually uv light). Since energy is absorbed, this process does not establish thermal equilibrium. However a steady state may be reached which generally corresponds to a predominance of the less stable isomer. Thus irradiation of *trans*-zearalenone with uv light led to a mixture containing 88% *cis*-zearalenone 43 (43).

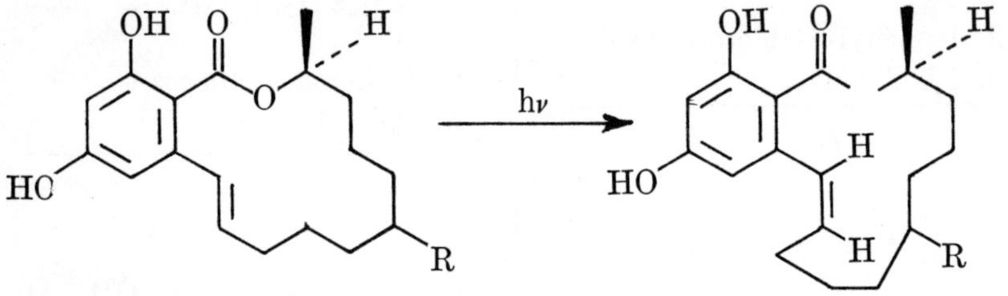

R = OH or =O   43

Miscellaneous Reactions. Several reactions of 6' ketone have been reported, such as: Grignard reactions (44), addition of hydrogen cyanide (45), Reformatsky reaction (46), chlorination with phosphorus penta-chloride (47), thioketal formation (48), and addition of acetylene (49).

Related Natural Macrolides

Compounds similar in molecular form to zearalenone, but perhaps not in biological activity, have reportedly been synthesized by fungi.

Radicicol (Monorden). This compound, an antibiotic, was first isolated in 1953 from *Monosporium bonorden* (50) and was named monorden (51). Ten years later McCapra et al. (51) and Mirrington et al. (52) independently proved that the structure of this compound was **44**. The compound was called radicicol since it was isolated from *Nectri radicicola* (52). Important chemical studies were carried out on radicicol by Mirrington et al. (53) who found that radicicol exhibited marked instability toward alkali. When it was treated with aqueous ethanolic potassium hydroxide, the solution instantaneously turned bright red. The reaction was reversed only if the alkaline solution was quickly quenched with an

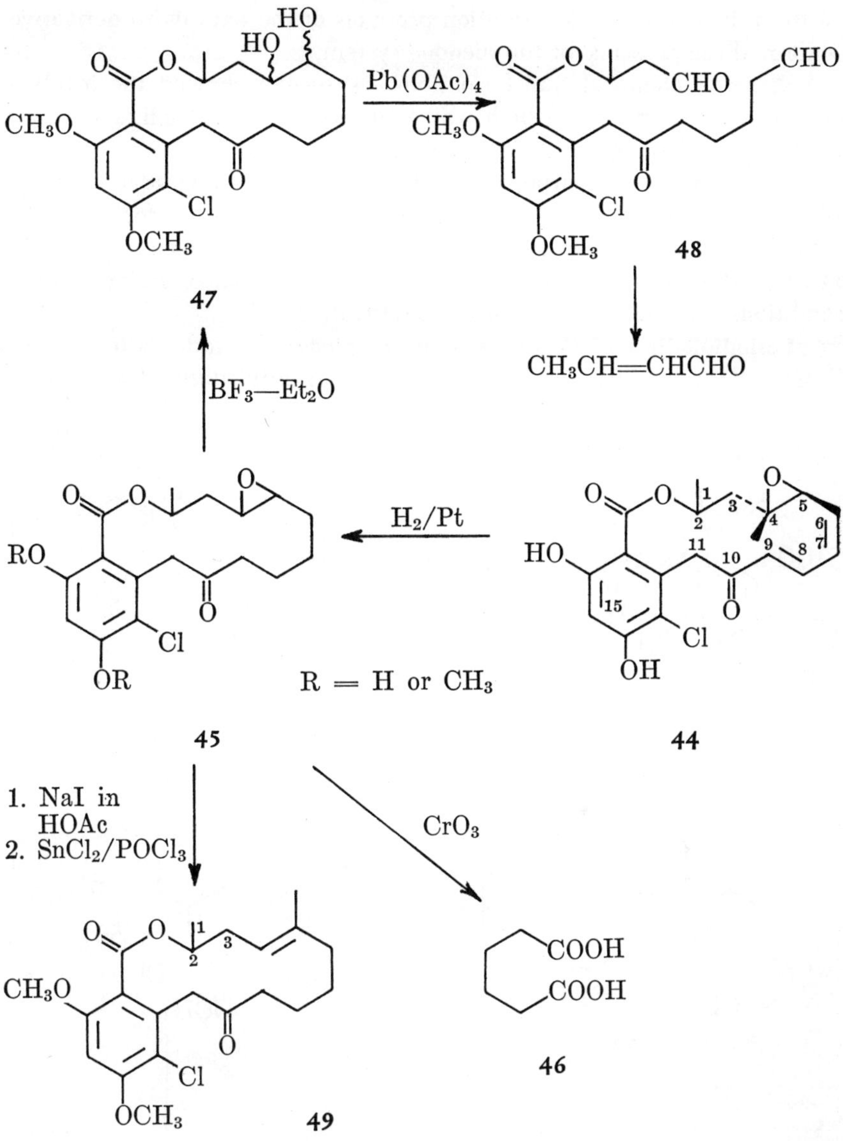

acid. However the tetrahydro derivative **45** obtained by catalytic hydrogenation of radicicol did not show such decomposition. The comparison
of the uv and NMR spectra of radicicol with those of tetrahydroradicicol
indicated the presence of an isolated, linear conjugated dienone

$$\overset{O}{\overset{\|}{(-C}}-CH=CH-CH=CH-)$$ system. Also the isolation of adipic acid

46 from the chromic acid oxidation products of the tetrahydro derivative confirmed the presence of the dienone system.

A series of chemical transformations (45 → 48) showed the involvement of an oxirane ring which was assigned the trans configuration on the basis of formation of the trans olefin 49 from 45.

It was mentioned earlier that radicicol undergoes degradation under alkaline conditions. Such degradation is initiated by the formation of the enolate anion 50 and gives rise to two isolable products: a phthalide 51 and an isocoumarin derivative 52. Tetrahydroradicicol under alkaline conditions also yields an isocoumarin derivative.

Lasiodiplodin and De-O-methyllasiodiplodin. Lasiodiplodin and de-O-methyllasiodiplodin are produced by *Lasiodiplodium theobromae.*

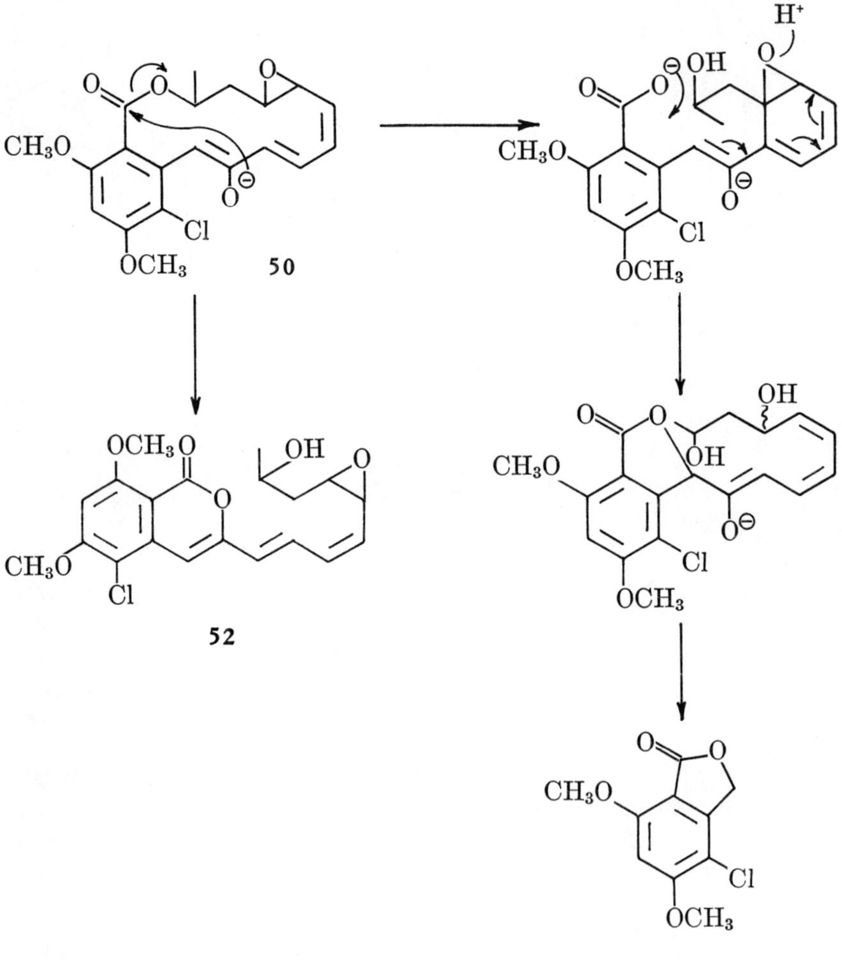

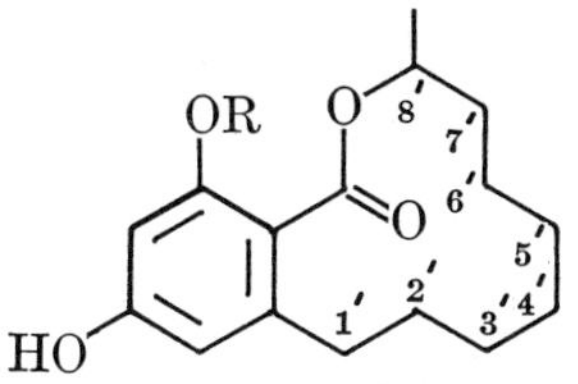

lasiodiplodin   R=CH$_3$

de-*O*-methyllasiodiplodin   R=H

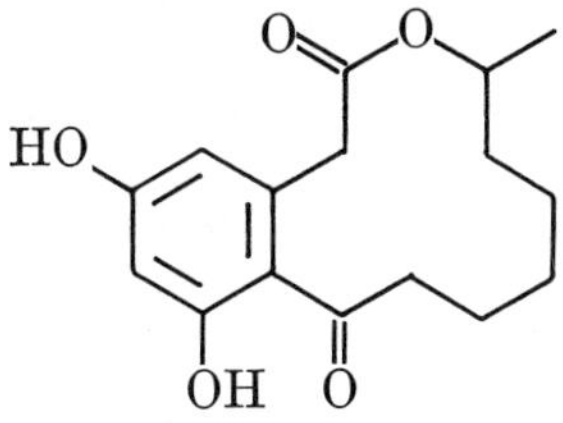

curvularin

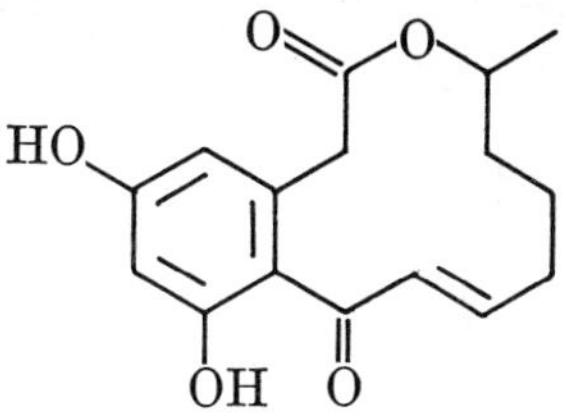

—dehydrocurvularin

Figure 5.   Naturally occurring macrolides

Based on the oxidation and spectral studies, Aldridge et al. (*54*) reported the structure of these macrolides. Oxidation of lasiodiplodin with Jones reagent gave the quinone indicating a resorcylic acid derivative. Further, the comparison of the related synthetic macrolide 76 with de-*O*-methyl-lasiodiplodin confirmed the structure of Lasiodiplodin (Figure 5).

Curvularin. Musgrave in 1956 (*55*) isolated two related metabolites from species of *Curvularia*. The metabolite, $C_{16}H_{20}O_5$, which appears to be a major metabolite, was named curvularin. The minor metabolite, $C_{16}H_{18}O_5$, was an α,β-dehydrocurvularin (*56*). Musgrave (*55, 57*) and Birch et al. (*58*) provided the proof for the structure of curvularin. Birch et al. (*58*) also demonstrated that curvularin is derived from the head to tail condensation of eight acetate units.

Naturally Occurring 3-4-Dehydroisocoumarins. Since zearalenone is a member of a class of natural products called the β-resorcylates, the naturally occurring dihydroisocoumarin derivatives, although not macrolides, are usually considered to be related to zearalenone. Table III lists some of these dihydroisocoumarins and appropriate references.

Synthetic Approaches to Macrolides (Zearalenone and Its Derivatives and Related Macrolides)

The first total synthesis of naturally occurring zearalenone together

Table III.   Naturally Occurring

Compound

3,4-Dihydro-6-methoxy,8-hydroxy-3-methylisocoumarin
3,4-Dihydro-6,8-dihydroxy-3-methylisocoumarin
3,4-Dihydro-6,8-dihydroxy-3-[β-(4-methoxyphenyl)ethyl]isocoumarin
3,4-Dihydro-6,8-dihydroxy-3,4,5-trimethylisocoumarin
3,4-Dihydro-6,8-dihydroxy-3,4,5-trimethylisocoumarin-7-carboxylic acid
Reticulol
Cladosporin

with its optical resolution was accomplished by a team of Merck chemists (*21*). The key feature involved in the synthesis (Scheme V) was the Witting condensation of an appropriately substituted aromatic nucleus **53** with an aliphatic component **54**. Noteworthy in this synthesis are the critical steps used to construct the aliphatic moiety **54** in which the C6 and C10 functionalities are mutually masked via internal ketal formation.

Girotra and Wendler (*65, 66*) were successful in condensing the aliphatic intermediate **56** with dimethoxyhomophthalic anhydride **57** to give lactonic acid **58** which undergoes decarboxylation to yield the seco acid **14**. Cyclization of the seco acid using trifluoroacetic acid anhydride in benzene and subsequent demethylation with boron tribromide yielded (±)-zearalenone. An approach at synthesis similar to that of Taub et al. (*21*) was made by Vlattas et al. (*67*); however the aromatic **59** and aliphatic **60** portions were constructed in a different manner (Scheme VI). Note that the specific cleavage of the ketal at C10 of the side chain of the acid **61** in aqueous acetone containing *p*-toluenesulfonic acid

6,8-Dihydroxyisocoumarin Derivatives

R_1	R_2	R_3	R_4	R_5	R_6	Ref
H	H	CH_3	H	H	CH_3	59
H	H	H	H	H	CH_3	60
H	H	H	H	H	CUT G CH_3CH⟨◯⟩OCH_3	61
H	H	H	CH_3	CH_3	CH_3	62
H	COOH	H	CH_3	CH_3	CH_3	62
H	OCH_3	H	H	H	CH_3	63
H	H	H	H	H	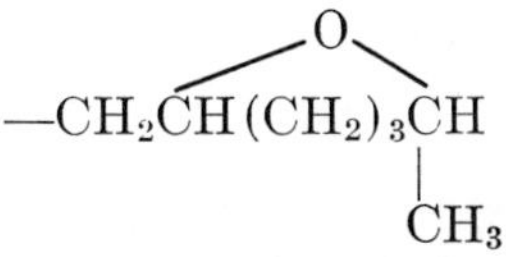	64

$$-CH_2CH(CH_2)_3\overset{\displaystyle O}{\overbrace{\quad\quad}}CH \atop CH_3$$

proceeded in 85% yield to give the required monoketal **62**. However
the corresponding ester of the acid was cleaved to a mixture of monoketals
and diketone.

Wehrmeister and Robertson (*36*) reported the synthesis of dideoxyzearalane **65**, a simple macrocyclic lactone having the same skeletal
structure as zearalenone. They synthesized the basic skeleton **63** required
for making the appropriate hydroxy acid **64** by condensation of 10-
undecenoic anhydride with phthalic anhydride in the presence of sodium
acetate. The hydroxy acid **64** was expected to lactonize to the desired
compound **65**; however the cyclization of the hydroxy acid **64** to dideoxyzearalane, which lacks zearalenone's double bond, ketone, and aromatic hydroxyls, was unexpectedly difficult. Similar difficulties were
reported in attempts to prepare di-*o*-methylcurvularin by cyclization of
the hydroxy acid **66** (*68, 69*). Several techniques, including use of

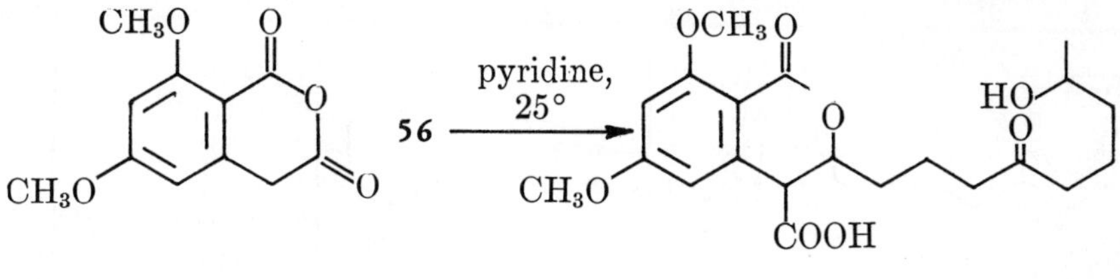

57   56 → pyridine, 25°   **58**

SCHEME V

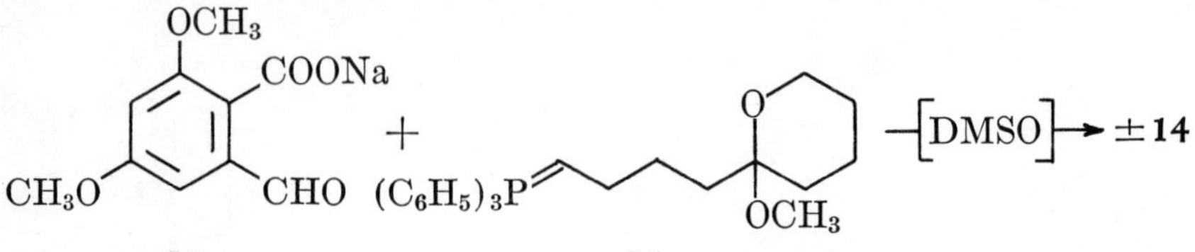

53 54

The Witting-Coupling with sodium salt of the acid **53** proceeded rapidly in good yield.

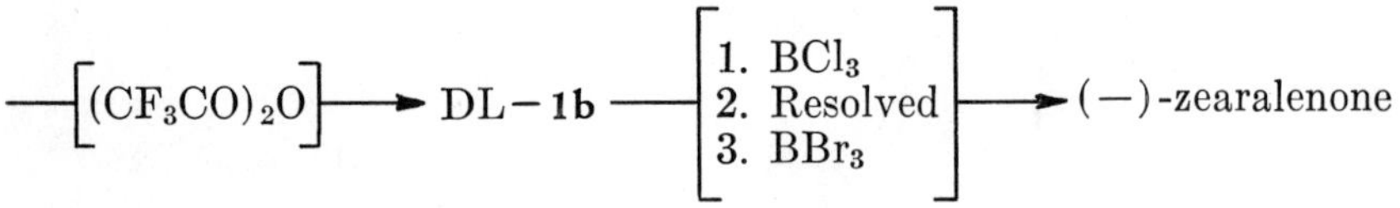

Synthesis of the aromatic nucleus **53**:

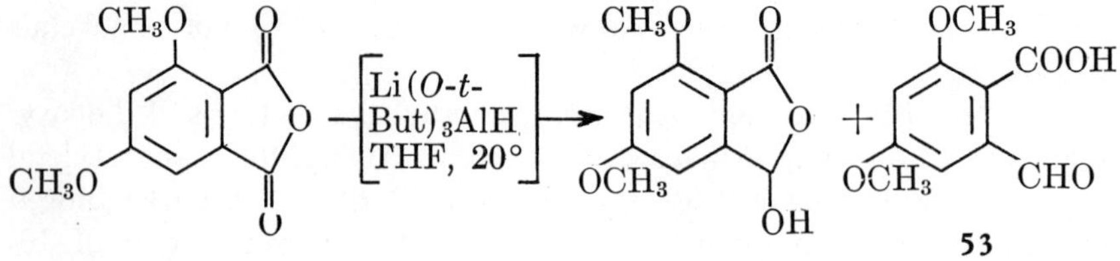

53

Synthesis of the aliphatic component:

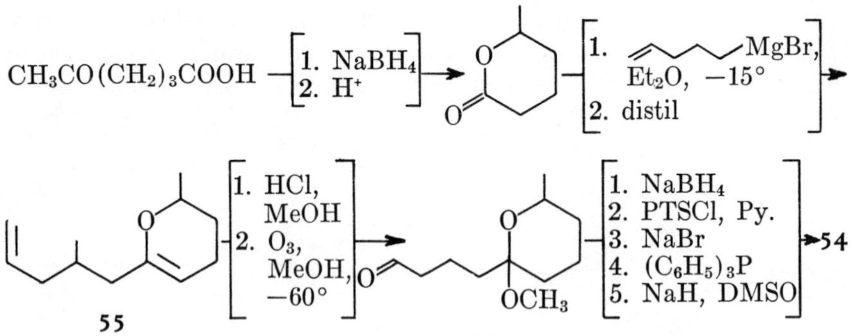

55 56

SCHEME VI

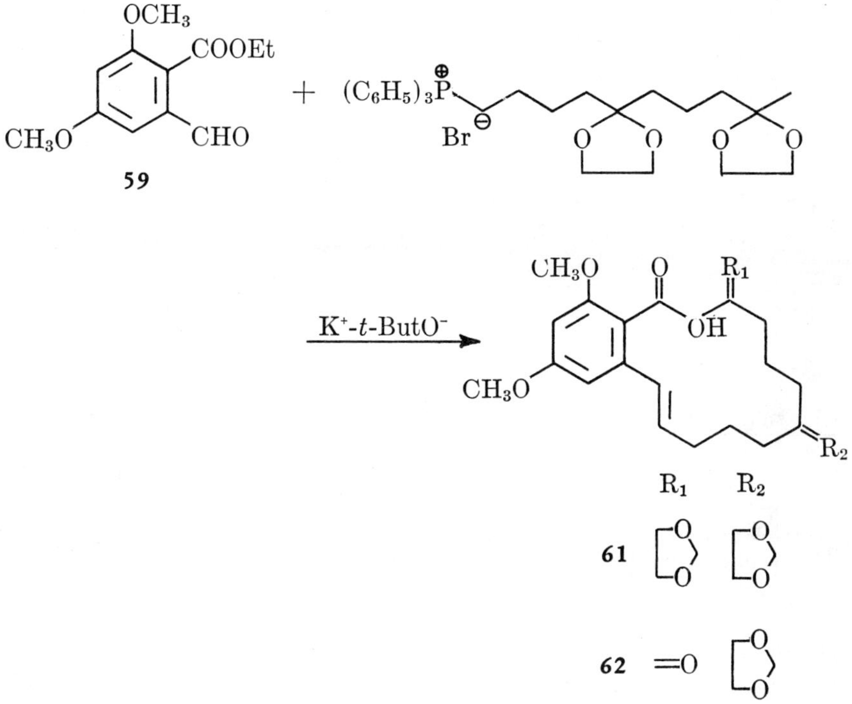

Synthesis of the aromatic component **59**:

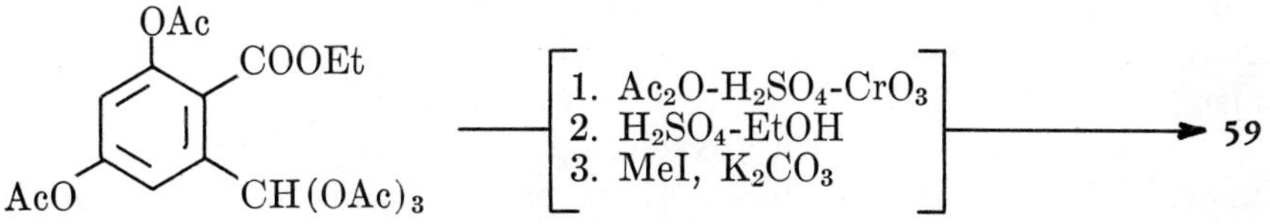

Synthesis of the aliphatic component **60**:

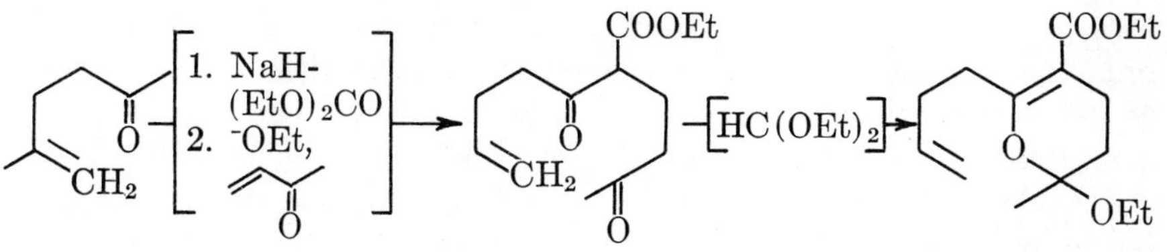

SCHEME VI (*Continued*)

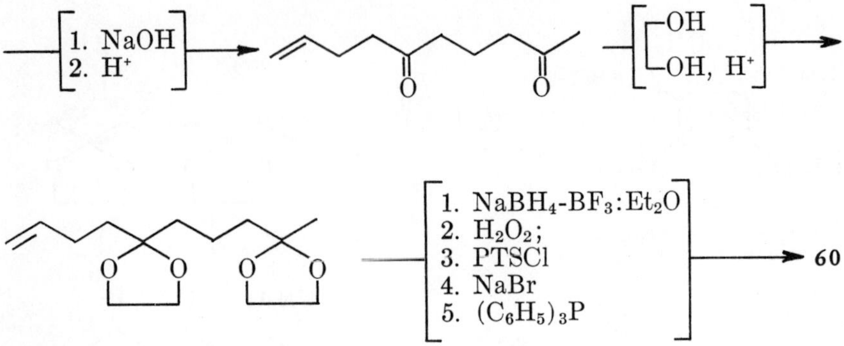

Ring closure:

61 — [Aqueous acetone containing PTS] → **62** — [1. CH_2N_2; 2. $NaBH_4$; 3. HO^-; 4. H^+; 5. BBr_3] → (+)-zearalenone

aluminum isopropoxide, sodium ethoxide with molecular sieves, sodium triphenylmethoxide, sodium hydride, polymeric dibutylin oxide, and trifluoroacetic acid anhydride were used to form the lactone of **64**. Finally it was lactonized to (±)dideoxyzearalane under high dilution conditions in the presence of phosgene and triethylamine in 25% yield. The ring closure of seco acid **14** under less dilute conditions provided zearalenone ether in as high as 80% yield (*21*). The presence of additional functional groups plays an important role in achieving the necessary steric requirements for such cyclizations.

A rather novel approach was developed by Hurd and Shah (*70, 71*) to cyclize macrocyclic structures. The approach essentially involved preparing an appropriately substituted α,ω diester (*see* Refs. *72* and *73*) **67** and its internal Dieckmann condensation to a desired macrolide **69** and **70.** A notable feature of this Dieckmann cyclization is the use of sodium bi(trimethylsilyl)amide, $[(CH_3)_3Si]_2$ NNa, as a base. The conventional base potassium *tert*-butoxide used in refluxing solvents did not appear promising to cyclize **67** because of the basic attack either on the lactone of **69, 70,** or on the ester function of **67.** Sodium bis(trimethylsilyl)amide permitted the cyclization to proceed smoothly in good yield.

A classical method to prepare a large-ring ketone using Thorpe–Ziegler cyclization was also attempted in order to synthesize the zearale-

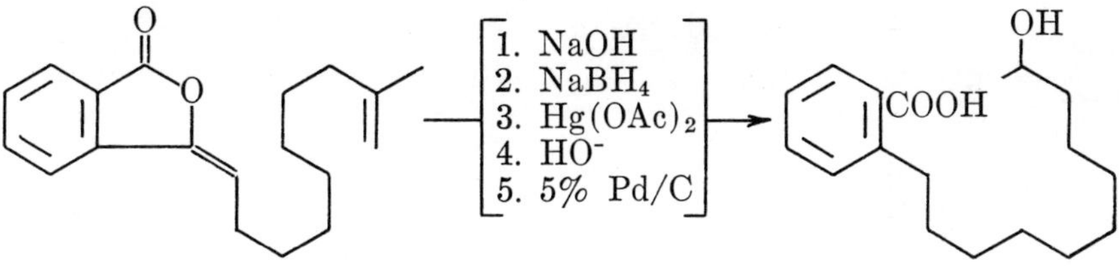

63

64

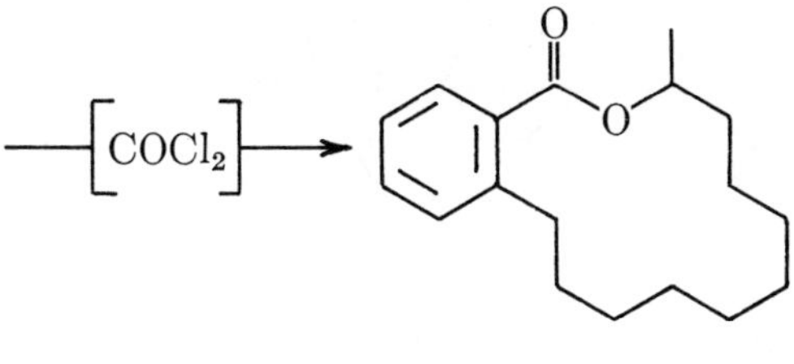

65

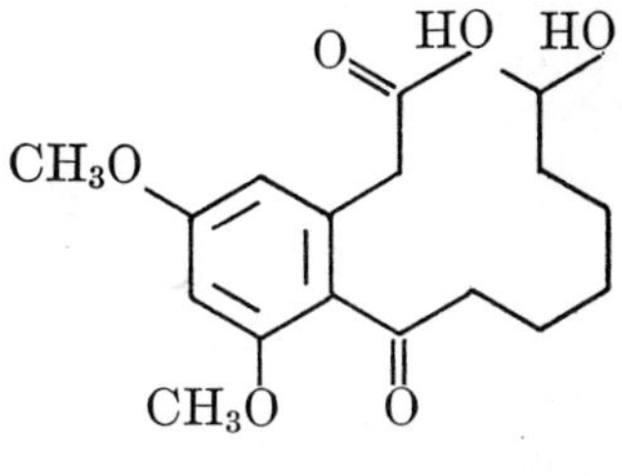

66

none skeleton (*70*). The dinitrile **68** in the presence of a suitable condensing agent [NaN(CH$_3$)C$_6$H$_5$ in ether] was expected to give a mixture of isomeric enamino nitriles **71** and **72** which upon hydrolysis and decarboxylation would yield a zearalenone skeleton. However the enamino nitriles in the presence of base rearranged to yield lactams **73** and **74**.

Synthesis of (±)-di-*o*-methylcurvularin has been reported by Baker et al. (*68*). Their attempts to lactonize the hydroxy acid **66**, as noted before, were unsuccessful. In an alternative route Baker et al. (*68*) obtained the desired macrolide in 14% yield from the acid **75** under the Friedel–Crafts reaction conditions.

Bagli and Immer (*74*) reported the synthesis of a macrolide, 4'-oxo-lasiodiplodin **76**. Since this type of macrolide was not reported to occur naturally at that time, 4'-oxolasiodiplodin was referred to as a biogeneti-

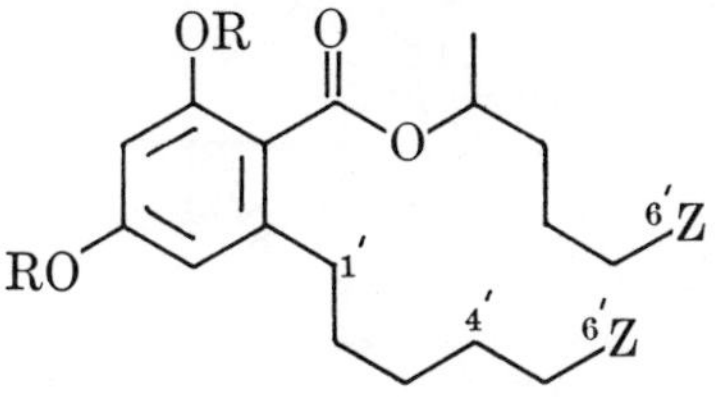

67   Z = COOCH$_3$
68   Z = CN
R = —CH$_2$C$_6$H$_5$

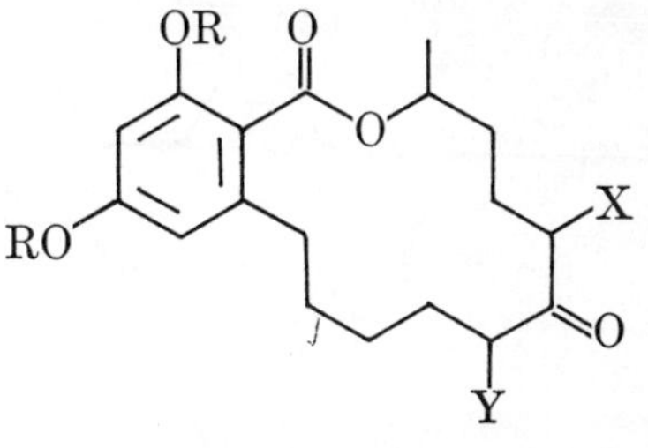

69 X = H, Y = COOCH$_3$
70 X = COOCH$_3$, Y = H

R = —CH₂C₆H₅

75

(CF₃CO)₂O → di-*O*-methylcurvularin

cally possible isomeric curvularin. The key feature in this synthesis (Scheme VII) is the ingenious device of the enole ether **77** which upon oxidation renders the desired macrolide.

Spectral Properties

PMR Spectroscopy of Zearalenone and Related Compounds. The PMR spectral characteristics of zearalenone and its derivatives, although not unique, are representative of the macrolides of the class of β-resorcylates and are presented in Table IV. Typically the aromatic protons of the macrolide constitute an AB system ($J_{AB} = 2.0$–2.5 Hz) and are observed at *ca.* 6.5 ppm. In general the undecenyl ring system is defined by the doublet ($J = 16$ Hz) observed at 6.3–7.1 because of C1' protons,

Table IV.   Chemical Shifts (δ Values) for Protons in Zearalenone and Its Derivatives[c]

	Position					
	C3	*C5*	*C1'*	*C2'*	*C10'*	*C11'*
Zearalenone	6.50d (2.5)	6.39d (2.5)	7.01d (16)	5.63m	5.00m	1.40d (6)
3-Formylzearalenone[a]	—	6.47s	7.04d (16)	5.88m	5.04m	1.45d (6)
5-Formylzearalenone[a]	6.42s	—	7.00d (16)	5.43m	5.20m	1.42d (6)
8'-Hydroxyzearalenone (F-5-3)	6.42d (2.5)	6.30d (2.5)	7.00d (16)	5.62m	5.29m	140d (6)
8'-Hydroxyzearalenone[a] (mp 172°–174°C)	6.51d (2.5)	6.32d (2.5)	7.08d (16)	5.86m	5.60m	1.43d (6)
Zearalen-6',8'-dione[a]	6.67d (2.5)	6.38d (2.5)	6.32d (16)	6.18m	5.44m	1.47d (6)
Zearalen-3',6'-dione[b]	6.43s	6.43s	7.67d (16)	6.47d (16)	—	1.27d (6)
7'-Zearalanone	6.32d (3)	6.25d (3)	—	—	—	1.37d (6)

[a] Ref. *18*.
[b] Ref. *38*.
[c] Coupling constants are given in (Hz): s = singlet, d = doublet, m = multiplet.

SCHEME VII

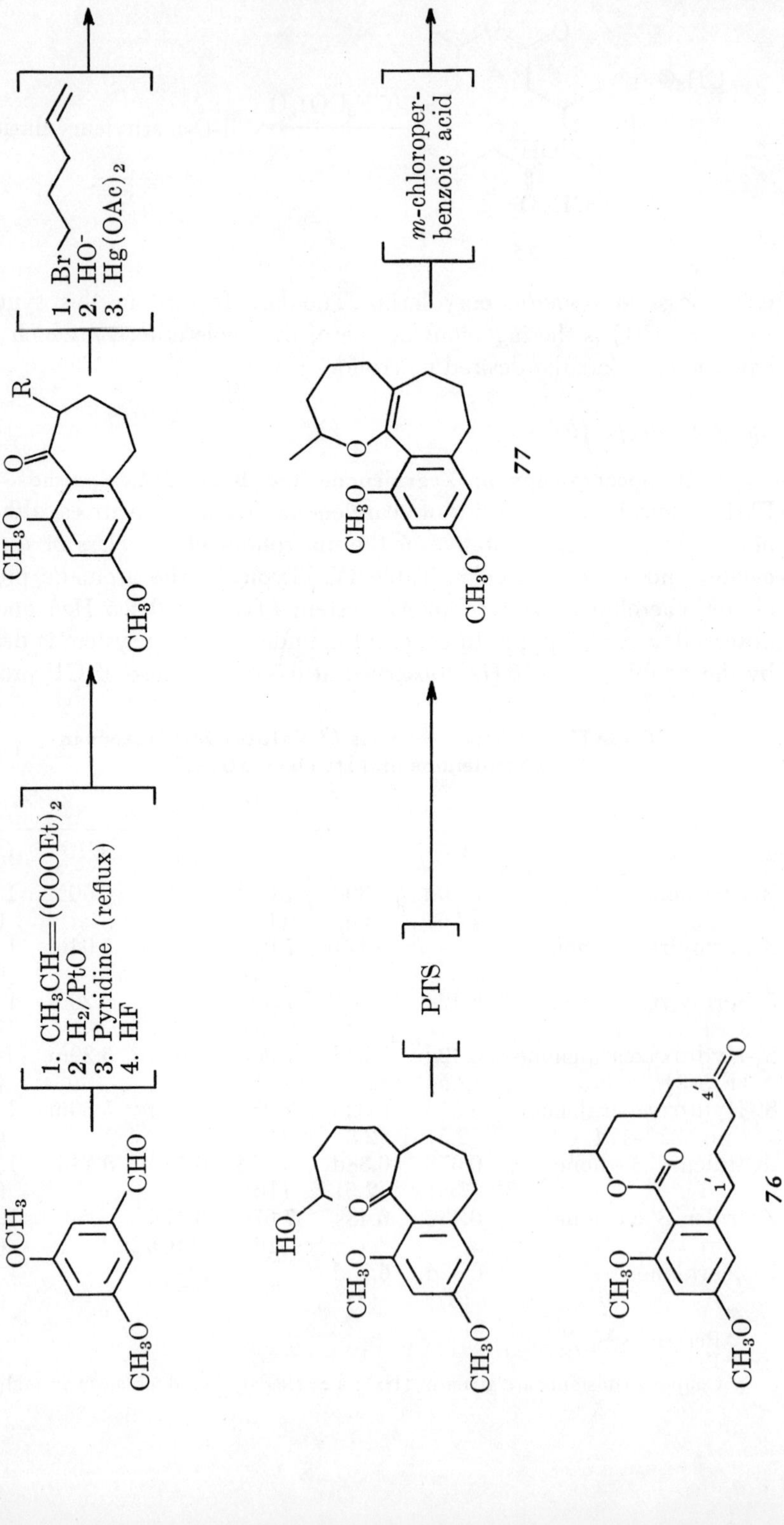

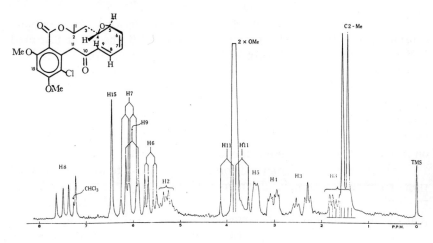

Figure 6.   NMR spectrum of the dimethyl ether of radicicol. (Data from Ref. 53.)

the mutliplet centered around 5.6 because of C2′ and C10′ protons, and a doublet of the C10′ methyl at 0.98 to 1.5 ppm ($J = 6$ Hz). Saturation of the double bond of zearalenone collapses the 1′-H doublet to yield a spectrum similar to that of lasiodiplodin. The benzylic protons of zearalanone and lasiodiplodin render a multiplet at *ca.* 2.5 ppm. This multiplet in the naturally occurring 3,4-dihydroisocoumarins, such as cladosporin, becomes an AB part of the ABX system because of the asymmetry at C3 position (*64*).

The spectrum shown in Figure 6 is that of the dimethyl ether of radicicol and is a rather complex spectrum among the β-resorcylate macrolides. Mirrington et al. (*52, 53*) and McCapra (*51*) during independent studies on the structure of radicicol interpreted the PMR spectra of radicicol and its derivatives. The notable features of the spectrum of radicicol are the presence of complex spin systems involving aliphatic protons at C2, C3, C4, and C5 and protons of the dienone system—*i.e.,* protons at C6, C7, C8, and C9.

The methine protons at C5 and 4 are observed as unresolved multiplets at 3.45 ppm and 3.05 ppm, respectively. The magnitude of the coupling constant ($J_{4,5} = 2.8$ Hz) between these two protons is consistent with the trans configuration of the epoxide. The doublet of triplets at 2.45 ppm together with a doublet of doublets at 1.8 ppm are attributed to C3 geminal protons ($J_{\text{gem}} = 15$ Hz) as revealed by spin decoupling experiments. Further it has been established that the proton resonating at 1–8 ppm is coupled to the C4 proton ($J_{3,4} = 8.6$ Hz).

The olefinic proton region in the spectrum is well resolved. Absorption at 7.5 ppm (doublet of doublets) can be assigned to the C8 proton.

This proton is located trans to the C9 proton as shown by the coupling constant $J_{9,8} = 16$ Hz. The protons at C7 and C6 absorb at 6.15 and 5.65 ppm, respectively. The splitting constant between the C7 and C6 protons is compatible with the cis configuration about the C_6–C_7 bond.

Mass Spectra. Mass spectrometry has proved indispensable in solving structural problems in natural-products chemistry. Considerable literature is available on the mass spectrometry of natural products such as steroids, terpenoids, and alkaloids (75, 76), but little has been published on macrolides such as zearalenone and its derivatives.

Zearalenone is a macrocyclic compound having a fourteen-membered ring. Examination of molecular models shows that the ring is flexible and resembles an aromatic ester in addition to being a lactone. It is expected that upon fragmentation the molecule would yield fragments derived from the aliphatic macrocyclic ring and those containing the aromatic nucleus. Peaks at m/e^+ 41, 51, 69, 122, 125, and 151 arise from the aliphatic moiety while those between m/e^+ 161 and 318 contain an aromatic ring (8). This has been demonstrated elegantly using a bromine-substitute derivative of zearalenone (17). The presence of bromine atoms in the fragment is quite diagnostic because of its isotopic doublet occurring

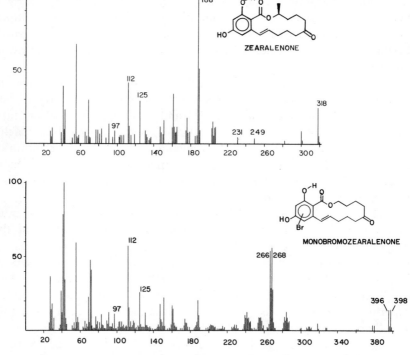

Figure 7.   Mass spectra of zearalenone and monobromozearalenone

in approximately equal abundance separated by two mass units. In addition a bromine substituted on an aromatic ring would not be expected to be lost readily during fragmentation in the mass spectrometer. Therefore the fragments involving an aromatic ring of zearalenone show the apparent shift in the mass spectrum of monobromozearalenone, *i.e.*, bromine on the aromatic ring (Figure 7). The shift in mass is demonstrated by m/e^+ 318 in the zearalenone spectrum; it is shifted to a clean doublet at m/e^+ 396 and 398 in monobromozearalenone. The fragment at m/e^+ 188 is shifted to m/e^+ 266 and 268, and m/e^+ 300 to m/e^+ 378 and 380.

Studies on some major fragments reveal that the differences observed among the spectra of derivatives of zearalenone are best rationalized on the basis of the stabilities of the ions and neutral species produced by fragmentation. The lactone carbonyl and the methyl protons are so oriented that the McLafferty rearrangement (*see* Ref. 77) smoothly converts zearalenone to the open-chain terminal olefin **78**. A simple α-cleavage of **78**, well known in the mass spectra of aliphatic ketones, generates fragment **79** which loses a molecule of water to give a fairly intense ion **80** at m/e^+ 231. A metastable ion observed at m/e^+ 214 substantiates the pathway.

When zearalenone loses an electron from the aromatic portion, it produces a radical cation capable of delocalizing the positive charge over the entire aromatic portion; it subsequently breaks down to **81** and **82**

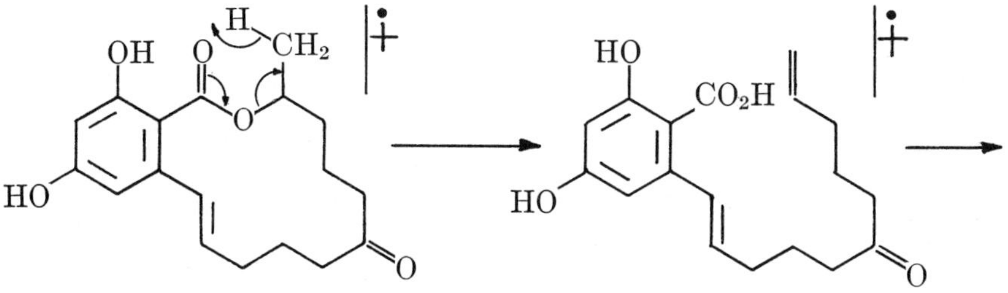

78

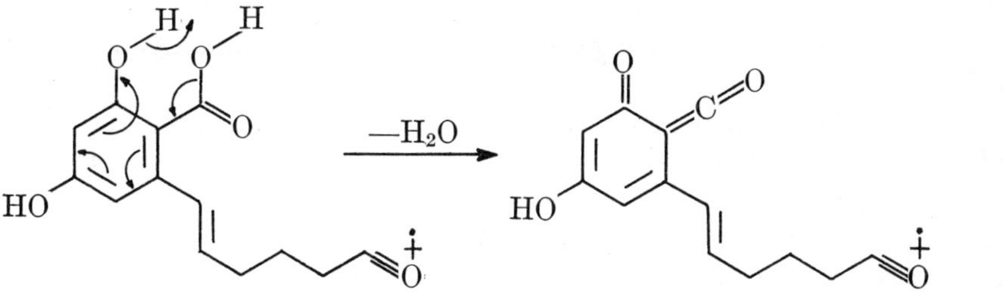

79   —H₂O   **80**

SCHEME VIII·

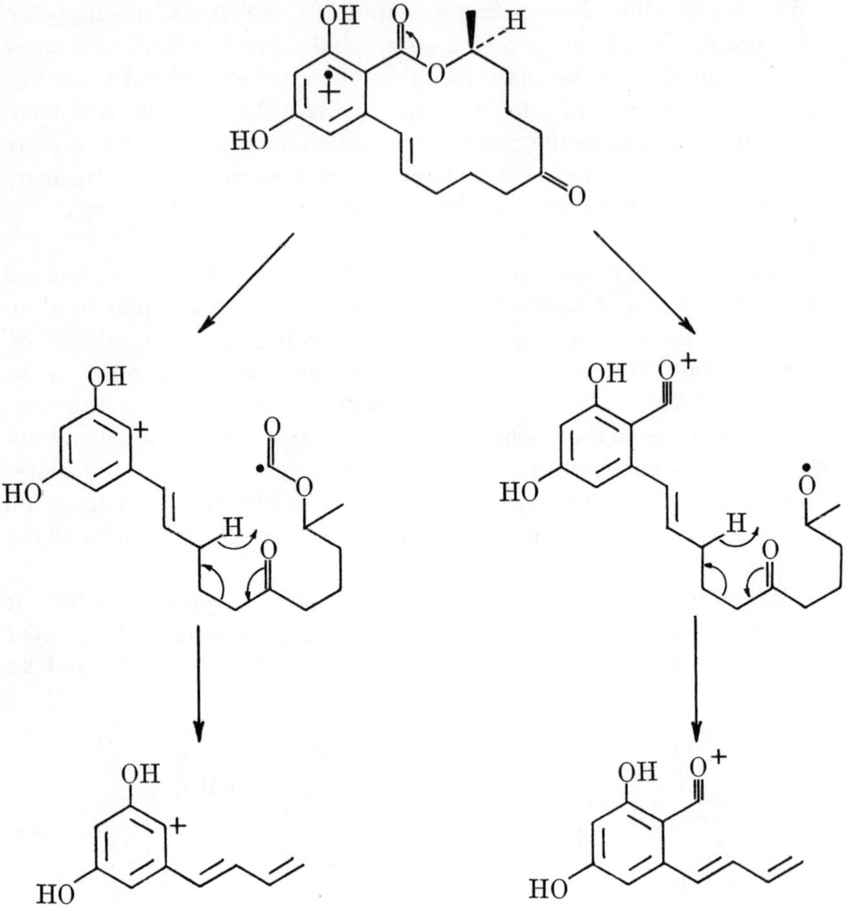

81   82

as shown in Scheme VIII. High resolution mass spectroscopy of zearalenone, monobromozearalenone, and other derivatives provides sufficient
evidence for the above fragmentation (Table V). The rearranged
molecular ion **78** also participates in another fragmentation process as
described in Scheme IX.

m/e^+ **179.** Formation of this fragment apparently requires overlap
of the π bonds of the carboxylic acid carbonyl and the C_1 olefin in the
ion **78.** When this condition is not satisfied, the formation of such a
fragment becomes an unimportant process. Zearalanone without the
olefinic bond gives an equivalent peak (at 181) of only 1% of the base
peak.

Table V.   Fragments Produced by Pathways in Scheme VIII

	Fragment 81 m/e	Fragment 82 m/e
Zearalenone	161	189
Monobromozearalenone	239, 241	267, 269
2,4-Dimethoxyzearalenone	189	217
2,4-Dideuteroxyzearalenone (d_2)	163	191
2,4-Di-trimethylsilyloxyzearalenone	305	333

SCHEME IX

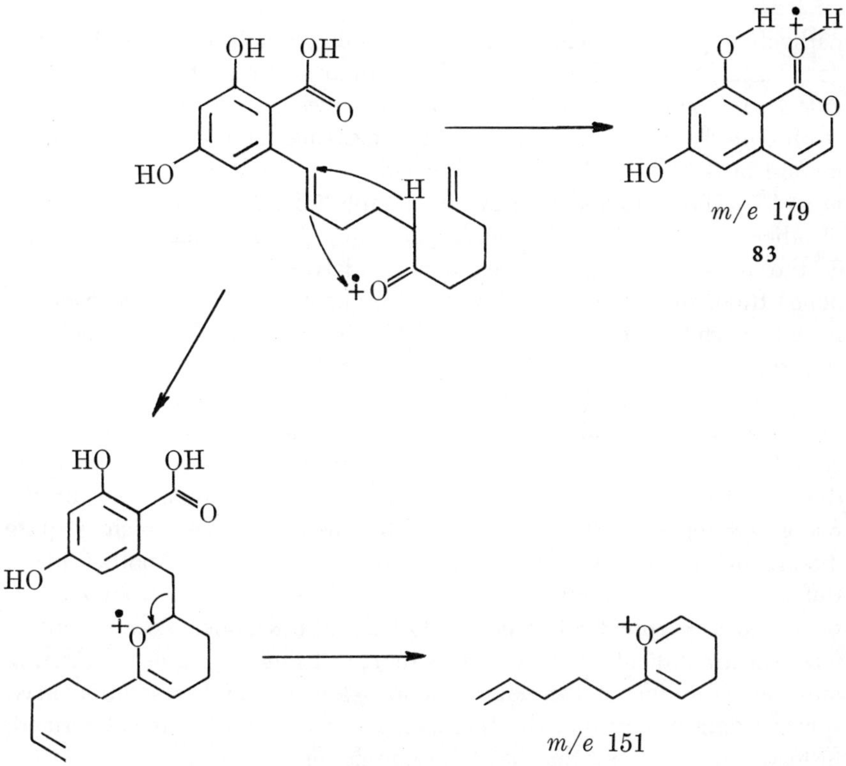

m/e 179

83

m/e 151

84

m/e$^+$ 151. This fragment arises from the aliphatic portion of the ion 78 and also requires the presence of a double bond. The fragment is absent in the mass spectrum of zearalanone. Evidence is provided by the high resolution mass spectroscopy of the deuterium-labeled zearalenone (Table VI).

Fragments with *m/e*$^+$ of 97, 112, and 125. These peaks arise by the

Table VI.   Fragments Produced by Pathways in Scheme IX

	Fragment 83		Fragment 84	
	Elemental Composition	m/e^+	Elemental Composition	m/e^+
Zearlanone-d_0	$C_{10}H_{15}O$	151.1122	$C_9H_7O_4$	179.0344
2,4,5,5,7,7,-Hexadeu- terozearalenone (86% d_6)	$C_{10}H_{12}OD_3$	154.1310	$C_9H_5O_4D_2$	181.0476
2,4-Dimethoxyzearale- none	$C_{10}H_{12}O$	151.1103	$C_{11}H_{11}O_4$	207.0656

pathway depicted in Scheme X. The rearranged molecular ion 78 undergoes basically three cleavages involving an aliphatic portion of the molecule zearalenone. Allylic cleavage at C3′ gives a fragment at m/e^+ 125; a McLafferty rearrangement causes a cleavage at C4′ to produce an intense peak at m/e^+ 112. In addition the usual α-cleavage at C5′ yields m/e^+ 97. These fragments provide valuable information on the location of other substituents on the macrocyclic ring. It was noted (17, 18) that in the naturally occurring zearalenone derivative (8′-hydroxyzearalenone) fragments m/e^+ 97, 112, and 125 in the zearalenone mass spectrum have been shifted to m/e^+ 95, 110 and 123, respectively. It was concluded that the hydroxyl group is located at C8′ (Scheme XI).

Modification of the lactone ring causes significant changes in the mass spectra of zearalenone (40), generally causing an increase in its complexity. Mass spectra of zearalanone derivatives have spectra quite different from the corresponding zearalenone derivatives. One of the major differences is the formation of fragment type 84 which is quite intense in the mass spectra of zearalenone derivatives. Another major difference is the formation of a fragment 81 at m/e^+ 161 from zearalenone and a fragment 86 at m/e^+ 163 from zearalanone. Low resolution mass spectra indicates that the peaks represent similar fragments differing only by saturation of the double bond. However high resolution mass spectral data proves that the fragment 86 at $m/e^+ = 163$ is not formed; instead a fragment 87 that has the same nominal mass as fragment 86 is formed as shown in Scheme XII (40).

Jensen et al. (38) noted that isomeric zearalanone (zearalan-7′-one) undergoes an initial McLafferty rearrangement at the lactone followed by α cleavage (b) to yield 88, or a McLafferty rearrangement at the ketone (a) to yield 89 as shown in the Scheme XIII. However we noticed a discrepancy in the fragments and their corresponding masses. Fragments 88 and 89 are not formed by the cleavages at (b) and (a), respectively, nor do they have corresponding values of $m/e^+ = 265$ and 98.

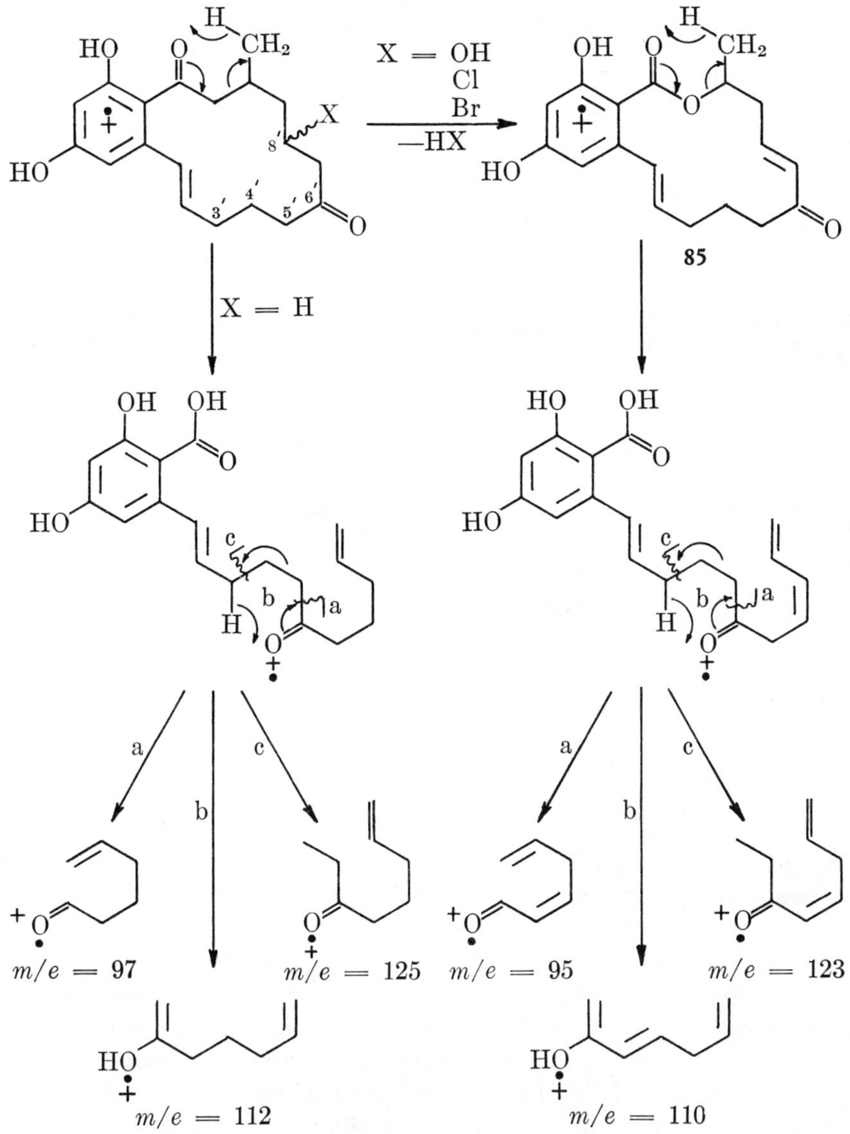

X = OH
Cl
Br

$\xrightarrow{-HX}$

85

X = H

a

b

c

m/e = 97

m/e = 125

m/e = 112

SCHEME X

a

b

c

m/e = 95

m/e = 123

m/e = 110

SCHEME XI

Instead fragments **90** (m/e^+ 265) and **91** (m/e^+ 98) are formed by a cleavage at (b) or (a) respectively. Nevertheless this mode of fragmentation provides valuable information regarding the location of the ketone group in the macrocyclic lactone. Thus peaks at m/e^+ 265 and 98 in the 7'-keto isomer are shifted to m/e^+ 237 and 126 in 5'-keto derivative.

SCHEME XII

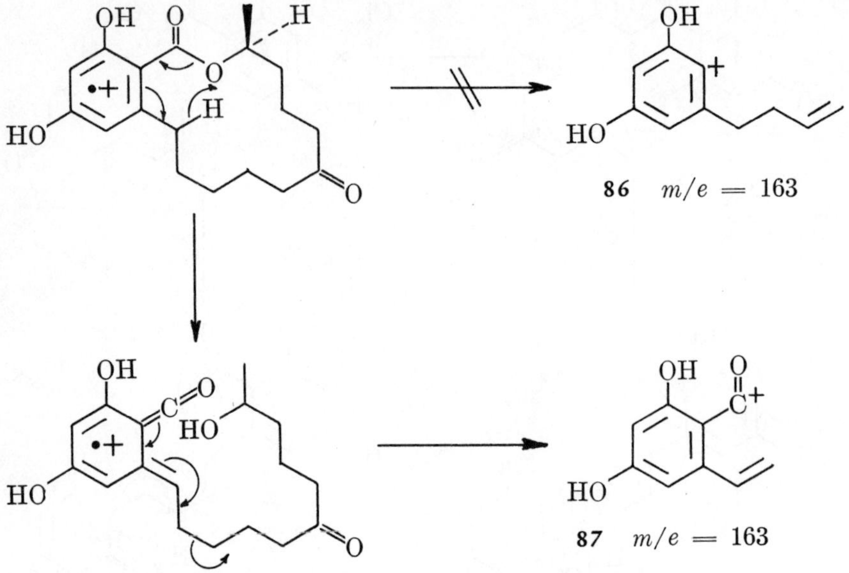

86 $m/e = 163$

87 $m/e = 163$

Since zearalenone and its derivatives exhibit similar uv, ir, and NMR spectral properties, distinction from each other using only these methods is usually difficult. Mass spectrometry is unique in providing a solution to the problem, and GC–MS offers even greater advantage in terms of sensitivity. For example, detection and identification of zearalenone in corn using TLC and GLC have been described (78); however the background interference becomes significant when the zearalenone level in the sample is too low (< 20 ppb), and precise identification becomes a critical problem. Such sample extracts, after proper clean-up, are converted into trimethylsilylether derivatives and are analyzed by GC–MS. An example of such an extract is illustrated in Figure 8a where multiple components are found, and zearalenone is buried among them. A mass spectral scan of the peak as shown in Figure 9 can be taken, and identification can be made by the fragmentation pattern. Alternatively, identification can be made by multiple ion detection, i.e., focusing on diagnostic fragments (m/e^+ 305, 333) of the TMS ether of zearalenone while it is being separated on the GLC column (Figure 8b).

Fluorescence

Zearalenone and its many derivatives exhibit fluorescence when irradiated by uv light. This property has been useful in identifying these compounds on TLC plates. Examination of derivatives of zearalenone

SCHEME XIII

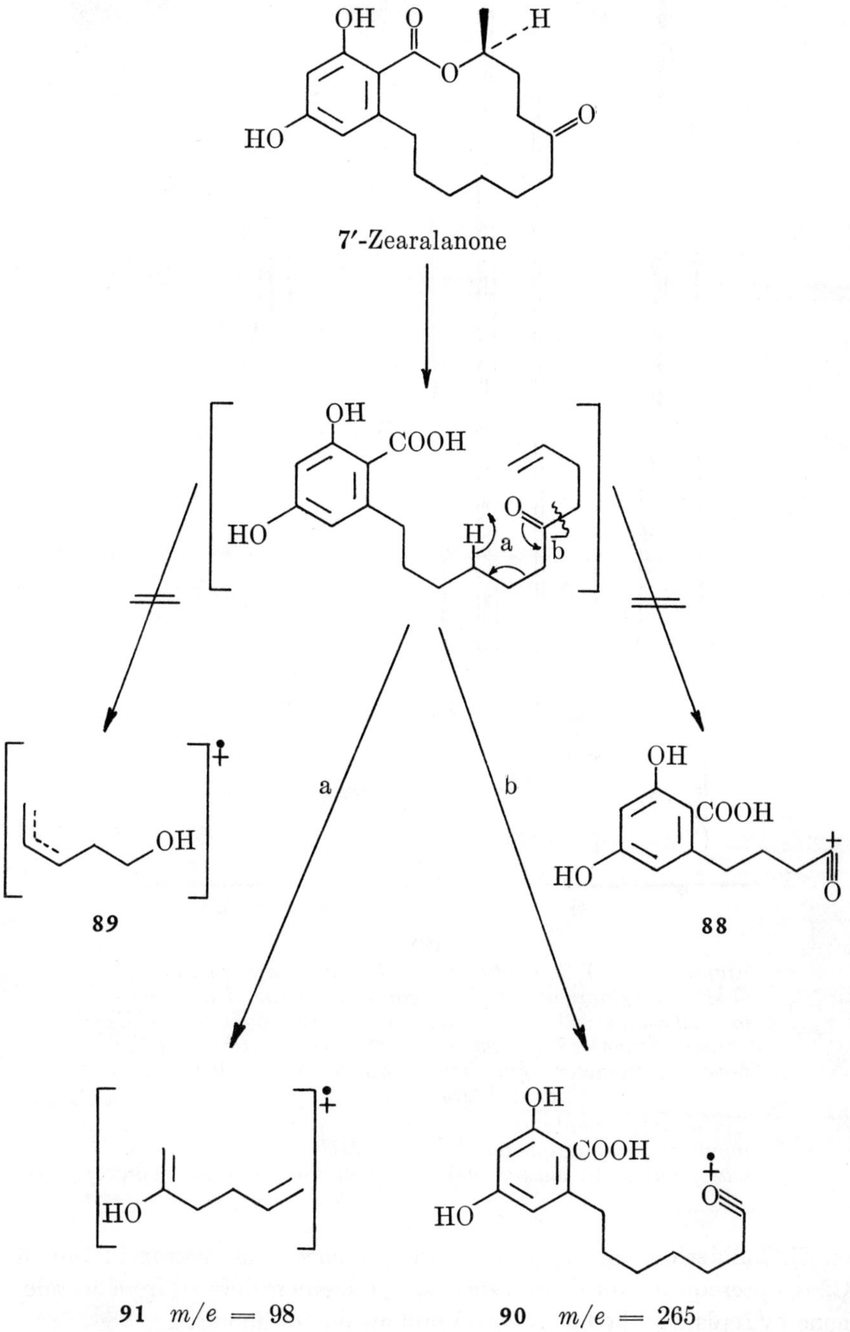

7'-Zearalanone

89

88

91 *m/e* = 98

90 *m/e* = 265

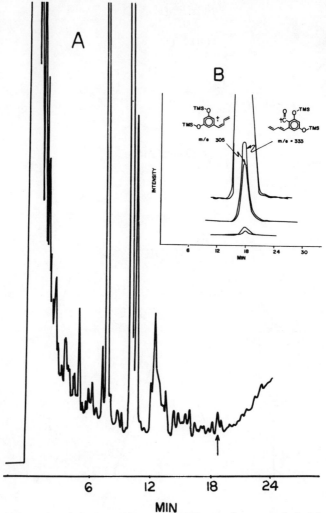

Figure 8. (A) Separation by GLC of the trimethylsilyl
(TMS) ether derivatives of the constituents found in a commercial swine ration. The response measured in the GLC
chromatogram is the total ion current as monitored by the
mass spectrometer. The arrow indicates a peak thought to
be di-TMS-zearalenone.

(B) Mass fragmentogram of the sample as shown in A when
monitored by multiple ion detection (MID). The ion monitor
was focused on masses 305 and 333; their structures are
shown.

on TLC under uv light showed that the presence of an hydroxyl group at
C2 is a prerequisite for fluorescence—i.e., the ethers derived from zearalenone by replacing the C2 hydroxyl protons do not fluoresce.

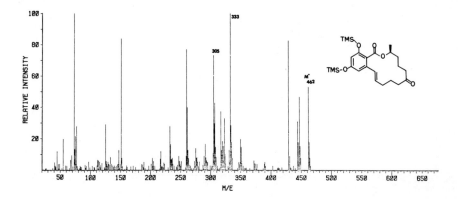

Figure 9.   Mass spectrum of the di-TMS-ether of zearalenone

The fluorescent properties of several simple compounds were examined on TLC plates under uv light. Salicylic acid and ethyl β-resorcylate appear blue fluorescent, and acetyl salicylic acid does not. Coplanarity of the lactone carbonyl and C2 hydroxyl group of zearalenone is also essential since any conformational change that destroys coplanarity eliminates fluorescence. A molecular model (Dreiding) of zearalenone reveals that the presence of a double bond in the 1′,2′ position is necessary to maintain the coplanarity of the lactone carbonyl and C2 hydroxyl group. Thus the removal of double bonds, as in zearalanone derivatives, renders them nonfluorescent.

Biosynthesis

The substitution pattern of the various macrolides discussed indicates that these metabolites are polyketides—*i.e.*, they are formed by condensation of acetyl or acyl units with malonyl units and concomitant decarboxylation as in fatty acid biosynthesis but without obligatory reduction of the intermediate β-dicarbonyl system (*79, 80*). The resulting poly-β-ketomethylene (polyketide) system has activated methylene groups that can take part in internal aldol-type condensation to give aromatic compounds.

In the study of the biosynthesis of zearalenone, acetate-1-^{14}C, diethyl malonate-2-^{14}C, shikimate-G^{14}C, senecioate-1-^{14}C, and DL-mevalonic-2-^{14}C-acid lactone were used in isotope incorporation studies, but only acetate and diethyl malonate were readily incorporated into zearalenone in as little as 1 min. ^{14}CO$_2$ was also readily fixed by *Fusarium roseum* and was incorporated into zearalenone in as short a time as 5 min. The mechanism involved in this incorporation is not known, but CO$_2$ is probably fixed into a dicarboxylic acid (*e.g.*, oxalacetic acid), cycled through the tri-

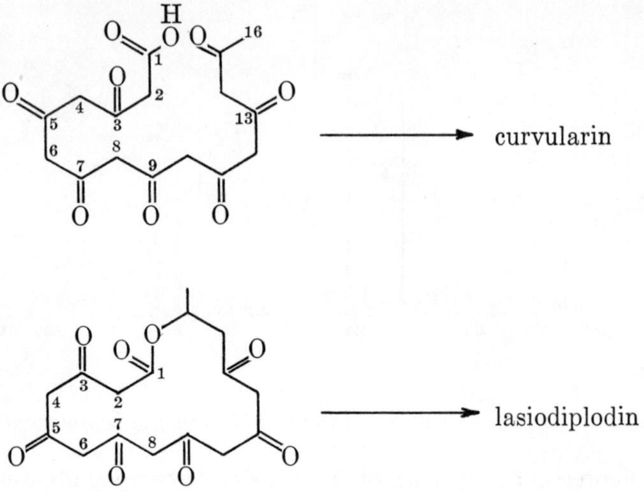

Figure 10. Cyclization of the octaketide chain to form curvularin and lasiodiplodin

carboxylic acid cycle, and then metabolized to acetate units which are then incorporated.

Malonate competes with acetate—*i.e.*, it lowers the incorporation of acetate into zearalenone when placed in competition. The data are consistent with the synthesis of zearalenone via the acetate–malonyl-CoA pathway. This was confirmed by studies of the incorporation of acetate-1-^{14}C followed by chemical degradation; the results are compatible with the polyketide pathway as shown in Figure 4.

Radicicol is also believed to be derived from nine acetate units (53). Similarly, curvularin, as noted before, has been shown to arise from eight acetate units (58). Lasiodiplodin, an octaketide, is derived by an alternative cyclization of the precursor of curvularin (Figure 10).

Structure and Biological Activity

The estrogenic activity of the various derivatives of zearalenone is listed in Table VII and is based on the increase in weight of the uterus of the mouse as described by Dorfman and Dorfman (*81*). As a basis of comparison the uterotropic activity of the various derivatives is compared with zearalenone and diethylstilbestrol (DES), respectively.

Zearalenone is approximately 0.0005 times as active as DES but is frequently encountered in nature in concentrations (0.1–200 ppm) sufficient to account for signs of hyperestrogenism in farm animals. One of its most active derivatives (epimer A of 7'-carboxyzearalane) is almost one-tenth as active as DES and 192 times more active than its parent compound. However the carboxy derivative has not been found in nature. Note that the formyl derivative (epimer B of 7'-formylzearalane) is almost as active as the 7'-carboxy derivative; this compound is less stable than the carboxy derivative, and this might explain its loss of activity. Also note that the functional group at the C6' position can be varied and moved on the undecenyl ring of zearalenone until optimum activity is achieved.

Simple reduction of the vinyl group of zearalenone and zearalenol will increase the uterotropic response, and this enhancement, although sometimes slight, appears to hold true throughout the series. As an example, substituting the 6'-ketone with a hydroxyl group concomitant with reduction of the 1',2' double bond yields two diasterioisomers identified by their differential melting points. The zearalanol isomer with the higher melting point (178°–180°C) is about 1.5 times more active than the isomer with the lower melting point (146°–148°C), and both are more active than zearalenone. Both isomers are slightly less active when the 1',2' double bond is not reduced. All estrogenic activity is lost when all functional groups are reduced as in dideoxyzearalane. On the other hand zearalane is just as active as zearalenone, which illustrates that the phenolic hydroxyl groups are necessary prerequisites for activity whereas the 6'-ketone is not.

Hurd and Shah (*71*) compared the uterotropic activity of S-zearalenone (naturally occurring) with the synthetic R,S-zearalanone. The S-zearalanone was about twice as active as the naturally occurring S-zearalenone; the R-zearalanone had about 0.6 the activity of S-zearalenone.

Peters (*42*) compared the activity of the cis and trans (naturally occurring) isomers of zearalenone and found that the cis isomer had about the same activity as the trans one. However in the zearalenol series the cis isomers of the diasterioisomers (high and low melting point) were significantly more active than their respective trans isomers.

Johnston et al. (*30*) studied the effect of the phenolic hydroxyls on the aromatic ring and on estrogenic activity. The 2,4-dideoxyzearalanone and 4-deoxyzearalanone derivatives retained less than 0.2 the activity of zearalenone, although 2-deoxyzearalanone was about 1.3 times more active. The 5-hydroxyzearalanone derivative retained less than 0.6 the activity of zearalenone. According to Johnston et al. (*30*) the greater activity of 2-deoxyzearalanone was somehow related to conformational restriction which H bonding of the lactone carbonyl imposed on the molecule. The 2,4-dimethoxy and 4-methoxy derivatives of zearalenone retained 6% of the activity of zearalenone, and 2-methoxyzearalenone retained about 20% (*82*).

Table VII.   Estrogenic Activity, Based on Uterotropic
Activity is Compared with

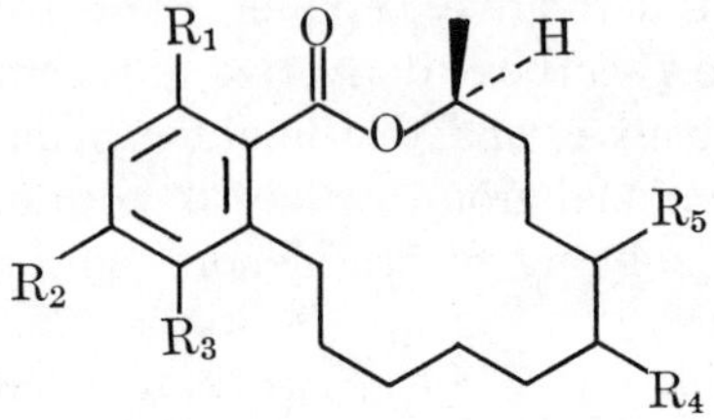

Compound	R_1	R_2
Zearalane	OH	OH
Zearalanol (HM) [a]	OH	OH
Zearalanol (LM) [b]	OH	OH
(S)-zearalanone	OH	OH
(R)-zearalanone	OH	OH
7'-Formyl zearalane (isomeric mixture)	OH	OH
7'-Formyl zearalane (epimer A,mp 141°–146°C)	OH	OH
7'-Formyl zearalane (epimer B,mp 148°–152°C)	OH	OH
7'-Carboxy zearalane (epimeric mixture)	OH	OH
7'-Carboxy zearalane (epimer A)	OH	OH
7'-Carboxy zearalane (epimer B)	OH	OH
2-Deoxyzearalanone	H	OH
4-Deoxyzearalanone	OH	H
2,4-Dideoxyzearalanone	H	H
5-Hydroxyzearalanone	OH	OH
5-Nitrozearalanone	OH	OH
2,4-Diacetoxyzearalanol	OAc	OAc
6'-Acetylzearalane	OH	OH
2,4-Dimethoxyzearalenone	—	—
4-Methoxyzearalenone	—	—
2-Methoxyzearalenone	—	—
Zearalenone 1	—	—
Diethylstilbestrol (DES)	—	—

[a] High melting point.
[b] Low melting point.

Conclusions and Discussion

The beta resorcylate macrolides, although not commonly encountered in nature, are extremely interesting because of their chemical
structure and physiological activity. Zearalenone, one of the structurally
less complex members of this class in spite of its large lactone ring, is
surprisingly stable to hydrolytic cleavage. This is partly attributed to

**Response in the Mouse of Various Derivatives of Zearalenone.
Zearalenone and Diethylstibestrol**

R_3	R_4	R_5	Uterotropic Activity Relative to: Zearalenone	DES	Ref
H	H_2	H_2	0.22-1.0	0.0001-0.0005	82
H	OH	H_2	4.8	0.0024	82
H	OH	H_2	2.7	0.0013	82
H	$=$O	H_2	2.0	0.0010	82
H	$=$O	H_2	0.63	0.0003	22
H	H_2	—CHO	50.0	0.025	83
H	H_2	—CHO	18.0	0.009	83
H	H_2	—CHO	94.0	0,047	83
H	H_2	—COOH	100.0	0.050	83
H	H_2	—COOH	192.0	0.096	83
H	H_2	—COOH	18.0	0.009	83
H	$=$O	H_2	1.26	0.00063	30
H	$=$O	H_2	< 0.2	< 0.0001	30
H	$=$O	H_2	< 0.2	< 0.0001	30
OH	$=$O	H_2	< 0.6	< 0.0003	30
NO_2	$=$O	H_2	1.4	0.0007	84
H	OH H	H_2	3.8	0.0019	84
H	OAc	H_2	2.0	0.0010	84
—	—	—	0.06	0.000003	82
—	—	—	0.06	0.000003	82
—	—	—	0.22	0.000017	82
—	—	—	1.0	0.0005	82
—	—	—	2000.0	1.0	82

the presence of a secondary methyl group that hinders the nucleophilic attack on the lactone carbonyl. The 1',2' trans double bond of zearalenone is electron poor as revealed by its resistance to bromination, epoxidation, and hydroboration. The allylic oxidation of zearalenone with chromium trioxide in pyridine was affected by the substituent (ketone or hydroxyl) at the C6' position. A ketone at C6' activates both alpha methylene positions (C5' and C7'). The base-catalyzed acylation (and alkylation) of zearalenone indicates that an enolate anion at C7' is preferentially formed. Although the reason (kinetic or thermodynamic) for such a preference is not known, it appears that the C7' position is sterically less hindered; therefore the proton abstraction and alkylation at C7' occur rapidly and preferentially. Base-catalyzed enolization of zearalenone needs to be explored in greater depth since these enolates serve as potential precursors of a variety of 7'-substituted zearalanes.

The approaches discussed for synthesis of zearalenone and related macrolides are based on conventional methods: the direct cyclization of a hydroxy acid and ester (21, 36, 67) and the peracid oxidation of bicyclic enole ethers (85). Successful synthesis of zearalenone by the latter method has not been described, although it holds promise as a successful mode of synthesis. Nevertheless Bagli and Immer (74) successfully synthesized an isomeric curvularin (4'-oxolasiodiplodin) using the peracid oxidation method. The synthesis developed by Hurd and Shah (70) is an extension of an intramolecular acetoacetic ester condensation called the Dieckmann condensation which leads to β keto esters. The reversibility of this condensation reaction normally restricts its use to diesters that can yield five- and six-membered ring products. However Hurd and Shah were able to cyclize the α,ω diester to the desired β keto ester 69, 70 successfully and in good yield.

Mass spectrometry has proved to be invaluable in elucidating the structure of zearalenone. Fragments such as 81 (m/e^+ 161) and 82 (m/e^+ 189) shown in Scheme VIII are useful in locating substituents on the aromatic ring. The fragments depicted in Scheme X provide information regarding the substituents at positions 4' through 9' together with the location of the ketone group. Thus fragments at m/e^+ 97, 112, and 125 are diagnostic for zearalenone, and those at 95, 110, and 123 are characteristic of the 8'-hydroxyzearalenones.

As far as we could determine no OH substituted, zearalenone derivative at C3', C4', or C5' has been found in nature; such substitution at C3' and C5' does not normally occur in the acetate, biosynthetic pathway. However the absence of a C4'-substituted derivative and the occurrence of C8' derivatives indicate that the hydroxylation reaction probably occurs after the formation of zearalenone rather than on the nascent polyketide chain.

Zearalenone is biosynthesized via the acetate–malonyl-CoA metabolic pathway, and this has been confirmed by studies involving degradation of the molecule after assimilation of ^{14}C from acetate. $^{14}CO_2$ is readily incorporated into the molecule, but the method of its fixation to accommodate such incorporation has not been studied.

The study of structure–activity relationships indicates that: (a) the hydroxyl at C2 is necessary for activity; (b) the cis isomers of the zearalenol series are more active than the trans isomers; (c) simple reduction of the vinyl group in the ring enhances activity; (d) all activity is lost in the dideoxyzearalane product; and (e) 7'-carboxyzearalane is the most active derivative of the series—*i.e.*, 192 times more active than zearalenone.

Literature Cited

1. Mirocha, C. J., Christensen, C. M., Nelson, G. H., "Microbial Toxins," VII, Chapter 4, Academic, New York, 1971.
2. Mirocha, C. J., Christensen, C. M., "Oestrogenic Mycotoxins Synthesized by *Fusarium*," in "Mycotoxins," I. F. H. Purchase, Ed., Elsevier, Amsterdam, 1974.
3. Buxton, E. A., *Vet. Med.* (1927) **22**, 451.
4. Legenhausen, A. H., *Vet. Med.* (1928) **23**, 29.
5. McNutt, S. H., Purwin, P., Murray, C., *J. Amer. Vet. Med. Ass.* (1928) **73**, 484.
6. Stobb, M., Baldwin, R. S., Tuite, J., Andrews, F. N., Gillette, K. G., *Nature* (1972) **196**, 1318.
7. Christensen, C. M., Nelson, G. H., Mirocha, C. J., *Appl. Microbiol.* (1965) **13**, 653.
8. Urry, W. H., Wehrmeister, H. L., Hodge, E. B., Hidy, P. H., *Tetrahedron Lett.* (1966) **27**, 3109–3114.
9. Wolf, J. C., Mirocha, C. J., *Can. J. Microbiol.* (1973) **19**, 725–734.
10. Wolf, J. C., "Studies on Regulation of Sexual Reproduction in *Fusarium roseum* 'Graminearum'," Ph.D. Thesis, University of Minnesota, 1975.
11. Nelson, R. R., "Morphological and Biochemical Events in Plant–Parasite Interaction," S. Akai, S. Ouchi, Eds., The Phytopathological Society of Japan, Tokyo, 1971.
12. Kuo, C. H., Taub, D., Hoffsommer, R. D., Wendler, N. L., Urry, W. H., Mullenbach, G., *Chem. Commun.* (1967) 761–762.
13. Morrison, J. D., Mosher, H. S., "Asymmetric Organic Reactions," pp. 30–34, Prentice-Hall, New Jersey, 1971.
14. Horeau, A., *Tetrahedron Lett.* (1961) 506.
15. Horeau, A., *Tetrahedron Lett.* (1962) 965.
16. Horeau, A., Kagan, H. B., *Tetrahedron* (1964) **20**, 2431.
17. Jackson, R. A., Fenton, S. W., Mirocha, C. J., Davis, G., *J. Agric. Food Chem.* (1974) **22**, 1015–1019.
18. Bolliger, G., Tamm, Ch., *Helv. Chim. Acta* (1972) **55**, 3030–3048.
19. Taylor, I. F. Jr., Watson, W. H., *Spg. Meetg. Amer. Crystallogr. Ass.* Abstract **G6**, Charlottesville, Va., 1975.
20. Steele, J. A., Ph.D. Thesis, University of Minnesota, 1974.
21. Taub, D., Girotra, N. N., Hoffsommer, R. D., Kuo, C. H., Slates, H. L., Weber, S., Wendler, N. L., *Tetrahedron* (1968) **24**, 2443–2461.
22. Peters, A. C., Hurd, R. N., *J. Med. Chem.* (1975) **18**, 215–217.
23. Wildholz, T. B., Brown, R. D., *J. Org. Chem.* (1972) **37**, 1647–1651.
24. Hodge, E. B., Hidy, P. H., Wehrmeister, H. L., U.S. Patent **3,373,028** (1968).
25. Parham, W. E., "Syntheses and Reactions in Organic Chemistry," pp. 355–356, John Wiley & Sons, New York, 1970.
26. Wynberg, H., *Chem. Rev.* (1960) **60**, 169.
27. Crounse, N. N., *Org. React.* (1949) **V**, 290.
28. Truce, W. E., *Org. React.* (1957) **IX**, 37.
29. Hodge, E. B., Hidy, P. H., Wehrmeister, H. L., U.S. Patent **3,373,039** (1968).

30. Johnston, D. B. R., Sanicki, C. A., Windholz, T. B., Patchett, A. A., *J. Med. Chem.* (1970) **13**, 941–944.
31. Hodge, E. B., Hidy, P. H., Wehrmeister, H. L., U.S. Patent **3,239,349** (1966).
32. *Ibid.* U.S. Patent **3,503,994** (1970).
33. Martin, J. L., U.S. Patent **3,373,031** (1968).
34. Abbott, R. L., U.S. Patent **3,373,037** (1968).
35. Bachman, M. C., Hidy, P. H., U.S. Patent **3,453,367** (1969).
36. Wehrmeister, H. L., Robertson, D. E., *J. Org. Chem.* (1968) **33**, 4173–4176.
37. Steele, J. A., Lieberman, J. R., Mirocha, C. J., *Can. J. Microbiol.* (1974) **20**, 531–534.
38. Jensen, N. P., Brown, R. D., Schmitt, S. M., Windholz, T. B., Patchett, A. A., *J. Org. Chem.* (1972) **37**, 1639–1647.
39. Jensen, N. P., Windhloz, T. B., U.S. Patent **3,621,036** (1971).
40. Jackson, R. A., "The Chemistry of Some Derivatives of the Macrolide, Zearalenone," Ph.D. Thesis, University of Minnesota, 1973.
41. Hassner, A., *J. Org. Chem.* (1968) **33**, 2684–2686.
42. Pathre, S. V., Mirocha, C. J., unpublished data.
43. Peters, A. C., *J. Med. Chem.* (1971) **15**, 867.
44. Hodge, E. B., Hidy, P. H., Wehrmeister, H. L., U.S. Patent **3,239,355** (1966).
45. *Ibid.* U.S. Patent **3,373,029** (1968).
46. *Ibid.* U.S. Patent **3,373,030** (1968).
47. *Ibid.* U.S. Patent **3,373,034** (1968).
48. *Ibid.* U.S. Patent **3,239,341** (1966).
49. *Ibid.* U.S. Patent **3,239,353** (1966).
50. Delmotte, P., Delmotte-Plaquee, J., *Nature* (1953) **171**, 344.
51. McCapra, F., Scott, A. I., Delmotte, P., Delmotte-Plaquee, J., Bhacca, N. S., *Tetrahedron Lett.* (1964) 869–875.
52. Mirrington, R. N., Ritchie, E., Shoppee, C. W., Taylor, W. C., Sternhell, S., *Tetrahedron Lett.* (1964) 365–370.
53. Mirrington, R. N., Ritchie, E., Shoppee, C. W., Sternhell, S., Taylor, W. C., *Aust. J. Chem.* (1966) **19**, 1265–1284.
54. Aldridge, D. C., Galt, S., Giles, D., Turner, W. B., *J. Chem. Soc. C:* (1971) 1623–1627.
55. Musgrave, O. C., *J. Chem. Soc. C:* (1956) 4301–4305.
56. Munro, H. D., Musgrave, O. C., Templeton, R., *J. Chem. Soc. C:* (1967) 947–948.
57. Musgrave, O. C., *J. Chem. Soc. C:* (1957) 1104–1108.
58. Birch, A. J., Musgrave, O. C., Rickards, R. W., Smith, H., *J. Chem. Soc. C:* (1959) 3146–3149.
59. Sondheimer, E., *J. Amer. Chem. Soc.* (1957) **79**, 5036–5039.
60. Curtis, R. F., Harries, P. C., Hassall, C. H., Levi, J. D., Phillips, D. M., *J. Chem. Soc. C:* (1966) 168–174.
61. Arakawa, H., Torimoto, N., Masui, Y., *Ann. Chem.* (1964) **728**, 152–157.
62. Curtis, R. F., Hassall, C. H., Nazar, M., *J. Chem. Soc. C:* (1968) 85–93.
63. Mitscher, L. A., Andres, W. W., McCrae, W., *Experientia* (1964) **20**, 258.
64. Scott, P. M., Walbeek, W., *J. Antibiot.* (1971) **24**, 747–755.
65. Girotra, N. N., Wendler, N. L., *Chem. Ind. (London)* (1967) 1493.
66. Girotra, N. N., Wendler, N. L., *J. Org. Chem.* (1969) **34**, 3192–3194.
67. Vlattas, I., Harrison, I. T., Tökes, L., Fried, J. H., Cross, A. D., *J. Org. Chem.* (1968) **33**, 4176–4179.
68. Baker, P. M., Bycroft, B. W., Roberts, J. C., *J. Chem. Soc. C:* (1967) 1913–1915.
69. Musgrave, O. C., Templeton, R., Munro, H. D., *J. Chem. Soc. C:* (1968) 250–255.

70. Hurd, R. N., Shah, D. H., *J. Org. Chem.* (1973) **38**, 390–394.
71. *Ibid.* (1973) **16**, 543–545.
72. *Ibid.* (1973) **38**, 607–609.
73. *Ibid.* (1973) **38**, 610.
74. Bagli, J. F., Immer, H., *Can. J. Chem.* (1968) **46**, 3115–3118.
75. Budzikiewicz, H., Djerassi, C., Williams, D. H., "Interpretation of Mass Spectra," Holden-Day, San Francisco, 1965.
76. Budzikiewicz, H., Djerassi, C., Williams, D. H., "Structural Elucidation of Natural Products by Mass Spectrometry, Part II Alkaloids," Holden-Day, San Francisco, 1964.
77. Kingston, D. G. I., Bursey, J. T., Bursey, M. M., *Chem. Rev.* (1974) **74**, 215–242.
78. Mirocha, C. J., Schauerhamer, B., Pathre, S. V., *J. Assoc. Off. Anal. Chem.* (1974) **57**, 1104–1110.
79. Turner, W. B., "Fungal Metabolites," Chapter 5, Academic, London–New York, 1971.
80. Richards, J. H., Hendrickson, J. B., "The Biosynthesis of Steroids, Terpenes, and Acetogenins," Benjamin, New York, 1964.
81. Dorfman, R. I., Dorfman, A. S., *Endocrinology* (1954) **55**, 65.
82. Commercial Solvents Corp., British Patent **1,152,678** (1969).
83. Brooks, J. R., Steelman, S. L., Patanelli, D. J., *Proc. Soc. Exp. Biol. Med.* (1971) **137**, 101–104.
84. Hurd, R. N., private communication.
85. Borowitz, I. J., Gonis, G., Kelsey, R., Rapp, R., Willaims, G. J., *J. Org. Chem.* (1966) **31**, 3032–3037.

RECEIVED November 18, 1974.

11

The Chemistry of the Epipolythiopiperazine-3,6-diones

C. LEIGH and A. TAYLOR

National Research Council of Canada, Atlantic Regional Laboratory,
Halifax, Nova Scotia, Canada

The 2,5-epipolythiopiperazine-3,6-dione system occurs in many natural products that have antiviral, antitumor, and antimicrobial properties as well as high mammalian toxicity. The chemistry of the epipolythiopiperazine-3,6-dione system is discussed in this review from five points of view. First, the unique reactions of the bridge of sulfur atoms are described, followed in the second section by a discussion of the complex stereochemistry of the system. An account of the syntheses of these compounds follows, illustrated by those of dehydrogliotoxin and sporidesmin. Our meager knowledge of the biosynthesis of these fungal metabolites is then summarized, and the review ends with a short section devoted to analytical methods that can be used for this structural moiety.

In 1932 Weindling (1) reported the production of a metabolite by *Gliocladium* spp. that inhibited the growth of other fungi. He obtained the material in crystalline form, but it was not until 1958 that its structure was elucidated, I (R = H) (2), and at about the same time the isolation of a second example of this class of mould metabolite (II) was reported (3). In the latter case however, Synge and White were pursuing a material that was thought to be toxic to sheep and cattle in New Zealand (4), a far cry from the antifungal behavior of gliotoxin (I). The next development occurred when screening techniques for compounds that inhibited the growth of virus were initiated by many of the large pharmaceutical companies. Quite rapidly several new specimens of the class III (5, 6), IV (7, 8), V (9, 10, 11), and VI (12) were isolated, and by a curious coincidence the enantiomer of IV was reported by a group primarily interested in compounds that were active against

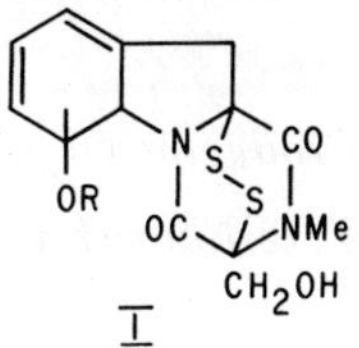

I

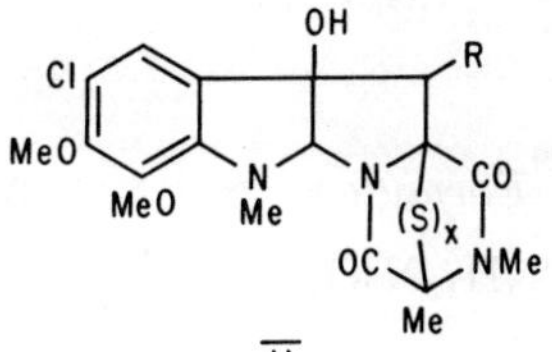

II

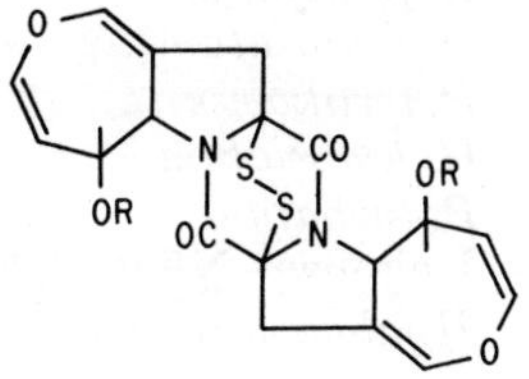

III

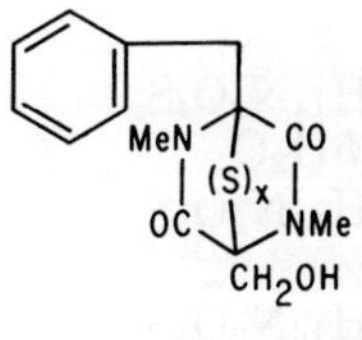

IV

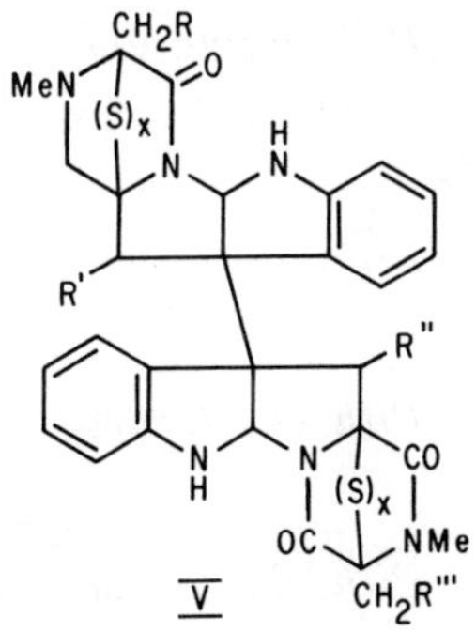

V

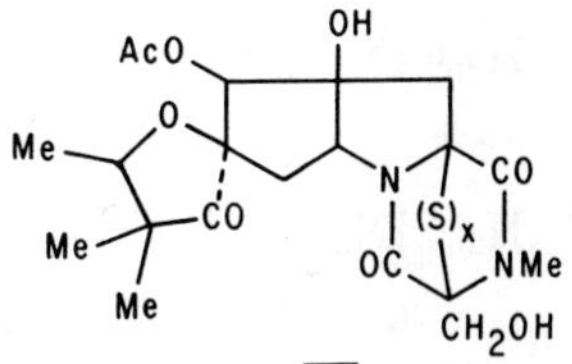

VI

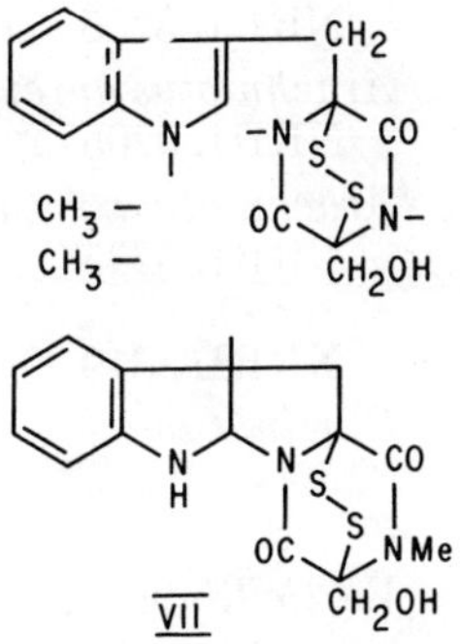

VII

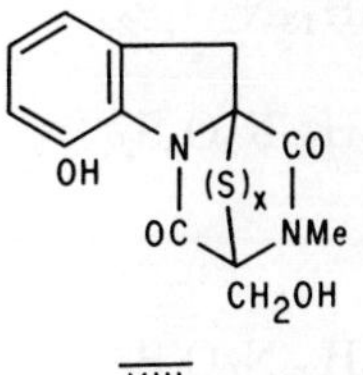

VIII

Table I.   Fungal Metabolites Having a

Formula	Name and Structure	Producing Organism[a]
$C_{13}H_{12}N_2O_4S_2$	Dehydrogliotoxin VIII, $x = 2$	P. terlikowskii
$C_{13}H_{14}N_2O_4S_2$	Gliotoxin I, R = H	P. terlikowskii A. terreus A. fumigatus G. fimbriatum
$C_{13}H_{14}N_2O_4S_2$ 0.5H$_2$O	Gliotoxin B I, R = H	P. terlikowskii G. fimbriatum
$C_{14}H_{16}N_2O_3S_2$	A26771A, IV, $x = 2$	P. turbatum Unknown, NRRL 3888
$C_{14}H_{16}N_2O_3S_2$	Hyalodendrin IV, $x = 2$	Hyalodendron sp.
$C_{14}H_{16}N_2O_3S_3$	IV, $x = 3$	Unknown, NRRL 3888
$C_{14}H_{16}N_2O_3S_4$	A26771C, IV, $x = 4$	P. turbatum
$C_{15}H_{16}N_2O_5S_2$	Gliotoxin acetate I, R = Ac	P. terlikowskii
$C_{18}H_{20}ClN_3O_5S_2$	Sporidesmin B II, R = H, $x = 2$	Pith. chartarum
$C_{18}H_{20}ClN_3O_6S_2$	Sporidesmin II, R = OH, $x = 2$	Pith. chartarum
$C_{18}H_{20}ClN_3O_6S_3$	Sporidesmin E (etherate) II, R = OH, $x = 3$	Pith. chartarum
$C_{18}H_{20}ClN_3O_6S_4$	Sporidesmin G II, R = OH, $x = 4$	Pith. chartarum
$C_{20}H_{18}N_2O_6S_2$	Apoaranotin	Arachniotus aureus NRRL 3205
$C_{20}H_{18}N_2O_7S_2$	Aranotin A21101 III, R = H, R = Ac	Arachniotus aureus NRRL 3205
$C_{22}H_{20}N_2O_8S_2$	Acetylaranotin LLS88α, R = Ac	Arachniotus aureus NRRL 3205 A. terreus NRRL 3319
$C_{30}H_{28}N_6O_6S_4$	Chaetocin V, R′ = R″ =, H R = R‴ = OH, $x = 2$	C. minutum
$C_{30}H_{28}N_6O_6S_4$	Verticillin A V, R′ = R″ = OH, R = R‴ = H, $x = 2$	Verticillium sp.

2,5-Epipolythiopiperazine-3,6-dione Functionality

mp, °C	[M]$_D$	nm	(log ϵ)	a	b	b^1	c	β
		$\lambda_{(max)}$		X-Ray Cryst. Data (K$_\alpha$)				
188°	−1310°	214	(4.34)					
		272	(3.73)					
		300	(3.67)					
221°	−840°	216	(3.97)	1.644	1.658	1.655	1.707	79°
		272	(3.80)					
	−840°			10.36	7.59		18.74	100°
105°	−285°			10.911	8.137		8.978	106.4°
101°	+84°	260 (Sh)	(3.00)					
130°	−726°							
170°–2°	−720°	268	(3.80)					
183°	+55°	218	(4.50)					
		256	(4.08)					
		307	(3.41)					
179°	+38°	218	(4.60)	9.64	10.58		23.88	
		254	(4.12)					
		302	(3.45)					
180°–5°	−666°	217	(4.52)					
		252	(4.22)					
		295	(3.50)					
148°–153°	−482°	219	(4.64)	15.160	21.369		9,978	
		252	(4.16)					
		300	(3.78)					
200°–205°	−2190°	265	(3.59)					
198°–200°								
201°–205°	−2640°	222 (Sh)	(4.01)	11.720	14.164		13.245	93.55°
		270 (Sh)	(3.26)					
240°	+5500°†	306	(3.78)	23.30	7.73		17.31	
199°–213°	+4910°	306	(3.78)					

Table I.

Formula	Name and Structure	Producing Organism[a]
$C_{30}H_{28}N_6O_7S_4$	Verticillin B V, R = H, R' = R'' = R'''=OH, x = 2	Verticillium sp.
$C_{30}H_{28}N_6O_7S_5$	Verticillin C V, R = H, R' = R'' = R''' = OH, x = 2, 3	Verticillium sp.
$C_{30}H_{28}N_6O_8S_4$	V, R = R' = R'' = R''' = OH, x = 2	Verticillium tenerum

[a] A. = Aspergillus, G = Gliocladium, P. = Penicillium, Pith. = Pithomyces, C. = Chaetomium.

other fungi (13). The biological investigations on sporidesmin, II, (R = OH, x = 2) (14), revealed its ability to inhibit the growth of lambs that otherwise did not appear to be ill. This result associated fungal metabolites with the well-known (15) poor growth of ruminants in the fall. A search of fungal isolates obtained from soil samples collected where such an ill-thrift condition was common resulted in the isolation of another metabolite of the epipolythiodioxopiperazine class (VII) which was probably the same as one of the earlier, highly active bacteriostatic materials isolated by Waksman (16, 17). Thus the compounds discussed in this review have a major role in theories of the etiology of poor growth in domestic animals and also in the attempt to find drugs capable of ameliorating RNA viral infections.

The 2,5-epipolythiopiperazine-3,6-dione unit is present in all of these metabolites mentioned, and the simplest example known, 1,4-dimethyl-2,5-epidithiopiperazine-3,6-dione (18), has many of the biological properties of its more complex, naturally occurring classmates. However, nothing is known of its long-term toxicology.

Gliotoxin, I, (R = H) and sporidesmin, II, (R = OH, x = 2) were investigated chemically before the nuclear magnetic resonance NMR, mass spectroscopic (MS), and circular dichroism (CD) behavior of compounds could be easily measured. Thus a great deal of degradative chemistry was done, and the structures were assembled by fitting the degradative pieces together into a harmonious whole. Indeed in the case of sporidesmin (II) the chemistry was complicated by an error in the x-ray crystallographic structure analysis (19). Most of this work has been summarized in a previous review (20) and is not repeated here. Here a list of the known compounds, their physical properties, and the names of the organisms that produce them are presented. The following

Continued

mp, °C	[M]$_D$	$\lambda_{(max)}$		X-Ray Cryst. Data (K$_\alpha$)				
		nm	(log ϵ)	a	b	b^1	c	β
230°–233°	+5020°	306	(3.75)					
230°–235°	+5790°	306	(3.74)					
232°–234°	+5520° ^{b}	308	(3.76)					

^{b} Rotation determined in dimethyl sulfoxide.

section of the review is directed to the chemistry that has been developed while investigating some of the newer antibiotics. One of the most interesting advances in the field in recent years has concerned the stereochemistry of the epipolythiopiperazine-3,6-dione system, especially with regard to the chirality of the chain of sulfur atoms and the theoretical interpretation of their complex CD spectra. A critical examination of this subject forms the third part of the review. Recently the biological activity of these compounds has stimulated much work on their synthesis; the several methods that have been developed are described next. Many of the natural products having the epipolythiodioxopiperazine function are biosynthesised from tryptophan or phenylalanine, and those that are not —*e.g.*, aranotins and sirodesmins—can be hypothetically elaborated from such precursors through oxepin intermediates. This subject forms the penultimate section. Finally a short section devoted to methods of analysis of compounds of this class is given.

Much of the information summarized in this chapter has been published as preliminary short papers with pious promises to publish full details later. We tended to take the authors' claims at their face value, but readers should refer to the original references and should write to the authors if experimental procedures are not obvious.

Production of Epipolythiodioxopiperazines by Fungi

Only two families of living organisms are known to produce epipolythiodioxopiperazines, and one of these is restricted to a single species— *Homo sapiens*—which is discussed later. For the remainder, this esoteric chemistry is restricted to the fungi. Reference to Table I shows, however, that this ability is widespread among the fungi, and there is good

Table II.   2,5-Epipolythiopiperazine-3,6-diones Whose Structures

Formula	Name and Structure	Producing Organism
$C_{20}H_{26}N_2O_8S_2$	Sirodesmin-A (VI, $x = 2$)	*Sirodesmium diversum* (Cooke) Hughes CMI 102519
$C_{20}H_{26}N_2O_8S_2$	Sirodesmin-G (VI, $x = 2$)	*Sirodesmium diversum* (Cooke) Hughes CMI 102519
$C_{20}H_{26}N_2O_8S_3$	Sirodesmin-C	*Sirodesmium diversum* (Cooke) Hughes CMI 102519
$C_{20}H_{26}N_2O_8S_4$	Sirodesmin-B[a]	*Sirodesmium diversum* (Cooke) Hughes CMI 102519
$C_{25}H_{30}ClN_2O_8S_2$	Oryzachlorin	*Aspergillus oryzae*
$C_{31}H_{30}N_6O_6S_4$	Chetomin (VII)	*Chaetomium cochliodes,* *C. globosum*
$C_{32}H_{30}N_6O_8S_4$	Melinacidin-III	*Acrostalagmus cinnabarinus*
$C_{34}H_{34}N_6O_6S_4$	Melinacidin-II	*Acrostalagmus cinnabarinus*
$C_{45}H_{45}N_9O_{12}S_6$	Melinacidin-IV	*Acrostalagmus cinnabarinus*

[a] Preliminary details of sirodesmins—D, E, F, H, and J have also been given in Netherland Patent No. 7312627.

evidence that the producing organisms use this synthetic activity in their natural habitat (*14*). The metabolites that have been thoroughly characterized, are given in Table I together with physical properties that can be used to estimate their purity. In Table II several other metabolites are listed that are also epipolythiodioxopiperazines but whose structures are either not established or have not been confirmed by synthesis or x-ray crystallography. In Table III the closely related 2,5-dithiomethyl-piperazine-3,6-diones that have been isolated from fungal cultures are given. In general, these compounds are not acutely toxic (*5, 6, 8, 21, 22,*

Table III.   Naturally Occurring

Formula	Producing Organism[a]	Compound
$C_{16}H_{22}N_2O_3S_2$	*H. victoriae* *P. turbatum* Unknown NRRL 3888	Gliovictin A26771E
$C_{16}H_{22}N_2O_3S_2$	*Hyalodendron* sp.	————
$C_{19}H_{22}ClN_3O_6S$	*Pithomyces chartarum*	Sporidesmin F
$C_{20}H_{26}ClN_3O_6S_2$	*Pithomyces chartarum*	Sporidesmin D
$C_{24}H_{26}N_2O_7S_2$	*Arachniotus aureus*	Bisdethiodi(thiomethyl) apoaranotin
$C_{24}H_{26}N_2O_8S_2$	*Arachniotus aureus*	Bisdethiodi(thiomethyl) acetylaranotin
	A. terreus	LL-S88β

[a] H. = Helminthosporium, P. = Penicillium, A. = Aspergillus.

Await Confirmation by Synthesis and/or X-Ray Crystallography

$[M]_D$	λ_{max} (nm)	Notes	Reference
		Desacetyl derivative mp 198°–201°	12
		Desacetyl derivative mp 195°–196°	12
			12
			12
	298		129
+2310	274		17
	285		
	293		
+776	300		130
+726	300		130
+718	301		130

23). They are included because, with one exception (*128*), they are found in extracts of cultures that produce the polysulfides and they are often useful to characterize mixtures of polysulfides.

Reactions of the 2,5-Epipolythiopiperazine-3,6-dione System

Figure 1 is a summary of the reactions that have been reported for the sulfur functionality in this system. The groups R, R', and R'' should not be interpreted as the same in all the reaction shown; no doubt most

2,5-Dithiomethylpiperazine-3,6-diones

$mg/l.$	mp	$[M]_D$	v_{max} (cm^{-1})	Ref.
40	134°	−230°	1650	128
4	135°	−166°	1655, 1640	8
				7
	140°	+227°	1657	23
0.02	65°–75°		1690, 1615	21
0.1	110°–120°	+292°	1680, 1665	21
	105°–107°	−907°		22
	213°–217°	−1505°	1685	5
	215°–236°		1678	6

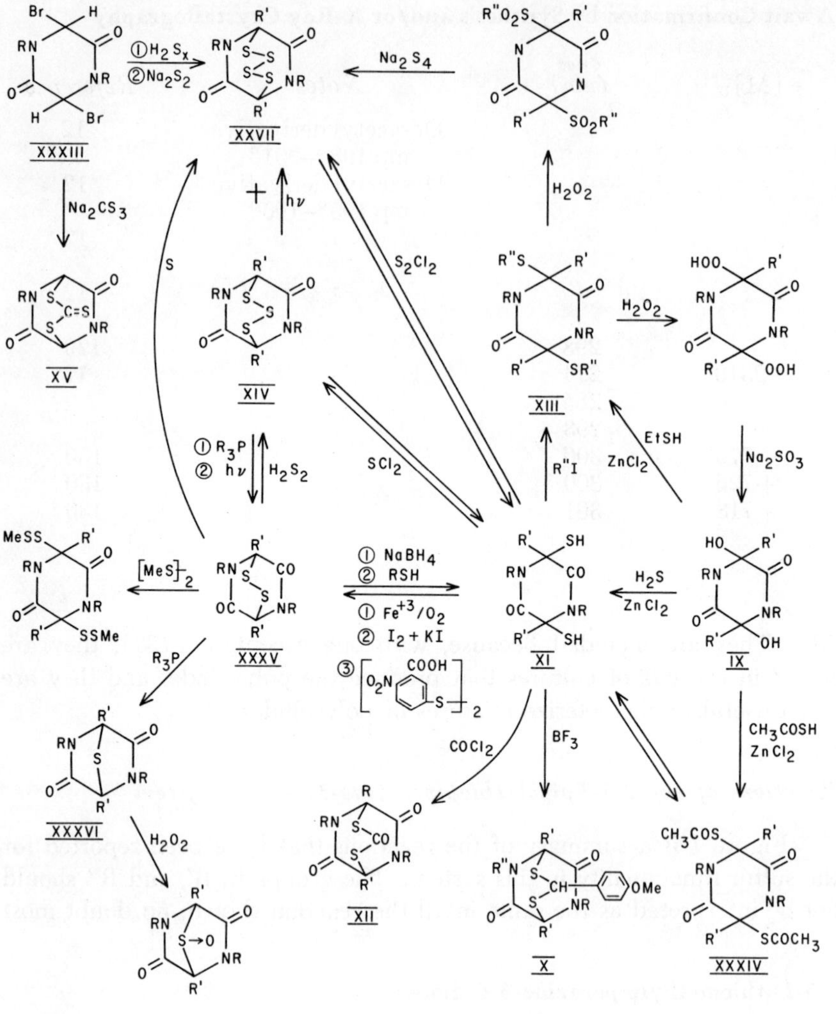

Figure 1.   Summary of the reactions reported for the sulfur functionality in the system (XI ⇄ XXXV)

of the transformations could be effected on all piperazine-3,6-diones. The compounds in Figure 1 are divided into those on the left which are oxidation products of those on the right. The reactions shown on the left of Figure 1 have been observed mostly in the sporidesmin and dehydrogliotoxin (VIII, $x = 2, 3, 4$) series. Thus sporidesmin (II, R = OH, $x = 2$) is converted into the trisulfide (II, R = OH, $x = 3$) with one mole of dihydrogen disulfide, but it is converted into a mixture of the tri- and tetrasulfides (II, R = OH, $x = 4$) with phosphorus pentasulfide or dihydrogen polysulfide, the tetrasulfide predominating. These reactions proceed without inversion at the asymmetric centers because sporidesmin (II, R = OH, x = 2) and dehydrogliotoxin (VIII, x = 2) can be obtained from the trisulfides so formed either photolytically or by reaction with trivalent phosphorus compounds (*e.g.*, triphenyl phosphine). Similarly (*12*) sirodesmins B and C (VI, x = 3, 4) are converted into sirodesmin A by treating with thionyl chloride in pyridine at 0°. However verticillin-C (V, R = H, R''' = R' = R'' = OH, x = 2, x = 3) was not converted into verticillin-B (V, R = H, R' = R'' = R''' = OH, x = 2) when treated with phosphine derivatives (*11*). The experimental facts have been interpreted by associating the sulfuration reaction with a specific insertion of the central sulfur atom(s) and the reverse reaction by their extrusion (*24, 25*).

The reactions may well proceed through intermediate branched isomers, *e.g.*,

$$\begin{array}{c}
\diagdown\text{S} \\
| \\
\diagup\text{S}
\end{array}
\xrightarrow{\text{H}_2\text{S}_2}
\text{H}_2\text{S} \;+\;
\begin{array}{c}
\diagdown\text{S}\rightarrow\text{S} \\
| \\
\diagup\text{S}
\end{array}
\;\rightleftharpoons\;
\begin{array}{c}
\diagdown\text{S} \\
\diagdown\!\!\diagup\text{S} \\
\diagup\text{S}
\end{array}$$

$$\text{R}_3\text{P}\!\rightarrow\!\text{S} \;+\;
\begin{array}{c}
\diagdown\text{S} \\
| \\
\diagup\text{S}
\end{array}
\quad\xleftarrow{\;\text{R}_3\text{P}\;}$$

for whose existance there is considerable support (*26, 27, 28*). When ^{35}S was inserted into the disulfide system by using $\text{H}_2{}^{35}\text{S}_2$ desulfurization of the trisulfide product by triphenyl phosphine or photolysis resulted in disulfide products whose radioactivity was lower than the detection limits. In the phosphine reaction, the triphenyl phosphine sulfide by-product contained 95% of the activity of the trisulfide. This result implies that if branched sulfur chains are involved in these reactions, the isomerization involves only —S—S— bonds—*i.e.*, —S—C— bonds remain intact as required by the retention of the chirality of the carbon centers (*24, 25*). Disulfides are not the end products of the reaction of phosphines with these sulfur bridged compounds. Episulfides can be isolated (*25*), and their CD show that inversion has occurred at the chiral centers. These episulfides, when treated with peracids, give products thought to be sulfoxides on the basis of their MS and the presence of an ir band @ ca. 1730 cm^{-1} analogous to that found in the strained ring system of their parents. These sulfoxides were racemates—*i.e.*, no asymmetric absorption bands were found at 210–400 nm. Presumably both sulfoxides enantiomeric at the sulfur atom are formed during the reaction (*29*), but such

racemization would not be expected to result in products without optical
activity. The mechanism of the observed racemization is not clear; the
reaction is similar in some respects to that between disulfides and dihydrogen disulfide. Hence an intermediate that has a linear sulfur–oxygen
bridge may be formed, and its formation would be expected to result in
racemization of the carbon centers:

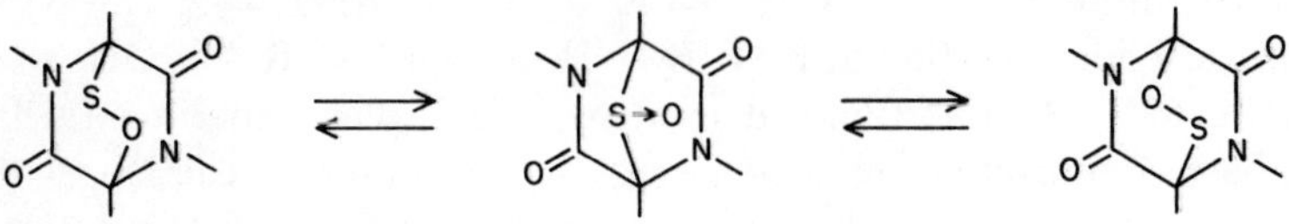

The right hand side of Figure 1 is concerned mainly with the reactions of piperazine-3,6-dione-2,5-dithiols (I). Their stability and many
of their reactions were unexpected. The smooth cyclization, in high yield
to the disulfide, with a variety of reagents was not predicted because of
the low dihedral angle of the —S—S— group (30, 31, 32, 33) (see Table
V); it implies that the system was, in some degree, strained. Secondly,
the conversion of piperazine-3,6-dione-*trans*-2,5-dithiols (*e.g.*, IX) to
epidisulfides (34) and the formation (35) of thioacetals (*e.g.*, X) from
trans dithiols (*e.g.*, XI) show that an unusual epimerization equilibrium
exists at the chiral centers (*cf.*, 131); presumably the ring closure reactions occur only with the *cis*-dithiols thus inducing further equilibrium of
the trans isomers. Even though the mechanism for this interesting change
is not known, one is impressed with the possibility of the sequence:

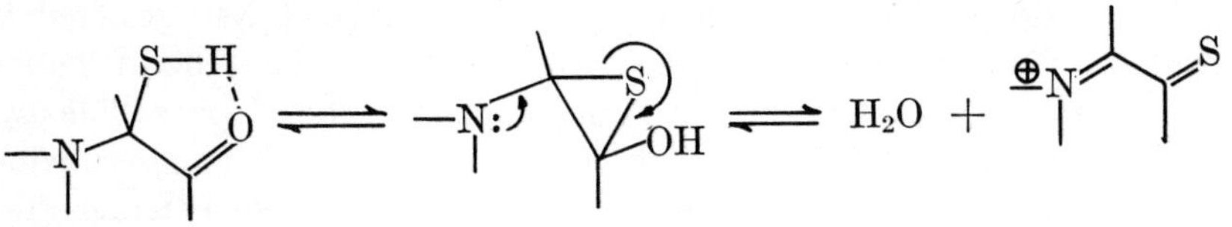

or alternatively with ring opening and closure of an hemithioacetal-like
species:

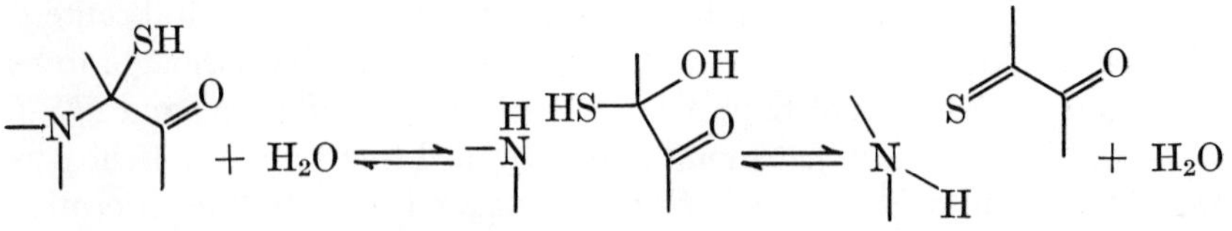

Such reactions are of course common in thiazolidine chemistry (36). By contrast, decarboxylation of compounds like (XXIX, R $= CO_2H$) gave predominently one stereoisomer (*37*).

The dithiols (XI) are readily alkylated with alkyl iodides in the presence of a weak base such as pyridine (*6, 21, 23*). This reaction is useful. The dimethylthio derivatives (*e.g.*, XIII, R″ $=$ Me) in particular often provide abundant molecular ions in their MS even in the case of such complex metabolites as chetomin (VII). Such behavior is in marked contrast to that of the corresponding disulfides whose principal fragmentation in the mass spectrometer is the loss of sulfur as S_8 with the result that molecular ions have been observed only in the cases of the gliotoxins, sporidesmins, and similar simple entities. Secondly, as shown in Tables I and II most of the organisms known to produce epipolythio-dioxopiperazines elaborate most of the known variations of the sulfur function. The separation of these complex mixtures is often tedious and can be circumvented by converting the mixture into a single dithiomethyl derivative by borohydride reduction and methylation. Finally the bio-synthesis of the dithiomethyl metabolites may be of some economic impor-tance, for these compounds have no known acute toxicity (*6, 21, 23*) as compared with, *e.g.*, the analogous disulfides. If, therefore, the fungus in the field could be induced to produce these metabolites at the expense of the toxic epipolysulfides, a way of controlling the effect of these com-pounds on animal growth might be open.

Basic conditions do not appear necessary for the formation of bridged tetrasulfides by the reaction of dithiols and dichlorodisulfide (*38*). The ring systems here are analogous to S_8, and these tetrasulfides are produced under a range of reaction conditions (*69*). The seven-membered ring system, *e.g.*, the trisulfides (XIV), the dithiocarbonate (XII), and the dithiothiocarbonate (XV), are all formed under mild basic conditions (*38*). These seven-membered ring sulfides are of considerable chemical interest. A discussion of the stereochemistry of the trisulfide group is deferred to a later section, and unfortunately structures XII and XV were symmetrical with respect to the sulfur bridge. However, the thioacetal (X, R′ $=$ H, R $=$ Me, R″ $=$ 2-methoxy-6-chloromethyl-phenyl) can be obtained in two diastereoisomeric forms; because only one isomer cyclizes to the indoline, it can be concluded (*35*) that the protons (R′) have acid-ities dependent on the stereochemistry of the bridge. This reaction of the dithiols (*e.g.*, XI) with anisaldehyde is general, and derivatives of formal-dehyde, acetaldehyde, and benzaldehyde have been made (*35*). How-ever only the anisaldehyde derivatives were converted into epidisulfides by oxidation with peracids presumably to sulfoxides and then acidic re-arrangement. This reaction is clearly an example of the sulfenate–sul-foxide rearrangement (*39, 40*) where solvolysis of the semithioacetal is favored by resonance stabilization of the intermediate carbonium ion.

Elimination of Sulfur from Epipolythiodioxopiperazines

Reductive Elimination. Sulfur has been replaced with hydrogen in these ketopiperazines either by treating with Raney nickel or aluminium amalgam. Apart from the sporidesmin group (*41*) useful products have been obtained by applying these reaction conditions to the naturally oc- curing epidisulfides. However, it is clear that usually mixtures of products were obtained and that their structures differed when the results from one group of metabolites were compared with another. Thus Raney nickel reduction of acetylaranotin (III, R = Ac) gave the dethio compound (*5*) with retention of configuration at the asymmetric centers. The prod- uct (XVI) gave an optically active octahydro derivative on catalytic

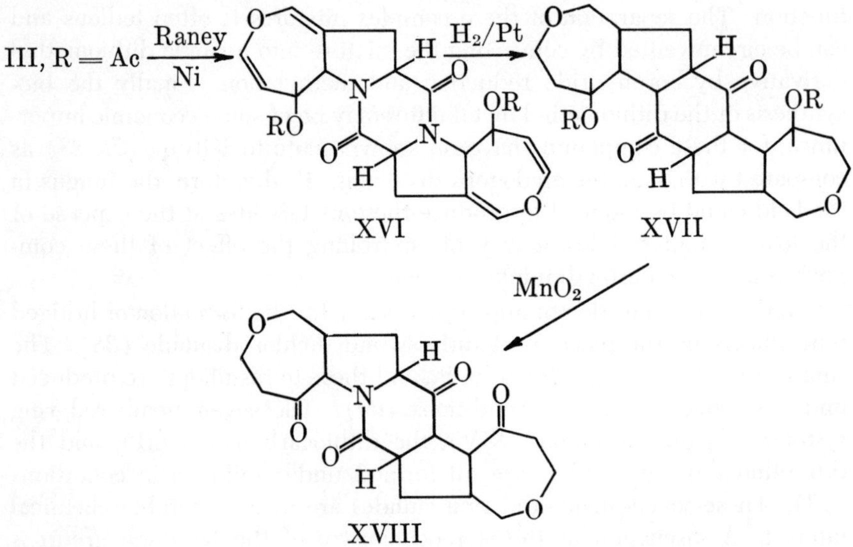

reduction with hydrogen (XVII, R = Ac). The latter on hydrolysis pro- vided a diol (XVII, R = H), and oxidation of this diol with manganese dioxide resulted in the isolation of the optically active diketone (XVIII). These reactions not only show that the hydroxyl (ester) groups in arano- tin are not functionalities of substituents of the dioxopiperazine ring (as occurs in many other groups of epipolythiodioxopiperazines) but also proves that the reductive desulfurization proceeded with retention of configuration. Johnson and Buchanan (*42*) obtained a dextrorotatory tetrahydrodethiogliotoxin (mp 194°C, $[\alpha]_D + 73°$) by Raney nickel de- sulfurization of gliotoxin (I, R = H); they reported that Dutcher also isolated this material together with an isomer (mp 155°, $[\alpha]_D + 50°$). Possibly both materials were mixtures since Raney nickel reduction of verticillin-A (V, R = R''' = H, R' =R'' = OH, x = 2) gave a mixture of products that were difficult to separate (*11*).

Reductions with aluminium amalgam have in general produced dethio compounds in the majority of examples studied, but the nature of the products differs. Thus gliotoxin (I, R = H) (*43, 44*) and hyalodendrin (*13*), (IV, x = 2) gave dihydrodethio products; however, although the product from gliotoxin appeared to retain its configuration, the product from hyalodendrin had $[\alpha]_D$ = 0°. (In some runs a diketopiperazine with low optical rotation was isolated). Chaetocin (V, R = R''' = OH, R' = R'' = H, x = 2) (*9*) gave the bisexocyclic, methylene derivative whose optical activity was not reported, and bisdethiodithiomethylacetyaranotin gave an optically active bisdethiomonothiomethylacetylaranotin. In the case of the verticillins, aluminium amalgam reduction provided the key to the structural elucidation of these complex molecules, which were very difficult to crystallize. The reactions are shown in Figure 2: verticillin-A (V, R = R''' = H, R' = R'' =OH) gave two tetrahydrodethio compounds (XIX), presumably stereoisomers, which when treated with alkali gave 3,3'-di-indolyl (XXIV). The monoacetate of verticillin-A when reduced under the same conditions gave two products XX and XXI, the former being analogous to the product obtained from chaetocin under the same reaction conditions. When these compounds were treated with dilute potassium carbonate solution, the indoles XXII and XXIII were obtained, the former having the same uv spectrum as chetomin (VII) (*17*). In addition, the 2-formylpiperazine (XXV) could be isolated from the reaction of XX and XXI with carbonate; this reaction had previously been observed under acid conditions in the sporidesmin series (*45*). The isolation of the aldehyde (XXV) is convincing evidence for the orientation of the hydroxyl groups in the verticillins.

Elimination of Sulfur under Acid or Basic Reaction Conditions. The elimination of sulfur from gliotoxins and sporidesmins under acidic and basic conditions has been reviewed (*20*). Generally speaking, the reaction proceeds in higher yield when the methyleneoxy or methinoxy substituents of the piperazine ring are esterified. When this procedure is adopted, sulfur is often smoothly eliminated merely by heating the compounds in pyridine solution. The reaction is best conducted under anhydrous conditions and also results in the elimination of the acyloxy group:

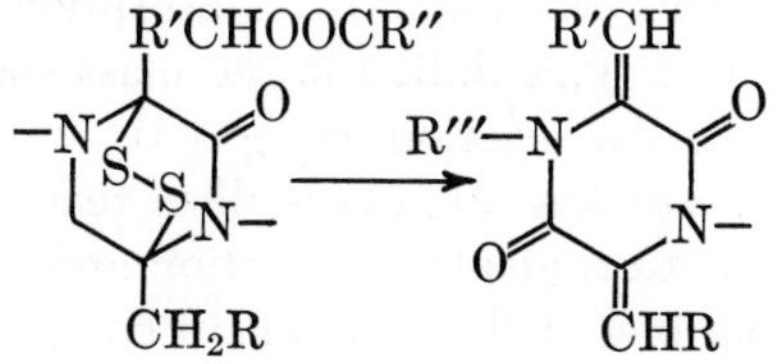

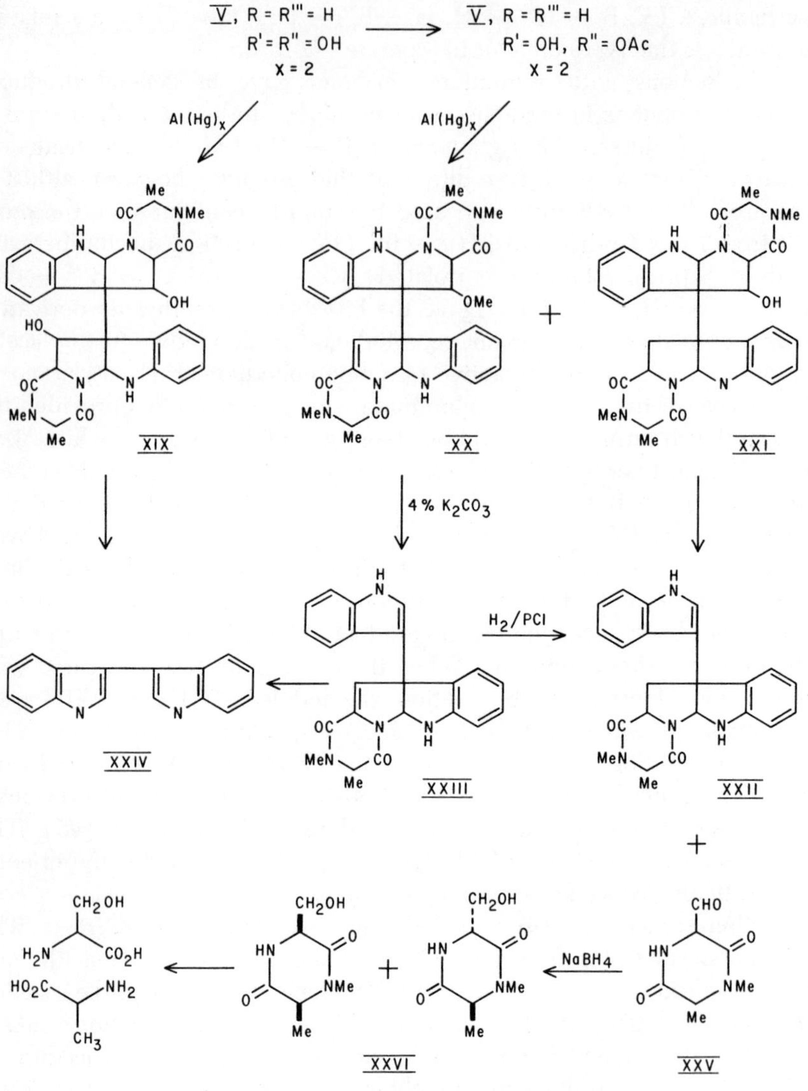

Figure 2.   Structural elucidation of the verticillins

This reaction is useful for several reasons. The olefinic products are easily detected because they have characteristic absorption in the visible spectrum and because their fragmentation in the mass spectrometer is highly characteristic (46); the ion reaction $M^+ \rightarrow (M - 67 - R' - R''')^+$ is highly probable. These olefins often crystallize readily, and if one of the unsaturated bonds is not conjugated, reduction and hydrolysis give valuable information about one of the amino acid components of the piperazine-3,6-dione moiety. In the work on chetomin (*17*) structure XXVIII was the most complex crystalline molecule obtained.

Stereochemistry of Epipolythiodioxopiperazines

In this section only problems associated with the 2,5-epipolythio-piperazine-3,6-dione group will be discussed. For this purpose the subject will be divided into parts dealing with disulfides, trisulfides, and tetrasulfides. A general background to problems of sulfur stereochemistry can be found in a recent review (*47*). In the past 10–15 years several x-ray crystallographic studies on piperazine-3,6-diones have been reported (*e.g.*, *48, 49, 50, 51*). In most cases the four atoms bonded to the nitrogen and carbon atoms of the amide groups are in a plane. Thus there are two planes of atoms in the dioxopiperazine ring, and the junction of the two planes lies along a line connecting the nonamide carbon atoms of the ring. The angle formed by this junction may be 180° when the dioxopiperazine ring is planar, or the value of the angle may be smaller when the dioxopiperazine ring is in the boat conformation. Only in the case of aranotin (*32*) are the amide groups nonplanar; there has only been one other case where the piperazine ring was in the chair conformation (*52*). In Table IV the molecular dimensions of a selected group of dioxopiperazines are given. The angle θ in Table IV indicates the angle formed between the two planes of atoms about the amide groups. It therefore indicates the degree of folding of the ring along the line joining the two chiral or potentially chiral carbon atoms. Generally, such folding is observed when the nonamide carbon atoms are substituted, but this is not always the case (*53*) and its presence or absence may depend on the chirality of the two asymmetric centers. In most cases when these centers have the same configuration, the ring is folded about 30° out of plane. If a source of ring strain is introduced, *e.g.*, by fusion of a pyrrolidine ring (XXIX, R + R' — $(CH_2)_3$, $R^3 = H$, $R^2 = Me_2CH \cdot CH_2$-), the angle of the planar junction is now about 140°. Finally, construction of a bridge of two sulfur atoms across the ring increases the deviation from planarity to about 50°, a surprisingly small increment (Table IV). Thus as Witkop and his co-workers pointed out (*54*), the geometry of the dioxopiperazine ring is only marginally affected by the presence of the epidithio bridge. When compounds with a bridge of four sulfur atoms are examined (Table IV), this trend is reversed, and the dioxopiperazine ring is more planar—*i.e.*, the plane of one amide bond is about 160° to the other.

Disulfides

In acyclic disulfides the dihedral angle of the group —C—S—S—C— usually lies at 74–105° (*47*), and the S—S bond length is 2.03–2.05 Å.

Table IV. Bond Angles and Bond Lengths in Some Piperazine-3,6-diones

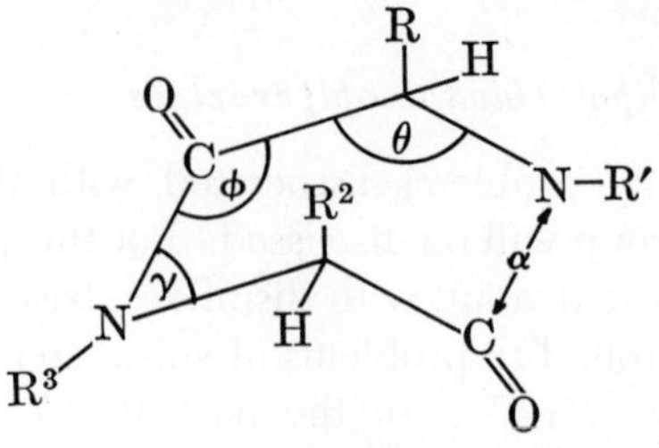

XXIX

Compounds and Structure	Peptide Bond Lengths $(A = a)$	Bond Angles °			Ref.
		γ	ψ	θ	
$R = R^1 = R^2 = R^3 = H$	1.325	126	118.9	180	48
$R = R^2 = H, R^1 = R^3 = Me$	1.348	124.6	118.1	180	49
$R = R^2 = Me, R^1 = R^3 = H$	1.344	126.05	116.8	154	50
	1.323				
$R = R^1 = (CH_2)_3, R^3 = H,$	1.341				
$R^2 = Me_2CHCH_2-$	1.367	123.25	114	143	51
$R + R^1 = R^2 + R^3 = (CH_2)_3$				159*	52
II, $x = 2$	1.35	115.1	113.5	135	30
	1.39	121.7	110		
I, R = H	1.35	118	114	130.5	31
V, R′ = R″ = H, R =					
R‴ = OH, $x = 2$		118	112	130	33
III, R = Ac	1.446	119	111	?	32
IV, $x = 2$	1.347	113.9	117.1	—	8
	1.369				
$R^1 = R^3 = Me, R + R^2 = S_4$	1.345	122.6	118	159	74
II, $x = 4$	1.35	124.2	117.5	157	73
	1.33				

* Calculated from NMR.

Reference to Table V shows that the S—S bond lengths of all the epidithiodioxopiperazines that have been determined lie outside this range and indeed are greater than that found (2.059 Å) in the strained cyclohexasulfur (55). The dihedral angles of the C—S—S—C bridge are also given in Table V where clearly the range found (8.8–18.2°) differs greatly from that found in acyclic disulfides. It is an interesting but unexplained fact that in two cases (31, 32) where two epidithiodioxopiperazine units are found in the crystal unit cell, the dihedral angles of the C—S—S—C groups are not the same, and each lies at one extreme of the range. The dihedral angle of about 90° in acyclic disulfides implies that if rotation

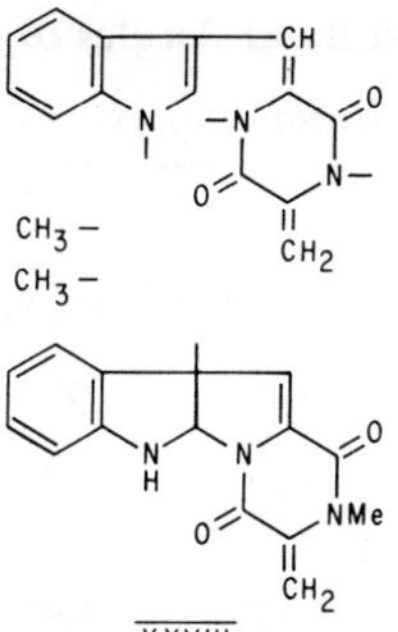

CH₃ —
CH₃ —

XXVIII

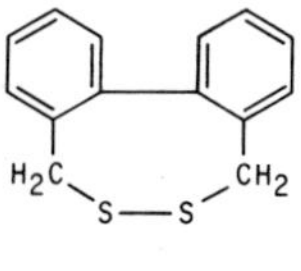

XXX

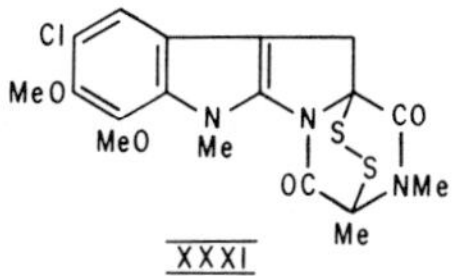

XXXI

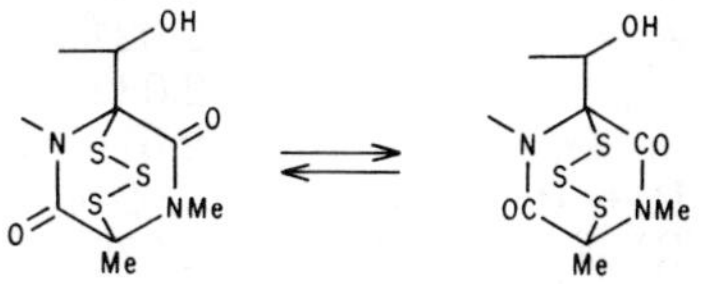

XXXII

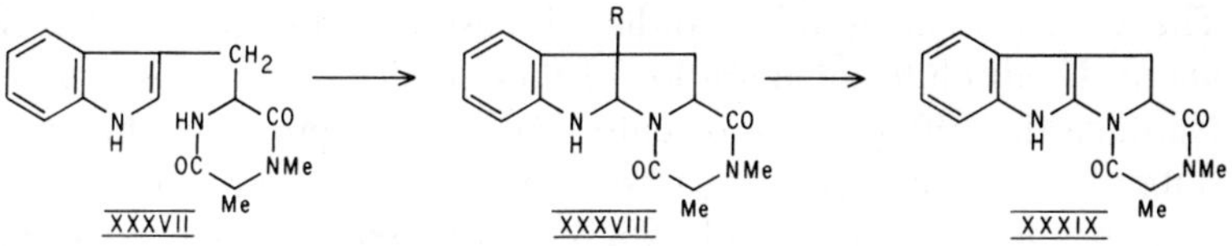

XXXVII

XXXVIII

XXXIX

about the S—S bond is restricted by, for example, repulsion between lone pairs of electrons on different sulfur atoms, then the compound is capable of existence in two enantiomeric forms. Such isomers have been shown to exist in a variety of cyclic disulfides of which 3,3,6,6-tetramethyl-1,2-dithian was one of the first examples (56). For simple cyclic compounds of this type it is possible to show that the energy barrier for intraconversion is about 10 kcal/mole. However, the geometry of the substituents can be manipulated to increase this energy barrier to the point where the enantiomers can be separated. An example of such a compound is XXX (57, 58) where the ΔG^{*} of inversion was estimated to be 28.8 kcal/mole. Thus the disulfide group is chiral and may be regarded as having a right-handed (P) screw sense or a left-handed (M) screw sense. Hence the stereochemistry of the epipolythiodioxopiperazine system involves not only the chirality of the nonamide carbon atoms but also the more unusual asymmetry of the chain of sulfur atoms. This fact is well illustrated in Table V where the dihedral angles C—S—S—C of those disulfides whose structures have been the subject of x-ray crystallographic studies

Table V.　Bond Lengths and Bond Angles of the

Structure	Bond Lengths (A)		Bond Angles		
	$-S-S-$	$-C-S-$	$\overset{\displaystyle O}{\overset{\displaystyle \|}{C}}-C-S$	$N-C-S$	$C-S-S$
II, $x = 2$	2.08	1.90	102°	112°	98°
I, R = H	2.08	1.89	103°	112°	98°
V, R′ = R″ = H R = R‴ = OH, $x = 2$	2.077	1.88	103°	112°	98°
III, R = Ac	2.082	1.882	103°	111°	97°
IV, $x = 2$	2.068	1.888	98.8°	111.6°	98.4°
II, $x = 4$	2.027 2.082 2.011	1.891 1.858	106.7°	112.7°	103°
XXIX, R = R² = S_4 R¹ = R³ = Me	2.0244 2.076	1.866	108.6°	113.9°	103.02°

are given. In these cases the dihedral angle is small, but both screw senses are known and are shown as + and − in Table V.

The x-ray crystallographic studies discussed so far give no information about the absolute configuration of these molecules and also have the disadvantage that the packing of chiral sulfur compounds in the crystalline state often involves packing forces sufficient to ensure that only one enantiomer is found in a crystal (25, 59). Therefore, it has been necessary to supplement the x-ray data with studies of optical rotatory dispersion and CD of these compounds in solution. The CD curves of epipolythiopiperazine-3,6-diones are complex (Figure 3), and at least three Cotton effects are observed (60). However the CDs of all the compounds examined so far (Table VI) are remarkably similar after allowing for the fact that some are mirror images of the others. Quite closely related metabolites, e.g., the epitrisulfides and the dethiodithiomethyl derivatives, have very different CD curves (21, 61). Further, as seen in Table VI, the results obtained in different laboratories and on different instruments show surprisingly good agreement. The CD of an epidithiodioxopiperazine therefore has excellent diagnostic value for the presence of this functionality in a newly isolated natural product. This conclusion receives reinforcement from the theoretical studies of Nagarajan and Woody (62). These authors investigated the CD of gliotoxin and acetylaranotin and attempted, from calculations of the rotational strengths of the various chromophores and pairwise combinations of them, to derive theoretical CD curves in agreement with the experimental data. The results for the two metabolites are shown in Figures 4 and 5. For the three asymmetric absorptions at ca. 230, 265, and 340 nm the theoretical curve predicts cor-

Sulfur Function in Epipolythiopiperazine-3,6-diones

	Dihedral Angles		
C–S–S–C	*C–S–S–S*	*S–S–S–S*	*S–S–S–C*
−10°			
−12° 8.8° 15.8°			
+11° −18.2° (−15.2°) −11.8°			
	−67.4°	107.1°	−71.7°
	68.63°	−105.33°	68.6°

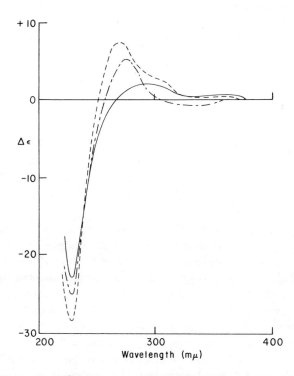

Figure 3.   The CD curves for sporidesmin ———, sporidesmen-B —·——·—, and gliotoxin - - - - -

Table VI. Circular Dichroism

Structure	Solvent	λ_{max} (nm)			
I, R = H	MeOH	338	312	272	234
	Dioxan	337	—	271	235
	EtOH	~335	—	274	233
VIII, $x = 2$	EtOH	340	300	282	230
IV, $x = 2$	MeOH	—	310	264	234
	MeOH	360	313	263	233
	Dioxan	362	316	265	237
XXXI	EtOH	—	325	285	230
II, $x = 2$, R = H	EtOH	360	300	268	232
II, $x = 2$, R = OH	EtOH	360	300	—	235
	MeOH	365	300	268	232
III, R = Ac	MeOH	344	310	266	228
	Dioxan	347	313	265	228
V, R′ = R″ = H, $x = S_2$	MeOH	—	304	270	239
R = R‴= OAc	MeOH	380	304	268	240
V, R = R′ = R″ = R‴ = OH, $x = S_2$	Me₂NCHO	372	307	274	253
V, R′ = R″ = H, $x = S_2$ R = R‴ = OH		375	307	272	236
V, R′ = R″ = R‴ = OH R = H, $x = S_2$	Dioxan	370	306	274	237
VII, (Diacetate)	Dioxan	—	303	272	238
VIII, $x = 3$	Dioxan	—	320	260	—
II, $x = 3$	MeOH	—	306	263	—
	CHCl₃	—	312	263	—
V, R = H, $x = S_2, S_3$ R′ = R″ = R‴ = OH	Dioxan	377	311	277	237.5
IV, $x = 4$	MeOH	328	297	263	255
VIII, $x = 4$	Dioxan	313	290	260	230
II, $x = 4$	Dioxan	313	302	276	253

rectly the wavelengths of the maxima and minima, but predictions of ellipticity, though of the right sign, were less accurate. Their final assignments were: the ~ 340 nm band was assigned to the $n\sigma^*$ disulfide transition; the ~ 270 nm band was assigned to the disulfide orbitals $n_2, n_3 \rightarrow \pi^*$ charge transfer bands (overlapping the $\pi \rightarrow \pi^*$ transition of the diene group in gliotoxin), and the 230 nm band is assigned to $n_2, n_3 \rightarrow \sigma^*$ disulfide transitions overlapping the peptide $n\pi^*$ transitions. The shoulder, frequently seen in the CD of these compounds at ~ 310 nm, was assigned to the $n_1 \rightarrow \pi^*$ charge transfer band where n_1 is the highest filled orbital of the disulfide and where π^* represents the antibonding π orbitals of the peptide groups. Thus the possible transitions of the disulfide group con-

of Epipolythiodioxopiperazines

	Δε			Ref.
−0.49	−0.19	+7.4	−33.5	62
−0.51	—	+6.6	−29.3	62
−0.45	—	+5.23	−25.33	60
−0.57	−0.86	+1.7	−20.0	60
—	+0.04	−8.63	+22.5	13
+0.32	−0.06	+8.8	−25.4	8
+0.24	−0.12	+7.1	−25.5	8
—	−5.8	+2.9	−20.0	60
+0.23	+2.05	+7.08	−28.6	60
+0.31	+1.80	—	−20.9	60
+0.3	+2.59	+5.88	−34.0	62
−0.67	−0.33	+8.2	−72.0	62
−0.81	−0.41	+8.2	−73.9	62
—	+14.3	−6.52	+73.8	9
−0.19	+14.7	−5.1	+76.7	62
−0.95	+19.4	−4.68	+47.8	10
−0.83	+17.43	−7.58	+100.46	11
−0.93	+18.76	−8.49	+106.09	11
—	+2.21	−0.33	+5.09	17
—	+7.69	−17.61	—	24
—	+0.27	−4.03	—	61
—	+0.76	−25.7	—	61
−0.42	+19.13	−7.79	+84.27	11
+0.9	−4.4	+13.6	+12.1	71
+13.34	−9.2	−24.55	−53.35	24
+1.03	+1.49	−1.19	−2.08	63

tribute to all the observed CD bands at wavelengths greater than 210 nm. From this discussion it might be concluded that the chirality of the disulfide group would be determined by the sign of the Cotton effect at 340 nm (*64*). Unfortunately such a conclusion is untenable since the magnitude of the rotational strength (-0.02 Debye–Bohr magnetons) is considerably less than that predicted for a dihedral angle of ~ 15° (*65*). One source of this reduction is the coupling of the $n_1\sigma^*$ disulfide transition with the dioxopiperazine peptide $\pi\pi^*$ transitions. In summary the CDs of epidithiodioxopiperazines are highly characteristic of this molecular group and also allow the natural products that have been isolated to be classified into two enantiomeric groups; however, the asymmetric ab-

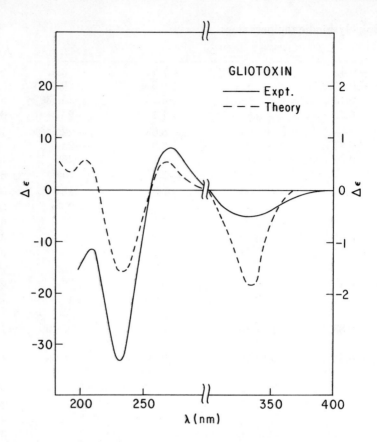

Figure 4.   Experimental and theoretical CD curves for gliotoxin

sorption bands cannot be simply assigned to unique asymmetric units.

The problem of the absolute configuration of the naturally occurring epidithiodioxopiperazines was solved by Herrmann and her colleagues (60). They were able to convert sporidesmin-B into anhydrosporidesmin-B (XXXI), a molecule in which the chiral centers have the same symmetry and are exclusively located in the epidithiodioxopiperazine moiety. Further, one of these asymmetric centers is located in the molecule in the same orientation to the indole chromophore as the asymmetric carbon atom is located in L-tryptophan whose absolute configuration is known. The optical rotatory dispersion curve of XXXI (Figure 6) had a negative Cotton effect at the same frequency and similar amplitude to that observed in L-tryptophan. Thus the absolute configuration of both asymmetric centers in anhydrosporidesmin-B was established, and from the x-ray crystallography the absolute configuration of the other chiral centers in sporidesmin could be deduced. In dehydrogliotoxin (VIII,

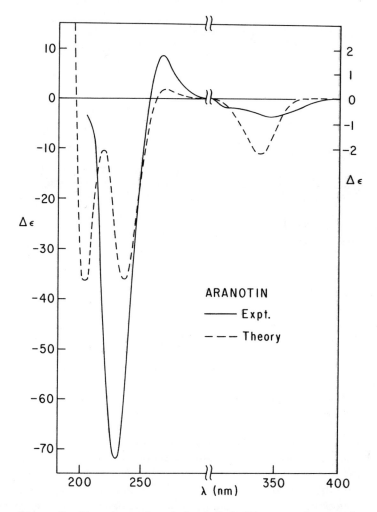

Figure 5.   Experimental and theoretical CD curves for acetyl-aranotin

$x = 2$), likewise, the epidithiodioxopiperazine moiety is the only asymmetric fragment in the molecule; this compound too has a negative Cotton effect in its optical rotatory dispersion curve. Herrmann et al. (*60*) concluded on this evidence and on the CD data (Table VI) that the absolute configurations of the sporidesmins and gliotoxins were the same so far as the epidithiodioxopiperazine units were concerned. This conclusion has been amply confirmed by many other groups of workers. Thus Fridrichsons and Mathieson (*31*) studied the intensity differences in the x-ray diffraction pattern of gliotoxin in 15 Bijvoet (*66*) pairs (associated with the sulfur atoms), $1k1$ and $1\overline{k}1$ ordered for a right-hand set of axes. The

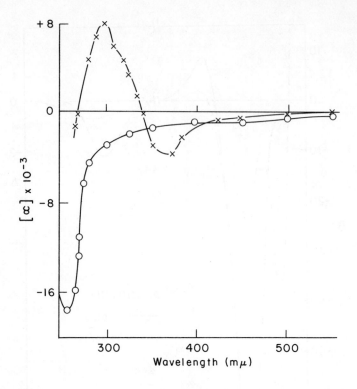

Figure 6. Optical rotatory dispersion curves for anhydro-sporidesmin-B ×—×—× *and dehydrogliotoxin* O—O—O

differences were in all cases of opposite sign, which showed that the absolute configuration of the epidithiodioxopiperazine group of gliotoxin belonged to the L series. Similar studies by Moncrief (67) showed that bisdethiodithiomethylacetylaranotin had the same absolute configuration, and the work of Weber (33) showed that chaetocin (V, R = R''' = OH, R' = R'' = H, x = 2) had the opposite configuration at the piperazine carbon centers with right-handed (P) helicity in the disulfide groups. These studies allow newly isolated epidithiodioxopiperazines to be assigned an absolute configuration from their CD properties if they belong to classes where the carbon chiral centers are L and the sulfur chain is M or where the carbon centers are D and the sulfur chain is P. X-ray analysis of the other two possible classes has not yet been reported.

Trisulfides

Five naturally occurring epitrithiodioxopiperazines have been reported; one of them, the trisulfide analogue of chetomin (VII, 68), has not yet been fully characterized. Two of the other compounds [IV, x =

3, (7) and V, R = R''' = H, R' = R'' = OH, $x = 2$, $x = 3$, (11)] have NMR spectra which suggest the presence of single conformational species or rapid interchange of one conformer to the other with respect to the NMR time scale. The remaining trisulfides, sporidesmin-E [II, $x = 3$, (61) and sirodesmin-C (12)] appeared on the basis of their NMR spectra to be mixtures of two isomers. Evidence that the two isomers of sporidesmin-E were interconvertible was obtained as follows. The relative intensities of the two sets of signals varied according to the solvent used for the NMR experiment. For example, in methanol the ratio 1:3 was observed, although in chloroform the relative intensity of one set of peaks compared with the other was 2:3. The signals observed in the spectrum were also temperature dependent; at 90°C most of the doublets collapsed, and single peaks having chemical shifts of the average of each doublet were observed. The phenomenon was reversible—*i.e.*, when the solution was cooled to room temperature, the original NMR spectrum was obtained. When sporidesmin-E was cooled to −40°C, and dissolved in chloroform at that temperature and its NMR spectrum recorded at the temperature, only one set of signals was seen (Figure 7A) (25). As the solution was

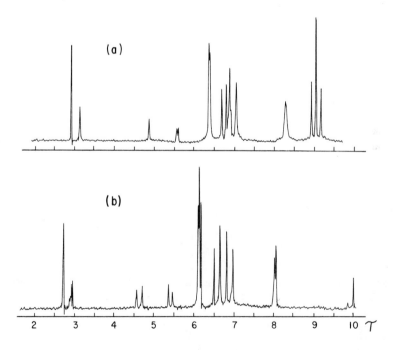

Figure 7. (a) The NMR spectrum of sporidesmin-E etherate (II, x = 3) crystals cooled to 233°K, dissolved in deuteriated chloroform and the spectrum measured at 233°K. (b) NMR spectrum of the same solution after being heated to 237°K and the ether removed.

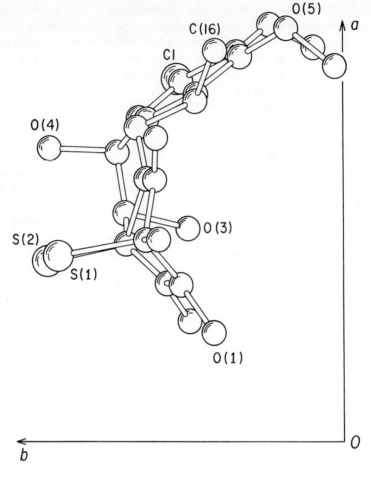

Figure 8.   View of the sporidesmin molecule down the C axis

allowed to warm to room temperature, the other set of signals appeared
(Figure 7B). However this group of peaks did not disappear when the
solution was cooled to −40°. These phenomena are typical of the effects
of changes in the conformation of sulfur chains on the chemical shifts of
hydrocarbon groups adjacent to the sulfur function (59, 69). A model of
sporidesmin-E (II, R = OH, $x = 3$) shows that the center sulfur atom
may be directed towards or away from the hinge of the book-like molecule (Figure 8) (30). Presumably interconversion of the two conformers
is slow enough at 25°C for the NMR spectra of both to be observed, but
at −40°C the rate of interconversion is small indeed. Since the reaction
rate of triphenyl phosphine with polysulfides is greater with sulfur atoms
bound to sulfur atoms other than with those bound to carbon and the

reaction is accompanied by inversion, it seemed possible that the reaction was bimolecular, and in the case of sporidesmin-E the assumed transition complex of such a reaction would be more easily formed with the conformer in which the central sulfur atom was directed away from the hinge of the molecule. We therefore examined the reaction of triphenyl phosphine with sporidesmin-E at $-40°C$ and found that the intensity of one set of signals decreased much more rapidly than the intensity of the other. There is therefore good evidence that sporidesmin-E exists as two stable conformers that differ only in the conformation of the trisulfide group. The difference in concentration of these two conformers in methanol and chloroform (*see* above) suggested that any differences in the CDs of the two conformers might be observable by comparing their CDs in the two solvents. Of course the amplitude of the Cotton effect is solvent dependent (*70*), but the wavelength of the asymmetric band at ~ 310 nm shifted from 306 nm in methanol to 312 nm in chloroform. Therefore it seems possible to conclude that the wavelength maximum where this asymmetric band is observed might indicate the screw sense of the trisulfide group.

Tetrasulfides

Four naturally occurring epitetrathiodioxiopiperazines are known. They include the epimers of (IV, $x = 4$) (*8, 71*) sirodesmin-B (VI, $x = 4$) (*12*) and sporidesmin-G (II, $x = 4$) (*63*). These compounds have considerable stereochemical and hence biological interest. Models can be made of these molecules where the dihedral angles of the sulfur chain do not deviate greatly from the values found in acyclic sulfides (*47*). Clearly as in the case of the disulfides, each of the two possible stereoisomers at the carbon centers can be associated with sulfur chains of P or M helicity. In addition given that —S—S— dihedral angles of $< 20°$ are stable, there are four additional conformations of the sulfur chain, where the central —S—S— dihedral angle is small, that might be expected to exist. The NMR spectrum of sporidesmin-G indicated the presence of only one conformer. Note that the sporidesmins are admirably suited for this kind of work since their NMR spectra consist only of singlets (*72*). The tetrasulfide obtained from the reaction of sporidesmin with $H_2 S_x$ had the same CD and NMR as the natural product. Therefore the question arose: what is the geometry of this conformation, and what is the reason for its apparent stability compared with other possible conformers? An x-ray crystallographic analysis was undertaken to answer these questions (*73*). An x-ray crystallographic analysis of the synthetic (*38*) compound (XXIX, $R^1 = R^3$ = Me, $R + R^2 = S_4$) has also been reported (*74*). The epitetrathiodioxopiperazine group in the latter crystals was enantiomeric to that of sporidesmin-G. Some of the crystallographic data is given in Tables IV and V.

In both cases the dioxopiperazine ring is in the boat conformation, but the ring is more planar than in the case of compounds with a disulfide bridge. In both of the tetrasulfides the S–S bond lengths alternate; the central S–S bonds are about the same lengths as those found in the epidisulfides, and the two terminal S–S bonds are about 2.5% shorter. Similar alternations in bond lengths of S–S bonds in sulfur chains have been observed in several other compounds (75, 76, 77). As seen from Table V, the dihedral angles of the three S–S bonds fall just outside the normal range, and the conformation of the sulfur chains in both compounds was that in which the central pair of sulfur atoms was directed towards the nitrogen atoms of the dioxopiperazine ring. Przybylska and Gopalakrishna (73) found that the interatomic distances between the central sulfur atoms and the nitrogen atoms of the peptide bonds were shorter (3.162 Å) than the sum of their van der Waal's radii (3.35 Å). They suggest that this might arise from donor–acceptor interactions and that this may be the reason for the stability of this conformation. However, these facts do not answer the question: Can the organisms whose metabolites these compounds are discriminate between P and M helicities in sulfur chains at the instant of biosynthesis? It is possible that the bridge is an oxidation artefact which occurs during the isolation procedure. The question is of considerable biological interest because the topography of many proteins depends on the presence of disulfide bonds of both P and M helicities (47). Are these artefacts of the crystallization process, and if so, can any conclusion about the mechanism of catalysis of enzymes, for instance, be made based on such derived topography? These questions might be answered if an epitetrathiodioxopiperazine could be isolated and shown by x-ray crystallography to possess a tetrasulfide chain of different conformation. Such a compound might be present in one of the two enantiomeric tetrasulfides (IV, $x = 4$) which have recently been reported (8, 71).

Synthesis of Epipolythiodioxopiperazines

The first successful synthesis of an epipolythiodioxopiperazine was discovered by Trown (18) who started with 1,4-dimethylpiperazine-3,6-dione and converted it into the dibromide (XXXIII, R = Me) which gave the thioacetate (XXXIV, R' = H, R = Me) with potassium thioacetate; then it was hydrolyzed to the dithiol and oxidized to the epidisulfide. The Lederle workers (78) and two other groups (38, 63) showed that the dibromide (XXXIII, R = Me) reacted with various sulfurating reagents, perhaps the best of which is dihydrogen polysulfide, to give the tetrasulfide (XXVII, R' = H, R = Me) in high yield. The tetrasulfide may then be reduced with borohydride to the dimercaptan and then oxidized to the disulfide—the overall yield from the dibromide is *ca.* 75%. Several N-substituted epidi- and tetrathiodioxopiperazines have been synthesized in this way; they include (XXXV, R = C_6H_5 R = *p*-MeO · C_6H_5). All these compounds showed antifungal properties, but unfortunately bromination of dioxopiperazines having a substituent at the two and/or five positions has been unsuccessful possibly due to the stereochemical parameters discussed above.

There are three obvious strategies that may be taken when starting a synthesis of epipolythiodioxopiperazines. One may start with piperazine-3,6-dione and introduce the possible substituents sequentially. Alternatively one may start with a 3,6-piperazinedione obtained from suitably chosen amino acids and then introduce the sulfur function. This procedure has the advantage that the chirality of the carbon centers is established at once. Finally the piperazine-3,6-dione complete with its sulfur bridge (or potential bridge) may be embellished with appropriate substituents. All of these strategies have been successfully exploited. Thus Poisel and Schmidt (*79*) found that L-prolyl-L-prolineanhydride [XXIX, R + R^1 = $(CH_2)_3$, R^2 + R^3 = $(CH_2)_3$] could be converted into its dianion with lithium di-isopropylimide and that its monoanion could be obtained with Na^+ $[CH_2 = SO · CH_3]^-$. The reactions of these anions with alkyl halides provided two and/or five substituted dioxopiperazines with retention of configuration. Hino and Sato (*80*) prepared the dianion of the ester (XXIX, R = R^2 = CO_2Et, R^1 = R^3 = Me) with NaH and found that its treatment with SCl_2 or S_2Cl_2 gave the epithio and epidithio derivatives (XXXV, R = Me, R' = CO_2Et and XXXVI, R = Me, R' = CO_2Et). Similar ionization could also be achieved by using sodium in liquid ammonia (*81*). Alternatively oxidizing piperazine-3,6-diones with lead tetraacetate gave the 2,5-diacetoxy compounds (*82*) which could then be easily transformed into epipolysulfides by the reactions shown in Figure 1.

Anions at the two and five positions of the piperazinedione ring can also be made when these positions bear a sulfur substituent (e.g., X) (*35*). Since such groups are readily converted into epidisulfides (*see* above), this constitutes a versatile approach to the synthesis of the naturally occurring epipolythiodioxopiperazines.

Although the synthesis of the gliotoxin and sporidesmin groups of antibiotics may be regarded as outside a discussion of the chemistry of the epipolythiodioxopiperazine group since it involves a good deal of indoline chemistry, it would be unsatisfactory not to include a summary of the considerable efforts that have been so successfully made. The synthesis of dehydrogliotoxin (*83*) has been reported briefly (*84*) and is shown in Figure 9. It illustrates the sequential introduction of substituents into the piperazine-3,6-dione ring, but probably the most remark-

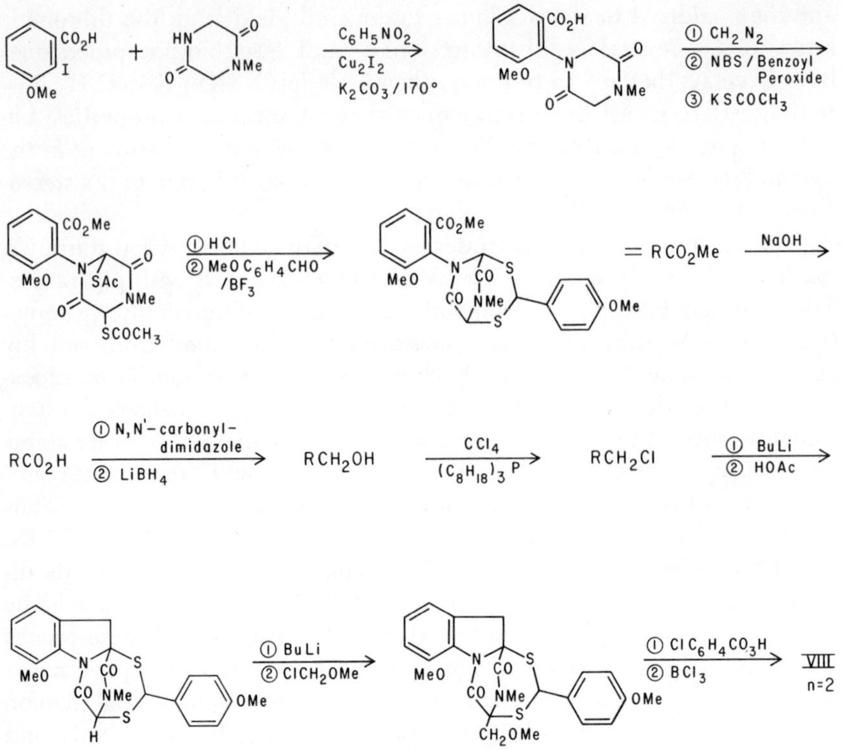

Figure 9. Synthesis of dehydrogliotoxin

able reaction is the first. An alternative approach to the synthesis of the fused indolinepyrazine system has been reported by Ottenheijm and his colleagues (135, 136, 137, 138). They showed that ethyl indoline-2-car-boxylates readily reacted with β- and γ-mercapto acids giving indolino-[2,1-b]-thiazolidones or tetrahydrothiazones. The latter compounds smoothly cyclized in excellent yield and high stereospecificity, to dioxo-piperazines having a —CH₂—S— bridge, i.e., to dehydrogliotoxin-like compounds where one sulfur atom is replaced with a methylene group (137). No biological activity was detected in these products. The synthesis of the sporidesmin group depends on the tedious synthesis of an indole derivative having the methyl, chlorine, and methoxy substituents in the right orientation and then on the correct stereochemical formation of the eserine ring system (the cis junction of the two five-membered rings). The orientation problem was solved (39, 85) when it was shown that chlorination of known (86) 6-7-dimethoxyoxindoles and 6,7-dimeth-oxyisatins gave the 5-chloro derivative. The formation of the eserine ring system has been achieved by three groups of workers. All depend on the oxidative generation of an indolenine radical at the three position of the indole ring:

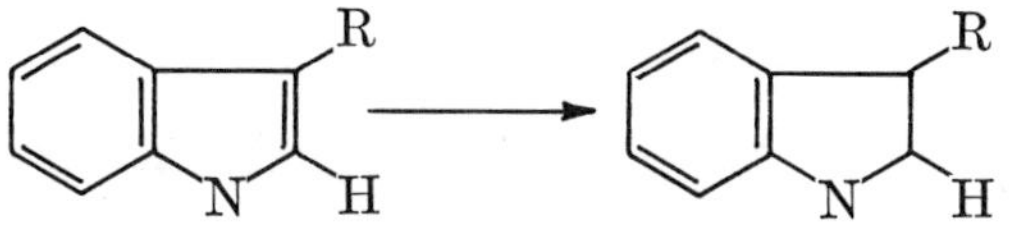

followed by addition to the enamine system. Witkop and his co-workers (*87*) were able to exploit much work done previously by his school (e.g., *88*) and show that lead tetraacetate, oxygen in the presence of platinum, or *t*-butyl hypochlorite oxidation of α-acylaminotryptamine derivatives resulted in cyclization to the tricyclic eserine system. The procedure suffers from the ready aromatization to the indole type (XXXIX) of the indoline intermediate (XXXVIII), but the reaction seems to be general and has been used recently to synthesize possible degradation products of chetomin. A photolytic oxidation of tryptophan and its derivatives has been reported (*89*). The intermediate hydroxyindoline (XL) was smoothly reduced to the hydroxyeserine (XLI) catalytically in the presence of a trace of hydrogen chloride. A third method involved the use of

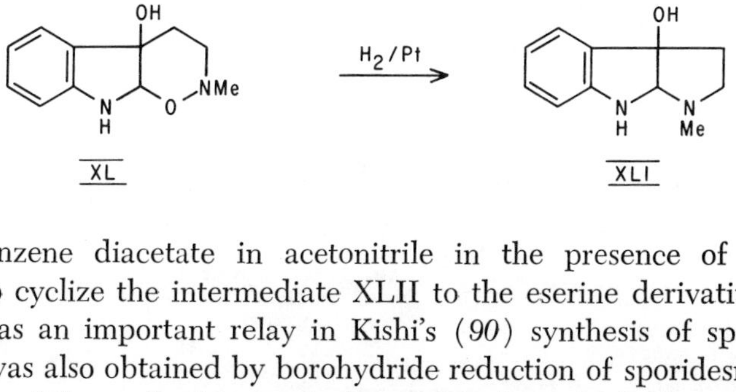

iodosobenzene diacetate in acetonitrile in the presence of dimethyl sulfide to cyclize the intermediate XLII to the eserine derivative XLIII. XLIII was an important relay in Kishi's (*90*) synthesis of sporidesmin since it was also obtained by borohydride reduction of sporidesmin (*21*), formation of the cyclic thioacetal of *p*-methoxybenzaldehyde, and acetylation. The synthesis of XLIII is shown in Figure 10. The intermediate acetate (XLII) was reduced to the methylene derivative (XLIV) which was cyclized to the eserine (XLV) by heating with benzoyl peroxide at 90°C for 2 hr in the presence of a trace of 4,4′-thiobis(-6-*t*-butyl-3-methylphenol). Only one of the possible isomers was formed, possibly because of the steric effects of the bulky *p*-methoxythiobenzal moiety. This product (XLV) was also prepared from sporidesmin-B (*72*) by a series of steps analogous to those shown in Figure 10 from sporidesmin (*91*). These procedures constitute formal syntheses of all the known

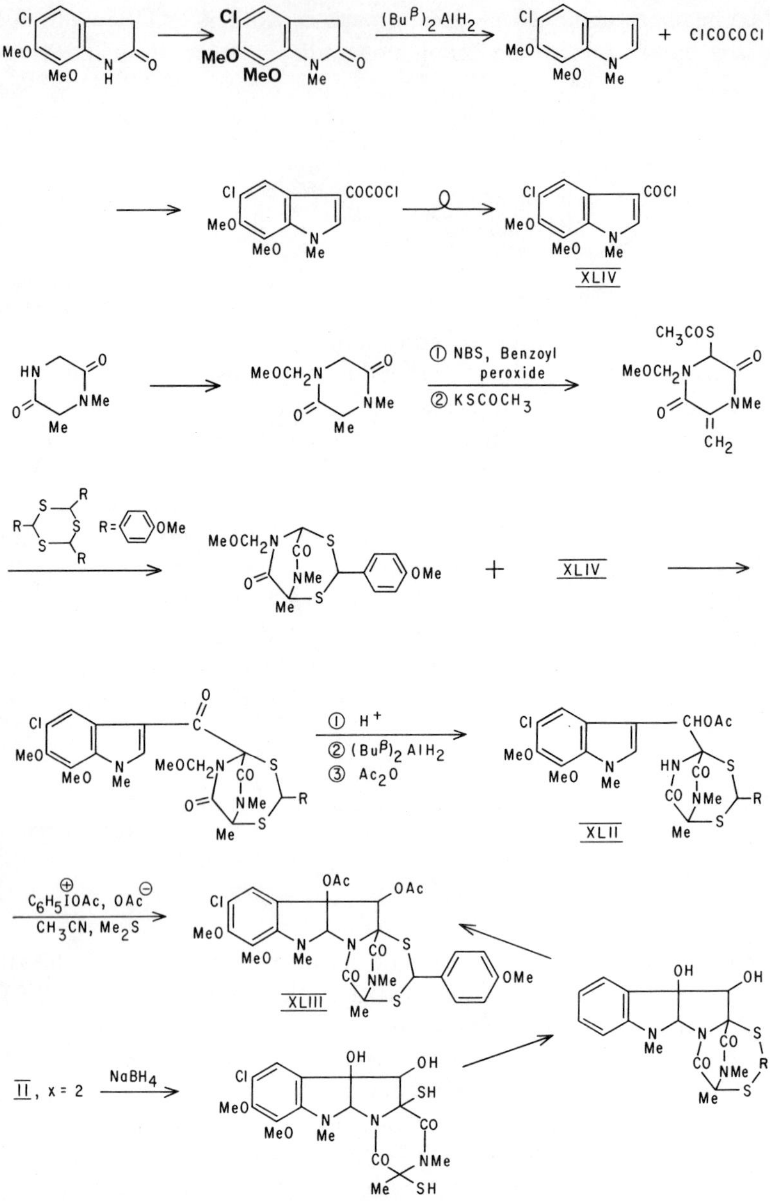

Figure 10.

sporidesmins except sporidesmin-F (*21*). They have also been successfully used in the total synthesis of hyalodendrin (IV, $x = 2$) (*92*).

One of the consequences of this synthetic activity has been to call
attention to the relationship between the epidithiodioxopiperazines and

the other great class of dipeptide antibiotics—the penicillins. One can envisage the transformation of one class into the other by such a reaction scheme as:

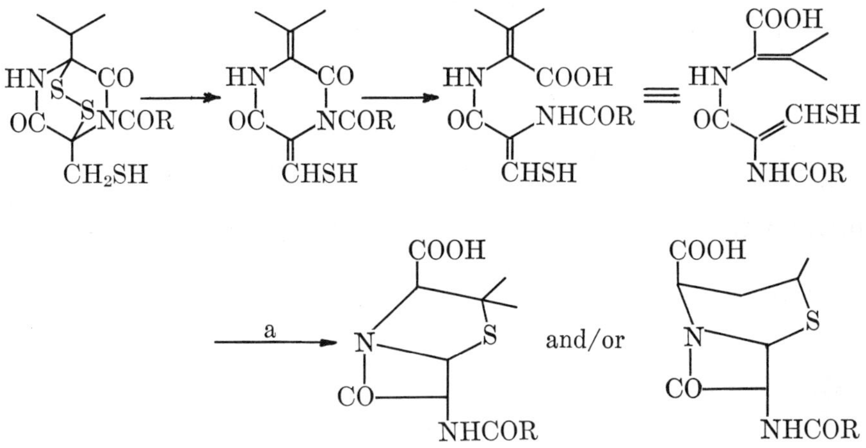

Transformations analagous to that shown at (a) have recently been described in a lecture by Y. Kishi at the I.U.P.A.C. symposium on natural products held in Ottawa, Canada, June 1974.

Biosynthesis

The earliest studies relating to the biosynthesis of gliotoxin concerned the optimization of its yield by adjusting the composition of the culture medium. Perhaps the most striking feature of the *Trichoderma viride* (*Gliocladium* spp.) fermentation is the low pH needed for maximum gliotoxin production (2–3.5) as opposed to maximum mycelial growth and sporulation (pH 6–7) (93, 94, 95). *Penicillium terlikowskii* and other fungi producing epipolythiodioxopiperazines have higher pH optima, e.g., *Chaetomium cochliodes*, pH 6.9 (16). Gliotoxin was one of the first antibiotics obtained by shake-flask (93) and semicontinuous (94) fermentation, and the high oxygen requirement of the fungus for its production was noticed early. It has been shown to have an optimum for oxygen significantly above that necessary for growth (96). A wide variety of carbon sources, e.g., glucose, can be utilized by *T. viride*. Ammonium was preferred to nitrate as a source of nitrogen and also gave rise to fewer chloroform-soluble gums than did peptone. Sulfate incorporation was apparently nonspecific, and no growth supplements were found that increased gliotoxin production (94). At least one group (97) has found augmented yields when an alternating cycle of 12 hr periods of light and dark were used.

With the introduction of radioactive and heavy isotopes, direct studies were made on the biosynthesis of gliotoxin. During the preparation of this review, it became clear that several, apparently conflicting results were recorded in the literature. We decided to present all of the results in Table VII and allow the reader to form an opinion. All of the groups of workers whose results are summarized in Table VII sought reproducible high yields of the antiobiotic but were not always successful. In addition, the precursors were generally added at a time judged to mark the highest biosynthetic activity in order that the dilution of the isotope be kept low. This consideration is especially important when isotopes that are not radioactive are used for labelling, for in these cases the detection techniques (MS and NMR) are less sensitive. It can be seen from the experiments using carboxyl-labelled phenylalanine that the mass of precursor fed also has a marked inverse relation to the dilution value. Thus in using nonradioactive labels one must feed rather high concentrations of precursor.

Using ^{14}C- and later ^{3}H-labelled precursors it was found that neither tryptophan nor acetate was a direct precursor of gliotoxin, although both were taken up into the cells. On the other hand phenylalanine and Me-labelled methionine were incorporated into the antibiotic in high yield (98, 99). Serine was also a biosynthetic precursor of gliotoxin (99, 100). Amino acid interconversions are a problem in such studies, and glycine was also incorporated in about the same yield as serine. In one of the first uses of MS for biosynthetic purposes Bose et al. (101) used the basic degradation product of gliotoxin (XLVI, R = H) to show that phenylalanine labelled with ^{14}C and ^{15}N can be incorporated directly in about 10% yield and that the nitrogen atom of phenylalanine appeared only in the indoline nitrogen atom of gliotoxin. By contrast ^{15}N-glycine, ^{15}N-aspartic acid, and ^{15}N-glutamic acid gave rise to unequal labelling of both nitrogen atoms of gliotoxin. When amino acids labelled with both ^{15}N and ^{14}C were fed, the dilution of the two isotopes differed; the ^{14}C:^{15}N ratio increased, thus suggesting deamination of the amino acid and amination of the corresponding α-ketoacid (102). Thus these precursor amino acids participate in the nitrogen pool, but the labelling experiments suggested that there was little exchange between, e.g., phenylalanine and serine. These experiments confirmed previous work (103) that the carbon skeleton of phenylalanine was incorporated intact. Since both D- and L-phenylalanines were equally good precursors, the phenylalanine fed was deaminated to an achiral intermediate.

By adding a constant amount of ^{35}S-L-methionine to a thousandfold greater concentration of various potential precursors of the sulfur function (that were not labelled), it was shown (104) that cysteine was preferred to methionine as a source of the sulfur in gliotoxin. In a similar way serine was found to be twenty times as effective a precursor of the carbon skeleton of gliotoxin as cysteine or alanine (*105*). Similar experiments in the aranotin series showed that both stereoisomers of phenylalanine were good precursors of bisdethiodithiomethyl acetylaranotin (BDA). Equimolar ^{35}S and C[^{3}H]$_3$ tagged L-methionine led to a higher incorporation of tritium than of ^{35}S, implying that the thiomethyl groups were not introduced in a single step. Also ^{35}S-labelled BDA was not transformed into acetylaranotin (*104*), though some evidence was obtained that the BDA was taken up into the cells.

Tryptophan, alanine, methionine, and serine brought about labelling of sporidesmin, but tryptophan greatly reduced the incorporation of serine. L-Cysteine and to a lesser extent ^{35}S-sodium sulfate and methionine labelled the disulfide bridge (*106*). The secondary hydroxyl group is probably introduced stereospecifically after formation of the eserine ring system (*132*).

Spurred by reports of exceedingly high incorporations of *m*-tyrosine into gliotoxin (*99*), three separate groups have attempted to repeat this work (*107, 108, 109*), but none has succeeded. However, some aspects of pyrrolidine ring formation in these antibiotics have been clarified in these investigations. All of the groups (Table VII) found that phenylalanine was incorporated better that Bz-oxygenated precursors, even though, e.g., *m*-tyrosine was found to accumulate in the cells (*109*). Perhaps most significantly, 3-^3H-phenylalanine was incorporated into gliotoxin and into BDA with retention of the label (*108*). On the basis of the oxepin structure of the aranotins, it was proposed (*22*) that pyrrolidine ring closure was achieved through attack of the lone pair on the nitrogen atom on the epoxide (XLVII), analogous to the intermediate in the "NIH shift" (*110*). The proposed scheme is shown in Figure 11. It is clear that the stereochemistry of the bridgehead protons with respect to the secondary hydroxyl groups in the aranotins and perhaps in the gliotoxins is correct for the trans opening of an epoxide. When totally deuteriated phenylalanine was incorporated into acetylaranotin; almost seven of the eight deuterium atoms which were carbon substituents were retained (*109*). Given that there is significant deamination of the amino acid, this result seems too good to be true; for only 4% of phenylalanine dideuteriated in the methylene groups was recovered in dideuteriated gliotoxin (*111*).

Much work has been done on the labelling of the methylene protons of phenylalanine with the object of obtaining information about the mechanism of addition of the sulfur bridge—there is some possibility that an olefinic intermediate like XLVI, R = H, was involved (*21*). Such a reaction can be realized chemically since the addition of ethanethiol to $\Delta^{2,3}$-prolineanhydride to give *cis*-2,5-dithioethylpiperazine-3,6-dione (XIII) has been reported (*112*). Such an intermediate would require the loss

Table VII.   Biosynthetic Feeding Experiments with

Precursor	Amount Fed (mg/l.)	Sp. Activity (mCi/mm)	Fed at (hr)
Tryptophan-7a-^{14}C	0.45	0.153	24–96
Sodium acetate-2-^{14}C	0.53	1.0	24–96
	0.62		
Methionine-^{14}CH$_3$	0.08	0.42	24–96
	0.17		
	0.65	1.96	42–65
Methionine-^{35}S (2S only)	1.56	526	72
Methionine-^{3}H$_3$C (2S only)	1.53	127	72
Glycine-2-^{14}C	0.08	1.68	23–50
Glycine-^{15}N	33.3	90–95% ^{15}N	60
Glycine-2-^{13}C	33.3	50–60% ^{13}C	60
Glycine-1-^{13}C	33.3	50–60% ^{13}C	60
Aspartate-^{15}N and -1-^{14}C	33.3	—	60
Glutamate-^{15}N	33.3	90–95% ^{15}N	60
Formate-^{13}C	33.3	50–60% ^{13}C	60
Alanine-3-^{14}C ^{a}	164	0.014	264 ^{a}
			312 ^{a}
Alanine-3-^{3}H ^{a}	163	0.169	264 ^{a}
Serine-3-^{14}C	0.043	2.02	44–53
Serine-1-^{14}C	0.18	1.77	31–52
2,3-DOPA-[4,5,6-^{3}H] ^{b}	0.83	18.5	20
3,5-DOPA-2-^{14}C $^{a,\, b}$	15	.422	48
	1.5		
ortho-Tyrosine-3,5-^{3}H	1.02	16.8	20
meta-Tyrosine-^{3}H	0.042 ml.	9.6μC/ml	27–65
meta-Tyrosine-[2,4,6-^{2}H$_3$]+ -1-^{14}C	185	84%D; 36.6	30
meta-Tyrosine-1'-^{14}C	0.96	0.33	30
	9.4		36
meta-Tyrosine-2'-^{14}C	14.2	0.536	48
meta-Tyrosine-2'-^{14}C ^{a}	15	0.536	48
	1.5		
meta-Tyrosine-[2,4,6-^{3}H]	2.87	—	0
meta-Tyrosine + DL-1- ^{14}C-phenylalanine	6.7 + 0.2	ratio 11.5	0
	3.2 + 3.1	ratio 11.9	
Phenylalanine-1'-^{14}C	0.33	0.422	24–59
			24–35
Phenylalanine-1'-^{14}C	9.5	0.174	36

Gliocladium spp (T. viride) and Penicillium terlikowski

Harvested at (hr)	Gliotoxin (mg/l.)	Incorporation (%)	Dilution[a]	Reference
120	94.6	0	—	98
120	65	0.02	1.53×10^5	98
	89	0.005	7.1×10^5	
120	95	0.16	3.26×10^5	98
	43	0.27	4.55×10^5	
120	44	3.39	9.1×10^3	99
	28	1.74	1.1×10^2	
96	—	10.2	—	104
96	—	13.3	—	
120	27	0.88–1.17	8.5–6.5×10^3	99
120	20–67	3.0–9.0	11–33	101
120	20–67	2.3–4.2	22–39	
120	20–67	4.0	23	
120	20–67	$2.7 + 0$	$37 + \infty$	102
120	20–67	2.7	37	
120	20–67	1.8–4.5	22–55	101
336	49.5	0.098	214	103
360	43.5	0.001	2320	
—	94.8	0.014	2450	
120	36	0.72	3.7×10^4	99
	72	2.74	1.9×10^4	
120	81	1.92	7.4×10^3	99
36	52	0.04	9.3×10^4	107
72	—	0.01	—	109
36	39	0.003	6.1×10^6	99
120	87	30.8	—	99
	.70	44.4	—	
72	33	$0 + 0.0024$	4×10^3	107
72	91	0.0043	1.2×10^6	107
	69	0.053	7.7×10^3	
72	—	0.04	—	
72	—	0.37	—	109
	—	0.12	—	
120	72	0.009	—	108
120	78	4.9 (^{14}C)	ratio 0.009	108
	53	1.6 (^{14}C)	ratio 0.13	
120	70	4.2	2600	98
	33	8.4	530	107
72	36	5.4	33	

Table VII.

Precursor	Amount Fed (mg/l.)	Sp. Activity (mCi/mm)	Fed at (hr)
Phenylalanine-1'-^{14}C	1.0	0.168	20
Phenylalanine-1'-^{14}C	219.7	0.0019	20
Phenylalanine-1'-^{14}C	22	0.017	20
Phenylalanine-1'-^{14}C	2.2	0.17	20
Phenylalanine-2'-^{14}C	0.95 0.18	0.84	47–69 45–47
Phenylalanine-3'-^{14}C	6.8	4.86	48
Phenylalanine-3'-^{14}C[a]	2	16.5	48
Phenylalanine-^{3}H	0.42 ml	5.5μCi/ml	27–47
Phenylalanine-^{15}N	33.3	90–95% ^{15}N	60
Phenylalanine + 2'S-1-^{14}C	33.3	90–95% ^{15}N	60
Phenylalanine + 2'R-1-^{14}C	33.3	90–95% ^{15}N	60
Phenylalanine-1'-^{14}C + -1'-^{13}C	33.3	50–69% ^{13}C	60
Phenylalanine-3'-^{14}C + -1'-^{13}C	33.3	50–60% ^{13}C	60
Phenylalanine[aryl-^{14}C][a]	100	0.066	192[a]
Phenylalanine[aryl-^{14}C][a]	700	0.023	216[a]
Phenylalanine-1'-^{14}C + -2-^{3}H	2.6	ratio 1:38.2	0
Phenylalanine-1'-^{14}C + -3-^{3}H	2.6	ratio 1:7.1	0
Phenylalanine-1'-^{14}C + -3-^{3}H	3.4	ratio 1:6.5	0
Phenylalanine-1'-^{14}C + -4-^{3}H	~10–3	ratio 1:4.7	0
Phenylalanine-[2,3,4,5,6-^{2}H$_5$]	231	85% ^{2}H	20
Phenylalanine-[3', 3'-^{2}H$_2$]	—	95% ^{2}H	20
Phenylalanine-[3'-^{3}H, 1'-^{14}C]	—	ratio 6.45	0
Phenylalanine-3'S-^{2}H + 1'-^{14}C	93	9.8 × 10^{-5}	20
Phenylalanine-3'S-^{2}H + 1'-^{14}C	218	2.0 × 10^{-4}	20
Phenylalanine-3'S-^{3}H + 1'-^{14}C	—	ratio 4.6	0
Phenylalanine-3'R-^{2}H + 1'-^{14}C	228	1.8 × 10^{-4}	20
Phenylalanine-3'R-^{2}H + ring-^{3}H	234	5.2 × 10^{-4}	20
Phenylalanine-3'R-^{3}H + 1'-^{14}C	— 2.9–3.6	ratio 5.01 ratio 12.2–13.7	0 0
XXIX, R' = R^3 = H R = PhCH$_2$, R^2 = CH$_2$OH	202	1.2 × 10^{-2}	0[a]
Dehydrogliotoxin-^{14}C[a] (VIII, $x = 2$)..	10	4.8 × 10^{-3}	192–264

Continued

Harvested at (hr)	Gliotoxin (mg/l.)	Incorporation (%)	Dilution[a]	Reference
36	46	11.0	200	
34	—	3.4	2.7	
34	—	3.7	28	107
34	—	6.5	107	
72	23	12.4	1000	98
	50	6.9	2050	
72	—	2.6	—	107
72	—	9.1	—	
120	53	14.2–17.6	—	
120	20–67	0.6–4.3	—	101
120	20–67	9.7 (^{15}N)	4.3 (^{14}C), 11.1 (^{15}N)	102
120	20–67	11.9 (^{15}N)	2.6 (^{14}C), 9.1 (^{15}N)	
120	20–67	6	8.4 (^{13}C) ; 8.1 (^{14}C)	102
120	20–67	5	10.0 (^{13}C) : 10.3 (^{14}C)	
—	20	9.6	1.9	103
336	54	2.4	3.8	
120	55	7.5	ratio 1:36.2	114
120	38	3.3	ratio 1:7.6	108
120	43	2.3	ratio 1:6.7	
120	67	7.5	ratio 1:4.9	114
34	23	—	5	107
34	—	—	43% ^{2}H$_2$, 4% ^{2}H$_1$	111
120	63	8.4	ratio 3.17	114
34	—	—	19 (^{2}H), 3.35 (^{14}C)	111
34	—	—	4.4 (^{2}H) 2.7 (^{14}C)	113
120	—	—	ratio 3.78	114
34	—	—	5.76 (^{2}H) ; 5.31 (^{14}C)	111
34	—	—	4.25 (^{2}H) ; 1.29 (^{3}H)	113
120	—	—	ratio 1.01	114
72	66	19–24	ratio 11.5–13.1	113
168	150–180	0.3	238–144	133
336	63	31	20	103

Table VII.

Precursor	Amount Fed (mg/l.)	Sp. Activity (mCi/mm)	Fed at (hr)
6-Hydroxypyrazinoindole-^{14}C (XLVI, R = OH)	20	4.8×10^{-3}	240–312
3-Methylenepyrazinoindole-^{14}C ^{a} (XLVI, R = H)	10	4.8×10^{-3}	192–264

[a] Experiment used *Penicillium terlikowskii.*
[b] DOPA = dihydroxyphenylalanine.

of one of the protons of the methylene group of phenylalanine. When phenylalanine dideuteriated at the methylene group was used as a precursor, 43% of the labelled species were monodeuteriated. This result led to an examination (*111*) of the fate of phenylalanine when the prochiral hydrogen atoms of the methylene group were sterospecifically labelled (*111, 113, 114*). In all cases both labels were retained to some extent, but the pro-S proton was retained in two to four times the amount of the pro-R proton—the earlier report (*111*) incorrectly reversed this result (*134*). It is possible that these incorporation studies merely reflect

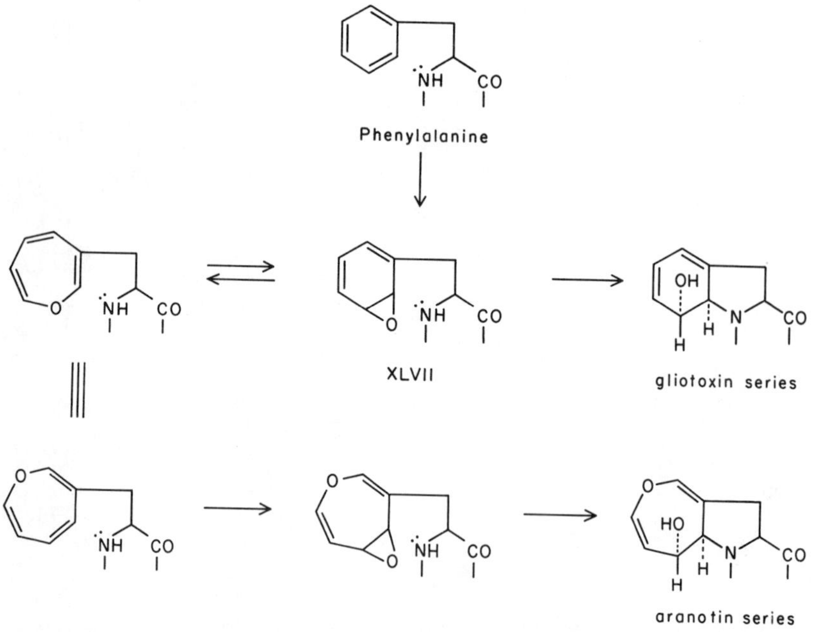

Figure 11.   Formulation of ring closure and trans opening of an epoxide

Continued

Harvested at (hr)	Gliotoxin (mg/l.)	Incorporation (%)	Dilution[a]	Reference
—	50	6	73	103
336	77	0	—	103

[a] dilution = specific activity of precursor/specific activity of product.
= $(x + y)/y$ where x and y refer to mass spectral intensities of selected peaks of mass M^+ and $M + 1^+$.

a stereospecific enolization of a substituted pyruvic acid since phenylalanine recovered from the mycelium from such precursor experiments also retained the pro-S proton preferentially.

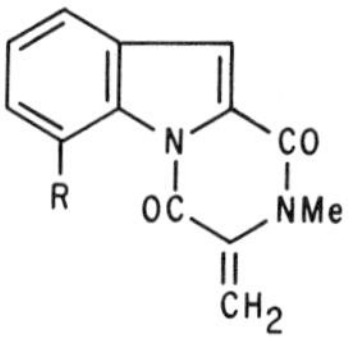

XLVI 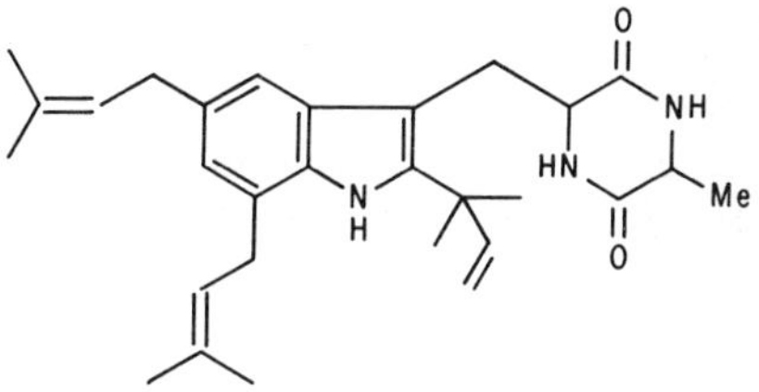   XLVIII

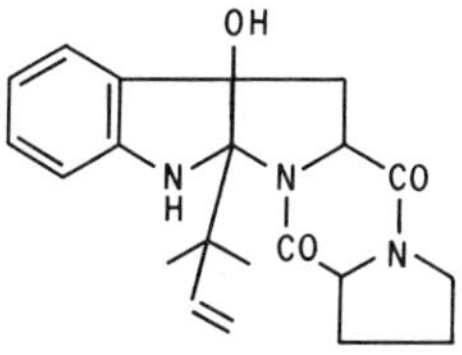

XLIX

Echinulin (XLVIII) and brevianamide-E (XLIX) have been shown to be biosynthesized from piperazine-3,6-diones (*115, 116*). Likewise DL-3-hydroxymethylene-L-6-(Bz-[³H])benzylpiperazine-2(¹⁴C),5-dione was incorporated into gliotoxin by *Gliocladium* sp. (*T. vidide*) in about 20% yield with an unchanged ¹⁴C:³H ratio (*113*). This result fits neatly with the benzoxepin theory of ring closure of the heterocyclic ring of the indoline moiety of gliotoxin. Witkop and his co-workers (*87*) have shown that the analogous dioxopiperazine of tryptophan and alanine (XXXVII) is smoothly cyclized to the eserine (XXXVIII) by radical oxidation. MacDonald and Slater (*133*) have also studied the incorporation of L-3-hydroxymethylene-L-6-benzylpiperazine-2,5(^{14}C)-dione by *Penicillium terlikowskii*. This precursor was shown to be taken up by the cultures, but was not incorporated into the gliotoxin produced by the cells, and was recovered unchanged from the culture filtrates. It is just possible that a different route of gliotoxin biosynthesis occurs in this organism, for most isolates also produce dehydrogliotoxin (*83*, VIII, $x = 2$) and the latter seems to be a precursor of gliotoxin, particularly in the later stages of the fermentation (*103*). There are precedents for this type of hydrogenation of aromatic rings (*117*).

In summary, the incorporation of D- and L-phenylalanine into gliotoxin or aranotins by *Gliocladium* spp., *P. terlikowskii, A. aureus* and *Aspergillus terrius* is established. It seems likely, under certain growth conditions, that the carbon and nitrogen skeleton of the amino acid is incorporated intact. Other aspects of these biosynthetic reactions are less certain. The isolation of apoaranotin (Table I) from cultures of *A. aureus* having both hydroxycyclohexadiene and hydroxybenzazepin moieties in the molecule, strongly supports the mechanism of formation of the indoline ring system proposed by the Lilly workers (*5*). However, much further work is required to resolve some of the apparent inconsistancies evident in the reported experimental results.

Analysis of Epipolythiodioxopiperazines

Chemical Methods. Epipolythiodioxopiperazines can be detected on paper chromatograms or thin layer chromatography plates by spraying the chromatograms with 5% aqueous silver nitrate solution. About 0.1 μg can be detected by this method, and the sensitivity can be increased to 0.02 μg by over spraying the silver sulfide spots with 0.01*N* sodium arsenite solution (*118*). Another method that is about as sensitive depends on spraying the chromatograms with a 1% solution of sodium azide in 0.01*N* iodine. The spray should be used very lightly, and the chromatograms are kept about five min and sprayed again with 1% soluble starch solution. Epidithiodioxopiperazines appear as colorless spots on a blue background (*119*).

Three methods have been used to quantitatively estimate epidithiodioxopiperazines. One that involves radioisotope dilution depends of course on the isolation of a pure sample of the metabolite of known specific activity. A second method used depended on a modification of the standard penicillin iodometric assay (*120, 121*). It suffers from the facts that spuriously high results are often obtained and that relatively large quantities ($\simeq$ 1 mg) of the polysufides are needed for accurate estimations. The third method uses the ability of the disulfides (but not always the tri- and tetrasulfides) to catalyze the decomposition of azide with iodine. These disulfides are efficient catalysts (*122, 123*) but the method requires careful standardization (*124, 125*). The method is very sensitive; 1 ml of 0.01*N* iodine is reduced by azide for each 0.055 mg of epidisulfide present, or alternatively 4 μl of nitrogen are evolved for each microgram of epidisulfide in the reaction mixture.

Biological Methods. These methods have been reviewed recently (*14*). Two techniques are generally applicable. Most of the epipolythio-dioxopiperazines described so far inhibit the growth of *Bacillus subtilis* (*126*). Of course the sensitivity of this organism to these metabolites varies (*127*), but in general there is a linear relationship over a concentration range of two or three orders of magnitude between a standard increment in the lag phase of growth of the organism and the concentration of the antibiotic. A more sensitive method (*121*) involves the growth of discontinuous layers of HeLa cells in the presence of these sulfur compounds. The effect can be measured either by determining the increase (or decrease) of the amount of protein in the cultures or by simply observing the spread of the cells on the glass surface of the culture vessel. In general in a twofold dilution series (with respect to the concentration of the antibiotic) a sharp end-point is usually seen between one concentration where the cells completely cover the surface of the culture vessels and the next higher concentration where the cell layer is discontinuous and the cells are pyknotic. In the case of the sporidesmins the method is extremely sensitive; about 1 ng of the toxin can be easily determined. Other epipolythiodioxopiperazines are less sensitive: chetomin is about 20 times less toxic, and gliotoxin is about 100 times.

Acknowledgments

We wish to thank Y. Kishi, G. M. Strunz, and W. B. Turner for sending us information not yet published and many other colleagues who have provided details of their experimental work. We also wish to thank G. M. Strunz who read the manuscript and made several helpful suggestions.

Literature Cited

1. Weindling, R., *Phytopathology* (1932) **22**, 837.
2. Bell, M. R., Johnson, J. R., Wildi, B. S., Woodward, R. B., *J. Amer. Chem. Soc.* (1958) **80**, 1001.
3. Synge, R. L. M., White, E. P., *N.Z. J. Agric. Res.* (1960) **3**, 907.
4. Hodges, R., Ronaldson, J. W., Taylor, A., White, E. P., *Chem. Ind.* (1963) 42.
5. Nagarajan, R., Huckstep, L. L., Lively, D. H., DeLong, D. C., Marsh, M. M., Neuss, N., *J. Amer. Chem. Soc.* (1968) **90**, 2980.
6. Miller, P. A., Trown, P. W., Fulmor, W., Morton, G. O., Karliner, J., *Biochem. Biophys. Res. Commun.* (1968) **33**, 219.

7. De Vault, R. L., Rosenbrook, W., J. Antibiot. (1973) **26**, 532.
8. Michel, K. H., Chaney, M. O., Jones, N. D., Hoehn, M. M., Nagarajan, R., J. Antibiot. (1974) **27**, 57.
9. Hauser, D., Weber, H. P., Sigg, H. P., Helv. Chim. Acta (1970) **53**, 1061.
10. Hauser, D., Loosli, H. R., Niklaus, P., Helv. Chim. Acta (1972) **55**, 2182.
11. Minato, H., Matsumoto, M., Katayama, T., J. Chem. Soc., Perkin Trans. 1 (1973) 1819.
12. Imperial Chemical Industries, Ltd., Netherland Patent 7312627 (March 18, 1974).
13. Strunz, G. M., Kakushima, M., Stillwell, M. A., Heissner, C. J., J. Chem. Soc., Perkin Trans. 1 (1973) 2600.
14. Atherton, L. G., Brewer, D., Taylor, A., "Mycotoxins," I. F. H. Purchase, Ed., Chapter 2, Elsevier, Amsterdam, 1974.
15. Brewer, D., Calder, F. W., MacIntyre, T. M., Taylor, A., J. Agric. Sci. (1971) **76**, 465.
16. Geiger, W. B., Conn, J. E., Waksman, S. A., J. Bacteriol. (1944) **48**, 531.
17. Safe, S., Taylor, A., J. Chem. Soc., Perkin Trans. 1 (1972) 472.
18. Trown, P. W., Biochem. Biophys. Res. Commun. (1968) **33**, 402.
19. Fridrichsons, J., Mathieson, A. McL., Tetrahedron Lett. (1962) 1265.
20. Taylor, A., "Biochemistry of Some Foodborne Microbial Toxins," R. I. Mateles, G. N. Wogan, Eds., p. 69, M.I.T. Press, Cambridge, Mass., 1967.
21. Jamieson, W. D., Rahman, R., Taylor, A., J. Chem. Soc., (C) (1969) 1564.
22. Neuss, N., Nagarajan, R., Molloy, B. B., Huckstep, L. L., Tetrahedron Lett. (1968) 4467.
23. Strunz, G. M., Heissner, C. J., Kakushima, M., Stillwell, M. A., Can. J. Chem. (1974) **52**, 325.
24. Safe, S., Taylor, A., J. Chem. Soc., (C) (1970) 432.
25. Safe, S., Taylor, A., J. Chem. Soc., (C) (1971) 1189.
26. Wieland, T., Schwahn, H., Chem. Ber. (1956) **89**, 421.
27. Barnard, D., Houseman, T. H., Porter, M., Tidd, B. K., Chem. Commun. (1969) 371.
28. Kuczkowski, R. L., J. Amer. Chem. Soc. (1964) **86**, 3617.
29. Lavine, T. F., J. Biol. Chem. (1947) **169**, 477.
30. Fridrichsons, J., Mathieson, A. McL., Acta Crystallogr., Sec. B (1965) **18**, 1043.
31. Fridrichsons, J., Mathieson, A. McL., Acta Crystallogr., Sec. B (1967) **23**, 439.
32. Cosulich, D. B., Nelson, N. R., van den Hende, J. H., J. Amer. Chem. Soc. (1968) **90**, 6519.
33. Weber, H. P., Acta Crystallogr., Sec. B (1972) **28**, 2950.
34. Öhler, E., Tataruch, F., Schmidt, U., Chem. Ber. (1973) **106**, 165.
35. Kishi, Y., Fukuyama, T., Nakatsuka, S., J. Amer. Chem. Soc. (1973) **95**, 6490.
36. Cook, A. H., Harris, G., Heilbron, I. M., J. Chem. Soc. (1948) 1060.
37. Kishi, Y., Nakatsuka, S., Fukuyama, T., Goto, T., Tetrahedron Lett. (1971) 4657.
38. Poisel, H., Schmidt, U., Chem. Ber. (1971) **104**, 1714.
39. Miller, E. G., Rayner, D. R., Mislow, K., J. Amer. Chem. Soc. (1966) **88**, 3139.
40. Braverman, S., Stabinsky, Y., Chem. Commun. (1967) 270.
41. Hodges, R., Ronaldson, J. W., Taylor, A., White, E. P., J. Chem. Soc. (1963) 5332.
42. Johnson, J. R., Buchanan, J. B., J. Amer. Chem. Soc. (1953) **75**, 2103.
43. Dutcher, J. D., Johnson, J. R., Bruce, W. F., J. Amer. Chem. Soc. (1945) **67**, 1736.

44. Elvige, J. A., Spring, F. S., *J. Chem. Soc.* (1949) 5139.
45. Hodges, R., Ronaldson, J. W., Shannon, J. S., Taylor, A., White, E. P., *J. Chem. Soc.* (1964) 26.
46. Ali, M. S., Shannon, J. S., Taylor, A., *J. Chem. Soc., C* (1968) 2044.
47. Rahman, R., Safe, S., Taylor, A., Quarterly Reviews, 1970, 24, 208.
48. Degeilh, R., Marsh, R. E., *Acta Crystallogr.* (1959) 12, 1007.
49. Groth, P., *Acta Chem. Scand.* (1969) 23, 3155.
50. Benadetti, E., Corradini, P., Pedone, C., *Biopolymers* (1969) 7, 751.
51. Karle, I. L., *J. Amer. Chem. Soc.* (1972) 94, 81.
52. Young, P. E., Madison, V., Blout, E. R., *J. Amer. Chem. Soc.* (1973) 95, 6142.
53. Sletten, E., *J. Amer. Chem. Soc.* (1970) 92, 172.
54. Karle, I. L., Ottenheym, H. C. J., Witkop, B., *J. Amer. Chem. Soc.* (1974) 96, 539.
55. Donnay, J. D. H., *Acta Crystallogr.* (1955) 8, 245.
56. Claseon, G., Androes, G., Calvin, M., *J. Amer. Chem. Soc.* (1961) 83, 4357.
57. Lüttringhaus, A., Hess, U., Rosenbaum, H. J., *Z. Naturforsch.* (1967) 22b, 1296.
58. Lüttringhaus, A., Rosenbaum, H. J., *Monatsh.* (1967) 98, 1323.
59. Bushweller, C. H., *J. Amer. Chem. Soc.* (1969) 91, 6019.
60. Herrmann, H., Hodges, R., Taylor, A., *J. Chem. Soc.* (1964) 4315.
61. Rahman, R., Safe, S., Taylor, A., *J. Chem. Soc., C* (1969) 1665.
62. Nagarajan, R., Woody, R. W., *J. Amer. Chem. Soc.* (1973) 95, 7212.
63. Francis, E., Rahman, R., Safe, S., Taylor, A., *J. Chem. Soc., Perkin Trans. 1* (1972) 470.
64. Beecham, A. F., Fridrichsons, J., Mathieson, A. McL., *Tetrahedron Lett.* (1966) 3131.
65. Linderberg, J., Michl, J., *J. Amer. Chem. Soc.* (1970) 92, 2619.
66. Bijvoet, J. M., Peerdeman, A. F., van Bommel, A. J., *Nature* (1951) 168, 271.
67. Moncrief, J. W., *J. Amer. Chem. Soc.* (1968) 90, 6517.
68. Brewer, D., Duncan, J. M., Jerram, W. A., Leach, C. K., Safe, S., Taylor, A., Vining, L. C., Archibald, R. McG., Stevenson, R. G., Mirocha, C. J., Christensen, C. M., *Can. J. Microbiol.* (1972) 18, 1129.
69. Kabuss, S., Lüttringhaus, A., Friebolin, H., Schmid, H. G., Mecke, R., *Tetrahedron Lett.* (1966) 719.
70. Djerassi, C., "Optical Rotatory Dispension," p. 29, McGraw-Hill, New York, 1960.
71. Strunz, G. M., Kakushima, M., Stillwell, M. A., *Can. J. Chem.* (1975) 53, 295.
72. Ronaldson, J. W., Taylor, A., White, E. P., Abraham, R. J., *J. Chem. Soc.* (1963) 3172.
73. Przybylska, M., Gopalakrishna, E. M., *Acta Crystallogr., Sect. B* (1974) 30, 597.
74. Davis, B. R., Bernal, I., *Proc. Natl. Acad. Sci. U.S.A.* (1973) 70, 279.
75. Ricci, J. S., Bernal, I., *J. Chem. Soc., B* (1971) 1928.
76. Davis, B. R., Bernal, I., Köpf, H., *Angew. Chem., Int. Ed. Engl.* (1971) 10, 921.
77. Barrick, J. C., Calvo, C., Olsen, F. P., *Chem. Commun.* (1971) 1043.
78. Svokos, S. G., Angier, R. B., Ger. Patent 2029306 (Cl. C 07d) (1970).
79. Poisel, H., Schmidt, U., *Chem. Ber.* (1972) 105, 625.
80. Hino, T., Sato, T., *Tetrahedron Lett.* (1971) 3127.
81. Öhler, E., Poisel, H., Tataruch, F., Schmidt, U., *Chem. Ber.* (1972) 105, 635.
82. Öhler, E., Tataruch, F., Schmidt, U., *Chem. Ber.* (1973) 106, 396.

83. Lowe, G., Taylor, A., Vining, L. C., *J. Chem. Soc.* (1966) 1799.
84. Kishi, Y., Fukuyama, T., Nakatsuka, S., *J. Amer. Chem. Soc.* (1972) **95**, 6492.
85. Hodges, R., Taylor, A., *J. Chem. Soc.* (1964) 4310.
86. Gulland, J. M., Robinson, R., Scott, J., Thornley, S., *J. Chem. Soc.* (1929) 2933.
87. Ohno, M., Spande, T. F., Witkop, B., *J. Amer. Chem. Soc.* (1970) **92**, 343.
88. Witkop, B., Patrick, J. B., *J. Amer. Chem. Soc.* (1951) **73**, 2188.
89. Nakagawa, M., Kaneko, T., Yoshikawa, K., Hino, T., *J. Amer. Chem. Soc.* (1974) **96**, 624.
90. Kishi, Y., Nakatsuka, S., Fukuyama, T., Havel, M., *J. Amer. Chem. Soc.* (1973) **95**, 6493.
91. Nakatsuka, S., Fukuyama, T., Kishi, Y., *Tetrahedron Lett.* (1974) 1549.
92. Strunz, G. M., Kakushima, M., *Experienta* (1974) **30**, 719.
93. Weindling, R., *Phytopathology* (1941) **31**, 991.
94. Brian, P. W., Hemming, H. G., *Ann. Appl. Biol.* (1945) **32**, 214.
95. Brian, P. W., Hemming, H. G., *Trans. Brit. Mycol. Soc.* (1950) **33**, 132.
96. Bu'Lock, J. D., Tse Hing Yuen, T. L. S., *Phytochemistry* (1971) **10**, 1835.
97. Morquer, R., Lacoste, L., Blaha, G., *C. R. Paris* (1967) **264** (D), 1840.
98. Suhadolnik, R. J., Chenoweth, R. G., *J. Amer. Chem. Soc.* (1958) **80**, 4391.
99. Winstead, J. A., Suhadolnik, R. J., *J. Amer. Chem. Soc.* (1960) **82**, 1644.
100. Suhadolnik, R. J., Fischer, A., Wilson, J., *Fed. Proc.* (1960) **19**, 8.
101. Bose, A. K., Das, K. G., Funke, P. T., Kugajevsky, I., Shukla, O. P., Khanchandani, K. S., Suhadolnik, R. J., *J. Amer. Chem. Soc.* (1968) **90**, 1038.
102. Bose, A. K., Khanchandani, K. S., Tavares, R., Funke, P. T., *J. Amer. Chem. Soc.* (1968) **90**, 3593.
103. Ali, M. S., Ph.D. Thesis, Dalhousie, 1968.
104. Neuss, N., Boeck, L. D., Brannon, D. R., Cline, J. C., DeLong, D. C., Gorman, M., Huckstep, L. L., Lively, D. H., Mabe, J., Marsh, M. M., Molloy, B. B., Nagarajan, R., Nelson, J. D., Stark, W. M., *Antimicrob. Agents Chemother.* (1968) 213.
105. Ryles, A. P., Ph.D. Thesis, Manchester, 1971.
106. Towers, N. R., Wright, D. E., *N.Z. J. Agric. Res.* (1969) **12**, 275.
107. Bu'Lock, J. D., Ryles, A. P., *Chem. Commun.* (1970) 1404.
108. Johns, N., Kirby, G. W., *Chem. Commun.* (1971) 163.
109. Brannon, D. R., Mabe, J. A., Molloy, B. B., Day, W. A., *Biochem. Biophys. Res. Commun.* (1971) **43**, 588.
110. Guroff, G., Daly, J. W., Jerina, D. M., Benson, J., Witkop, B., Udenfriend, S., *Science* (1967) **157**, 1524.
111. Bu'Lock, J. D., Ryles, A. P., Johns, N., Kirby, G. W., *Chem. Commun.* (1972) 100.
112. Machin, P. J., Sammes, P. G., *J. Chem. Soc., Perkin Trans. 1* (1974) 698.
113. Leigh, C., Ph.D. Thesis, Manchester, 1973; Bu'Lock, J. D., Leigh, C., *J. Chem. Soc., Chem. Commun.*, 1975, 628.
114. Johns, N., Ph.D. Thesis, Loughborough, 1972.
115. Slater, G. P., MacDonald, J. C., Nakashima, R., *Biochemistry* (1970) **9**, 2886.
116. Baldas, J., Birch, A. J., Russell, R. A., *J. Chem. Soc., Perkin Trans. 1* (1974) 50.
117. Dutton, P. L., Evans, W. D., *Biochem. J.* (1969) **113**, 525.
118. Rahman, R., Safe, S., Taylor, A., *J. Chromatogr.* (1970) **53**, 592.
119. Russell, G. R., *Nature* (1960) **186**, 788.
120. Claire, N. T., "Microbiological Aspects of Facial Eczema," No. 37, p. 15, N.Z. Dept. Sci. and Ind. Res., Information Series, 1964.

121. Done, J., Mortimer, P. H., Taylor, A., Russell, D. W., *J. Gen. Microbiol.* (1961) **26**, 207.
122. Dahl, W. E., Pardue, H. L., *Anal. Chem.* (1965) **37**, 1382.
123. Marbrook, J., *N.Z. J. Agric. Res.* (1964) **7**, 596.
124. Brewer, D., Taylor, A., *Can. J. Microbiol.* (1967) **13**, 1577.
125. Clare, N. T., Gumbley, J. M., *N.Z. J. Agric. Res.* (1962) **5**, 36.
126. Brewer, D., Hannah, D. E., Taylor, A., *Can. J. Microbiol.* (1966) **12**, 1187.
127. Taylor, A., The Toxicology of Sporidesmins and Other Epipolythiadioxo-piperazines, in "Microbial Toxins," Vol. 7, S. Kadis, A. Ciegler, S. J. Ajl, Eds., p. 363, Academic Press, New York, 1971.
128. Dorn, F., Arigoni, D., *Experienta* (1974) **30**, 134.
129. Kako, A., Saeki, T., Suzuhi, S., Ando, K., Tamura, G., Arima, K., *J. Antibiot.* (1969) **22**, 322.
130. Argoudelis, A. D., Reusser, F., *J. Antibiot.* (1971) **24**, 383; *ibid.* (1972) **25**, 171.
131. Eguchi, C., Kakuta, A., *J. Amer. Chem. Soc.* (1974) **96**, 3985.
132. Kirby, G. W., Varley, M. J., *Chem. Commun.* (1974) 833.
133. MacDonald, J. C., Slater, G. P., *Can. J. Biochem.* (1975) **53**, 475.
134. Johns, N., Kirby, G. W., Bu'Lock, J. D., Ryles, A. P., *J. Chem. Soc. Perkin Trans. I*, 1975, 383.
135. Ottenheijm, H. C. J., Vermeulen, N. P. E., Breuer, L. F. J. M., Justus Liebigs Ann. Chem. (1974) 206.
136. Ottenheijm, H. C. J., Spande, T. F., Witkop, B., *J. Amer. Chem. Soc.* (1973) **95**, 1989.
137. Ottenheijm, H. C. J., Hulshof, J. A. M., Nivard, R. J. F., *J. Org. Chem.* (1975) **40**, 2147.
138. Ottenheijm, H. C. J., Potman, A. D., van Vroonhoven, T., *Rec. Trav. Chim.* (1975) **94**, 135, 138.
139. Ottenheijm, H. C. J., Kerkhoff, G. P. C., Bijen, J. W. H. A., Spande, T. F., *Chem. Commun.* (1975), 765.

RECEIVED November 8, 1974.

12

The Ochratoxins and Other Related Compounds

STANLEY NESHEIM

Division of Chemistry and Physics, Food and Drug Administration, 200 "C" Street, S. W., Washington, D.C. 20204

The ochratoxins are toxic metabolites elaborated by several species of Aspergillus ochraceus *as well as by* Penicillium viridicatum. *The discovery, chemistry, history, sources, occurrence, toxicology, and fate in foods and feeds of these metabolites are reviewed. Emphasized are the analytical methods for the detection and estimation of the ochratoxins with reference to their applicability in commodities such as grains, nuts, beer, and animal tissues. Similarities and differences in sampling procedures, extraction methods and solvents, extract purification, toxin detection and estimation, and chemical and biological techniques of confirmation of identity are described. Other metabolites which interfere with current methods are listed. Suggestions to direct further efforts in developing analytical methods of ochratoxins are proposed.*

In a screening program to determine possible causes of certain animal diseases in South Africa, Scott showed that three of five strains of *Aspergillus ochraceus* Wilh isolated from local domestic legumes and cereal products were toxigenic (*1*). The toxic metabolites were later isolated and chemically characterized (*2, 3, 4*). The major toxic compound was named ochratoxin A; several related compounds were also isolated and identified (Figure 1). More recently one or more of the ochratoxins have been isolated from various mold species of the *Aspergillus* and *Penicillium* genera (*5–14*). These molds are commonly found in soils and on food and feed commodities such as nuts, dried fish, grains, beans, peas, coffee, spices, alfalfa, and meats (*9, 10, 12, 15–24*). Ochratoxin A, the 7-carboxy-5-chloro-8-hydroxy-3,4-dihydro-3-R-methyl isocoumarin amide of L-β-phenylalanine (Figure 1), is the most toxic of the ochratoxins (*25*) and is produced in highest yield (*26*). Its chemical structure has been confirmed by synthesis (*27, 28*). Both it and ochratoxin B, its dechloro analog, are acidic compounds and fluoresce intensely under ultraviolet light. They are relatively heat stable, resisting autoclaving in oatmeal and cereal (*29*). However, they are largely destroyed in coffee by heating to 200°C for 5 min or more under simulated coffee roasting conditions (*21*). Both ochratoxins A and B have been found as natural contaminants of food and feeds such as wheat, barley, oats, coffee beans, corn, rye, and dried white beans (*9, 10, 12, 14, 29–39*). The levels detected ranged from <10 μg/kg to 28 mg/kg. The higher levels were found in lower grade or moldy materials. In Denmark, where samples were taken from districts experiencing a high incidence of swine nephropathy, 58% of 33 samples were contaminated, and averaged 3 mg/kg. In other surveys there and elsewhere involving nonselected samples the incidence and degree of contamination was low. To control, reduce or eliminate ochratoxin contamination, factors which can modify mold development (including moisture, temperature, aeration, time, and substrate) have been investigated (*21, 40, 41*). The fate of ochratoxin in the normal use of contaminated products has also been studied. As mentioned above, under simulated coffee roasting conditions the ochratoxins are largely destroyed (*21*), but 30% remained intact in oatmeal or rice cereals after 3 hr of autoclaving (*29*). On malting and brewing beer from barley contaminated with 1–5000 μg/kg ochratoxin A the beer contained from 6–20 μg/l.; this corresponds to a 2–7% transmission (*42*).

Several investigators studied the toxicological and pathological effects produced by the ochratoxins. The LD_{50} for ochratoxin A administered *per os* varies from 2.1–4.67 mg/kg for the chick, swine, and trout to 22 mg/kg for the female rat (*12, 25, 30, 33, 43–57*). Ochratoxin A has been reported as teratogenic to mice and rats (*51, 59, 59*) and to the chicken embryo (*60*); other investigators however report no teratogenic effects in chicken embryos (*61, 62*). A dose of 200 μg ochratoxin A/kg body weight has been reported to produce nephrosis in pigs (*31, 52*).

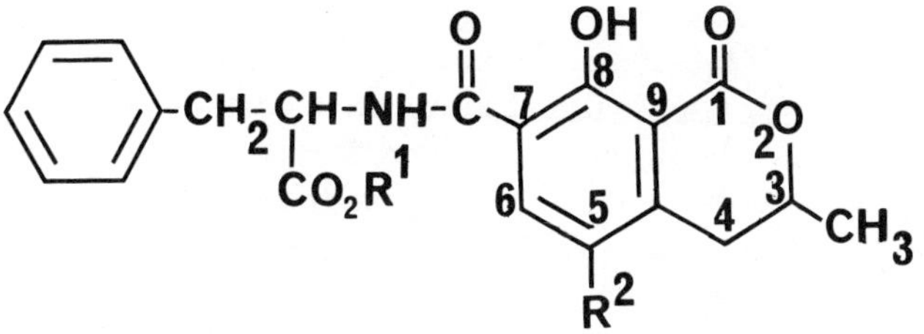

Figure 1.   Ochratoxin A: $R^1 = H$, $R^2 = Cl$; ochratoxin B: $R^1 = R^2 = H$; ochratoxin C: $R^1 = -CH_2-CH_3$, $R^2 = Cl$

The deposition of ochratoxin A in the liver, kidney, fat, and muscle tissues of swine and the excretion of ochratoxin A in cows' milk have been reported (30, 63, 64).

To help detect, control, and eliminate ochratoxin from human and animal foods and feeds, sensitive analytical methods including some screening methods have been developed. Some of these have been used for the surveillance of various commodities and to detect the natural occurrence of ochratoxins. Two of the ochratoxin methods have been tested in interlaboratory collaborative studies (65, 66) and were adopted "official first action" for inclusion in "Official Methods of Analysis" of the Association of Official Analytical Chemists (67). Such adoption means that the method has been validated by testing in several laboratories on identical sets of samples containing ochratoxins at unknown levels occurring both as a natural contaminant and as an added contaminant.

Although several good general reviews covering broad areas of the subject (1, 12, 14, 33, 47, 68–71) and reviews of some of the methods (25, 72, 73) have been prepared, no in-depth review of the methodology has been made. This chapter attempts to summarize all the work on methodology including much that has been scattered as parts of reports in other areas, fields, or disciplines.

Most of the published ochratoxin methods described below apply only to the analysis of ochratoxins A and B. A few methods have been applied to the analysis of the methyl and ethyl esters (2–4, 15, 26, 43, 65, 67, 74–78). Although the esters of ochratoxin A are as toxic as the parent compounds (47), they have been found only in substrates molded under laboratory conditions and at much lower concentrations than those of ochratoxins A and B (4).

All ochratoxin methods consist of two or more of the following basic steps: lot sampling, analytical sample preparation, extraction of the toxins, purification or concentration, detection, quantitation, and confirmation of identity of the toxin. The methods differ in commodity applicability, sensitivity (or minimum detection level), accuracy, precision, amount of validation data supporting the method, cost of materials, equipment, time, and labor.

The choice of a method is dictated by factors such as type and number of samples to be analyzed and information required for the particular study. The analyst should not be limited to any specific method. For a survey, for example, he can and should use the simplest reliable method available (i.e., a screening method) to eliminate the many negative samples and then perhaps apply another, more rigorous method to the positive samples. Of course the screening method should have a sensitivity adequate to the needs of the survey.

Methods are continually improved as new techniques appear and are applied to old problems. The annual report of the General Referee on Mycotoxins of the Association of Official Analytical Chemists is published every year in the March issue of the *Journal of the Association of Official Analytical Chemists* and provides a continuing review of developments in methodology. Associate Referees are assigned to separate topics such as "Ochratoxins," "Aflatoxins in Coffee," "Mycotoxins in Grains," to name a few, under the review of the General Referee. The Associate Referees also report progress in their assignments but on a less regular basis.

Lot Sampling

For mycotoxins in general or for ochratoxins specifically, the contamination in the commodity may be in small pockets or in a few of many units of the commodity. A. *ochraceus* is known to produce as high as 1.3–1.5 mg ochratoxin A/kg on chopped corn, polished rice, or wheat bran (29) and 3.9 g/kg on shredded wheat (79). These high levels can be associated with very small portions of a total lot. Therefore, large samples must be taken to increase the probability of including contaminated portions of heterogeneous lots. Common practice for aflatoxin analysis is to take a 25 kg sample for larger kernel materials such as nuts and a five kg sample for commodities such as small grains. The considerations involved in sampling peanuts have been published (80–82).

Analytical Sample Preparation

The effectiveness of some approaches to reduction of the lot sample to an analytical sample, 10–350 g, has been studied (83, 84). Generally 10 g is considered too small for adequate analytical sampling; currently a 100-g sample is recommended. For small samples ($\leq$ 1 kg) the entire quantity can be extracted. It is ground finely enough for efficient extraction—i.e., to pass a 1–2 mm screen. If it is too fine, problems can arise in filtration steps subsequent to extraction. Larger samples must be ground similarly and blended thoroughly before sample selection. When it is not practical to grind finely the entire sample lot (as in the case of cottonseed lintels for example), a compromise can be made by first coarsely grinding the sample to pass through a 2–5 mm screen and then blending and removing a 1–1.5-kg subsample. This subsample is ground, blended, and sampled for analysis.

Extraction

The methods for which quantitative data have been published, the extraction solvent used, and representative commodities for which they

Table I. Quantitative Ochratoxin Methods

Commodity	Extraction Solvent[a]	Recovery[b] %	Sensitivity[b] μg/kg	Reference
Culture media and mycelia	CHCl₃–MeOH, 1:1		10–100	31, 49, 85, 86
Wheat, flour, corn meal, cooked barley, rice	MeOH–H₂O– Hexane, 55:45:40	63–102	25, 20	10, 87, 88
Cereal, beans, peanuts, feces	MeOH–H₂O– Hexane, 55:45:40 + 1% H₂SO₄ (20%)	90–100		10
Maize, peanuts, sorghum	CHCl₃–MeOH– Hexane, 8:2:1	80–100	20	81
Capsicum pepper, barley, green coffee	CHCl₃	79–103	40	15
Corn meal, rice, cereal, wheat bran, oat meal	(1) Hexane (defat) (2) CHCl₃– MeOH, 1:1	73–165	10–50	85
Barley, oats, beer, coffee, tissue	CHCl₃–H₂O (0.1M H₃PO₄) 10:1	55–117	2–20	32, 42, 52, 65–67, 74, 89
Nuts, grains, beans, fruit, coffee, cocoa, coconut, meats, potatoes, dairy products, sugar, candy	CHCl₃–H₂O, 10:1	40–60	50	35–39, 75, 90, 91
Grains, sausage	CH₃CN–H₂O (4% KCl) 9:1	86–100	50–100	7, 76, 92
Grains	CH₃CN–H₂O (4% KCl, 2% H₂SO₄) 9:1	85–113	10	10, 41

[a] Solvents (v/v): HOAc = acetic acid; n-BuOH = butanol, Et₂O = ethyl ether; EtOAc = ethyl acetate; Formic acid = formic acid (90%); i-PrOH = 2-propanol; MeOH = methanol; MiBK = methyl isobutyl ketone; Pet. ether = petroleum ether; T = toluene.

[b] Recovery of ochratoxin A as obtained using the entire procedure described in references.

were developed or to which they have been applied are shown in Table I. In general, three extraction techniques are used: (a) Soxhlet extraction, the most time-consuming; (b) shaking the commodity for 10–30 min. with solvent; and (c) blending with solvent in a Waring type blender for 1–3 min. All extractants are organic solvents or mixtures of these; water, acid, or both are added in some cases. The recoveries shown in Table I are for ochratoxin A only. It can be assumed that similar results would be obtained for ochratoxin B. The recoveries tabulated are for the entire method and not for the extraction step alone.

Table II lists the methods for which only qualitative information is available. Often these are methods for isolating the toxins rather than methods of analysis.

Extract Purification

The extract obtained from a material containing more than $\mu g/kg$ amounts of ochratoxin can be taken directly for analysis, but for the more general case further purification is necessary to remove interfering components. The extract, after filtration, may be concentrated or dissolved in a different solvent and purified by one or more of the following tech-

Table II.   Qualitative Methods for Ochratoxin Analysis

Application	Extractant[a]	References
Shredded wheat cereal, yeast extract, mold culture media, dry mold mycelium, animal tissue	$CHCl_3$, pH 1.5–7	7, 13, 18, 26, 32, 35, 42, 45, 52, 62, 69, 89, 90, 93–102
Corn, dry mycelium	$CHCl_3$–MeOH, 1:1	2–4, 103
Grain	$CHCl_3$–MeOH, 7:3	5
Urine	$CHCl_3$–MeOH, 4:1	88
Liquid culture medium, mycelium	$CHCl_3$–MeOH, pH 1	104
Rice, liquid culture medium	EtOAc, pH $\leq$ 3	14, 105
Corn, peanut sorghum	Acetone–H_2O, 85:15	75
Corn, wheat	CH_3CN–H_2O–hexane, 9:1:5	8
Liquid sucrose yeast extract	Dowex 1-X8 resin (formate form) 200-400 mesh	105
Starter medium	Dowex 1 formate, 50 mesh	53, 106
Urine	$NaHCO_3$ (sat soln)	106

[a] *See* note *a,* Table I.

Table III.   Quantitative Methods of Extract Purification

Liquid/Liquid Partition in Separatory Funnel or on Diatomaceous Earth Column

Solvent Pairs[a]	References
$CHCl_3$/0.1 or $0.5M$ $NaHCO_3$ $NaHCO_3$ + excess acid/$CHCl_3$	75, 85, 86, 103
Hexane/MeOH–H_2O, 55:45/$CHCl_3$–hexane, 1:1	9, 10, 87
(1) Hexane/MeOH–H_2O, 85:15 (2) MeOH–H_2O, 1:1/$CHCl_3$	75
Hexane–acetone–formic acid/$0.2N$ NaOH NaOH + HCl to pH 2.5/$CHCl_3$	15
Solid extract/1% $NaHCO_3$ $NaHCO_3$ + HCl to pH 2.5/$CHCl_3$	85
CH_3CN–H_2O (4% KCl) 9:1/i-octane (fat) CH_3CH–H_2O/$CHCl_3$	76, 92
CH_3CH–H_2O/$CHCl_3$ CH_3CN–H_2O/$CHCl_3$	7

Chromatography

Adsorbent	Eluting Solvent[a]	References
Silica gel	(1) Pet. ether–Et_2O, 3:1 (2) MeOH–$CHCl_3$, 3:97 (3) C_6H_6–HOAc, 9:1	75
Silica gel	(1) Hexane (2) Acetone–C_6H_6, 5:95 (3) MeOH–HOAc, 3:97 (4) HOAc–C_6H_6, 1:9	35–39, 90, 91
Florisil	(1) MeOH–$CHCl_3$, 1:9 (2) Acetone–hexane, 1:1 (3) Hexane–acetone–formic acid, 59:40:1	15
Diatomaceous earth-$0.1N$ $NaHCO_3$	(1) Hexane (2) $CHCl_3$ (3) Formic acid–$CHCl_3$, 1:99 or HOAc–C_6H_6, 2:98	21, 32, 42, 52, 65, 67, 74
Sephadex LH-20	(1) $CHCl_3$ (2) MeOH or MeOH–$CHCl_3$, 1:1	43, 85, 107

[a] *See* note *a*, Table I.

niques: (a) liquid–liquid partition of toxins and interfering materials between immiscible liquids; (b) formation of water-soluble salts and subsequent recovery of toxins after acidification by extraction with an organic solvent; (c) column chromatography or preparatory thin layer chromatography (TLC). Several partition systems, adsorbents, and eluting solvents which have been used are shown in Tables III and IV.

Table IV.   Qualitative Methods of Extract Purification

Liquid/Liquid[a] Partition in Separatory Funnel

Partitioning Solvents	References
$CHCl_3/0.5M$ NaHCO$_3$; NaHCO$_3$+ excess acid/CHCl$_3$	2, 3, 13, 18, 19, 26, 89, 98, 102
(1) 10M Formic acid in MeOH–H$_2$O, 1:1/CHCl$_3$	53, 106
(2) HOAc–C$_6$H$_6$, 12:88/0.5M NaHCO$_3$; NaHCO$_3$/CHCl$_3$	

Column Chromatography

Adsorbents	Eluting Solvents[a]	References
Acidic silica gel	C$_6$H$_6$–CHCl$_3$, 3:1	2, 3
Silica gel	HOAc–C$_6$H$_6$, 1:9	5, 43, 107
Silica gel	HOAc–C$_6$H$_6$, 12:88	53, 106
Silica gel	(1) C$_6$H$_6$ (2) C$_6$H$_6$–CHCl$_3$, 1:1 (3) CHCl$_3$ (4) CHCl$_3$–MeOH, 19:1 (5) C$_6$H$_6$–AcOH, 9:1	13
Silica gel	HOAc–C$_6$H$_6$, 0:100 to 15:85	26
Silica gel	EtOAc–CHCl$_3$, 1:3	62, 108
Silica gel	C$_6$H$_6$–CHCl$_3$–HOAc, 12:3:1	28
Silica gel	CHCl$_3$–MeOH, 50:1	27
Silica gel–oxalic acid, 95:5	(1) C$_6$H$_6$ (2) CHCl$_3$–acetone, 100:0 to 90:10	98, 102
Silica gel–oxalic acid, 95:5	CHCl$_3$–acetone, 100:0 to 85:15	102
Silica gel–oxalic acid, 95:5	C$_6$H$_6$–EtOAc, 100:0 to 30:70	102
Silica gel–oxalic acid, 95:5	C$_6$H$_6$–acetone, 100:0 to 85:15	102
Alumina, acid	(1) C$_6$H$_6$ (2) C$_6$H$_6$–CHCl$_3$, 1:3 (3) CHCl$_3$ (4) CHCl$_3$–HOAc, 20:1 (5) CHCl$_3$–HOAc, 10:1	13
Sephadex G-25	0.01M NaCl–0.1M phosphate	109

Table IV. Continued

Column Chromatography

Adsorbents	Eluting Solvents[a]	References
"Dowex 1 × 8" 200-400 mesh (formate form)	buffer, pH 7.2 3.5–10N formic acid in MeOH–H_2O, 1:1	3, 53, 106

Miscellaneous	References
Dissolve in $CHCl_3$ and precipitate ochratoxins A and B by adding hexane	26
Chill at 5° for 18 hr in $CHCl_3$ and remove solid impurities	13
Preparatory TLC on silica gel	4, 9, 13, 18, 27, 28, 49, 100, 102–104, 110
Preparatory TLC on silica gel sheets	99
Preparatory TLC on 0.25 mm or 2 mm Channel plates (Kontes Glass Co., K 41603)	15
Membrane diffusion	34

[a] See note a, Table I.

Separation, Detection and Quantitation

The most sensitive techniques for quantitation of ochratoxins are ultraviolet spectrophotometry and visual estimation or spectrofluorodensitometry of TLC plates. However, the uv determination requires several micrograms of material and is therefore used mainly to quantitate standard solutions of pure ochratoxins. The fluorescence determination can be made on a few nanograms. The toxins as isolated by all methods of analysis consist of microgram or smaller quantities of one or more toxins dissolved in extraneous material which may amount to > 100 mg from 10-g samples of commodities such as grains or nuts. This mixture is therefore further fractionated (usually by TLC), and the toxins are determined by visual or instrumental comparison on thin layer plates of the fluorescence intensities of the unknown spots with spots of the TLC standards. The many solvents and absorbents which have been used for the TLC detection and estimation of ochratoxins and some typical R_f values are listed in Table V. It should be emphasized that nearly all the methods depend on good TLC resolution of the toxins from each other and from interfering materials. The TLC R_f values are not very reproducible, and unknown spots are best identified by chromatography with known ochratoxin standards added to the extract either in solution or on the origin spot on the TLC plate. Identical R_f values of unknown and standard, even in several TLC systems, do not positively identify the unknown. Usually further confirmation of identity must be made. This is discussed below.

Table V. R_f Values[a] of Ochratoxins for Their Separation, Detection and Quantitation

	Ochratoxins: Esters[c] of				
Solvent[b]	A	B	A	B	References
Thin Layer Chromatography (Silica Gel)					
C_6H_6–HOAc, 25:1			55	30	4, 27
C_6H_6–HOAc, 9:1	45	24	67	46	1, 5–9, 13, 26, 37, 75, 79, 90
C_6H_6–HOAc, 8:2					111, 112
C_6H_6–HOAc, 3:1	50	35	65		78, 86, 110
C_6H_6–HOAc, 4:1	69	45			27, 62, 104, 108, 111, 113
C_6H_6–HOAc–H_2O 90:10:1	32				35–38, 96
C_6H_6–MeOH–HOAc, 18:1:1	65	50	100	100	8, 21, 35, 36, 67, 74, 76, 77, 96, 117
C_6H_6–MeOH–HOAc, 12:2:1	60	52			1–3, 86, 111
C_6H_6–MeOH–HOAc, 24:2:1	60	35			9, 10, 85, 87, 100, 115–117
C_6H_6–CCl_4–nBuOH–EtOAc–formic acid, 35:25:20:19:1					15
C_6H_6–MeOH–EtOAc, 15:3:1	31	14	74		14, 97, 105
C_6H_6–EtOAc–formic acid, 70:30:1	50				28
C_6H_6–acetone–formic acid, 80:20:1	46				28
C_6H_6–BuOH–EtOAc–formic acid, 69:15:12:4	74	65	81		15
C_6H_6–BuOH–EtOAc–formic acid, 50:15:33:2	71	63	80		15
Toluene–EtOAc–formic acid, 5:4:1	70				13, 18, 21, 28, 35, 36, 75, 87, 90, 91, 94–96, 99–102, 111, 118
Toluene–EtOAc–formic acid, 6:3:1	55–70				6, 7, 9, 10, 98, 116
EtOAc–i-PrOH–H_2O, 5:2:1	42	25	95		97
Et_2O–MeOH–H_2O–formic acid, 95:4:1:1	27				10
$CHCl_3$–acetone, 93:7					91
$CHCl_3$–EtOAc–formic acid, 60:40:1					119
$CHCl_3$–acetone–i-PrOH, 85:12.5:2.5					15

Table V.   Continued

Solvent[b]	Ochratoxins: Esters[e] of				References
	A	B	A	B	
CHCl₃–acetone–formic acid, 80:20:1	65				28, 102
CHCl₃–MiBK, 4:1 (Oxalic acid impregnated silica)	48	20			1, 120
Di-isopropyl ether (Oxalic acid impregnated silica)	35				28
Hexane–acetone–HOAc, 18:2:1				50	67, 74, 76

Thin Layer Chromatography (Alumina)

CHCl₃–acetone, 4:1					9

Paper Chromatography

i-PrOH–3N (NH₄)₂CO₃, 3:1	65				2, 3, 86
Hexane (formamide impregnated paper)			50	18	4

Silica Gel Mini-Column Chromatography Detection[d]

Toluene–EtOAc–formic acid, 5:4:1				89	

[a] Rfx100.
[b] See a, Table I.
[e] Methyl or ethyl esters of ochratoxins A and B.
[d] Fluorescent band detected on 4 mm × 7 cm silica gel column.

The method of visual comparison of fluorescence intensities suffers from poor precision ($> \pm 20\%$) (65) and depends greatly on the analyst's ability and experience. The TLC densitometry is more objective but suffers more from instrumental problems, interferences, and poor resolution in TLC. The types of TLC scanning instruments, linear ranges and sensitivities obtained with them are shown in Table VI. Also listed in Table VI are other analytical methods. These are less sensitive or more complicated to use but have been used in special circumstances as indicated in references listed in the table.

Chemical Confirmation of Identity

The presence of ochratoxins in a sample is initially based on the identity of the R_f values of the unknowns with those of standard ochratoxins. Additional proof is most frequently obtained by developing chromatograms in several solvent systems. This is conclusive evidence only in a negative sense—i.e., that the initial suspect spots are not ochratoxins. For positive proof the toxins are separated and purified by pre-

Table VI. Instrumental Methods for Quantitation of Ochratoxins
(ng/spot)

Instrument	Linear Range	Sensi-tivity	CV[b]	References
TLC Fluorodensitometry[a]				
Photovolt, model 530	10–100		7.1	15, 26, 91, 101
Ozumor, SD-91, Asuka Kogyo Co., Tokyo	0–5000	170		14, 105
Hitachi Fluoro spec-trometer, MPF-2A, TLC accessory 018-0057				65, 74
Schoeffel, SD 3000	3–10			65, 77
Aminco-Bowman spectro photo fluorometer	0–10	0.5–1.0	3.6	5, 43, 85, 114, 121
Aminco-Bowman spectro photo fluorometer (after exposing TLC spots to NH₃)	0.25–5	0.25		52, 117
Four different instru-ments (Photovolt, Schoeffel, Aminco-Bowman and Hitachi)			6.4	32, 42, 52, 65, 67, 74
Miscellaneous Techniques				
UV spectrophotometry		sensitivity 0.5–5 µg/ml		15, 18, 26, 28, 43–45, 67, 74, 85, 98, 103, 109, 110, 112, 118, 121–123
UV spectrophotometric dialysis and titration				121
Phosphorescence and fluorescence				118
Hydrolysis followed by GLC analysis for phenylalanine				43, 121
Radiochemical methods				62, 99, 108, 110

[a] In acid medium: excitation maximum 310–340 nm, emission maximum 440–475 nm; in basic medium: excitation maximum 360–390 nm, emission maximum 427–445 nm.

[b] Coefficient of variation $= \dfrac{\text{standard deviation} \times 100}{\text{average}}$

paratory TLC and identified by one or more of the physical chemical or bioassay techniques (Table VII).

Almost every instrument for measuring physical parameters has been applied to the identification of ochratoxins (ir, uv, NMR, and mass spectrometry). Physical and chemical properties such as melting points, elemental analysis, and chemical derivative formation have also been used. The basic TLC sprays listed in Table V change the fluorescence of ochratoxins A and B from green to blue by forming a salt with the phenolic functional group.

Table VII.   Chemical Confirmation of Identity of Ochratoxins

TLC Sprays	References
NH$_4$OH or NH$_3$ fumes	5–7, 10, 13, 35, 36, 87, 90, 91, 93, 94, 99–101, 117, 119
Triethylamine	87
NaHCO$_3$	67, 74
FeCl$_3$	7, 104, 120
KOH (20%)	75
AlCl$_3$	6, 7
Repeated TLC with up to 10 different solvent systems	4, 9, 27, 28, 35, 36, 86, 87, 90, 95
Solubility in NaHCO$_3$ solution	9, 90, 94, 35–38
Chemical derivatives	
Methyl esters and ethers	2–4, 7, 10, 26, 31, 35, 37, 38, 94, 99, 104
Ethyl esters	4, 26, 65, 67, 52, 74
Acetates	15, 100
Trifluoroacetates	15
Trimethylsilyl ether	15
Spectral methods	
Visual comparison under short and long uv light	76, 94
Fluorescence spectrophotometry, acid-base	5
Ultraviolet spectrophotometry	2–4, 9, 15, 18, 26, 28, 44, 98, 100, 102, 122
Infrared spectrophotometry	2–4, 13, 15, 26–28, 102
Optical rotatory dispersion and polarimetry	2–4, 13, 27, 28, 104
Nuclear magnetic resonance	2–4, 13, 26, 27, 31, 69, 102, 104, 124
Mass spectrometry	2–4, 26–28, 69, 104, 125
Melting points, C,H,N analysis	2–4, 13, 26, 27, 98, 102, 124

A TLC identification may be made by preparing the esters or ethers of both the unknown and standard ochratoxins and comparing the TLC characteristics (R_f's) of these derivatives.

Biological Tests

Table VIII lists some of the more sensitive tests which have been devised to test ochratoxin for biological activity. These are for the most part qualitative in nature. In conjunction with other physical and chemical data some of the biological tests are occasionally used for confirming the identity of ochratoxins.

Ochratoxin-Related Metabolites (Table IX)

The few chemically related derivatives of the ochratoxins reported so far include, besides the ethyl and methyl esters of ochratoxins A and

Table VIII.   Biological Tests for Ochratoxin A

System	Type Response	Sensitivity	Reference
Chicken embryo	death	LD_{50} 0.01– 17 μg/egg	25, 60–62, 70, 78, 126
Zebra fish larva	death	LC_{50} 1.7 μg/ml	129
Brine shrimp	death	20% mortality 1 μg/ml	70, 130
Brine shrimp larvae	death	LC_{50} 10 μg/ml; 17% mortality 0.2 μg/disc	131
Bacillus megaterium	growth inhibition	1 μg/disc	35, 36, 127, 128
Bacillus cereus mycoides	growth inhibition	1.5 μg/disc	127
Tetrahymena pyriformis HSM	growth inhibition	1% 200 μg/ml	132
HeLa cell	cytotoxicity	10 μg/ml	22, 68, 97
Tracheal organ culture	death	LC_{50} 1.7 μg/ml	133
Day old duckling	death	150 μg/duckling	1–4
Day old chick	death	LD_{50} 135–166 μg/chick	107, 122, 134

B, 4-hydroxy-ochratoxin A and ochratoxin α and β (Figure 1). Methods for one or more of the methyl and ethyl esters have been published (*4, 65, 74–77*). They are as toxic as the parent compounds (*25*) but are produced in rather low yield by the mold (*4*). Ochratoxin D reported by Scott is synonymous with 4-hydroxyochratoxin A. Ochratoxin α is derived from ochratoxin A by removing the phenylalanine moiety. Several of the other compounds shown in Table IX are related to the ochratoxins only in that they are produced by the same molds and hence can interfere both in chemical analyses, tests, and in biological assays or toxicity studies. The derivatives for the most part are relatively nontoxic (*25*). Methods of analysis are available for some of these substances but have not been referenced because they are beyond the scope of this review.

Conclusion

The multiplicity of methods in use as outlined here indicates the lack of a single method adequate for all tasks. Methodology will probably be greatly improved in the near future when the promising technique of high efficiency liquid chromatography (already successfully applied to the analysis of the mycotoxins, aflatoxins, patulin, and sterigmatocystin) is applied to ochratoxins. It is hoped that the future will bring reliable, rapid, inexpensive, and even automated methods to effectively and economically protect the food and feed supply.

Table IX. Ochratoxins, Related Metabolites and Derivatives
Produced by Two Major Ochratoxin-Producing Fungi

Compound	A. ochra-ceus	P. viridi-catum	Reference
Ochratoxin A and B	+	+	1, 12, 13, 93, 98, 119
Methyl and ethyl esters of ochratoxins A and B	+		4
4-Hydroxy ochratoxin A	+	+	12, 98, 104
Ochratoxin $T_A{}^a$ and $T_C{}^a$			78
Ochratoxin α and β^b	+	+	29, 44, 88, 99, 104, 107, 111, 112, 113, 117
L-Alanine and L-leucine derivatives of ochratoxin α			136
4-Hydroxyaspergillic acid	+		4, 97
Aspocracin	+		137, 138
Brevianamide A and B		+	139
Citrinin		+	9, 10, 12, 31, 50, 119
Emodin	+		14
3-(1,2-Epoxypropyl)-5,6-dihydro-5-hydroxy-6-methyl-2-one	+		140
Ergosterol	+		13, 14
Erythritol	+		14
Griseofulvin		+	141
Mellein (ochracin)	+		1, 22, 125
4-Hydroxymellein	+		96, 135
Oxalic acid		+	9, 50
Penicillic acid	+	+	4, 5, 14, 22, 91, 93, 97, 103, 119, 142, 143
L-Prolyl-L-leucine anhydride	+		1
L-Prolyl-L-valine anhydride	+		1
Secalonic acid	+		14, 145
Viridicatin		+	146
Viridicatol		+	147
Viridicatum toxin		+	141
Unidentified toxins	+	+	11, 16, 23, 93, 97, 119, 144, 148–152

[a] Ochratoxins A and C in which the phenylalanine moiety has been replaced with tyrosine.
[b] Ochratoxins in which the phenylalanine moiety has been removed.

Literature Cited

1. Steyn, P. S., "Microbial Toxins," Vol. VI, A. Ciegler, S. Kadis, S. J. Ajd, Eds., pp. 179–205, Academic Press, New York, 1971.
2. Van der Merwe, K. J., Steyn, P. S., Fourie, L., Scott, de B., Theron, J. J., *Nature* (1965) **205**, 1112.
3. Van der Merwe, K. J., Steyn, P. S., Fourie, L., *J. Chem. Soc.* (1965) 7083.

4. Steyn, P. S., Holzapfel, C. W., *J. S. Afr. Chem. Inst.* (1967) **20**, 186.
5. Ciegler, A., *Can. J. Microbiol.* (1972) **18**, 631.
6. Ciegler, H., Fennel, D. J., Mintzlaff, H. J., Leistner, L., *Naturwissenschaften* (1972) **59**, 365.
7. Ciegler, A., Mintzlaff, H. J., Machnik, W., Leistner, L., *Fleischwirtschaft* (1972) **52**, 1311.
8. Hesseltine, C. W., Vandegraft, E. E., Fennell, D. I., Smith, M. L., Shotwell, O. J., *Mycologia* (1972) **64**, 539.
9. Scott, P. M., van Walbeek, J. W., Harwig, J., Fennell, D. I., *Can. J. Plant Sci.* (1970) **50**, 583.
10. Scott, P. M., van Walbeek, W., Kennedy, B., Anyeti, D., *J. Agric. Food Chem.* (1972) **20**, 1103.
11. Semeniuk, G., Harshfield, G. S., Carlson, C. W., Hesseltine, C. W., Kwolek, W. F., "Proceedings First U.S.-Japan Conference on Toxic Micro-Organisms," U.S. Department of Interior, Washington, D.C. (1970) 185–190.
12. van Walbeek, W., *Can. Inst. Food Technol. J.* (1973) **6**, 96.
13. van Walbeek, W., Scott, P. M., Harwig, J., Lawrence, J. W., *Can. J. Microbiol.* (1969) **15**, 1281.
14. Yamazaki, M., "Mycotoxins in Human Health," I. F. H. Purchase, Ed., p. 107, Macmillan Press Ltd., London, 1971.
15. Broce, D., Ph.D. Thesis, Louisiana State University, Baton Rouge, 1970.
16. Doupnik, B., Jr., Bell, D. K., *Appl. Microbiol.* (1971) **21**, 1104.
17. Leistner, L., Mintzlaff, H. J., Maing, I. Y., Abstracts of the 2nd International Union of Pure and Applied Chemistry Sponsored International Symposium Mycotoxins in Food, Pulaway, Poland (1974) July 23-25.
18. Moore, J. H., Ph.D. Thesis, Auburn University, Auburn, Ala., 1971.
19. Nesheim, S., *J. Ass. Offic. Anal. Chem.* (1967) **50**, 370.
20. Tsunoda, H., "Proceedings First U.S.-Japan Conference on Toxic Micro-Organisms," U.S. Department of Interior, Washington, D.C. (1970) 143.
21. Levi, C. P., Trenk, H. L., Mohr, H. K., *J. Ass. Offic. Anal. Chem.* (1974) 866.
22. Umeda, M., Yamashita, T., Saito, M., Sekita, S., Takahashi, C., Yoshihira, K., Natori, S., Kurata, H., Udagawa, S., *Jap. J. Exp. Med.* (1974) **44**, 83.
23. Saito, M., Ohtsuba, K., Umeda, M., Enomoto, M., Kurata, H., Udagawa, S., Sakabe, F., Ichinoe, M., *Jap. J. Exp. Med.* (1971) **40**, 1.
24. Saito, M., Ishiko, T., Enomoto, M., Ohtsubo, K., Umeda, M., Kurata, H., Udagawa, S., Taniguchi, S., Sekita, S., *Jap. J. Exp. Med.* (1974) **44**, 63.
25. Chu, F. S., *Crit. Rev. Toxicol.* (1974) **2**, 499.
26. Nesheim, S., *J. Ass. Offic. Anal. Chem.* (1969) **52**, 975.
27. Steyn, P. S., Holzapfel, C. W., *Tetrahedron* (1967) **23**, 4449.
28. Roberts, J. C., Woollven, P., *J. Chem. Soc., C* (1970) 278.
29. Trenk, H. L., Butz, M. E., Chu, F. S., *Appl. Microbiol.* (1971) **21**, 1032.
30. Krogh, P., Abstracts of the 2nd International Union of Pure and Applied Chemistry Sponsored International Symposium Mycotoxins in Food, Pulaway, Poland (1974) July 23-25.
31. Krogh, P., Hald, B., Pedersen, E. J., *Acta Pathol. Microbiol. Scand., Sect. B* (1973) **81**, 689.
32. Krogh, P., Hald, B., Englund, P., Rutqvist, L., Swahn, O., *Acta Pathol. Microbiol. Scand. Sect. B* (1974) **82**, 301.
33. Munro, I. C., Scott, P. M., Moodie, C. A., Willes, R. F., *J. Amer. Vet. Med. Ass.* (1973) **163**, 1269.
34. Patterson, D. S. P., Roberts, B. A., Abstracts of the 2nd International Union of Pure and Applied Chemistry Sponsored International Symposium Mycotoxins in Food, Pulaway, Poland (1974) July 23-25.

35. Shotwell, O. L., Hesseltine, C. W., Goulden, M. L., *Appl. Microbiol.*
    (1969) **17**, 765.
36. Shotwell, O. L., Hesseltine, C. W., Goulden, M. L., *J. Ass. Offic. Anal.
    Chem.* (1969) **52**, 81.
37. Shotwell, O. L., Hesseltine, C. W., Goulden, M. L., Vandegraft, E. E.,
    Cereal Chem. (1970) **47**, 700.
38. Shotwell, O. L., Hesseltine, C. W., Vandegraft, E. E., Goulden, M. L.,
    Cereal Sci. Today (1971) **16**, 266.
39. Shotwell, O. L., Goulden, M. L., Fennell, D. I., Hesseltine, C. W., 88th
    Ann. Meetg., Association of Analytical Chemists, Washington, D.C.,
    Oct. 14-17, 1974.
40. Lillehoj, E. B., *J. Amer. Vet. Med. Ass.* (1973) **163**, 1281.
41. Harwig, J., Chen, Y.-K., *Can. J. Plant Sci.* (1974) **54**, 17.
42. Krogh, P., Hald, B., Gjertsen, P., Myken, F., *Appl. Microbiol.* (1974) **28**,
    31.
43. Chu, F. S., *Biochem. Pharmacol.* (1974) **23**, 1105.
44. Doster, R. C., Sinnhuber, R. O., *Food Cosmet. Toxicol.* (1972) **10**, 389.
45. Doster, R. C., Arscott, G. H., Sinnhuber, R. O., *Poultry Sci.* (1973) **52**,
    2351.
46. Elling, F., Moeller, T., *Bull. World Health Org.* (1973) **49**, 411.
47. *Food Cosmet. Toxicol.* (1973) **11**, 903.
48. Galtier, P., Moré, J., Bodin, G., *Ann. Rech. Veter.* (1974) **5**, 233.
49. Huff, W. E., Wyatt, R. D., Tucker, T. L., Hamilton, P. B., *Poultry Sci.*
    (1974) **53**, 1585.
50. Krogh, P., Hasselager, E., Friis, P., *Acta Pathol. Microbiol. Scand. Sect. B*
    (1970) **78**, 401.
51. Moré, J., Galtier, P., *Ann. Rech. Veter.* (1974) **5**, 167.
52. Krogh, P., Axelsen, N. H., Elling, F., Gyrd-Hansen, N., Hald, B., Hyld-
    gaard-Jensen, J., Larsen, A. E., Madsen, A., Mortensen, H. P., Moeller,
    T., Petersen, O. K., Ravnskov, U., Rostgaard, M., Aalund, O., *Acta
    Pathol. Microbiol. Scand. Sect. A* (1974) Supplement 246, 1.
53. Meisner, H., Chan, S., *Biochemistry* (1974) **13**, 2795.
54. Munro, I. C., Moodie, C. A., Kuiper-Goodman, T., Scott, P. M., Grice,
    H. C., *Toxicol. Appl. Pharmacol.* (1974) **28**, 180.
55. Szczech, G. M., Carlton, W. W., Tuite, J., *Toxicol. Appl. Pharmacol.*
    (1973) **25**, 456.
56. Szczech, G. M., Carlton, W. W., Tuite, J., *Vet. Pathol.* (1973) **10**, 219.
57. Szczech, G. M., Carlton, W. W., and Tuite, J. *Vet. Pathol.* (1973) **10**, 135.
58. Hayes, A. W., Hood, R. D., *Toxicol. Appl. Pharmacol.* (1973) **25**, 457.
59. Hayes, A. W., Hood, R. D., Lee, H. L., *Teratology* (1974) **9**, 93.
60. Verrett, M. J., unpublished data (1974).
61. Mintzlaff, H. J., Christ, W., *Fleischwirtschaft* (1972) **52**, 1174.
62. Yamazaki, M., Suzuki, S., Sakakibara, Y., Miyaki, K., *Jap. J. Med. Sci.
    Biol.* (1971) **24**, 245.
63. Madsen, A., Mortensen, H. P., Larsen, A. E., Flengmark, P., Hald, B.,
    Krogh, P., Elling, F., *Ugeskr. Agron. Hort.* (1973) **6**, 100.
64. Ribelin, W. E., Smalley, E. B., Strong, F. M., Abstract of the 2nd Int.
    Cong. Plant Pathol., Minneapolis, Minn. (1973) Sept. 5-12.
65. Nesheim, S., *J. Ass. Offic. Anal. Chem.* (1973) **56**, 822.
66. Levi, C. P., Presented at the 88th Annual Meeting of the Association of
    Official Analytical Chemists, Washington, D.C. (1974) Oct. 14-17.
67. "Changes in Methods," *J. Ass. Offic. Anal. Chem.* (1973) **56**, 486.
68. Enomoto, M., Saito, M., *Annu. Rev. Microbiol.* (1972) **26**, 279.
69. Ferreira, N. P., "Biochemistry of Some Foodborne Microbiological Toxins,"
    Mateles, R. I., Wogan, G. N., Eds., p. 157, MIT Press, Cambridge,
    Mass. 1967.

70. Brown, R. F., "Proceedings First U.S.-Japan Conference on Toxic Micro-Organisms," U.S. Department of Interior, Washington, D.C., (1970) pp. 12-18.
71. Mirocha, C. J. Christensen, C. M., *Ann. Rev. Phytopathol.* (1974) **12**, 303.
72. Fishbein, L., Falk, H. L., *Chromatogr. Rev.* (1970) **12**, 42.
73. Stoloff, L., *Clin. Toxicol.* (1972) **5**, 465.
74. Nesheim, S., Hardin, N. F., Francis, O. J., Jr., Langham, W. S., *J. Ass. Offic. Anal. Chem.* (1973) **56**, 817.
75. Vorster, L. J., *Analyst* (1969) **94**, 136.
76. Stoloff, L., Nesheim, S., Yin, L., Rodricks, J. V., Stack, M., *J. Ass. Offic. Anal. Chem.* (1971) **54**, 91.
77. Stoloff, L., "Quantitative Thin-Layer Chromatography," J. Touchstone, Ed., p. 95, John Wiley & Sons, New York, 1973.
78. Wei, R., Chu, F. S., Experientia (1974) **30**, 174.
79. Schindler, A. F., Nesheim, S., *J. Ass. Offic. Anal. Chem.* (1970) **53**, 89.
80. Tiemstra, P. J., *J. Amer. Oil Chem. Soc.* (1971) **46**, 1307.
81. Whitaker, T. B., Dickens, J. W., Wiser, E. H., *J. Amer. Oil Chem. Soc.* (1970) **47**, 501; Whitaker, T. B., Dickens, J. W., Monroe, R. J., *ibid.* (1974) **51**, 214.
82. Whitaker, T. B., Wiser, E. H., *J. Amer. Oil Chem. Soc.* (1969) **46**, 377.
83. Stoloff, L., Dantzman, J., *J. Amer. Oil Chem. Soc.* (1972) **49**, 264.
84. Stoloff, L., Campbell, A. D., Beckwith, A. C., Nesheim, S., Winbush, J. S., Jr., Fordham, O. M., Jr., *J. Amer. Oil Chem. Soc.* (1969) **46**, 678.
85. Chu, F. S., Butz, M. E., *J. Ass. Offic. Anal. Chem.* (1970) **53**, 1253.
86. Steyn, P. S., van der Merwe, K. J., *Nature* (1966) **211**, 418.
87. Scott, P. M., Hand, T. B., *J. Ass. Offic. Anal. Chem.* (1967) **50**, 366.
88. van Walbeek, W., Moodie, C. A., Scott, P. M., Harwig, J., Grice, H. C., *Toxicol. Appl. Pharmacol.* (1971) **20**, 439.
89. Hald, B., Krogh, P., *J. Ass. Offic. Anal. Chem.* (1975) **58**, 156.
90. Eppley, R. M., *J. Ass. Offic. Anal. Chem.* (1968) **51**, 74.
91. Escher, F. E., Koehler, P. E., Ayres, J. C., *Appl. Microbiol.* (1973) **26**, 27.
92. Yin, L., *Ass. Offic. Anal. Chem.* (1969) **52**, 880.
93. Bullerman, L. B., *J. Milk Food Technol.* (1974) **37**, 1.
94. Davis, N. D., Searcy, J. W., Diener, U. L., *Appl. Microbiol.* (1969) **17**, 742.
95. Lai, M., Semeniuk, G., Hesseltine, C. W., *Appl. Microbiol.* (1970) **19**, 542.
96. Moore, J. H., Davis, N. D., Diener, U. L., *Appl. Microbiol.* (1972) **23**, 1067.
97. Natori, S., Sakaki, S., Kurata, H., Udagawa, S., Ichine, M., Saito, M., Umeda, M., *Chem. Pharm. Bull.* (1970) **18**, 2259.
98. Scott, P. M., Kennedy, B., van Walbeek, W., *J. Ass. Offic. Anal. Chem.* (1971) **54**, 1445.
99. Searcy, J. W., Davis, N. D., Diener, U. L., *Appl. Microbiol.* (1969) **18**, 622.
100. van Walbeek, W., Scott, P. M., Thatcher, F. S., *Can. J. Microbiol.* (1968) **14**, 131.
101. Wu, M. T., Ayres, J. C., *J. Agric. Food Chem.* (1974) **22**, 537.
102. Galtier, P., *Ann. Rech. Veter.* (1974) **5**, 155.
103. Bacon, C. W., Sweeney, J. G., Robbins, J. D., Burkick, D., *Appl. Microbiol.* (1973) **26**, 155.
104. Hutchison, R. D., Steyn, P. S., Thompson, D. C., *Tetrahedron Lett.* (1971) **43**, 4033.
105. Yamazaki, M., Maebayashi, Y., Miyaki, K., *Appl. Microbiol.* (1970) **20**, 452.
106. Davis, N. D., Sansing, G. A., Ellenburg, T. V., Diener, U. L., *Appl. Microbiol.* (1972) **23**, 433.
107. Chu, F. S., Chang, C. C., *J. Ass. Offic. Anal. Chem.* (1971) **54**, 1032.

108. Maebayashi, Y., Miyaki, K., Yamazaki, M., *Chem. Pharm. Bull.* (1972) 20, 2172.
109. Pitout, M. J., *Toxicol. Appl. Pharmacol.* (1968) 13, 299.
110. Wei, R., Strong, F. M., Smalley, E. B., *Appl. Microbiol.* (1971) 22, 276.
111. Nel, W., Purchase, I. F. H., *J. S. Afr. Chem. Inst.* (1968) 21, 87.
112. Pitout, M. J., *Biochem. Pharmacol.* (1969) 18, 485.
113. Steyn, P. S., Holzapfel, C. W., Ferreira, N. P., *Phytochemistry* (1970) 9, 1977.
114. Lemieszek, K., Abstracts of the 2nd International Union of Pure and Applied Chemistry Sponsored International Symposium Mycotoxins in Food. Pulaway, Poland (1974) July 23-25.
115. Chu, F. S., *J. Ass. Offic. Anal. Chem.* (1970) 53, 696.
116. Scott, P. M., Lawrence, J. W., van Walbeek, W., *Appl. Microbiol.* (1970) 20, 839.
117. Trenk, H. L., Chu, F. S., *J. Ass. Offic. Anal. Chem.* (1971) 54, 1307.
118. Neely, W. C., West, A. D., *J. Ass. Offic. Anal. Chem.* (1972) 55, 1305.
119. Ciegler, A., Fennell, D. I., Sansing, G. A., Detroy, R. W., Bennett, G. A., *Appl. Microbiol.* (1973) 26, 271.
120. Steyn, P. S., *J. Chromatogr.* (1969) 45, 473.
121. Shu, F. S., *Arch. Biochem. Biophys.* (1971) 147, 359.
122. Chu, F. S., Noh, I., Chang, C. C., *Life Sci.* (1972) 11, Part I, 503.
123. Pitout, M. J., "Mycotoxins in Human Health," I. F. H. Purchase, *Ed.*, p. 53, Macmillan, London, 1971.
124. Yamazaki, M., Maebayashi, Y., Miyaki, K., *Tetrahedron Lett.* (1971) 25, 2301.
125. Doster, R. C., Sinnhuber, R. O., Wales, J. H., *Food Cosmet. Toxicol.* (1972) 10, 85.
126. Choudhury, H., Carlson, C. W., *Poultry Sci.* (1973) 52, 1202.
127. Broce, D., Grodner, R. M., Killebrew, R. L., Bonner, F. L., *J. Ass. Offic. Anal. Chem.* (1970) 53, 616.
128. Clements, N. L., Abstracts of the American Association of Cereal Chemists —American Oil Chemists Society Joint Meeting, Washington, D.C. (1968).
129. Abedi, Z. H., Scott, P. M., *J. Ass. Offic. Anal. Chem.* (1969) 52, 963.
130. Brown, R. F., *J. Amer. Oil Chem. Soc.* (1969) 46, 119.
131. Harwig, J., Scott, P. M., *Appl. Microbiol.* (1971) 21, 1011.
132. Hayes, A. W., Melton, R., Smith, S. J., *Bull. Environ. Contam. Toxicol.* (1974) 11, 321.
133. Cardeilhac, P. T., Nair, K. P. C., Colwell, W. M., *J. Ass. Offic. Anal. Chem.* (1972) 55, 1120.
134. Peckham, J. C., Doupnik, B., Jr., Jones, O. H., Jr., *Appl. Microbiol.* (1971) 21, 492.
135. Cole, R. J., Moore, J. H., Davis, N. D., Kirksey, J. W., Diener, U. L., *J. Agric. Food Chem.* (1971) 19, 909.
136. Pawlowski, N. E., Doster, R. C., Lee, D. J., Nixon, J. E., Sinnhuber, R. O., "Abstracts of Papers," 167th National Meeting, ACS, March 31-April 5, 1974, Los Angeles, Calif.
137. Myokei, R., Sakurai, A., Chang, C., Kodaira, Y., Takahashi, N., Tamura, S., *Tetrahedron Lett.* (1969).
138. Myokei, R., Sakurai, A., Chang, C., Kodaira, Y., Takahashi, N., Tamura, S., *Agric. Biol. Chem.* (1969) 33, 1491.
139. Wilson, B. J., Yang, D. T. C., Harris, T. M., *Appl. Microbiol.* (1973) 26, 633.
140. Moore, J. H., Murray, T. P., Marks, M. E., *J. Agric. Food Chem.* (1974) 22, 697.
141. Hutchison, R. D., Steyn, P. S., van Rensburg, S. J., *Toxicol. Appl. Pharmacol.* (1973) 24, 507.

142. Udagawa, S., Ichinoe, M., Kurata, H., "Proceedings First U.S.-Japan Conference on Toxic Micro-Organisms," U.S. Department of Interior, Washington, D.C. (1970) pp. 174–187.
143. Wu, M. T., Ayres, J. C., Kohler, P. E., *Appl. Microbiol.* (1974) **27**, 427.
144. Budiarso, I. T., Carlton, W. W., Tuite, J. F., *Vet. Pathol.* (1970) **7**, 531.
145. Yamazaki, M., Maebayashi, Y., Miyaki, K., *Chem. Pharm. Bull.* (1971) **19**, 199.
146. Cunningham, K. G., Freeman, G. G., *Biochem. J.* (1953) **53**, 328.
147. Luckner, M., Mohammed, Y. S., *Tetrahedron Lett.* (1964) **29**, 1987.
148. Carlton, W. W., Tuite, J., Caldwell, R., *J. Amer. Vet. Med. Ass.* (1973) **163**, 1295.
149. McCracken, M. D., Carlton, W. W., Tuite, J., *Food Cosmet. Toxicol.* (1974) **12**, 79.
150. *Ibid.*, 89.
151. *Ibid.*, 99.
152. Zwicker, G. M., Carlton, W. W., Tuite, J., *Food Cosmet. Toxicol.* (1973) **11**, 989.

RECEIVED December 16, 1974.

13

Phytopathogenic Toxins from Fungi:
An Overview

H. H. LUKE

U.S. Department of Agriculture, Plant Pathology Dept., University of Florida, Gainesville, Fla. 32611

R. H. BIGGS

Fruit Crops Department, University of Florida, Gainesville, Fla. 32611

Phytopathogenic toxins that are produced by plant pathogens are classified into two types: nonspecific, those that affect a greater number of plant species than the pathogen that produces them; and specific, those that affect only the same hosts as the pathogen. Evidence indicating that plant pathogens induce disease by toxigenic action has been established by using specific toxins produced in vitro. *It is difficult to isolate toxins from infected plants and therefore it is hard to show that toxins produced* in vivo *incite disease. Most phytopathogenic toxins are produced by species of* Alternaria *or* Bipolaris *(formerly* Helminthosporium*). Similarities in the molecular structure of mycotoxins and some phytopathogenic toxins indicate that the latter may be toxic also to animals. Moreover some phytotoxins occur in higher concentrations in infected plants than mycotoxins.*

Phytopathogenic toxins are produced by plant pathogens, induce disease development, and may be considered as pathogenic agents (2). Many fungal metabolites are toxic to plants but do not initiate disease development. Toxins that do not initiate disease or that have a minor influence on disease are referred to as phytotoxins (2). Phytotoxins are usually produced during the later part of the disease syndrome. Some phytotoxins that are produced *in vitro* have not been found *in vivo*. The

296

idea that plant pathogens produce toxins that cause plant disease originated about a century ago (*1*). Currently only 10 known toxins initiate disease, and their precise mode of action is not known. One of the major reasons for limited progress on this topic is the lack of knowledge of the chemical structure of these toxins. The exact structure of only a few toxins is known, and unfortunately most of those that have been described chemically either do not cause disease or have only a minor influence on disease development. We hope in this discourse to alert chemists to the need to determine the structures of phytopathogenic toxins.

Most toxins that incite diseases of higher plants are produced by species of *Bipolaris* (formerly *Helminthosporium*) or *Alternaria*. Some toxins produced by these two genera are specific and some are nonspecific. A few fungi other than species of *Bipolaris* or *Alternaria* also produce toxins. Therefore this discourse is subdivided into six categories: specific and nonspecific *Bipolaris* toxins, specific and nonspecific *Alternaria* toxins, and other toxins. In the sixth section we discuss similarities between mycotoxins and phytopathogenic toxins. Several toxins from each category are discussed.

Specific Bipolaris *Toxins*

Specific toxins are those that affect the same hosts as the pathogen that produces them. Specific toxins have been termed pathotoxins (*2*) and host-specific toxins (*3*). These terms are synonymous because they denote a substance produced by a plant pathogen that initiates disease. The most conclusive evidence that toxins produced by plant pathogenic fungi incite disease has been obtained with specific toxins (*2, 32*). We believe that there are many specific toxins that occur only *in vivo*, but it is difficult to extract them from the infected host. Therefore the most conclusive evidence that toxins initiate plant disease has been obtained by using specific toxins produced in artificial media.

Bipolaris victoriae. This fungus (formerly *Helminthosporium victoriae*) causes a devastating disease of oat cultivars that have the Victoria gene for crown rust resistance (*4*). The fungus causes necrosis at the base of the stem and striping or reddening of leaves. Leaf striping and discoloration progress upward from the lower leaves. Plants show blighting and discoloration at nodal areas and severe lodging at the base and upper nodes. Because the pathogen could not be isolated from the discolored leaves, it was suggested that this symptom resulted from a toxin that originated at the site of infection (*5*). This observation was confirmed and extended to show that culture filtrates were toxic to cultivars that were susceptible to the pathogen. Oat cultivars resistant to the pathogen were uniformly resistant to the toxin (*6*). Further study revealed that nonpathogenic cultures of the fungus did not produce the toxin. Differences in degree of pathogenicity among cultures were positively correlated with differences in toxin production, and toxin production was directly related to the growth rate of the fungus (7). Thus this toxin, given the trivial name victorin (8), was established as a specific toxin that is the causal agent of Victoria blight of oats.

The intact victorin molecule does not react with ninhydrin, but hydrolysis yields two compounds that do react with ninhydrin. One was reported to be a tricyclic secondary amine (victoxinine, empirical formula of $C_{17}H_{29}NO$), and the other was a peptide composed of five amino acids (9). Victoxinine was said to be the toxic principle, and the small peptide supposedly conveyed specificity to the intact molecule (10). Another report however stated that victoxinine was not the toxic moiety of victorin (3). In a later discussion Pringle appeared reluctant to concede that a peptide linkage occurs in the intact toxin molecule (11). Unfortunately the chemistry of the intact toxin has not been studied successfully. Emphasis was placed on victoxinine which may not be involved in the disease caused by B. victoriae. As a result, the chemistry of victoxinine is not presented in this discourse. A reliable molecular structure for victorin would certainly be useful to determine the mode of action of this toxin.

Although the precise mode of action of victorin is not known, various forms of circumstantial evidence suggest that the toxin causes an irreversible physiological malfunction of the plasma membrane (12, 13). This conclusion is based on five different lines of evidence:

(a) Small quantities of toxin caused electrolyte leakage within 5 min after treatment, and there was a strong positive correlation between electrolyte leakage and toxin concentration (14).

(b) Electron micrographs showed that victorin caused partial separation of the plasma membrane from the cell wall resulting in blister-like formations. Such separation disrupted the osmotic properties of the membrane and caused the loss of cellular components and cell turgor (12, 15).

(c) When cell walls were removed, victorin caused bursting of protoplasts from susceptible cultivars, but protoplasts from resistant cultivars seemed to burst at a slower rate (16).

(d) Treatment with toxin caused leakage of phosphorylated hexoses from susceptible tissue. Phosphorylated sugars do not pass through membranes that function normally, and therefore victorin appears to disrupt the physiological function of the plasma membrane (13).

(e) Victorin induced leakage of ^{86}Rb and ^{45}Ca from susceptible but not from resistant root tissue. If victorin and calcium compete for negatively charged sites on the plasma membrane, the removal of calcium from negatively charged sites may result in a repulsion between negative charges on the membrane and the cell wall (17). Repulsion forces would result in blister-like formations observed with the electron microscope (*12*).

The exact manner by which victorin causes dysfunction of the plasma membrane is not known, nor is it known if the action on the plasma membrane is a primary or secondary one. The speed (5 min) with which victorin disrupts the function of the plasma membrane suggests that the action is direct, but a firm conclusion to this effect should be supported by direct evidence. The unstable nature of the purified toxin has prevented successful labeling experiments that could show the site of action of victorin.

Bipolaris zeicola. This fungus (formerly *Helminthosporium carbonum*) causes a leaf blotch on certain inbred lines of corn (*Zea mays*). In the early stages of disease, water soaking of leaf tissues is pronounced. Lesions become elongated and develop a yellowish-brown color. The margins are irregular, and in advanced stages the lesions show a definite zonate pattern (*18, 19*).

Although the structural configuration of the *B. zeicola* toxin has not been determined, its empirical formula is considered to be $C_{32}H_{50}N_6O_{10}$. This formula is considered approximate because of the unstable nature of the molecule. Data from ion exclusion columns indicated that the toxin has a molecular weight of less than 700 (*11*). However the unreliable nature of data obtained from ion exclusion columns suggests that more study of the molecular properties of this toxin is needed. IR spectrometry revealed that the *B. zeicola* toxin is a substituted polyamid. A complete acid hydrolysis resulted in five different ninhydrin-reacting products, all of which appeared to be on aliphatic carbons. Because none of these compounds reacted with *p*-nitrobenzylchloride, none appear to have methylamino groups (*11*). The intact toxin did not react with ninhydrin or with 2,4-dinitrofluorobenzene. This toxin contains 11 rings, double bonds, or both (*11*). Thus either the intact toxin has ring structure, or the terminal amino groups are acylated.

Low levels of the toxin (45 μg/ml) inhibit root elongation of other nonhost plants. If the toxin concentration is low enough, cultivars susceptible to *B. zeicola* are more sensitive to the toxin than cultivars that are resistant to the fungus (*20*). Therefore the toxin may be considered specific if the proper concentration is used.

Although the mode of action of the *B. zeicola* toxin is not known, some information on physiological changes induced by this toxin is available. The toxin stimulates respiration, induces electrolyte leakage, and increases dark fixation of CO_2. But amino acid and uridine incorporation is decreased. The uptake of *B. zeicola* toxin seems to require energy (*20*).

Bipolaris maydis. This fungus (formerly *Helminthosporium maydis*) causes a severe leaf blight of corn cultivars that have the Texas male-sterile cytoplasm and a minor leaf spot on cultivars that do not have this cytoplasm. The symptoms of the disease are characterized by small, light-green, water-soaked spots. After five to six days the symptoms on resistant and susceptible cultivars differ distinctly. Lesions on leaves of resistant cultivars are small (2–5 mm) and have brown-to-tan necrotic centers circumscribed by reddish borders and chlorotic margins. Blotches on leaves of susceptible cultivars range from 10 to 40 mm and have light tan necrotic centers without defined pigmented borders. After 10 days blotches on susceptible cultivars have dark brown borders but little or no chlorosis (18, 19).

B. maydis produces four toxins in vitro referred to as toxins I, II, III, and IV. Three of these have been isolated from leaf tissue of susceptible corn plants infected with the fungus. The toxicity and specificity of all four are similar. Toxins I, II, and III, which can be biologically derived from mevalonic acid, have been reported to be two terpenoids and a terpenoid glycoside (21). Toxins I and II are highly saturated and give proton magnetic resonance spectra similar to spectra emitted by tetra-cyclic triterpenoids. Toxin III may be a glycoside of a compound similar to toxins I and II, but toxin III contains a larger number of hydroxyl groups. The molecular weight of toxin III, about 162, is greater than the weights of toxins I and II. Toxin III has properties similar to those of a reducing hexose sugar, indicating that toxin III is a glycoside. Data seem to indicate that the completely saturated carbon skeleton is similar to tetracyclic triterpenoids or the pentacyclic triterpenoids (21).

The production of toxin by B. maydis was first reported by Orsenigo and Sina (22). Toxins reported by them and those reported by Quimo and Quimo (23) were slightly toxic and nonspecific. Later reports how-ever showed that B. maydis produced a specific toxin (24, 25). These researchers indicated that toxins were produced in vivo and in vitro.

Isolated mitochondria from resistant cultivars were not affected by B. maydis toxin, but mitochondria from Texas male-sterile cultivars were severely affected by it (26). A later report suggested that the mitochon-dria were not the primary site of action of the toxin (27). This con-clusion was based on two observations. First, toxin treatment inhibited root growth in 30 min, but 2 hr of toxin treatment was required to inhibit respiration. Second, prolonged treatments with high toxin con-centrations were required to decrease cellular ATP. However a current report indicated that the mitochondria from susceptible cultivars are perhaps the site of action of this toxin (28). These researchers also re-ported that the close agreement between susceptibility to B. maydis and the suppression of respiratory control of isolated mitochondria indicated that either measurement could be used to predict the other (28). Mito-chondria isolated from cultivars resistant to B. maydis race T are not affected by toxin treatment. This fact raises some question on how mitochondria affect disease development because resistant cultivars are not immune to the fungus or the toxin (29). However, isolated organelles may not react *in vitro* as they do *in vivo*.

The toxin produced by B. *maydis* causes electrolyte leakage of cultivars susceptible to the fungus, but resistant cultivars also leak electrolytes when high concentrations of the toxin are used (30). This observation is consistent with the reaction of the fungus and the toxin. A later study with toxin on excised roots did not indicate a large or rapid ion leakage. The workers reported that root growth was inhibited in 30 min after toxin treatment. This was the earliest effect of the toxin that could be detected (31). Roots do not leak electrolytes as rapidly as leaves, and therefore root tissue is not adequate for permeability studies. In another study these researchers could not detect any damage to membranes of susceptible cultivars treated with the toxin (31). Other researchers however suggested that toxins may cause physiological disruptions of membranes or that the physical damage is below the resolution of the electron microscope (12, 32). Arntzen et al. (31) could not determine the site of action of the B. *maydis* toxin, but they suggested that neither the mitochondria nor the plasma membrane was involved. The site and mode of action of the B. *maydis* toxins have been difficult to resolve for two reasons. First, one or more of the four toxins that the fungus produces may act as a nonspecific toxin. Second, nuclear genes modify the cytoplasmically-inherited reaction to the toxin and the fungus (29). This modification may explain the lack of agreement among various scientists working on the mode of action of the B. *maydis* toxins. Gracen (29) speculated that the site of action of this toxin is a component that is a structural unit of membranes. This fungus appears to initiate disease in a wide variety of genotypes, and the toxin amplifies an abnormality in the structure of membranes in cultivars with the Texas male-sterile cytoplasm.

Bipolaris sacchari. This fungus (formerly *Helminthosporium sacchari*) causes eyespot disease of certain clones of sugarcane. Early symptoms on leaves consist of elongated lesions with red centers circumscribed by narrow chlorotic margins. A few days after infection reddish-brown streaks may lengthen to 8 cm (33).

Lee first suggested that a toxin was involved in the disease (34). The absolute structure of the specific toxin produced by B. *sacchari* is not known; however, much is known about the chemistry of this toxin which was named helminthosporoside (2-hydroxycyclopropyl-α-D-galactopyranoside) (35). The location of the hydroxyl group on the cyclopropane ring indicated that positions 2 and 3 were identical. The conclusion that galactose is the glycone portion of the toxin was based on chromatography after acid hydrolysis and the incorporation of galactose-1-^{14}C into the glycone portion of the toxin. NMR spectral data indicated that the aglycone portion of the toxin is 2-hydroxycyclopropane. The presence of a hydroxyl group on the aglycone was confirmed by detecting acrolein as an end product of acid hydrolysis (35).

Details of the mode of action of helminthosporoside were established in a series of papers published by Strobel and associates. The first experiments indicated that clones susceptible to *B. sacchari* had a membrane protein that binds helminthosporoside whereas membranes from resistant clones did not have binding properties. Moreover clones that had an intermediate reaction to the toxin also had an intermediate binding capacity. These results were confirmed *in vivo* with radioactive toxin. The binding protein was isolated, and a molecular weight of about 45,000 was determined. It consisted of four subunits, each with a molecular weight of about 11,700. The two binding sites that were reported appeared to have different binding affinities (36).

Later reports indicated that the protein from susceptible clones that binds helminthosporoside is on the external surface of the plasma membrane (37, 38). This conclusion was based on three kinds of data: (a) The application of antiserum prepared to membranes from susceptible plants resulted in the protection of leaf tissue susceptible to the toxin. (b) The application of the antiserum to the binding protein agglutinated protoplasts from susceptible clones. (c) Pyridoxal phosphate reacts with the surface of the plasma membrane. Sugarcane cells were treated with pyridoxal phosphate that had been reduced with ^{3}HNaBH$_4$. Binding protein was isolated from treated tissue and was found to be labeled suggesting that the protein that binds the toxin is on the surface of the plasma membrane (39).

The toxin binding protein binds the toxin and increases ATPase activity. Increased ATPase activity causes a net increase in K$^+$ uptake. Disruptions of enzymes in the plasma membrane may cause ion efflux to be greater than ion influx; thus the osmolarity of the plasma membrane is partially lost. Increased osmotic pressure or general loss of membrane integrity may cause cells to burst. These suppositions need to be supported by direct evidence showing that membranes from which the binding protein was extracted were indeed pure plasma membrane preparations. Evidence showing how the binding of the toxin to binding protein activates the potassium–magnesium–ATPase system is also needed. Although we do not know the precise mode of action of this toxin, it appears that the site of action of helminthosporoside is on the plasma membrane. This assumption is consistent with an earlier report indicating that the site of action of victorin is the plasma membrane (12). Therefore the plasma membrane may be the site of action of many specific toxins that incite abrupt electrolyte leakage.

Nonspecific Bipolaris Toxins

Nonspecific toxins are toxins produced by plant pathogens that do not affect the same hosts as the pathogens that produce them. Emphasis on specific toxins has left the impression that nonspecific toxins have little importance in disease development. Although some nonspecific toxins have been shown to be unrelated to disease development, we believe that some are disease-inducing agents. Sometimes, nonspecific toxins are vital to the entry of the host by the pathogen. Moreover some toxins produced *in vitro* may not show specificity or adequate toxicity because compounds that regulate entry of the toxin into plant cells are not produced *in vitro*. Also some toxins may not show specificity because administering the correct concentration of the toxin to the host is difficult.

Bipolaris oryzae. This fungus (formerly *Helminthosporium oryzae*) causes a seedling blight and leaf blotch of rice. Small elliptical leaf spots enlarge and have reddish-brown margins with gray centers. During severe epidemics infected leaves dry out before plants mature. Brown necrotic areas result in shriveled kernels and broken panicles. When the disease is severe, small brown lesions occur on bracts and seeds causing discoloration of the grain (33).

The first toxin isolated from *B. oryzae* was called cochiobolin (41). Another group named the toxin ophiobolin (42). A later report proposed the trivial names ophiobolin A, B, C, and D. Ophiobolin A is a sesquiterpenoid with an empirical formula of $C_{25}H_{36}O_4$ (43). The molecule appears to have two double bonds and four rings, and its molceular structure has been proposed. Ophiobolin was the first of the new family of C_{25} terpenes to be discovered, and its biosynthesis is being determined. No correlation was possible between ophiobolins and other naturally-occurring compounds because of their peculiar structures. The structures of ophiobolins A, B, C, and D are similar. Excellent reviews on the structure and biosynthesis of this unique group of compounds are now available (44, 45).

In 1939 it was first reported that *B. oryzae* produces a toxin that may initiate disease (46). At the onset of infection the pathogen produces two or more toxins that are structurally similar to ophiobolin. These toxins kill host cells in advance of hyphal development suggesting that analogs of ophiobolin are responsible for the penetration of the host by the pathogen. After invasion the pathogen produces ophiobolin which causes a malfunction of the polyphenol metabolism of the host (47). Another assumption about the mode of action of ophiobolin is that the toxin depresses regulatory factors that maintain the normal enzyme synthesis in healthy plants (48). Another worker suggested that ophiobolin irreversibly damages cytoplasmic membranes (41).

Bipolaris sorokinianum. This fungus (formerly *Helminthosporium sativum*) causes a seedling blight and spot blotch of barley and attacks other gramineous species. Dark brown lesions occur on the coleoptile and progress inward. Seedling leaves become dark green with dark lesions near the soil that extend into the leaf blade. Seedling development is retarded, and tillering becomes excessive. In the later stages of disease, tissue rots at or below the soil surface (33).

Although the role of the toxin helminthosporal in plant disease is dubious, much is known about the chemistry of toxins produced by *B. sorokinianum*. First attempts to identify helminthosporal indicated that it is a sesquiterpenoid with an empirical formula of $C_{15}H_{22}O_2$ (49). Its structure has been described (44), and its biosynthesis appears to involve mevalonic acid (50). Another toxin, helminthosporol, with growth-promoting properties has been isolated from *B. sorokinianum*. The structure of helminthosporol is similar to that of helminthosporal, but strains of the fungus that produce helminthosporol do not produce helminthosporal (51).

Helminthosporol inhibits respiration, and the site of action appears to be between flavoprotein dehydrogenase(s) and cytochrome C. This toxin also disrupts oxidative phosphorylation (52). Helminthosporol acts as a growth-promoting substance similar to the cytokinins (53).

Specific Alternaria Toxins

Toxins produced by *Alternaria citri, A. kikuchiana,* and *A. mali* have been reported to have the same host range as the pathogens that produce them. Little is known about the toxins produced by *A. citri* and *A. mali*, but toxins produced by *A. kikuchiana* have been studied more extensively.

Alternaria citri. This fungus causes a distinctive dark brown spot with a light tan center on young leaves and fruits of Emperor mandarin, calamondin, and *Citrus reticulata* cv. Sovereign. Leaves of susceptible cultivars become more resistant as they approach maturity. Many cultivars of citrus are resistant to *A. citri*. When the disease is severe, young fruits drop from the tree within three days after infection (54).

Histological studies showed that *A. citri* did not penetrate young fruits and leaves of susceptible cultivars. Nevertheless inoculation with the pathogen resulted in typical brown spots indicating that a toxin initiated disease. Culture filtrates from pathogenic isolates diluted 100-fold caused typical brown spot symptoms. Other results showed that nonpathogenic strains of *A. citri* did not produce the toxin. Thus three lines of evidence suggest that *A. citri* causes disease through toxigenic action. The last report available to us was published in 1966 (*54*), and recent correspondence indicated that additional work with this toxin has not been initiated (*55*). Hopefully additional research will be carried out with this system. We know that the toxin produced by *A. citri* causes disease through toxigenic action and that old tissue is resistant to the toxin. Therefore genetic variability in the host would not be a problem as it is in other toxin-host combinations.

Alternaria kikuchiana. This fungus produces a small, black necrotic spot surrounded by a yellow halo on fruits and leaves of certain cultivars of Japanese pears (*56*). It is highly pathogenic on Nijisseiki pears but does not cause disease on European and North American pears (*57*).

Three different toxins, phytoalternarian A, B, and C were isolated by Hiroe and Aoe (*58*) from the culture filtrates of this fungus. Although phytoalternarian A affects the same hosts as *A. kikuchiana,* little is known about the chemistry of these toxins. The phytoalternarians give a negative Fehling reaction but express a positive ninhydrin reaction, indicating that they have peptide linkages (*59*).

There is little information concerning the mode of action of these toxins. Information recently received indicated that arbutin and chlorogenic acid may be responsible for the brown spot symptom that is characteristic of the disease (*60*). Another report indicated that the toxin inhibited β-glucosidase in susceptible cultivars but not in resistant cultivars; thus β-glucosidase activity is responsible for resistance (*61*). Details of other aspects of the phytoalternarians were reviewed by Templeton (*62*).

Altenin is another toxin that has been isolated from *A. kikuchiana.* Little has been reported on its toxicity and specificity. It has been identified as ethylhydroxy-5-(1-hydroxyethyl)-4-oxotetrahydrofuronate with an empirical formula of $C_9H_{14}O_6$ (*63*). This structure was also synthesized, and the active portion of altenin was reported to be in the endiol carboxyl grouping (*64*).

Alternaria mali. This fungus causes brown necrotic spots on Indo and Ralls apple varieties, but the pathogen and toxic culture filtrate do not affect Jonathan or McIntosh varieties. A toxin produced by the fungus killed cells of young apple leaves in advance of the invading pathogen. Moreover culture filtrates from highly virulent strains of *A. mali* were more toxic than those from moderately virulent strains. Culture filtrates from nonvirulent strains were nontoxic. These two observations strongly suggest that *A. mali* causes disease by toxigenic action. Other evidence indicated that *A. mali* also produced a nonspecific toxin which caused wilting and vein-banding necrosis in several plants (*65*).

Recent papers indicated that the specific toxin alternariolide produced by *A. mali* has an empirical formula of $C_{23}H_{31}N_3O_6$. The structure that has been proposed for alternariolide indicated that this toxin is a cyclic tripeptide lactone. The three amino acids were reported to be 2-hydroxyisovaleric acid, alanine, and one designated as alternamic acid (*66*). Now that some chemistry is known about this phytopathogenic toxin, studies on its mode of action should yield conclusive results.

Nonspecific Alternaria Toxins

A recent report lists 19 toxic compounds produced by various species of *Alternaria* (*62*). However only a few toxins produced by *A. solani*, *A. tenuis*, and *A. zinniae* will be discussed. The phytotoxic compounds produced by these species of *Alternaria* vary chemically—a carboxylic acid, a cyclic pentapeptide, and a penta-substituted benzene.

Alternaria solani. This fungus causes a devastating blight of the tomato and potato. Symptoms first appear on leaves as small (1–4 mm), dark brown spots. Later a chlorotic ring appears around the necrotic spot. Sometimes leaflets next to the necrotic spot become chlorotic. When the disease is severe, leaflets wither and drop off (*67*).

Although this toxin may play only a minor role in disease, its chemistry has been studied. Alternaric acid has an empirical formula of $C_{21}H_{30}O_8$. Its structure was reported to be 12-(5,6-dihydro-4-hydroxy-6-methyl-2-oxopyran-3-yl)-4,6-dehydroxy-3-methyl-9-methylene-12-oxododec-6-ene-5-carboxylic acid (*68, 69*). Alternaric acid has a low level of toxicity, and it is toxic to many plants not parasitized by *A. solani*. No detailed data on its mode of action have been reported.

Alternaria tenuis. This fungus causes a variegated seedling chlorosis on cotton, citrus, and many other plants. Symptoms are characterized by chlorotic spots sharply delineated from normal green areas. Chlorosis is irreversible, and seedling growth is retarded. Cotton seedlings with more than 35% chlorosis usually die. The fungus appears to produce a toxin while growing on the seed coat or soil refuse. The toxin diffuses into the cotyledons either through injury during germination or when the seed coat ruptures (*70*).

The toxin produced by *A. tenuis*, tentoxin, has a molecular weight of 414.5 and an empirical formula of $C_{22}H_{30}N_4O_4$. Its structure has been described as cyclo-*N*-methyldehydrophenylalanyl-L-leucylglycyl-L-*N*-methylalanyl (*62*). Because the structure is cyclic, the intact toxin gives a negative reaction to ninhydrin. NMR data have indicated the amino acid sequence. The optical rotary dispersion spectrum shows optical activity.

Although the precise mode of action of this toxin is not known, it appears that tentoxin inhibits chlorophyll formation in specific tissues of certain plant species. Only the cotyledons and primary leaves of sensitive species become chlorotic when seeds or very young plants are treated with the toxin. Except in tomato and the crucifers, old primary leaves are not affected by the toxin. Most dicotyledonous plants are sensitive to the toxin, but sorghum and crabgrass are the only monocots that have been found to be sensitive. Tentoxin does not interfere with the conversion of protochlorophyll to chlorophyll. Moreover it appears that this toxin causes a reduction in chlorophyll synthesis within each chloroplast rather than a nonuniform expression of toxicity among plastids (71).

Alternaria zinniae. This fungus causes a leaf spot and seedling blight of zinnia, sunflower, and marigolds (72, 73). Small brown spots occur on cotyledons, leaves, stems, and flowers. Initial symptoms are characterized by a necrotic fleck surrounded by a chlorotic halo. Later spots enlarge and become irregular and reddish brown. Plants that have severe stem lesions wilt rapidly even though the lesion does not girdle the stem. This reaction seems to suggest that a toxin is involved in the disease syndrome (74).

The toxin produced by *A. zinniae*, zinniol, is a penta-substituted benzene with an empirical formula of $C_9H_{21}O_4$. A structure of zinniol has been suggested (73). Moreover two isomeric phthalides obtained from zinniol have been used to resynthesize and confirm its structure.

The mode of action of zinniol is not known. It does not appear to incite disease development, but it may be involved in some of the secondary symptoms because 500–1000 ppm of the toxin are required to cause severe symptoms; also it is not specific.

Other Toxins

Numerous toxins have been reported; therefore it would be unrealistic to include the remainder of the phytopathogenic toxins in this section. Only a few that are known to initiate disease and those that have been recently discovered are included. Moreover the presence of a toxin in this section does not imply that it is relatively unimportant. The toxins discussed in this section are produced by *Periconia, Phyllosticta, Didymella,* and *Fusicoccum.*

Periconia circinata. This fungus is a soil inhabitant that invades the subterranean parts of milo-type sorghums (75). The foliage of diseased plants turns yellow, wilts, and shows typical blight symptoms. If the infection is severe, the plants commonly bloom early, grow stunted, and die prematurely (76). Culms appear red near the base of the plant (77). Leukel (77) first reported that a toxin produced the same symptoms as the pathogen and that they had the same host range. The observations were confirmed in 1961 (78).

Although two toxins were isolated from culture filtrate of *P. circinata,* only one of these has been studied, and little information on its nature has been reported. It has a molecular weight of less than 2000 and reacts positively to ninhydrin. The first report indicated that acid hydrolysis yielded five amino acids (aspartic, glutamic, alanine, serine, and one of the leucines) (3). A later paper reported four amino acids (aspartic, glutamic, alanine, and serine) (11). Assuming that leucine does not occur in the molecule, it appears that the toxin may be a small peptide that yields 6 moles alanine, 4 moles aspartic, and 2 moles each of glutamic acid and serine (11).

Limited studies of the mode of action of the toxin produced by *P. circinata* revealed that the toxin and the fungus cause increased respiration, electrolyte leakage, and decreased ability to incorporate amino acids and uridine (79). The toxin did not affect the activities of mitochondria in cell-free preparations. The physiological disruptions caused by the toxin produced by *P. circinata* are similar to those caused by victorin thus suggesting that the site of action is the plasma membrane (79). These conclusions were not adequately substantiated; therefore the site of action and an explanation for host-specificity need to be determined before the mode of action can be ascertained.

Phyllosticta maydis. This fungus produces a yellow leaf blight of corn which first appears as yellow blotches on the lower leaves. Blotches expand rapidly resulting in general yellowing. Necrotic, buff-colored lesions are elliptical (7–10 × 15–25 mm) running parallel with, but not entirely delineated by, the veins. Severely diseased leaves die and turn brown; eventually all but the topmost leaves become severely blighted. Lesions on the upper leaves are long and narrow and are usually concentrated near the midvein. The necrotic lesions of yellow leaf blight are similar to those of southern leaf blight (80), and the presence of Texas male-sterile cytoplasm greatly increases susceptibility to *P. maydis.*

Nothing is known about the chemistry of the toxin(s) produced by *P. maydis,* but electrolyte leakage, disruption of mitochondrial function, and root inhibition caused by the *P. maydis* toxin are similar to physiological malfunctions incited by *Bipolaris maydis* race T toxin (81, 82).

Didymella applanata. This fungus causes a stem and bud disease of the raspberry characterized by defective budding in the axils of the leaf stalks. The fungus enters the stem through insect wounds and causes dark discoloration near the buds. Discolored spots become lighter in the summer. Damage to stems kills buds and severely damages fruits (83).

The toxin produced by *D. applanata* is a monosaccharide derivative oligosaccharide with a molecular weight of 1682 ± 150, and no or very little reducing power. One of the monosaccharides is glucose. Monosaccharides were found after trimethylsiylation. Groups other than monosaccharides are attracted to some members of the monosaccharide nucleus (*83*).

Although the toxin appears to cause symptoms similar to those caused by the pathogen, one experiment failed to yield information on its phytotoxicity (*83*). Nevertheless these workers indicated that unpublished results of Kerling and Schipper established that *D. applanata* produces a phytotoxin in culture that causes small interveinal necrotic spots on the leaves and sprout wilting.

Fusicoccum amygdali. This fungus causes a leaf blight and wilt of almond and peach trees. The fungus enters through a bud or leaf scar and causes, some distance from the point of infection, wilt within a few days. Eight to 10 days after invasion, gum materials occur in the bark and xylem tissue next to the lesion site. When gummosis occurs, the pathogen behaves as a local parasite and becomes limited to the tissue that was first invaded. Then corky layers that formed around the lesion cause canker formation (*84*).

The toxin fusicoccin produced by *F. amygdali*, is a small diterpenoid with an empirical formula of $C_{36}H_{56}O_{12}$ and a molecular weight of 680. Labeled mevalonalactone incorporated into fusicoccin indicated that fusicoccin aglycone has a diterpenic tricyclic skeleton. Thus fusicoccin is a glucoside of a carbotricyclic terpene (*85*). Fusicoccin has been synthesized, and its absolute structure has been determined. Moreover 16 different derivatives of fusicoccin have been prepared. Perhaps more is known about the chemistry of the phytopathogenic toxin than about any of the others that have been studied (*44, 85*).

Fusicoccin is not specific and is highly toxic to many plant species at 2 μg/ml, but it appears to cause wilting at some distance from the point of invasion. Therefore if the water-transport system is not physically blocked, fusicoccin would appear to be an exceptional non-specific toxin that is important in disease.

Various derivatives were prepared to study the portion of the molecule responsible for the toxicity of fusicoccin (*86*). Removal of the *tert*-pentenyl or the glucosidic moiety drastically reduced toxicity. Fusicoccin increases water uptake of pea seedlings, and derivatives from which the *tert*-pentenyl group has been removed also stimulate water uptake of pea seedlings. This uptake is significant because the *tert*-pentenyl group is needed for toxicity. Therefore fusicoccin appears to be active in both the water-uptake and water-transport systems. More evidence indicated that fusicoccin causes irreversible extension of the cell wall (*87*).

Also fusicoccin causes abnormal opening of the stomata. This observation led to the conclusion that unusual stomatal opening resulted in excessive water loss (*88*). It has also been suggested that fusicoccin causes permeability changes in the plasma membrane of plant cells (*89*).

Others observed that stomata treated with fusicoccin could be closed with abscisin, but tomato cuttings after this treatment wilted. It was therefore concluded that the toxin decreases the resistance of the plasma membrane to water passage and that stomatal opening is a secondary effect (90). It appears that disruption of the function of the plasma membrane of subepidermal cells would result in loss of cell turgor. Loss of cell turgor of these cells would result in a loss of pressure on guard cells, a loss that could culminate in stomatal opening. Fusicoccin could cause wilting in this manner.

Fusarial Phytotoxic Mycotoxins

Fusarium species produce numerous toxins, but a few species produce both mycotoxins and phytotoxins. Although some toxins affect both plants and animals, none of the mycotoxins that affect plants initiate plant disease. Many of the mycotoxins (trichothecenes) produced by *Fusarium* species have a molecular structure similar to that of the sesquiterpenoids. Moreover some phytopathogenic toxins produced by different fungi are diterpenoids or sesquiterpenoids. Unfortnuately little is known about the animal toxicity of the phytopathogenic terpenoids that are important in plant disease. The objective of this section is to discuss the relationship between mycotoxins and phytotoxins.

The phytotoxic materials produced by fungi are referred to as phytotoxins (2). Phytopathogenic toxins differ from phytotoxins in initiating plant disease. Phytotoxins do not initiate disease, but they are involved in a minor way during the later part of the disease syndrome. In this discourse a mycotoxin is considered a toxin produced by a fungus that is toxic to animals.

Brian et al. (91) first observed that compounds (trichothecenes) produced by plant pathogens are toxic to plants and animals. The same trichothecenes that caused skin irritation, nerve damage, and hemorrhage in animals also cause wilting and necrosis in pea seedlings (92). The trichothecenes also inhibit plant growth by interfering with the action of indoleactic acid (91). The interaction between the trichothecenes and growth hormones has not been reported in animals. Moreover the trichothecenes are very toxic to both plants and animals. Concentrations as low as 0.1 μg/ml inhibit growth of certain plant species (91). Moniliformin is a toxin recently isolated from a plant pathogenic fungus (*Fusarium moniliforme*) that is toxic to plants and animals (93).

Some phytotoxins cause physiological disturbances in plants similar to those that mycotoxins cause in animals. For example fusicoccin (a diterpenoid) causes permeability changes and necrosis in many plant species whereas certain sesquiterpenoids cause increased vascular permeability in rats (*94*). This observation may explain the edema and hemorrhaging in animals which is characteristic of the trichothecene-type toxins. Moreover the trichothecenes are chemically similar to fusicoccin. The specific mechanism by which the trichothecene toxins affect membrane systems in animals is not known.

The similarities in molecular structure and physiological response between certain phytopathogenic toxins and some mycotoxins indicate that some phytopathogenic toxins may also be toxic to animals. Some of the phytopathogenic toxins have not been isolated from diseased plants because of their labile nature or because of low concentrations; therefore these types of toxins would not injure animals in nature. Some toxins that cause plant disease (fusicoccin, helminthosporoside) have been isolated from infected plants. Moreover some of these have chemical structures similar to those of various mycotoxins, and the phytopathogenic toxins occurred in relatively large quantities. On the other hand certain mycotoxins (trichothecenes) have not been isolated from naturally infected plants or stored grain. Because it has not been established that a given trichothecene was responsible for mycotoxicosis in the field, it has been suggested that naturally occurring mycotoxicosis may result from different substances produced by several fungi (*95*). This assumption adds significance when it is realized that some of the phytotoxins and phytopathogenic toxins occur in higher concentrations in naturally infected plants than do the mycotoxins. Therefore some of these phytotoxic compounds may be involved in the naturally occurring mycotoxicosis complex. This involvement would suggest that the animal toxicity of phytotoxic compounds isolated from infected plants should be studied. Little attention has been given to this subject.

Discussion

Although toxins have been implicated in plant disease for almost a century, only 10 are considered to induce disease. Evidence that these 10 incite disease hinges on two forms of circumstantial evidence: the toxin has the same host range as the pathogen, and a positive correlation exists between toxin production and pathogenicity.

Although indirect evidence suggests that a few toxins induce plant disease, their precise mode of action is unknown. Plant scientists have had little success in this area. The explanation, mainly conjecture, rests on three major points. The first concerns concentrations and stability of the toxin. Many toxins are produced in small quantities *in vivo*, and some of major importance are not stable when purified. Sometimes, two or more toxins of similar constitution are produced, and thus it is difficult to ascertain which toxin incites disease development.

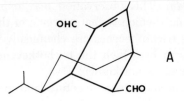

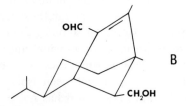

*Figure 1.   Chemical structure of helmin-
thosporol A and helminthosporol B*

The second point involves interactions between the host and the toxin(s). Sometimes the host produces toxins that cause necrosis. Such toxins are produced in response to infection or injury. When toxins produced by the host and the pathogen are produced only *in vivo*, it is difficult to determine the origin of a given toxin or one that triggers disease. Occasionally both resistant and susceptible cultivars inactivate toxins at different rates. Many compounds are not readily transported in plants, and it is difficult to detect cellular damage somewhat removed from the point of infection. Such detection (5–10 mm) from the invading pathogen should be used as a primary criterion to implicate a toxin as a disease-inducing agent. This criterion would be most useful when the toxin is produced only *in vivo*. We believe that many disease-inducing toxins are commonly produced only *in vivo* and that scientists who are interested in the toxigenic nature of phytopathogens should turn their attention to toxins produced *in vivo*.

The third and perhaps the foremost reason for the slow progress with phytopathogenic toxins is the lack of knowledge of the chemical structures of these compounds. Until recently very little was known about the structures of phytopathogenic toxins. Most of the toxins that attracted the attention of chemists were not the causal agents of plant disease. Much credit to elucidate the modes of action of antibiotics and mycotoxins must be given to chemists who determined the structures and functional groups of these compounds. Once these are known, the site of action is more easily ascertained. Knowledge of this kind would be helpful to biologists who wish to determine the mode of action of toxigenic compounds. Hopefully this symposium will stimulate the interest of chemists in phytopathogenic toxins. Their expertise is sorely needed.

Since this symposium emphasizes mycotoxins or toxins that affect animals, it is interesting to note similarities between mycotoxins and toxins that affect plants. Some of the important mycotoxins (trichothecenes) are known to be the primary agents that incite plant disease. That is, some mycotoxins are of only minor importance to symptom development in plants, or their toxicity to plants may be coincidental. This point of view may be in error because some mycotoxins cause severe reactions and death in certain plants at very low concentrations. Several phytotoxins and mycotoxins have chemical structures that are terpenic in origin. Structural relationships and pathways of synthesis allow classification as sesquiterpenoid, diterpenoid, and sesterterpenoid.

Several well known sesquiterpenoids are fomannosin, helminthosporal, helminthosporol (*see* Figure 1), and diacetoxyscirpenol. Some compounds that have the 12,13-epoxytrichothecene nucleus have similar chemical structures and biological properties of toxicity to plant and animal cells (*44*). In a recent review, 22 naturally occurring 12,13-epoxytrichothecenes were listed, and their chemical structures were compared (*95*). Experiments with labeled compounds showed that the nuclei of these substances are derived from mevalonic acid (*96, 97*).

A well-known, diterpenoid, phytopathogenic toxin is fusicoccin. Its structure is known and is well documented in a recent review (*44*). The absolute structure for fusicoccin is shown in Figure 2. Incorporation of

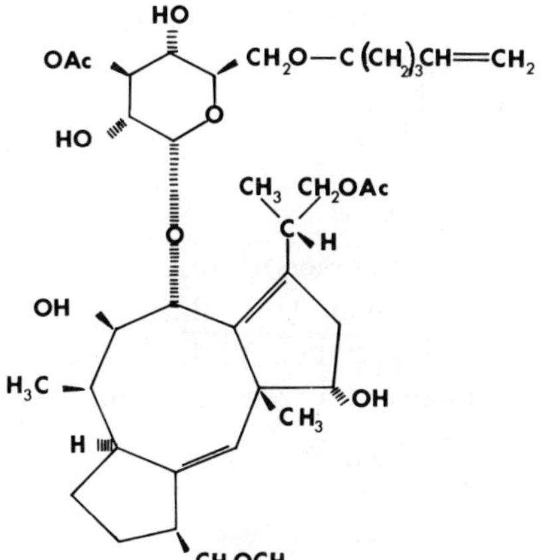

Figure 2.   Chemical structure of fusicoccin

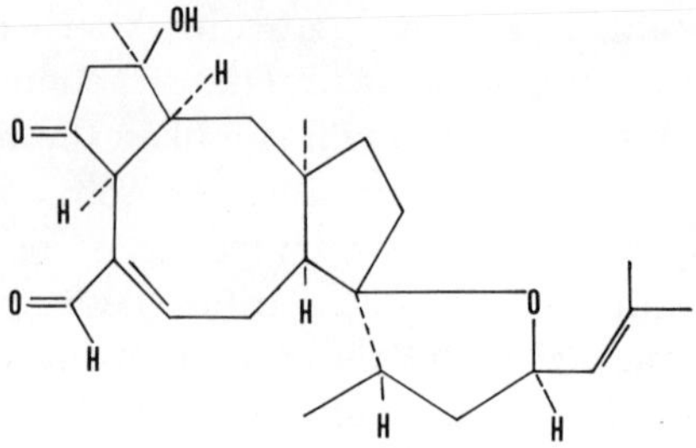

Figure 3.   Chemical structure of ophiobolin A

labeled mevalonolactone in the compound indicated that the fusicoccin aglycone had a diterpenic tricyclic skeleton. Other evidences from oxidation and addition reactions, x-ray analysis of derivatives, and NMR spectra substantiate the structure. The same basic ring system that occurs in fusicoccin occurs in the ophiobolins (Figure 3). Because the additional isoprene unit yielded $C_{25}H_{40}$ there has been formal international agreement that substances like zizanins and ophiobolins constitute a new class of terpenoids, sesterterpenes, with the term ophiobolane proposed for the fundamental hydrocarbon (98). The essential evidence to elucidate the structural relationships have been reviewed by Casinovi (44). Geranyl farnesol seems to be an intermediate in the biosynthesis of the ophiobolins (99).

Because some phytopathogenic toxins and mycotoxins are terpenic in origin and have portions of their biosynthetic pathways the same as those for phytohormones (gibberellins) and animal hormones (various steroids), continued work on elucidating biosynthetic pathways, chemical structures of active components, and modes of action are much needed. It may be significant that several phytotoxins and several plant and animal hormones seem to alter membrane physiology, but the actual sites of action are not known.

Acknowledgments

We acknowledge the assistance of S. A. Morey in the preparation of this manuscript, T. E. Freeman, J. A. Bartz, and R. E. Stall for their helpful reviews, and G. A. Strobel, V. E. Gracen, Jr., K. G. Pegg, K. Sawamura, and M. Ohkawa for recent unpublished information and current reprints.

Literature Cited

1. deBary, A., *Bot. Zt.* (1886) **44**, 337.
2. Wheeler, H., Luke, H. H., *Ann. Rev. Microbiol.* (1963) **17**, 223.

3. Pringle, R. B., Scheffer, R. P., *Ann. Rev. Phytopathol.* (1964) **2**, 133.
4. Meehan, F., Murphey, H. C., *Phytopathology* (1946) **36**, 406.
5. Meehan, F., Murphey, H. C., *Science* (1946) **104**, 413.
6. *Ibid.* (1947) **106**, 270.
7. Luke, H. H., Wheeler, H. E., *Phytopathology* (1955) **45**, 453.
8. Wheeler, H. E., Luke, H. H., *Phytopathology* (1954) **44**, 334.
9. Pringle, R. B., Braun, A. C., *Phytopathology* (1957) **47**, 369.
10. Braun, A. C., Pringle, R. B., "Plant Pathology: Problems and Progress," C. S. Holton, Ed., pp. 88-99, University of Wisconsin, Madison, Wis., 1959.
11. Pringle, R. B., "Phytotoxins in Plant Disease," R. S. K. Wood, A. Ballio, A. Graniti, Eds., pp. 139-155, Academic, New York, 1972.
12. Luke, H. H., Warmke, H. E., Hanchey, P., *Phytopathology* (1966) **56**, 1178.
13. Luke, H. H., Freeman, T. E., Garrard, L. A., Humphreys, T. E., *Phytopathology* (1969) **59**, 1002.
14. Wheeler, H., Black, H. S., *Amer. J. Bot.* (1963) **50**, 686.
15. Hanchey, P., Wheeler, H., Luke, H. H., *Amer. J. Bot.* (1968) **55**, 53.
16. Sammadar, K. R., Scheffer, R. P., *Plant Physiol.* (1968) **43**, 21.
17. Gracen, V. E., Jr., West, S. H., Luke, H. H., Wallace, A. T., *Can. J. Bot.*, in press.
18. Ullstrup, A. J., *Phytopathology* (1941) **31**, 508.
19. *Ibid.* (1944) **34**, 214.
20. Scheffer, R. P., Yoder, O. C., "Phytotoxins in Plant Disease," R. S. K. Wood, A. Ballio, A. Graniti, Eds., pp. 251-272, Academic, New York, 1972.
21. Karr, A. L., Jr., Karr, D. B., Strobel, G. A., *Plant Physiol.* (1974) **53**, 250.
22. Orsenigo, M., Sina, P., *Nuovo G. Bot. Ital.* (1961) **68**, 64.
23. Quimo, T. H., Quimo, A. J., *Philipp. Agric.* (1966) **49**, 778.
24. Smedegar–Petersen, U., Nelson, R. R., *Can. J. Bot.* (1969) **47**, 951.
25. Hooker, A. L., Smith, D. R., Lim, S. M., Beckett, J. B., *Plant Dis. Rep.* (1970) **54**, 708.
26. Miller, R. J., Koeppe, D. E., *Science* (1971) **173**, 67.
27. Arntzen, C. J., *Biochem. Biophys. Acta* (1972) **283**, 539.
28. Krueger, W. A., Josephson, L. M., Hilty, J. W., *Phytopathology* (1974) **64**, 735.
29. Gracen, V. E., Jr., personal communication, 1974.
30. Gracen, V. E., Jr., Grogan, C. O., Fortes, M. J., *Can. J. Bot.* (1972) **50**, 2167.
31. Arntzen, C. J., Koeppe, D. E., Miller, R. J., Peverly, J. H., *Physiol. Plant Pathol.* (1973) **3**, 79.
32. Luke, H. H., Gracen, V. E., Jr., "Microbial Toxins," Vol. VIII, S. Kadis, A. Ciegler, S. Ajl, Eds., pp. 139-168, Academic, New York, 1972.
33. Dickson, J. G., "Diseases of Field Crops," McGraw-Hill, New York, 1956.
34. Lee, A., *Plant Physiol.* (1929) **8**, 193.
35. Steiner, G. W., Strobel, G. A., *J. Biol. Chem.* (1971) **246**, 4350.
36. Strobel, G. A., *J. Biol. Chem.* (1973) **248**, 1321.
37. Strobel, G. A., *Proc. Nat. Acad. Sci. U.S.A.* (1973) **70**, 1693.
38. *Ibid.* (1974) **71**, 1413.
39. Strobel, G. A., *Ann. Rev. Plant Physiol.* (1974) **25**, 541.
40. Strobel, G. A., *Proc. Nat. Acad. Sci. U.S.A.* (1974) **71**, 4232.
41. Orsenigo, M., *Phytopathol. Z.* (1957) **29**, 189.
42. Nakamura, S., Ishibashi, K., *J. Agric. Chem. Soc. Jap.* (1958) **32**, 732.
43. Camonica, L., Fiecchi, A., Galli, K. M., Ranzi, B. M., Scala, A., *Tetrahedron Lett.* (1966) 3035.
44. Casinovi, C. G., "Phytotoxins in Plant Disease," R. S. K. Wood, A. Ballio, A. Graniti, Eds., pp. 105-122, Academic, New York, 1972.

316   MYCOTOXINS

45. Canonica, L., "Phytotoxins in Plant Disease," R. S. K. Wood, A. Ballio, A. Graniti, Eds., pp. 157-174, Academic, New York, 1972.
46. Yoshii, H., *Ann. Phytopathol. Soc. Jap.* (1939) **9**, 170.
47. Oku, H., "The Dynamic Role of Molecular Constituents in Plant–Parasite Interaction," C. J. Mirocha, I. Uritani, Eds., pp. 237-255, Amer. Phytopathol. Soc., St. Paul, Minn., 1967.
48. Oku, H., "Biochemical Regulation in Diseased Plants or Injury," pp. 253-260, Phytopathol. Soc. Jap., 1968.
49. deMayo, P., Spencer, E. Y., *J. Amer. Chem. Soc.* (1962) **84**, 494.
50. deMayo, P., Robinson, J. R., Spencer, E. Y., White, R. W., *Experientia* (1962) **18**, 359.
51. Tamura, S., Sakurai, A., Kainuma, K., Takai, M., *Agric. Biol. Chem. Tokyo* (1963) **27**, 738.
52. Taniguchi, T., White, G. A., *Biochem. Biophys. Res. Commun.* (1967) **28**, 819.
53. Mori, S., Inoue, Y., Mitso, K., *Plant Cell Physiol. Tokyo* (1969) **7**, 503.
54. Pegg, K. G., *Queensl. J. Agric. Anim. Sci.* (1966) **23**, 15.
55. Pegg, K. G., personal communication, 1974.
56. Tanaka, S., *Mem. Coll. Agric. Kyoto Univ.* (1933) **28**, 1.
57. Hiroe, I., Nishamura, S., Sato, M., *Trans. Tottori Soc. Agric. Sci.* (1958) **11**, 291.
58. Hiroe, I., Aoe, S., *J. Fac. Agric. Tottori Univ.* (1954) **2**, 1.
59. Mohri, R., Kashima, C., Gasha, T., Sugiyama, N., *Ann. Phytopathol. Soc. Jap.* (1967) **33**, 289.
60. Ohkawa, M., Torikata, A., *J. Jap. Soc. Horti. Sci.* (1972) **41**, 119.
61. *Ibid.* (1972) **41**, 245.
62. Koncewicz, M., Mathiaparanam, P., Uchytil, T. F., Saprapano, L., Tam, J., Rich, D. H., Durbin, R. D., *Biochem. Biophys. Res. Commun.* (1973) **53**, 653.
63. Sugiyama, N., Kashima, C., Hosoi, Y., Ikeda, T., Mohhi, R., *Bull. Chem. Soc. Jap.* (1966) **39**, 2470.
64. *Ibid.* (1967) **40**, 2594.
65. Sawamura, K., *Bull. Horti. Res. Stn. Ser. C* (1966) **4**, 1.
66. Okuno, T., Ishita, Y., Nakayama, S., Sawai, K., Fujita, T., Sawamura, K., *Ann. Phytopathol. Soc. Jap.*, in press.
67. Walker, J. C., "Diseases of Vegetable Crops," McGraw-Hill, New York, 1952.
68. Bartels–Keith, J. R., Grove, J. F., *Proc. Chem. Soc.* (1959) 398.
69. Grove, J. F., *J. Chem. Soc.* (1952) 4056.
70. Fulton, N. D., Ballenbacher, K., Templeton, G. E., *Phytopathology* (1965) **55**, 49.
71. Halloin, J. M., DeZoeten, G. A., Gaard, G., Walker, J. C., *Plant Physiol.* (1970) **45**, 310.
72. White, G. A., Starratt, A. N., *Can. J. Bot.* (1967) **45**, 2087.
73. Starratt, A. N., *Can. J. Chem.* (1968) **46**, 767.
74. Dimock, A. W., Osborn, J. H., *Phytopathology* (1943) **33**, 372.
75. Karper, R. F., Quinby, J. R., *J. Amer. Soc. Agron.* (1946) **38**, 441.
76. Quinby, J. R., Karper, R. E., *Agron. J.* (1949) **41**, 188.
77. Leukel, R. W., *J. Agric. Res.* (1948) **77**, 201.
78. Scheffer, R. P., Pringle, R. B., *Nature* (1961) **191**, 912.
79. Gardner, J. M., Mansour, I. S., Scheffer, R. P., *Physiol. Plant Pathol.* (1972) **2**, 197.
80. Arny, D. C., Worf, G. L., Ahrens, R. W., Lindsay, M. F., *Plant Dis. Rep.* (1970) **54**, 281.
81. Comstock, J. C., Martinson, C. A., Gengenbach, B. G., *Phytopathology* (1973) **63**, 1357.
82. Yoder, O. C., *Phytopathology* (1973) **63**, 1361.

83. Schuring, F., Salmink, C. A., "Microbial Toxins," Vol. VIII, S. Kadis, A. Ciegler, S. Ajl. Eds., pp. 193-209, Academic, New York, 1972.
84. Graniti, A., *Phytopathol. Mediterr.* (1962) **1**, 182.
85. Ballio, A., Brufani, M., Casinovi, C. G., Cerrim, S., Fedeli, W., Pellicciani, R., Santurbano, B., Vaciago, A., *Experientia* (1968) **24**, 631.
86. Ballio, A., Bottalico, A., Framondino, M., Graniti, A., Randazzo, G., *Phytopathol. Mediterr.* (1971) **10**, 26.
87. Lado, P., Pennachioni, A., Caldogno, F. R., Russi, S., Silano, V., *Physiol. Plant Pathol.* (1972) **2**, 75.
88. Graniti, A., Turner, N. C., *Phytopathol. Mediterr.* (1970) **9**, 160.
89. Ballio, A., Bottalico, A., Buonocore, V., Carilli, A., DiVittorio, V., Graniti, A., *Life Sci.* (1968) **7**, 751.
90. Chain, E. B., Mantle, P. G., Milborrow, B. V., *Physiol. Plant Pathol.* (1971) **1**, 495.
91. Brian, P. W., Curtis, P. J., Hemming, H. G., Jeffreys, E. G., Unwin, C. H., Wright, J. M., *J. Exp. Bot.* (1961) **12**, 1.
92. Bolton, A. T., Nuttall, V. W., *Can. J. Plant Sci.* (1968) **48**, 161.
93. Cole, J. R., Kirksey, J. W., Cutler, H. G., Doupnik, B. L., Peckham, J. C., *Science* (1973) **179**, 1324.
94. Kosuri, N. R., Ph.D. Thesis, University of Wisconsin, Madison, Wis., 1969.
95. Bamburg, J. R., Strong, F. M., "Microbial Toxins," Vol. VIII, S. Kadis, A. Ciegler, S. Ajl, Eds., pp. 207-292, Academic, New York, 1972.
96. Jones, E. R. H., Lowe, G., *J. Chem. Soc.* (1960) 3959.
97. Achilladelis, B., Adams, P. M., Hanson, J. B., *Chem. Commun.* (1970) 511.
98. Tsuda, K., Nozoe, S., Morisaki, M., Hirai, R., Itai, A., Okuda, S., *Tetrahedron Lett.* (1967) 3369.
99. Rios, T., Perez, C., *Chem. Commun.* (1969) 214.

RECEIVED November 8, 1974. Mention of a trademark or proprietary product does not constitute a guarantee or warranty of the product by the U. S. Department of Agriculture and does not imply its approval to the exclusion of other products that may also be suitable.

14

Helminthosporium, Drechslera, and Bipolaris Toxins

ODETTE L. SHOTWELL and J. J. ELLIS

Northern Regional Research Laboratory, Agricultural Research Service, U.S. Department of Agriculture, Peoria, Ill. 61604

Metabolites produced by Helminthosporium *and* Drechslera *(Bipolaris) species include: pigments—polyhydroxyanthraquinones and polyhydroxyxanthones; antibiotics—ophiobolins, monocerins, siccanin, and helmintin; mycotoxin—sterigmatocystin; phytotoxin—helminthosporal; pathotoxins from* Drechslera carbonum, D. victoriae, D. maydis, *and* D. sacchari, *and teratogenic compounds—cytochalasins. Most of these compounds are toxic either to animals or plants. Others such as the polyhydroxyanthraquinones and polyhydroxyxanthones belong to classes of compounds known to be toxic. With the exception of the pathotoxins there is little evidence for the natural occurrence of* Helminthosporium *and* Drechslera *toxins. The mycotoxin sterigmatocystin has been found in moldy grain collected on a farm in Canada.*

Many biologically active compounds are produced by species of *Helminthosporium* Link and *Drechslera* Ito (*Bipolaris* Shoem.). Toxins include the pigments described by Raistrick and co-workers in a series of papers beginning in 1933. Almost all the pigments, polyhydroxyanthraquinones and polyhydroxyxanthones, came from molds implicated in plant diseases. Much later *Helminthosporium* and *Drechslera* species were found to produce antibiotics, but these were too toxic for human therapy. Although the pathotoxins have been studied extensively, the structure of only one has been elaborated—helminthosporiside. Helminthosporal, one of the better known *Helminthosporium* phytotoxins, damages cereal crops. Sterigmatocystin, a carcinogen whose metabolic pathway is related to that an aflatoxin B_1, is formed by an unidentified species of the genus. The cytochalasins form one of the more important groups of metabolites because of their teratogenic properties and are considered to be mycotoxins. Cytochalasins are produced by Aspergilli, *Phoma, Zygosporium,* and probably *Phomopsis* as well as by *Helminthosporium* species.

Species in this group of molds include the genera *Helminthosporium* and *Drechslera* (*Bipolaris*). The sexual stages of the group are *Ophiobolus* Riess, *Trichometasphaeria* Munk, *Cochliobolus* Drechsler, *Pyrenophora* Fr., and *Leptosphaeria* Ces. *et* de Not. When examining the literature for secondary metabolites and toxins produced by *Helminthosporium* you must look under all these names. There are reviews that cover much of the earlier work on these phytotoxins, pathotoxins, and secondary metabolites (*1, 2, 3, 4*). Work since then will be emphasized here.

Pathotoxins are phytotoxins produced by plant disease fungi that are host specific (*3*). That is, a pathotoxin causes all the symptoms of a given disease even if its producing fungus is not present. Resistance or susceptibility in a given plant strain applies to both the fungus and the pathotoxin it forms. Of the seven known host-specific toxins, four are produced by *Helminthosporium* species: *D. victoriae* (Meehan *et* Murphy) Subram. *et* Jain, *H. carbonum* Ullstrup (the *Drechslera* conidial state of *Cochliobolus carbonus* Nelson), *H. maydis* Nisik *et* Miyake [*Drechslera* conidial state of *Cochliobolus heterostrophus* (Drechsler) Drechsler], and *H. sacchari* Butler [synonym of *Drechslera sacchari* (Butler) Subram. *et* Jain] (*2*).

The best known pathotoxin, victorin formed by *D. victoriae,* is the causative agent for leaf blight of the Victoria variety of oats (*5*). It has been isolated and partially characterized. The toxin is a polypeptide complex that can be broken down by mild alkali treatment into two components: a pentapeptide and a basic tricyclic compound, victoxinine (*5*). Hydrolysis of the pentapeptide yields the common amino acids— aspartic, glutamic, valine, glycine, and leucine. The pentapeptide is nontoxic. Victoxinine is toxic to oats, rye, barley, wheat, and grain sorghum lacking the selectivity or host specificity of the complete toxin (*6*). Evidently the specificity of the complete toxin is a function of the pentapeptide moiety. Victorin (active at 0.01 μg/ml) is about 7500 times as toxic as victoxinine on a weight basis to susceptible oat species. Although victoxinine has been characterized, the structure of the pentapeptide and the nature of its attachment to victoxinine in the pathogen remains to be determined. The mechanism of the action of victorin in plants depends on the complete structure. Sophisticated techniques exist that should make the elucidation of the complete structure possible.

For structural studies victoxinine $C_{17}H_{29}NO$ was isolated from culture filtrates of *H. sativum* Pammel, King *et* Bakke [the *Drechslera*

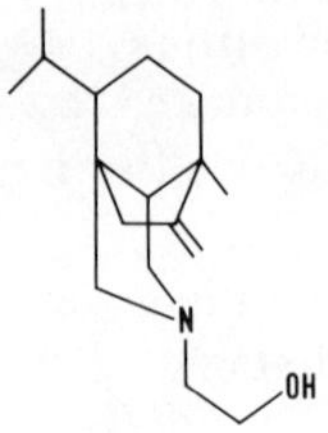

I. Victoxinine 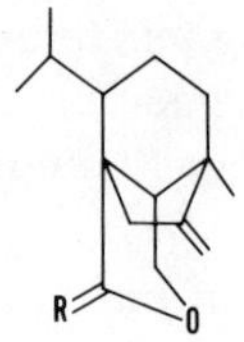   II. R = H,OH Prehelminthosporol
                      III. R = O

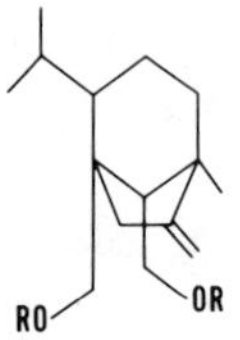

IV. R = H   VI.
V. R = MeSO₂

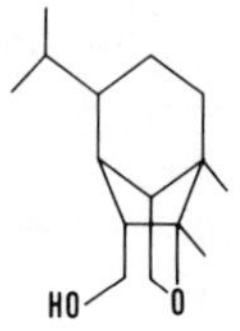

*Figure 1. Victoxinine and related
compounds*

conidial state of *Cochliobolus sativus* (Ito *et* Kuribayashi) Drechsler
et Dastur] in 8–12 mg quantities (*7*). The acetylated derivative, NMR
spectrum, and biogenetic relationship to other terpenoid metabolites
suggested Structure I as a possible structure for victoxinine (Figure 1).
The structure was confirmed by its partial synthesis from prehelminthosporol (Structure II). Prehelminthosporol was converted into the lactone
(Structure III) and then into the diol (Structure IV) with lithium aluminum hydride. Acid treatment cyclized Structure IV to the saturated
isomer Structure VI. The dimethyl sulfonate (Structure V) from Structure IV was treated with ethanolamine in dioxan to give victoxinine.
Structures IV and VI were subsequently found as major metabolites in
culture filtrates of *D. victoriae* (*7*).

A metabolite belonging to a completely different class of compounds
was isolated in 1974 from culture filtrates of *D. victoriae* (*8*). The new
metabolite, gliovictin VII, belongs to a series of microbial sulfur-containing compounds such as gliotoxin (Structure VIII) and sporidesmin D
(Structure IX) whose origin can be explained by a diketopiperazine
precursor (Figure 2). Gliovictin is not as toxic as gliotoxin. Apparently
the disulfide group present in gliotoxin is responsible for the difference
in toxicity. Also methylated sulfide groups are not as toxic.

The pathotoxin from *H. carbonum* (a *Drechslera*) causes leaf spots
and ear rots on certain kinds of corn and is toxic to susceptible corn at
0.5 mg/ml. The impure toxin is stable but becomes unstable when

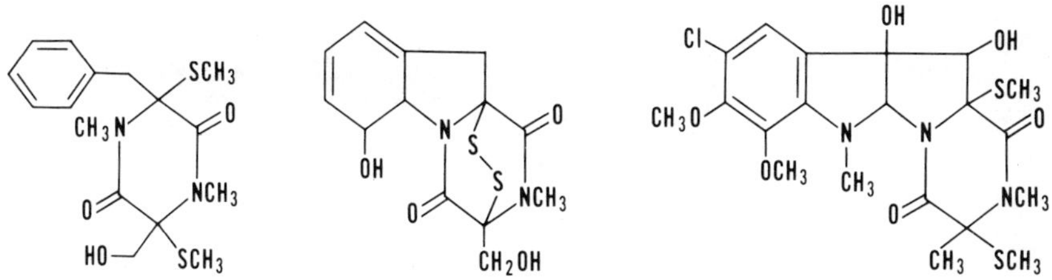

VII. Gliovictin   VIII. Gliotoxin   IX. Sporidesmin D

Figure 2. *Microbial sulfur-containing compounds*

purified and crystallized and loses activity at $-20°C$. Acid hydrolysis yields five ninhydrin-reacting compounds: alanine, proline, and three unidentified ones. Because the toxin is soluble in organic solvents, it is probably a cyclic peptide (9).

Helminthosporoside (Figure 3) is the first host-specific plant toxin to have a structure (Structure X) proposed for it (10). The compound is produced by *H. sacchari* (*D. sacchari*), the causal organism of eye spot disease in sugar cane. Sugarcane leaves treated with the pure toxin exhibit symptoms identical to those produced by the fungus. A light green spot forms, which develops into reddish brown runners. Acid hydrolysis of helminthosporoside resulted in galactose and a hydroxylated cyclopropane. On the basis of spectral and chemical properties the proposed structure for the toxin is 2-hydroxycyclopropyl-α-D-galactopyranoside (Structure X).

A pathotoxin produced by *H. maydis* (*D. maydis*) causes blight symptoms on corn (11). Evidence indicates that the toxin is a fairly stable, low-molecular-weight polypeptide. Several phytotoxins have been reported as metabolites of species of *Helminthosporium*. *Helminthosporium sativum* (a *Drechslera*) produces a toxin responsible for widespread seedling blight, foot and root rot, and leaf spot in cereals in North America that has brought about financial losses, particularly in western Canada (12, 13). The toxin helminthosporal (Structure XI) is not host-specific (Figure 4). A closely related sesquiterpenoid compound, helminthosporol (Structure XII), is also formed by *H. sativum*. Structure XI

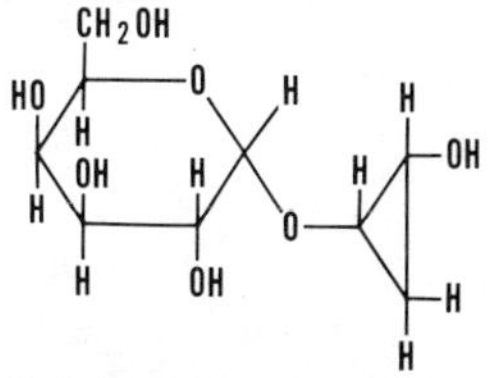

X. Helminthosporoside

Figure 3. *2-Hydroxycyclopropyl-α-D-galactopyranoside, helminthosporiside*

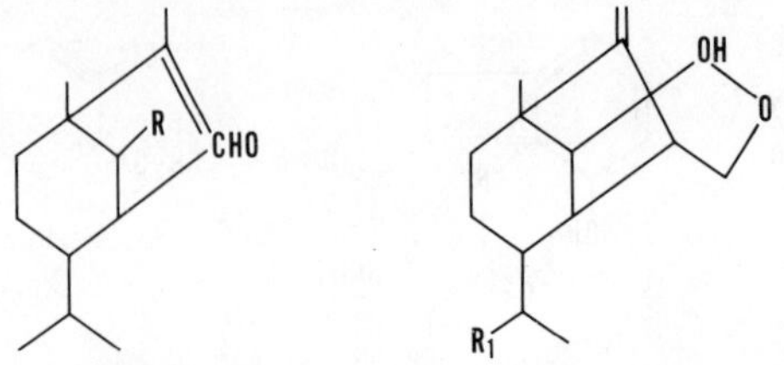

XI. R = CHO Helminthosporal   XIII. R_1 = CH_3 Prehelminthosporol
XII. R = CH_2OH Helminthosporol   XIV. R_1 = CH_2OH
                                           9-hydroxyprehelminthosporol

Figure 4. Sesquiterpenoid compounds

has been determined, and the compound, a dialdehyde, has been synthesized. Helminthosporol (Structure XII), the compound in which one of the aldehyde groups is reduced to an alcohol, stimulates the elongation of leaf sheaths of rice seedlings.

Biosynthetic studies indicate that these compounds are probably formed by nonhead-to-tail linking of three terpene units followed by a cyclization of the precursor (*14*). Probably helminthosporal and helminthosporol do not exist as such in culture liquors, but they are formed during isolation procedures from acetals of compounds designated as prehelminthosporal (Structure XIII) and prehelminthosporol (Structure II). Prehelminthosporol and 9-hydroxyprehelminthosporol (Structure XIV) have been isolated from culture filtrates of fermentations of *Cochliobolus sativus* (Ito *et* Kuribayashi) Drechsler *ex* Dastur [the perfect stage of *H. sativum* (the *Drechslera* conidial state of *C. sativus*)] (*15*). Prehelminthosporal has not been detected in culture liquors of *H. sativum*.

Some of the first secondary metabolites of molds studied were the polyhydroxyanthraquinone pigments isolated and characterized by Raistrick and his associates (*16, 17, 18, 19, 20, 21*). These compounds are closely related (Table I). For example tritosporin is indeed ω-hydroxycatenarin and can be synthesized from catenarin; cynodontin has been synthesized from helminthosporin. *Helminthosporium* and *Drechslera* strains that produce polyhydroxyanthraquinones have been isolated as causative agents of plant diseases (Table I). The compounds are highly colored pigments that fluoresce and are probably responsible for the discolorations noticed on diseased leaves. In 1974 chrysophanol and emodin, polyhydroxyanthraquinones, were isolated from culture liquors of *Drechslera catenaria* (Drechsl.) Ito (*H. catenarium* Drechsler) (*22*). These naturally occurring quinones have cathartic properties (*23*).

A polyhydroxyxanthone, ravenelin (Structure XV, Figure 5), is produced by *H. turcicum* (*D. turcica*), the causative agent of northern corn blight, and *H. ravenelii* Curt. [synonym of *Drechslera ravenelii* (Curt.)

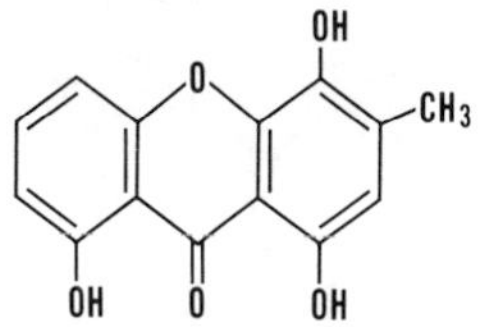

XV. Ravenelin

Figure 5.   Ravenelin

Subram. *et* Jain], a parasite growing on grasses in North and South America and in China (*24*). Myycelia of *D. leersiae* (Atk.) Subram. *et* Jain contain luteoleersin ($C_{26}H_{38}O_7$) and alboleersin ($C_{26}H_{40}O_7$) which are closely related and readily interconvertible (*25*). Luteoleersin is thought to be a substituted quinone or semiquinone and alboleersin, the phenol corresponding to luteoleersin.

Although the structures of polyhydroxyanthraquinones and polyhydroxyxanthones indicate possible toxicity, actual toxicities of these compounds to animals have never been determined. No information exists on the possible effects on animals grazing on grasses infected with *Drechslera* strains producing these compounds. Because of the number of animal deaths attributed to mycotoxicoses, it would be important to determine whether these compounds are responsible for any deaths or, if not, any toxic effects.

Several metabolites of species of *Helminthosporium* and *Drechslera* have antimicrobial properties and were discovered in searches for new antibiotics. The species were selected for screening programs for new antibiotics because of their known toxicity against plants. Members of a family of antibiotics known as ophiobolins have been isolated as metabolites of the fungi that are responsible for southern corn blight [*Cochliobolus heterostrophus* (Drechsler) Drechsler] and northern corn blight [*D. turcica* (Pass.) Subram. *et* Jain, the conidial state of *Trichometasphaeri turcica* Luttrell]. Nomenclature of the compounds was clarified in a joint paper by a group of Japanese and Italian workers (*26*) who studied them. Their structures and biological properties are summarized in Table II. The structure of ophiobolin A (Structure XVI) was determined independently by Nozoe et al. (*27*) and by Canonica et al. (*28*). Nozoe and his co-workers based their conclusions on x-ray crystallographic analysis and on ir and NMR spectra of the bromomethoxy derivative. Canonica and his associates studied NMR, ir, and uv spectra of several derivatives and reaction products. Three other compounds structurally related to ophiobolin A were isolated from cultures of *Ophiobolus heterostrophus* Drechsler [synonym of *Cochliobolus heterostrophus* Drechsler (*H. maydis* Nisik. *et* Miyake, the

Table I.

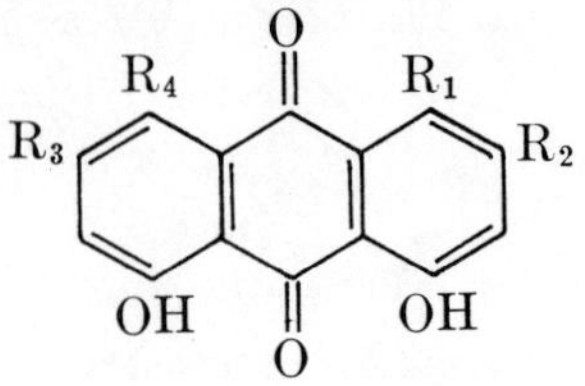

Compound	R_1	R_2	R_3	R_4	Color and Crystal Form
Catenarin	OH	CH_3	OH	H	deep red plates
Cynodontin	OH	CH_3	H	OH	bronze plates
Helminthosporin	H	CH_3	H	OH	dark red needles
Tritisporin	OH	CH_2OH	OH	H	brown needles

Polyhydroxyanthraquinones

Producing Species	Plant Disease Associated with Producing Species	Reference
Drechslera catenaria (Dreschsler) S. Ito		*16, 17, 18*
Drechslera graminea (Rabenh. *ex* Schlecht.) Shoem. [conidial state of *Pyrenophora graminea* Ito *et* Kuribayoshi]	leaf stripe of barley	
Helminthosporium velutinum Link *ex* Ficinus *et* Schubert		
Helminthosporium tritici-vulgaris Nisikado [*Drechslera* conidial state of *Pyrenophora tritici-repentis* (Died.) Drechsler]	yellow spot disease of wheat	
Penicillium islandicum Sopp		
Aspergillus amstelodami (Mang.) Thom *et* Church		
Drechslera cynodontis (Marignoni) Subram. *et* Jain [conidial state of *Cochliobolus cynodontis* Nelson]	parasite on Bermuda, durba, and teosinte grasses	*16, 17, 19*
Drechslera euchlaenae (Zimm.) Subram. *et* Jain		
Pyrenophora avenae Ito *et* Kuribayashi [conidial state is *Drechslera avenae* (Eidam) Scharif = *Helminthosporium avenae* Eidam]	leaf spot of oats	
Drechslera victoriae (Meehan *et* Murphy) Subram. *et* Jain [conidial state of *Cochliobolus victoriae* Nelson]		
Drechslera graminea (Rabenth. *ex* Schlecht.) Shoem.	leaf stripe of barley	*19, 20*
Drechslera cynodontis (Marignoni) Subram. *et* Jain	parasite on Bermuda, durba, and teosinte grasses	
Drechslera catenaria (Drechsler) S. Ito		
Helminthosporium tritici-vulgaris Nisikado [a *Drechslera, see* above]	yellow spot disease of wheat	
Helminthosporium tritici-vulgaris Nisikado [a *Drechslera*]	yellow spot disease of wheat	*21*

Table I.

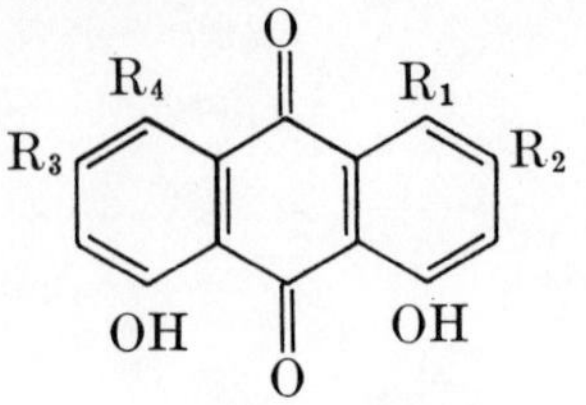

Compound	R_1	R_2	R_3	R_4	Color and Crystal Form
Chrysophanol	H	H	CH$_3$	H	dark yellow leaflets
Emodin	H	OH	CH$_3$	H	orange needles

Table II.

Ophiobolin	Other Names
A	cochliobolin
	ophiobolin
	ophiobalin
	cochliobolin A

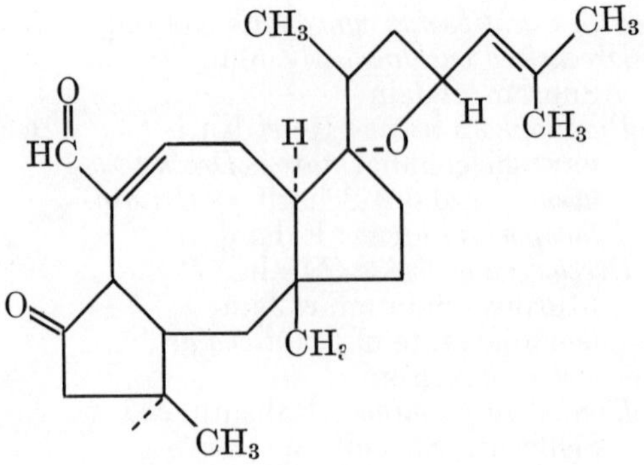

XVI

Continued

Producing Species	Plant Disease Associated with Producing Species	Reference
Drechslera catenaria (Drechsler) S. Ito		*22, 23*
Penicillium islandicum Sopp *Trichoderma polysporum* (Link *ex* Pers.) Rifai [*Pachybasium candidum* (Sacc.) Peyron.] *Drechslera catenaria* (Drechsler) S. Ito		*22, 23*

Ophiobolins

Producing Organisms	Antimicrobial Activity	Toxicity	Reference
Drechslera turica (Pass.) Subram. *et* Jain [conidial state of *Trichometasphaeria turcica* Luttrell]	active at levels of 1–5 µg/ml against *Trichophyton*, *Glomerella*, *Gleosporium*,	to mice, LD$_{50}$: 12 mg/kg i.v.; 238 mg/kg, subcutaneously; 73 mg/kg i.p.	*26, 27*
Drechslera zizaniae (Nisikado) Subram. *et* Jain	*Trichomonas vaginalis* Donne, and phytotoxic		*28, 29*
Drechslera leersiae (Atk.) Subram. *et* Jain	fungi		
Drechslera panici– miliacei (Nisikado) Subram. *et* Jain			
Cochliobolus heterostrophus (Drechsler) Drechsler [the sexual stage of *Drechslera maydis* (Nisik. *et* Miyake) Subram. *et* Jain]		pathogenic to rice	

Table II.

Ophiobolin   Other Names

    B   zizanin

           ophiobolosin A

           zizanin B

           cochliobolin B

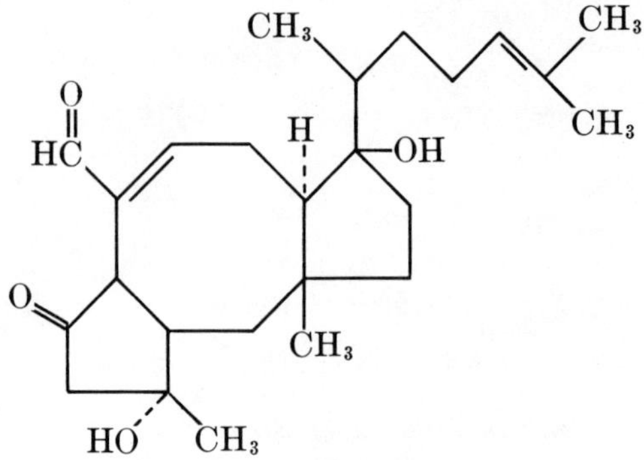

XVII

    C   zizanin A

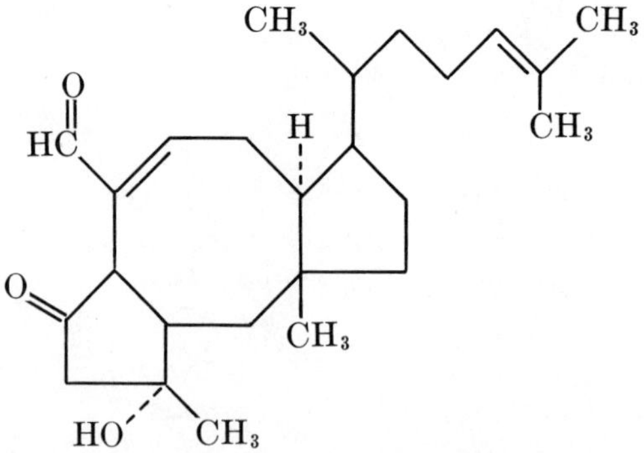

XVIII

    D   cephalonic acid

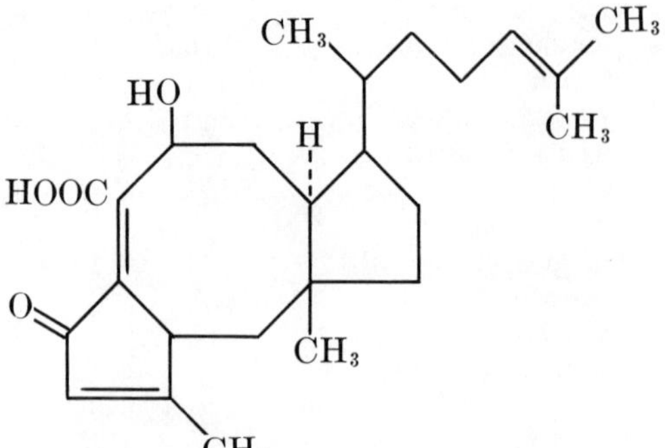

XIX

Continued

Producing Organisms	Antimicrobial Activity	Toxicity	Reference
Cochliobolus heterostrophus (Drechsler) Drechsler	active against *Trichophyton interdigitale*, *Macrosporium*	to mice, LD_{50}: 4.4 mg/kg i.p.	*29, 30*
Drechslera zizaniae (Nisikado) Subram. et Jain	*bataicola*, *Glomerella fructigena*, and *Gleosporium kaki*		*31, 32*
Cochliobolus miyabeanus (S. Ito et Kuribayashi) Drechsler ex Dastur [conidial state is *Drechslera oryzae* (Breda de Haan) Subram. et Jain		pathogenic to rice	
Drechslera zizaniae (Nisikado) Subram. et Jain			*31*
Cephalosporium caerulens Matsuamae, Kamio et Hata [name not validly published]	Slightly active against *Staphylococcus aureus* Rosenbach		*33, 34*

Drechslera conidial state)] and *D. zizaniae* (Nisikado) Subram. *et* Jain (*29, 30, 31, 32*). These were ophiobolin B (Structure XVII), ophiobolin C (Structure XVIII), and anhydroophiobolin. Ophiobolosin B was isolated from the mycelium of *Cochliobolus miyabeanus* (Ito *et* Kuribayashi) Drechsler *ex* Dastur [conidial state is *D. oryzae* (Breda de Haan) Subram. *et* Jain] which also formed ophiobolin B (*32*). Although the structure of ophiobolosin B has not been elaborated, the compound has the same effect on rice seedlings and fungi as ophiobolin B. Cephalonic acid (Structure XIX), a compound closely related to the ophiobolins, has been isolated as a minor metabolite of *Cephalosporium caerulens* Matsuamae, Kamio *et* Hata (name not validly published) (Table II) (*33, 34*).

The novel skeletons of the ophiobolins are formed biosynthetically by the head-to-tail condensation of five isoprene units (*35*). These are the first examples of C_{25} terpenoids. Evidence for the formation of the skeleton was established by culturing *C. miyabeanus* in a synthetic medium containing (2-^{14}C) mevalonic acid lactone (*14*). Labels appeared in carbons 4, 8, 12, 16, and 24 (or 25) in ophiobolin A (Figure 6). Both Nozoe et al. (*35*) and Canonica (*14*) proposed that in the biosynthesis of ophiobolin A and B molecular oxygen may be directly incorpo-

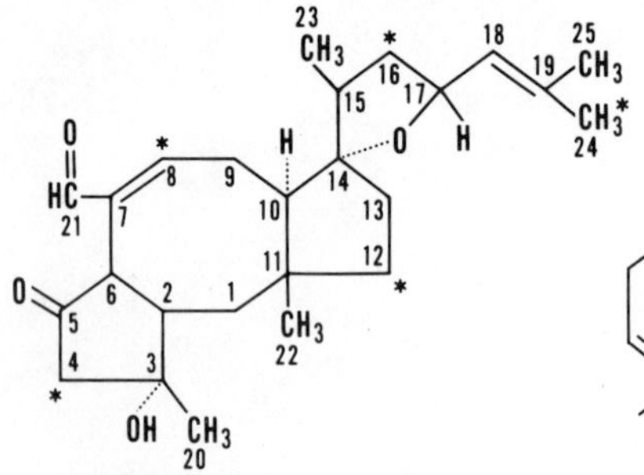

XVI. Ophiobolin A

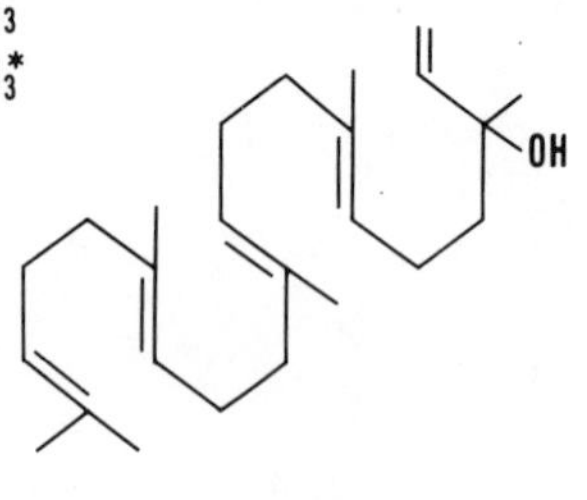

XXI. Geranylnerolidol

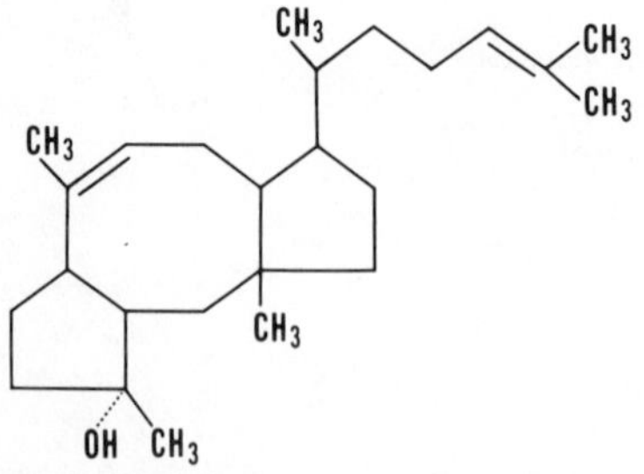

XX. Precursors

Figure 6.   Compounds involved in biosynthesis of ophiobolins

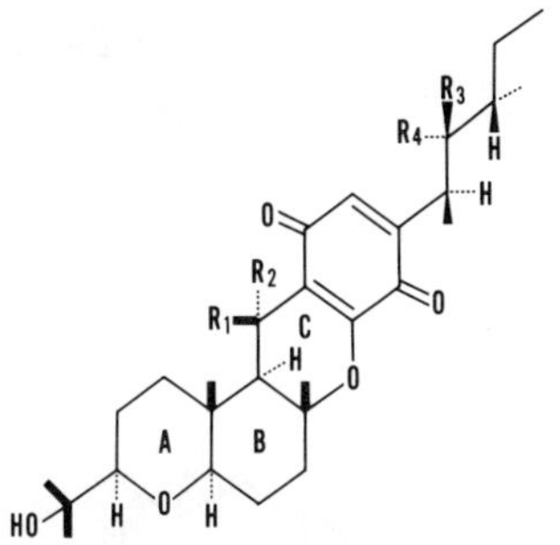

XXII. $R_1 = R_3 = H$; $R_2 = OH$; $R_4 = OAc$ Cochlioquinone A
XXIII. $R_1 = R_2 = H$; $R_3R_4 = O$ Cochlioquinone B

Figure 7.   Cochlioquinones

rated into the C14 and that the oxygen on the C3 comes from the medium. The pathway for the formation of ophiobolins is precursor Structures XX → XVIII → XVII → XVI. The probable course of cyclization of the biological equivalent of geranyl farnesyl pyrophosphate was studied by incorporating tritium-labeled and doubly labeled (tritium and ^{14}C) mevalonic acid lactone into fermentations of *C. miyabeanus* and *C. hetero-strophus* (*14, 36*).

Two compounds, geranylnerolidol (Structure XXI) and a proposed precursor of the ophiobolins (Structure XX), have been isolated from *C. heterostrophus* (*37*). In the same study Nozoe and co-workers detected by gas–liquid chromatography diterpene and sesterterpene hydrocarbons, a sesterterpene alcohol, and squalene. Any one of these compounds could be involved in the biosynthesis of ophiobolins.

When the mold that produces the ophiobolins, *C. miyabeanus,* is grown under suitable conditions, two yellow pigments can be isolated from the mycelium and medium (*38*). These pigments can be extracted with hexane and purified by fractional crystallization and chromatography. Structures XXII and XXIII (Figure 7) were established for the two pigments cochlioquinones A and B by chemical, spectroscopic, and crystallographic evidence. Cochlioquinones A and B contain a sesquiterpenoid unit. Studies show that the biosynthesis of A and B occurs through the introduction of a farnesyl unit onto an aromatic precursor (*39*). Labeled mevalonic acid lactone is incorporated exclusively into the C_{15} terpenoid unit (Rings A, B, and C). The nonterpenoid precursor is aromatic and has secondary methyl groups derived from methionine.

In screening *Helminthosporium* and *Drechslera* species pathogenic to plants for antimicrobial activity, several metabolites other than the ophiobolins have been isolated and described (Table III). *Pyrenophora avenae* Ito *et* Kuribayashi [*H. avenae* Eidam is a synonym of the *Drechslera* conidial state, *D. avenae* (Eidam) Scharif], a pathogen of

Table III.   Metabolites of

Metabolite   *Structure*

Siccanin

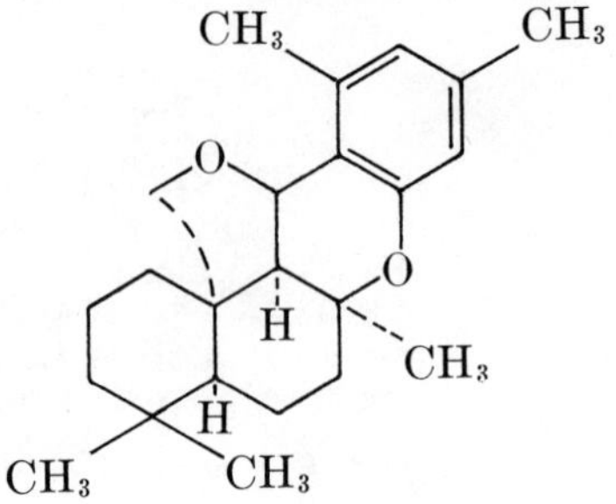

XXIV

Helmintin $C_{11}H_8O_2N_2$

Pyrenophorin

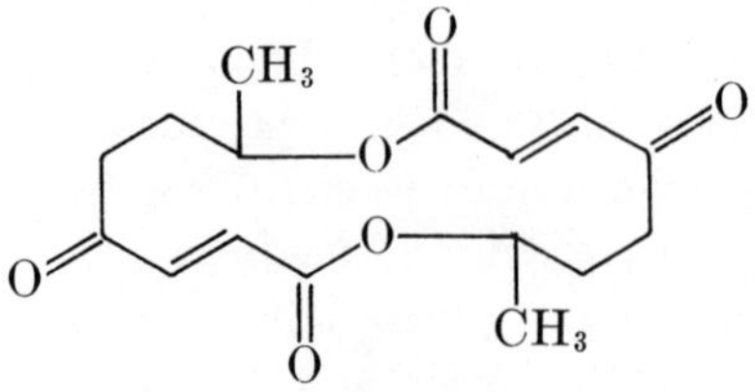

XXV

Monocerin

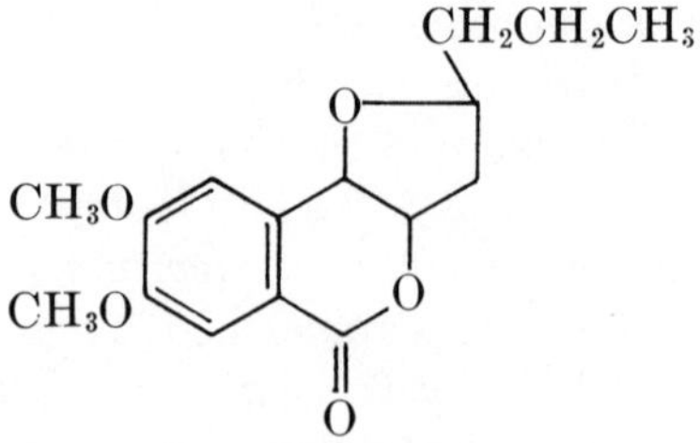

XXVI

Helminthosporium Species

Producing Organisms	Antimicrobial Activity	Toxicity	Reference
Pyrenophora avenae Ito *et* Kuribayashi [conidial state is *Drechslera avenae* (Eidam) Scharif = *H. avenae* Eidam] *Drechslera siccans* (Drechsler) Shoem.	*Tichophyton*, 0.1 μg/ml *Gibberella*, Aspergilli, Penicillia, *Alternaria*; 5–12 μg/ml	no adverse effect in mice at 500 mg/kg i.p.	*40, 41*
Drechslera siccans (Drechsler) Shoem.	*Trichophyton*, 5 μg/ml *Microsporum gypseum* (Bodin) Guiart *et* Grigorakis, 10 μg/ml; *Rhizopus stolonifer* (Ehrenb. *ex* Fr.) Vuill. [*R. nigricans* Ehrenb.], 10 μg/ml		*42*
Pyrenophora avenae Ito *et* Kuribayashi (*see* above)	antitumor, some yeast, pathogenic plant fungi, *Trichomonas*	LD$_{50}$ for mice: 44.1 mg/kg i.p.	*43, 44*
Drechslera monoceras (Drechsler) Subram. *et* Jain	inhibits powdery mildew (*Erysiphe graminis* DC.) of wheat		*45*

Table III.

| *Metabolite* | *Structure* |

3'-Amino-
3'-deoxyadenosine

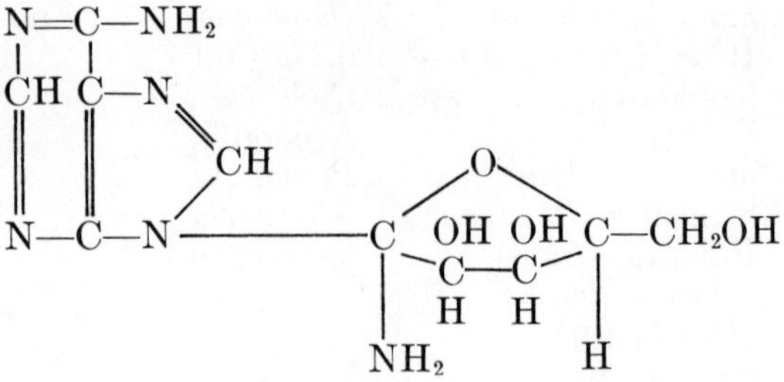

XXVII

Heveadride

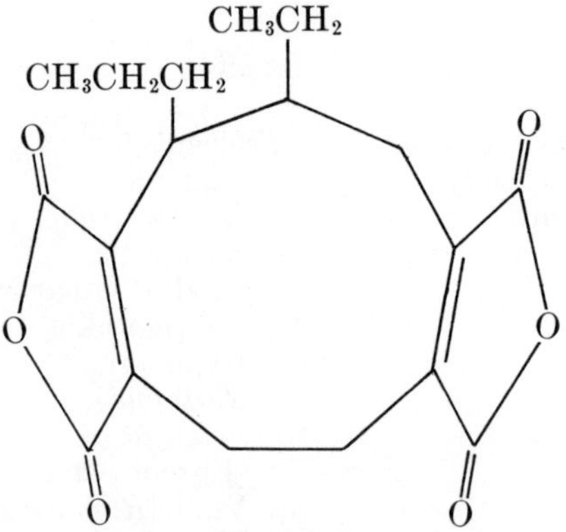

XXVIII

oats, forms siccanin (Structure XXIV) and pyrenophorin (Structure XXV). *Drechslera siccans* (Drechsler) Shoem., the fungus responsible for leaf spot on rye grass, forms siccanin and helmintin. Other compounds such as monocerin (Structure XXVI), 3'-amino-3'-deoxyadenosine (Structure XXVII), and heveadride (Structure XXVIII) have been isolated from culture filtrates and mycelium of *Helminthosporium* species (Table III). Heveadride (Structure XXVIII) is an isomer of byssochlamic acid.

The biosynthetic pathway of siccanin (Structure XXIV) has been established through intact and cell-free systems of *D. siccans* (Drechsler) Shoem. (*49*) (Figure 8). It involves the following steps: (a) Formation of *trans*-γ-monocyclofarnesol (Structure XXIX) from mevalonic acid lactone or farnesyl pyrophosphate; (b) coupling reaction of the terpenic precursor with orsellinic acid; (c) oxidative conversion of presiccanochromenic acid (Structure XXX) into siccanochromenic acid (Structure

Continued

Producing Organisms	Antimicrobial Activity	Toxicity	Reference
Helminthosporium sp.	Antitumor, inhibits yeast	LD$_{50}$ for mice: 28 mg/kg i.p.	*46, 47*

48

XXXI); (d) decarboxylation of Structure XXXI to siccanochromen A (Structure XXXII), and (e) epoxy–olefin type of cyclization of siccanochromen B (Structure XXXIII) to siccanin. The precursors of siccanin have previously been isolated from cultures of *H. siccans* Dreschler (synonym of *D. siccans*) during biosynthetic studies and characterized as triprenyl phenol derivatives. They include Structures XXX (*50*), XXXI (*51*), XXXII, and XXXIII (*52, 53*). Previously *trans*-α-monocyclofarnesol has been isolated as a minor constituent of *H. siccans* mycelia (*54*).

Sterigmatocystin (Structure XXXIV, Figure 9), a carcinogenic compound structurally related to the aflatoxins, was reported to be produced by an unidentified species of *Bipolaris* by Holzapfel *et al.* (*55*). In 1970 Aucamp and Holzapfel (*56*) discovered that three polyhydroxyanthraquinones—bipolarin (Structure XXXV), versicolorin C (Structure XXXVI), and averufanin (Structure XXXVII)—were produced by *Bipolaris*. In the same study curvularin (Structure XXXVIII), a macro-

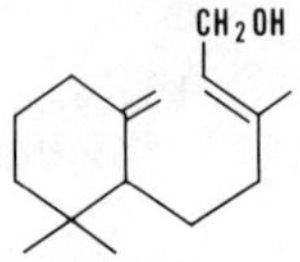

XXIX. *trans*-γ-monocyclofarnesol 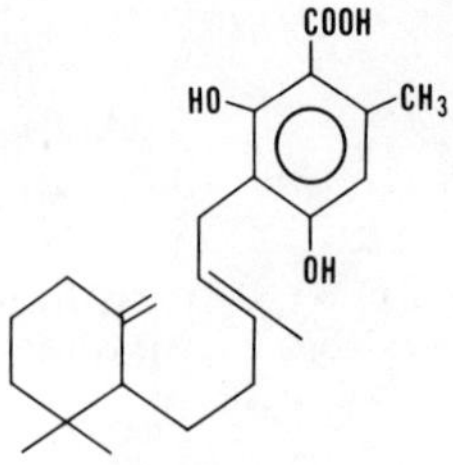   XXX. Presiccanochromenic acid

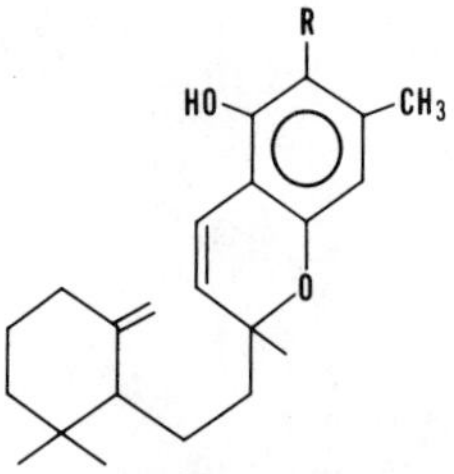

XXXI. R = COOH, Siccanochromenic acid   XXXIII. Siccanochromen B
XXXII. R = H, Siccanochromen A

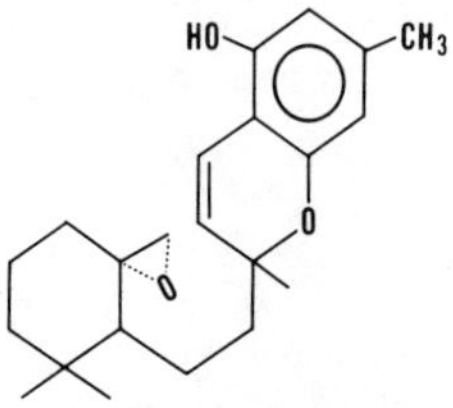

Figure 8.   Precursors of siccanin

cyclic lactone, was also isolated from *Bipolaris*. Sterigmatocystin has
been known as a metabolite of *Aspergillus versicolor* (Vuill.) Tiraboschi.
Versicolorin C is produced by *A. fllavus* Link *ex* Fr., *A. versicolor*, and
A. nidulans (Eidam) Wint. These compounds are significant because
their biosynthetic pathways are closely related to those of the aflatoxins,
potent carcinogens elaborated by strains of the *A. flavus* series.

Versicolorin C, an orange-red pigment, and averufanin have also
been isolated as metabolites from a strain of *A. flavus* that produces
aflatoxin B_1 (Structure XXXIX) (57). Aucamp and Holzapfel (56) proposed that bipolarin may bridge the gap in biosynthetic pathways
between a hypothetical C_{18}-polyketide on the one hand and versicolorin
C, sterigmatocystin, and aflatoxin B_1 on the other. The polyketide would
be formed by the condensation of acetate units after which it would
cyclize to an anthraquinone (58). In 1973 the conversion of sterigmatocystin to aflatoxin B_1 by the resting mycelium of *A. parasiticus* Speare
was reported (59).

Sterigmatocystin was produced by *Bipolaris* on corn meal in yields
as great as 1.2 g/kg. This high yield raises the possibility that sterigmatocystin could be a dangerous mycotoxin. The LD_{50} of the mycotoxin
administered intraperitoneally in dimethyl sulfoxide or wheat germ oil
was 60–65 mg/kg in albino rats. Necrosis of kidney and liver cells was

revealed by histopathological examinations of tissues (55). Another study (60) showed that sterigmatocystin caused not only local sarcomas but also liver tumors and had about 1/100–1/250 of the activity of aflatoxin. Subcutaneous injections of sterigmatocystin in rats (0.5 mg twice weekly for 24 weeks) induced local sarcomas and after 47 weeks induced liver tumors in two rats. Large doses of aflatoxin B_1 subcutaneously did not produce liver tumors although they caused many more local sarcomas. Oral administration of sterigmatocystin also produced liver tumors in rats (61). Tumors of other types were noticed.

Besides sterigmatocystin one other mycotoxin has been reported as a product of *Helminthosporium* (62). The unknown mycotoxin may in fact be several toxic compounds. It is formed on a high-protein cereal medium by *H. carbonum* (a *Drechslera*) and is toxic to mice.

Cytochalasins A (Structure XL), B (Structure XLI), and F (Structure XLII) produced by *H. dematioideum* Bubák *et* Wróblewski [synonym of *D. dematioidea* (Bub. *et* Wrób.) Subram. *et* Jain] (Figure 10) belong to a series of related biologically active compounds studied by groups in three countries. The compounds have an effect on cellular functions and morphology and are considered to be mycotoxins. They

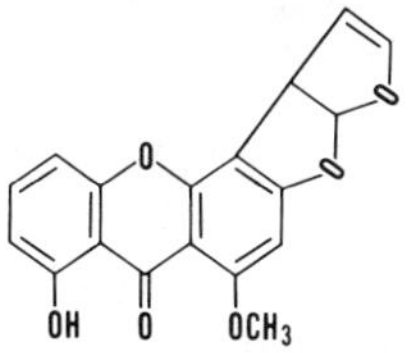

XXXIV. Sterigmatocystin

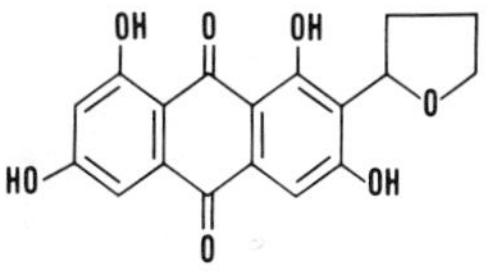

XXXV. Bipolarin

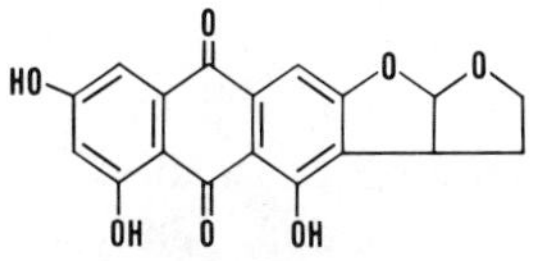

XXXVI. Versicolorin C

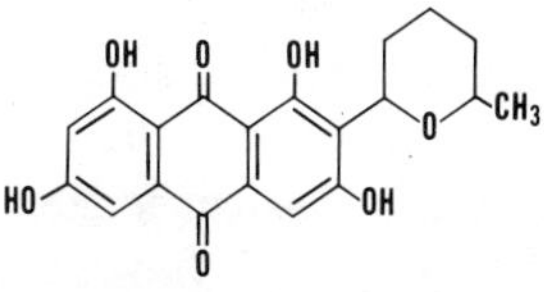

XXXVII. Averufanin

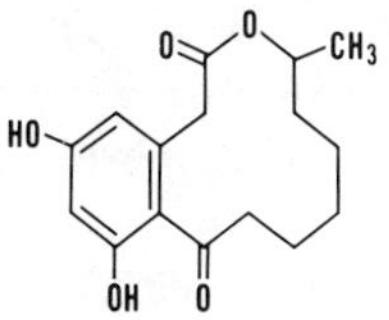

XXXVIII. Curvularin

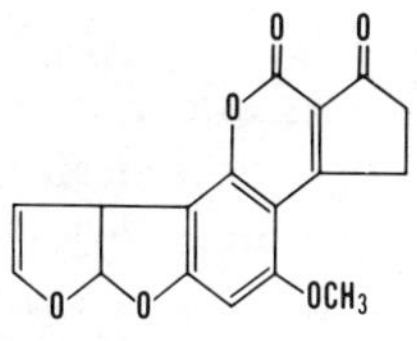

XXXIX. Aflatoxin B_1

Figure 9. Helminthosporium *metabolites with biosynthetic pathways related to aflatoxin* B_1

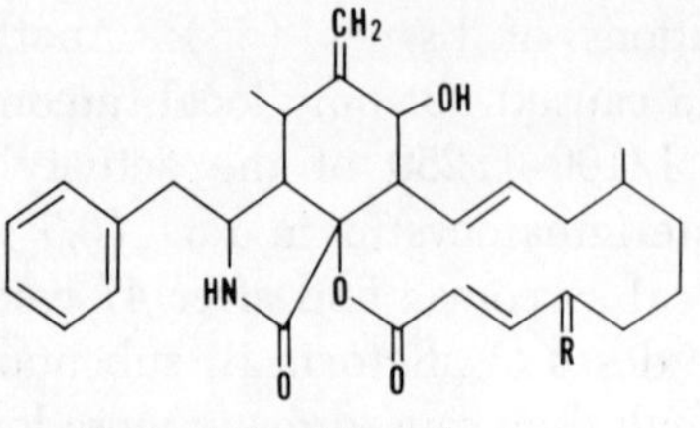

XL. R = O Cytochalasin A
XLI. R = H,OH Cytochalasin B

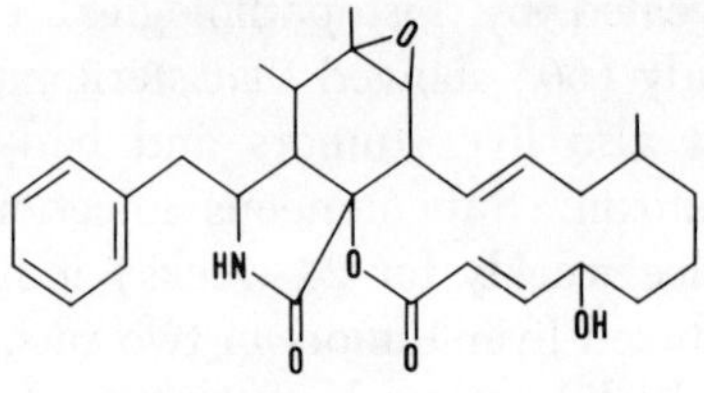

XLII. Cytochalasin F

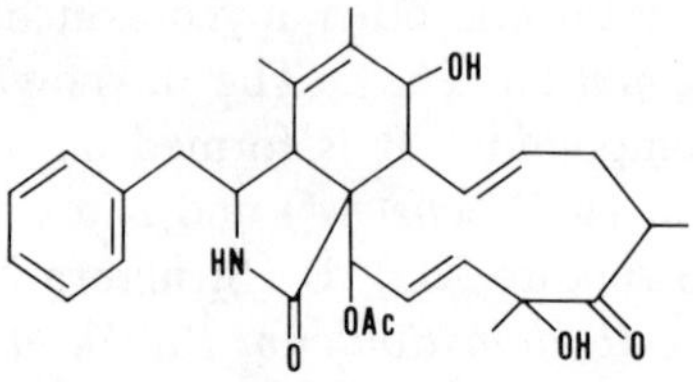

XLIII. Cytochalasin C

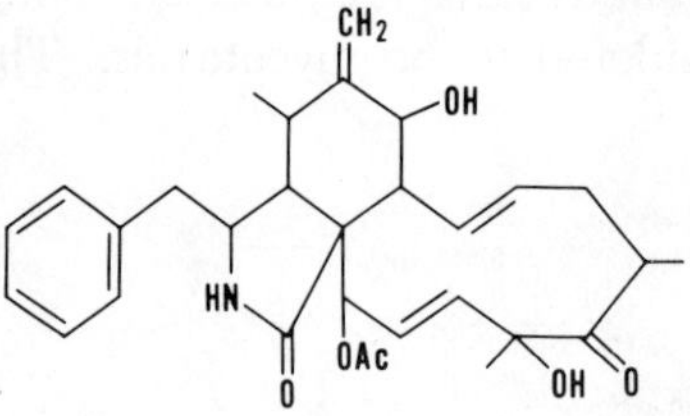

XLIX. Cytochalasin D

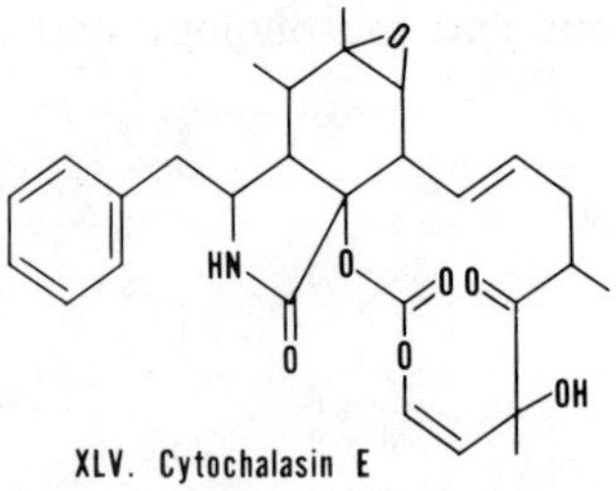

XLV. Cytochalasin E

Figure 10.   Cytochalasins

are characterized by a substituted, hydrogenated isoindole group to which is fused a macrocyclic ring that is either a carbocyclic compound, a lactone, or a cyclic carbonate. The metabolites isolated by the Swiss from a *Phoma* species have been called phomins. Those from *Zygosporium masonii* Hughes were named zygosporins by the Japanese. The English described their metabolites from *Helminthosporium* species as cytochalasins (cytos = cell; chalasis = relaxation). The three groups proposed a systematic nomenclature based on the generic name cytochalasan for the cytochalasins, phomins, and zygosporins (63).

Phomin (phomine, cytochalasin B), the first cytochalasin reported, was described in 1966 as a macrolide antibiotic with cytostatic activity produced by a *Phoma* species (64). Later in a more detailed investigation of the *Phoma* metabolites a closely related compound with similar activity, dehydrophomin (cytochalasin A), was isolated (65). Structures were first determined by a series of degradations; later ir, NMR, and mass spectroscopy of the compounds confirmed these degradation products. X-ray analysis of the phomin–silver fluoroborate complex established the absolute stereochemistry of phomin (66).

In 1967 Aldridge and co-workers (67) isolated cytochalasins A and B from *H. dematioideum* (*Drechslera dematioidea*) and C and D from *Metarrhizium anisopliae* (Metsch.) Sorok. Subsequently they established Structures XL and XLI as the structures of A and B (68). C. Tamm of Basel, Switzerland and D. C. Aldridge's group determined the structure of cytochalasin B (phomin) about the same time based on almost completely independent evidence, but the degradations they designed differed. Earlier a French patent reported two fungicidal compounds produced by *H. dematioideum* (*Drechslera dematioidea*) that contained nitrogen. They were intraconvertible by oxidation–reduction reactions, had the empirical formulas of $C_{29}H_{35}NO_5$ and $C_{29}H_{37}NO_5$, and almost certainly were cytochalasins A and B (69).

Cytochalasins C and D are produced in low yields by *M. anisopliae* and are difficult to separate. Because he had particular difficulty obtaining cytochalasin D, almost all of Aldridge's degradative studies were done on C (70). He determined that cytochalasins C (Structure XLIII) and D (Structure XLIV) have lactone groups in the macrocyclic ring. Simultaneously Minato and Matsumoto (71) reported the isolation of a cytotoxic antibiotic, zygosporin A, from culture filtrates of *Zygosporium masonii*. Their studies revealed Structure XLIV for zygosporin A which is identical to cytochalasin D. Later Minato and Katayama (72) isolated and characterized minor metabolites of *Z. masonii*, zygosporins D, E, F, and G that were related to the cytochalasins in structure and biological activity.

Structures were proposed in 1972 for cytochalasin E produced by *Rosellinia necatrix* (Hartig) Berl. *et* Prill. and for F, a minor metabolite of *H. dematioideum* (*Drechslera dematioidea*) (73). Since then alternate structures that seem correct have been established for cytochalasin E (Structure XLV) and F (Structure XLII) (74). The cyclohexane rings in E and F contain epoxides rather than the previously suggested double bond and hydroxyl group. Perhaps more importantly, the cytochalasin E studied was produced by *Aspergillus clavatus* Desm. collected from mold-damaged rice in a Thai household where a young boy died of an unidentified toxicosis. The cytochalasin E produced on rice inoculated with *A. clavatus* had an LD_{50} in rats of 2.6 mg/kg i.p. or 9.1 mg/kg orally. Death in mice was attributed to circulatory collapse caused by massive extravascular effusion of plasma.

In India a compound that is considered closely related to cytochalasin D was produced by a newly identified fungus, *Phomopsis paspali* Pendse (name not validly published) (75). The fungus had been isolated from the food grain, millet (*Paspalum scrobiculatum* Linn.), which is consumed by the poorest section of the rural population. The grain's toxicity to man and animals has been known for centuries, and extracts reportedly have a tranquilizing effect on animals. Bhide and Pendse also reported that cytochalasins given by ip injection to dogs at 1–2 mg/kg produced tranquility along with tremors and depressed motor activity.

Cytochalasins affect cellular functions and possess teratogenic properties that may present potential hazards to animals and man. So many studies have been made on the biological properties of cytochalasins that a complete presentation cannot be made here. The activities of cytochalasins A, B, C, and D are essentially similar but vary in potency. Almost all work has been on B because it is more available than A, C, and D. Carter (76) first found that cytochalasins inhibit movement and cytoplasmic cleavage in cultured cells leading to multinucleated cells. At higher concentrations nuclear extrusion takes place.

The effect of cytochalasin B on morphogenesis has been further studied with mouse salivary-gland epithelium cells (77), mouse embryos (78), onion roots (79), and the water mold *Achlya ambisexualis* J. R. Raper (80). Embryonic development of mice cells was extremely limited after cytochalasin treatment and did not proceed into organogenesis. Defendi and Stoker (81) studied the general polyploid produced by cytochalasin B. Cytochalasins also affect hexose and sucrose transport in cells (82, 83, 84). Earlier Wessels and co-workers (85) summarized the effects of cytochalasin on microfilaments in cellular and developmental processes. One report has been made on the mode of action of tritium-labeled cytochalasin B of high specific activity (86).

The cytochalasins may be one of the more important mycotoxins, and the extent to which they present a problem to man and animals should be evaluated. The work in Thailand on cytochalasin E (74) and in India on cytochalasin D (75) implicates them as possibly occurring naturally on foods that comprise an important part of the diets of people in these countries. When cases of mycotoxicosis arise, consideration should be given to the cytochalasins as causative agents.

Most of the antibiotics described as being produced by *Helminthosporium* and *Drechslera* species are known to be toxic—too toxic to be useful therapeutically. These antibiotics might turn out to be mycotoxins. Of the mycotoxins now considered to present serious problems, several were originally described as toxic antibiotics (*e.g.*, patulin and penicillic acid).

Literature Cited

1. Scott, P. M., Somers, E., *J. Agric. Food Chem.* (1969) **17**, 430–436.

2. Hesseltine, C. W., Ellis, J. J., Shotwell, O. L., *J. Agric. Food Chem.* (1971) **19**, 707–717.
3. Wood, R. K. S., Ballio, A., Graniti, A., "Phytotoxins in Plant Disease," Academic, New York, 1972.
4. Scheffer, R. P., Samaddar, K. R., *Recent Advan. Phytochem.* (1970) **3**, 123–142.
5. Pringle, R. B., Braun, A. C., *Phytopathology* (1960) **50**, 324–325.
6. Scheffer, R. P., Pringle, R. B., *Phytopathology* (1963) **53**, 558–561.
7. Dorn, F., Arigoni, D., *Chem. Commun.* (1972) 1342–1343.
8. Dorn, F., Arigoni, D., *Experientia* (1974) **30**, 134–135.
9. Pringle, R. B., "Phytotoxins in Plant Disease," R. K. S. Wood, A. Ballio, A. Graniti, Eds., pp. 146–151, Academic, New York, 1972.
10. Steiner, G. W., Strobel, G. A., *J. Biol. Chem.* (1971) **246**, 4350–4357.
11. Smedegard-Petersen, V., Nelson, R. R., *Can. J. Bot.* (1969) **47**, 951–957.
12. de Mayo, P., Spencer, E. Y., White, R. W., *J. Amer. Chem. Soc.* (1962) **84**, 494–495.
13. Spencer, E. Y., Ludwig, R. A., de Mayo, P., White, R. W., Williams, R. E., ADVAN. CHEM. SER. (1966) **53**, 106–111.
14. Canonica, L., "Phytotoxins In Plant Disease," R. K. S. Wood, A. Ballio, A. Graniti, Eds., pp. 157–173, Academic, New York, 1972.
15. Aldridge, D. C., Turner, W. B., *J. Chem. Soc. (C)* (1970) 686–688.
16. Raistrick, H., Robinson, R., Todd, A. R., *Biochem. J.* (1934) **28**, 559–572.
17. Anslow, W. K., Raistrick, H., *Biochem. J.* (1940) **34**, 1124–1133.
18. Anslow, W. K., Raistrick, H., *Biochem. J.* (1941) **35**, 1006–1010.
19. Raistrick, H., Robinson, R., Todd, A. B., *Biochem. J.* (1933) **27**, 1170–1175.
20. Charles, J. H. V., Raistrick, H., Robinson, R., Todd, A. R., *Biochem. J.* (1933) **27**, 499–511.
21. Neelakantan, S., Pocker, A., Raistrick, H., *Biochem. J.* (1956) **64**, 464–469.
22. van Eijk, G. W., *Phytochem. Rep.* (1974) **13**, 650.
23. Thomson, R. H., "Naturally Occurring Quinones," pp. 179, 191, Academic, New York, 1957.
24. Raistrick, H., Robinson, R., White, D. E., *Biochem. J.* (1936) **30**, 1303–1304.
25. Ashley, J. N., Raistrick, H., *Biochem. J.* (1938) **32**, 449–454.
26. Tsuda, K., Nozoe, S., Morisaki, M., Hirai, K., Itai, A., Okuda, S., Canonica, L., Fiecchi, A., Galli Kienle, M., Scala, A., *Tetrahedron Lett.* (1967) 3369–3370.
27. Nozoe, S., Morisaki, M., Tsuda, K., Iitaka, Y., Takahashi, N., Tamura, S., Ishibashi, K., Shirasaka, M., *J. Amer. Chem. Soc.* (1965) **87**, 4968–4970.
28. Canonica, L., Fiecchi, A., Galli Kienle, M., Scala, A., *Tetrahedron Lett.* (1966) 1211–1218.
29. Canonica, L., Fiecchi, A., Galli Kienle, M., Scala, A., *Tetrahedron Lett.* (1966) 1329–1333.
30. Ishibashi, K., *J. Antibiot. Ser. A* (1962) **15**, 88–92.
31. Nozoe, S., Hirai, K., Tsuda, K., *Tetrahedron Lett.* (1966) 2211–2216.
32. Ohkawa, H., Tamura, T., *Agric. Biol. Chem.* (1966) **30**, 285–291.
33. Itai, A., Nozoe, S., Tsuda, K., Okuda, S., Iitaka, Y., Nakayama, Y., *Tetrahedron Lett.* (1967) 4111–4112.
34. Nozoe, S., Itai, A., Tsuda, K., Okuda, S., *Tetrahedron Lett.* (1967) 4113–4117.
35. Nozoe, S., Morisaki, M., Tsuda, K., Okuda, S., *Tetrahedron Lett.* (1967) 3365–3368.
36. Nozoe, S., Morisaki, M., Okuda, S., Tsuda, K., *Tetrahedron Lett.* (1968) 2347–2349.
37. Nozoe, S., Morisaki, M., Fukushima, K., Okuda, S., *Tetrahedron Lett.* (1968) 4457–4458.

38. Carruthers, J. R., Cerrini, S., Fedeli, W., Casinovi, C. G., Galeffi, C., Torracca Vaccaro, A. M., *Chem. Commun.* (1971) 164–166.
39. Canonica, L., Ranzi, B. M., Rindone, B., Scala, A., Scolastico, C., *Chem. Commun.* (1973) 213–214.
40. Ishibashi, K., *J. Antibiot., Ser. A* (1962) **15**, 161–167.
41. Hirai, K., Nozoe, S., Tsuda, K., Iitaka, Y., Ishibashi, K., Shirasaka, M., *Tetrahedron Lett.* (1967) 2177–2179.
42. Inagaki, N., *Chem. Pharm. Bull. (Japan)* (1962) **10**, 152–154.
43. Ishibashi, K., *J. Agric. Chem. Soc. Jap.* (1961) **35**, 257–262.
44. Nozoe, S., Hirai, K., Tsuda, K., Ishibashi, K., Shirasaka, M., Grove, J. F., *Tetrahedron Lett.* (1965) 4675–4677.
45. Aldridge, D. C., Turner, W. B., *J. Chem. Soc. C* (1970) 2598–2600.
46. Gerber, N. N., Lechevalier, H. A., *J. Org. Chem.* (1962) **27**, 1731–1732.
47. Pugh, L. H., Lechevalier, H. A., Solotorovsky, M., *Antibiot. Chemother.* (1962) **12**, 310–317.
48. Crane, R. I., Heddon, P., MacMillan, J., Turner, W. B., *J. Chem. Soc., Perkin Trans. 1* (1973) 194–200.
49. Suzuki, K. T., Nozoe, S., *Bioorg. Chem.* (1974) **3**, 72–80.
50. Nozoe, S., Suzuki, K. T., *Tetrahedron Lett.* (1969) 2457–2460.
51. Shoyama, Y., Yamauchi, T., Nishioka, I., *Chem. Pharm. Bull. (Jap.)* (1970) **18**, 1327.
52. Nozoe, S., Suzuki, K. T., Okuda, S., *Tetrahedron Lett.* (1968) 3643–3646.
53. Nozoe, S., Suzuki, K. T., Tetrahedron (1971) **27**, 6063–6071.
54. Suzuki, K. T., Suzuki, N., Nozoe, S., *Chem. Commun.* (1971) 527.
55. Holzapfel, C. W., Purchase, I. F. H., Steyn, P. S., Gouws, L., *S. Afr. Med. J.* (1966) **40**, 1110–1111.
56. Aucamp, P. J., Holzapfel, C. W., *J. S. Afr. Chem. Inst.* (1970) **23**, 40–56.
57. Heathcote, J. G., Dutton, M. F., *Tetrahedron* (1969) **25**, 1497–1500.
58. Heathcote, J. G., Dutton, M. F., Hibbert, J. R., *Chem. Ind.* (1973) 1027–1030.
59. Hsieh, D. P. H., Lin, M. T., Yao, R. C., *Biochem. Biophys. Res. Commun.* (1973) **52**, 992–997.
60. Dickens, F., Jones, H. E. H., Waynforth, H. B., *Brit. J. Cancer* (1966) **20**, 134–144.
61. Purchase, I. F. H., van der Watt, J. J., *Food Cosmet. Toxicol.* (1970) **8**, 289–295.
62. Hamilton, P. B., Nelson, R. R., Harris, B. S. H., *Appl. Microbiol.* (1968) **16**, 1719–1722.
63. Binder, M., Tamm, C., Turner, W. B., Minato, H., *J. Chem. Soc., Perkin Trans. 2* (1973) 1146–1147.
64. Rothweiler, W., Tamm, C., *Experientia* (1966) **22**, 750–752.
65. Rothweiler, W., Tamm, C., *Helv. Chim. Acta* (1970) **53**, 696–724.
66. McLaughlin, G. M., Sim, G. A., Kiechel, J. R., Tamm, C., *Chem. Commun.* (1970) 1398–1399.
67. Aldridge, D. C., Armstrong, J. J., Speake, R. N., Turner, W. B., *Chem. Commun.* (1967) 26–27.
68. Aldridge, D. C., Armstrong, J. J., Speake, R. N., Turner, W. B., *J. Chem. Soc. C* (1967) 1667–1676.
69. Imperial Chemical Industries, Ltd., Fr. Patent 1,437,461 (May 6, 1966); *Chem. Abstr.* (1967) **66**, 9972e.
70. Aldridge, D. C., Turner, W. B., *J. Chem. Soc. C* (1969) 923–928.
71. Minato, H., Matsumoto, M., *J. Chem. Soc. C* (1970) 38–45.
72. Minato, H., Katayama, T., *J. Chem. Soc. C* (1970) 45–47.
73. Aldridge, D. C., Burrows, B. F., Turner, W. B., *Chem. Commun.* (1972) 148–149.

74. Buchi, G., Kitaura, Y., Yuan, S. S., Wright, H. E., Clardy, J., Demain, A. L., Glinsukon, T., Hunt, N., Wogan, G. N., *J. Amer. Chem. Soc.* (1973) **95**, 5423–5425.
75. Pendse, G. S., *Experientia* (1974) **30**, 107–108.
76. Carter, S. B., *Nature* (1967) **213**, 261–264.
77. Spooner, B. S., Wessels, N. K., *Proc. Nat. Acad. Sci.* (1970) **66**, 360–364.
78. Snow, M. H. L., *Nature* (1973) **244**, 513–514.
79. Thomas, D. des S., Lager, N. M., Manavathu, E. K., *Can. J. Bot.* (1973) **51**, 2269–2273.
80. Thomas, D. des S., Lutzac, M., Manavathu, E. K., *Nature* (1974) **249**, 140–142.
81. Defendi, U., Stoker, M. G. P., *Nature, New Biol.* (1973) **242**, 24–26.
82. Kletzien, R. F., Perdue, J. F., Springer, A., *J. Biol. Chem.* (1972) **247**, 2964–2966.
83. Mizel, S. B., Wilson, L., *J. Biol. Chem.* (1972) **247**, 4102–4105.
84. Thompson, R. G., Thompson, A. D., *Can. J. Bot.* (1973) **51**, 933–936.
85. Wessels, N. K., Spooner, B. S., Ash, J. F., Bradley, M. O., Luduena, M. A., Taylor, E. L., Wrenn, J. T., Yamada, K. M., *Science* (1971) **171**, 135–143.
86. Lin, S., Santi, D. V., Spudich, J. A., *J. Biol. Chem.* (1974) **249**, 2268–2274.

RECEIVED November 8, 1974.

15

The Structure and Toxicity of the *Alternaria* Metabolites

D. J. HARVAN and R. W. PERO[1]

National Institute of Environmental Health Sciences, P.O. Box 12233, Research Triangle Park, N. C. 27709

The Alternaria *are a common field fungi responsible for a variety of plant diseases including tobacco brown spot, tomato blight, and citrus seedling chlorosis. They have been implicated in diseases of poultry and have been demonstrated lethal to mammals. The metabolites of the* Alternaria *represent several structural classes: dibenzo-pyrones, anthraquinones, tetramic acids, and polypeptides. The metabolites are discussed with regard to: structure; mammalian, plant, and cytotoxicity; methods of analysis; synthesis, and biosynthetic pathways.*

The *Alternaria* are common plant pathogens which infest a wide variety of food crops. Grain crops, hay, and silage are often contaminated with this fungus, generally as a field infection (*1, 2*). Black spot of Japanese pear (*3*), tobacco brown spot (*4*), early blight of tomato and potato, and citrus seedling chlorosis are all caused by *Alternaria spp.* (*5*).

The toxicity of the *Alternaria* has been well established. Grains which had been infected with *A. humicola* and *A. alternata* (Fries) Keissler (*A. tenuis, Auct.* and *A. longipes*) (*6*) were believed the source of several outbreaks of moldy grain toxicosis in man in the U.S.S.R. during World War II (*7*). Of the *Alternaria* isolates tested from a variety of food crops, 90% were lethal to rats when fed in a corn-rice mixture (*2*). Doupnik and Sobers (*8*) reported that 33% of the isolates tested were lethal to chicks. Slifkin and Spalding (*9*) found that *A. mali* was toxic to HeLa cells and mice in feeding studies. The *Alternaria* have been implicated as toxins to geese and other poultry (*10, 11*). Of 212 *Alternaria* isolates from tobacco, 60% were lethal to mice following intraperitoneal injection (*12*). Several workers attempted to establish a correlation between pathogenicity

---

[1] Current address: University of Lund, Lund, Sweden.

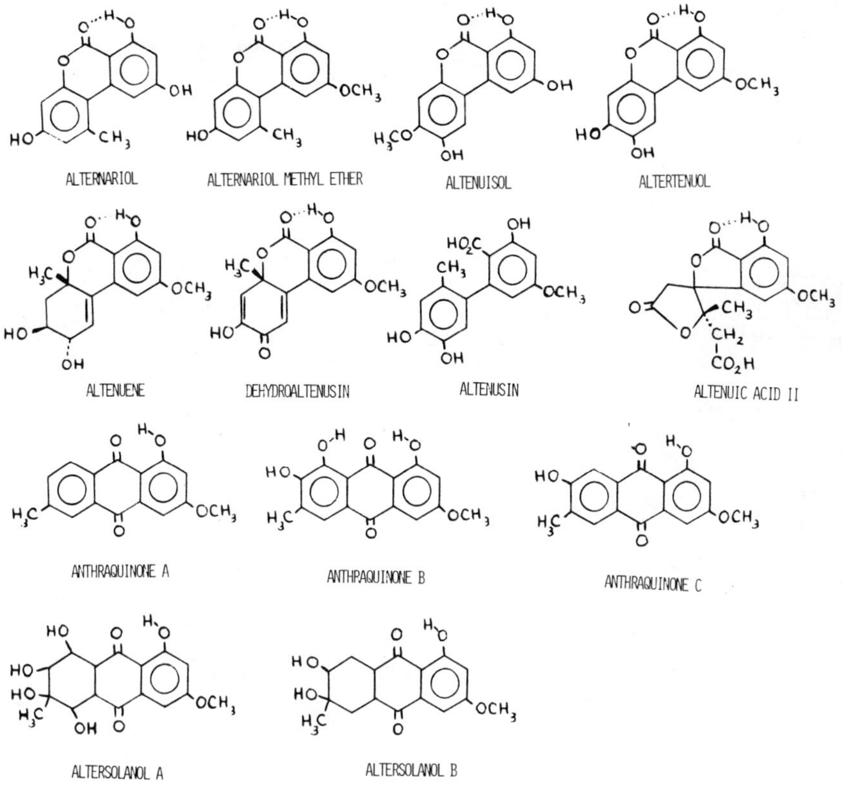

Figure 1. Structures of the metabolites of Alternaria spp.

to tobacco leaves and toxicity of the isolates (13). In these studies 74% of the pathogenic isolates were toxic to chicks, and 75% of the nonpathogenic isolates were nontoxic. The *Alternaria* possess a wide range of antibiotic activity. Of 127 isolates 86 were active against either bacteria, yeast, or molds (14).

Structure of the Metabolites

The structures of the known *Alternaria* metabolites are presented in Figures 1 and 2. The most commonly occurring class of compounds are the dibenzo-pyrones and their derivatives: alternariol, alternariol methyl ether, altenuisol, altertenuol, altenuene, dehydroaltenusin, altenusin, and the altenuic acids.

Alternariol and the methyl ether are produced by most *A. alternata* isolates as well as many other *Alternaria* species; both are colorless, crystalline compounds. Alternariol has a melting point of 350°C (dec); the methyl ether melts at 267°C. Because of their phenolic nature, they exhibit

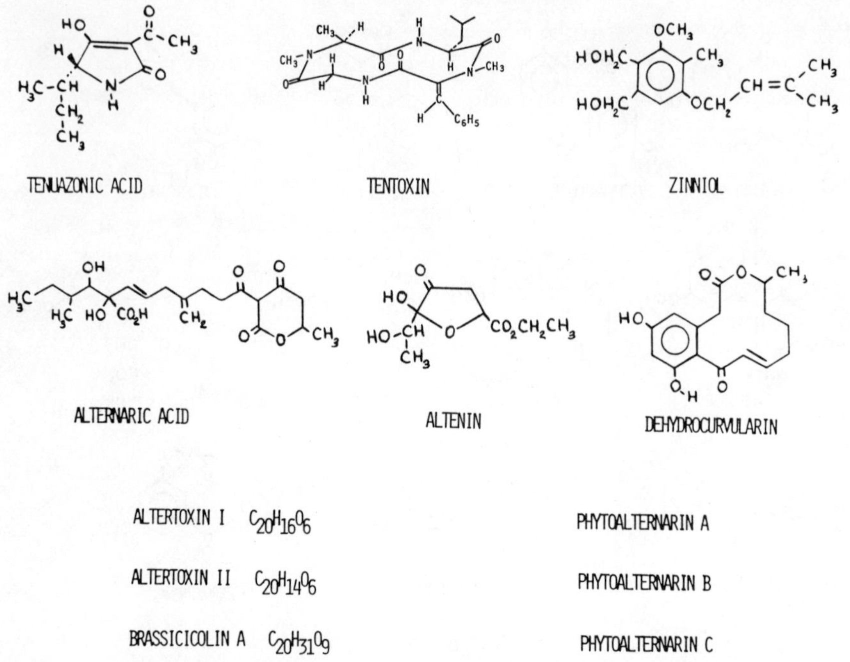

TENUAZONIC ACID   TENTOXIN   ZINNIOL

ALTERNARIC ACID   ALTENIN   DEHYDROCURVULARIN

ALTERTOXIN I $C_{20}H_{16}O_6$ PHYTOALTERNARIN A

ALTERTOXIN II $C_{20}H_{14}O_6$ PHYTOALTERNARIN B

BRASSICICOLIN A $C_{20}H_{31}O_9$ PHYTOALTERNARIN C

Figure 2.   Structures of the metabolites of Alternaria spp.

intense purple ferric reactions and fluoresce bright blue under uv irradiation. They are produced in rather large quantities accounting for up to
13% of the dry mycelial weight of some isolates (*15*). Their biosynthesis
is the best studied of the metabolites (*16, 17*). Several synthetic methods
have been reported for alternariol (*18, 19*), and the selective methylation
of alternariol to the methyl ether has been described (*20*).

Altenuisol and altertenuol are closely related metabolites of *A. alternata* and in fact may be identical compounds. Thomas (*20*) postulated
the altertenuol structure based mainly on the empirical formula and biosynthetic arguments. Altertenuol is a crystalline material (mp = 284°–
285°C) which forms a triacetate (mp = 245°C). Pero et al. (*21*) isolated altenuisol (mp = 277°–282°C; triacetate mp = 210°–213°C) and
proposed this differing structure based on the fact that altenuisol failed to
react with a molybdate ion, a property common to orthodihydric phenols
(*22*), but did react after demethylation with hydriodic acid. The position
of the methoxyl group was established by comparing the NMR shifts of
altenuisol and its triacetate with scopoletin and its acetate. Further work
is necessary to resolve the structure of these two metabolites.

Altenuene, dehydroaltenusin, and altenusin are closely related metabolites whose structures have been determined by x-ray crystallography.
Altenuene was isolated by silica gel chromatography of *A. alternata* ex-

tracts and was crystallized as colorless needles, melting point = 190°–191°C. Its original structure postulation (23) has been revised (24). Dehydroaltenusin was isolated by the adsorption of *A. alternata* culture medium on charcoal, followed by ethanol extraction. The resulting solution yielded dehydroaltenusin as yellow plates melting at 189°–190°C. The original structure postulation was incorrect (25) and has been recently revised (26). Altenusin crystallized from chloroform extracts as colorless prisms, melting at 202°–203°C. It is interconvertible with dehydroaltenusin by oxidation with ferric chloride or reduction with sodium dithionite (27).

Altenuic acid II is one of three isomeric acids isolated from *A. alternata* (27). It was separated from acids I and III by its limited solubility in ether, and crystallized from aqueous dioxane as colorless plates melting at 245°–246°C. Altenuic acid I and II are converted into altenuic acid III by treatment with dilute sodium hydroxide. The structure of altenuic acid II has been established by x-ray crystallography (28). The structures of altenuic acids I and III are undetermined.

A second class of metabolites are the anthraquinone pigments isolated from *A. solani* (29, 30). The pigments were isolated by silica gel chromatography of the chloroform extracts of the fungus. Anthraquinones A, B, and C are substituted xanthopurpurins, and the altersolanols are partially reduced anthraquinones. Altersolanol A is converted to anthraquinone B upon dehydration at moderate temperatures, and altersolanol B furnishes anthraquinone A upon aromatization with thionyl chloride in pyridine. Anthraquinone C is identical to the previously identified macrosporin, a metabolite of *Macrosporium porri* (31).

Tenuazonic acid is a tetramic acid derivative which is produced by a large variety of *Alternaria spp.* (32). It is also a metabolite of *Pyricularia oryzae* (33), *Sphaeropsidales,* and some *Aspergilli* (34). It was first isolated by Rosett in 1957 (27), and its structure was elucidated by Stickings in 1959 (35). It has been found in naturally infected rice plants at 2.6 mg/kg plant tissue (36). Tenuazonic acid is an optically active liquid which loses activity upon long standing or with treatment in a base. This is attributed to the formation of isotenuazonic acid, a crystalline solid which is believed to be a mixture of diastereoisomers. Tenuazonic acid forms a crystalline salt with *N,N'*-dibenzylethylenediamine which is a convenient method for storage of the compound. The synthesis of the compound has been described (37); a series of analogs was prepared, and their biological activities were assessed (38).

Zinniol is a penta-substituted benzene derivative produced by *A. zinniae* (42). The structure is believed to be 1,2-bis-(hydroxymethyl)-5-(3,3'-dimethylallyloxy)-3-methoxy-4-methylbenzene, although the position of the methoxy and dimethylallyloxy substituents is not absolutely established (*43*). It is quite similar in structure to the antifungal agent quadrilineatin, a metabolite of *Aspergillus quadrilineatus.*

Alternaric acid is produced by strains of *A. solani* which are noted for their specific antifungal activity. The compound is purified by recrystallization from benzene, giving colorless plates and melting at 138°C (*44, 45*). Its structure was established by Bartels–Keith and Grove in 1959 (*46*).

Altenin is an optically active, yellow liquid that is produced by *A. kikuchiana.* It is isolated from the culture filtrate and purified by chromatography on alumina and silica gel. It is unstable at higher temperatures; it loses its biological activity in ten minutes at 80°C and in 1 hr at 60°C. The assigned structure is believed to be the most probable of several tautomeric forms (*3*).

α,β-Dehydrocurvularin is a metabolic product of *A. cucumerina,* the causative agent of leaf spot on cucurbits, particularly muskmelon and watermelon (*47*). It is a colorless, crystalline solid, melting point 230°–232°C, with an optical rotation of −85°. It is also a metabolite of several *Curvularia spp.* (*48*).

Altertoxins I and II are metabolites of unknown structure and are produced by *A. mali* (*49*) and *A. alternata.* Altertoxin I ($C_{20}H_{16}O_6$) is a yellow, amorphous solid with an undefined melting point; it decomposes at *ca.* 210°C. It fluoresces bright yellow under irradiation, and this property has been used as a method of analysis (*50*). Altertoxin II ($C_{20}H_{14}O_6$) is an orange, crystalline solid which decomposes at 185°–195°C. It is closely related to Altertoxin I and is probably the dehydro derivative. Under irradiation it appears as a dark, quenching spot. Both compounds are highly aromatic materials, possessing neither methoxyl nor carbon–methyl groups. They both have carbonyl absorptions at 1650 cm^{-1} which indicates hydrogen-bounding by adjacent hydroxyls. Their structure is being investigated by x-ray crystallography.

Brassicicolin A is a metabolite isolated from *A. brassicicola.* The material is a colorless oil, with $[\alpha]_D = 20.1°$. Its elemental composition has been reported to be $C_{20}H_{31}O_9$. The compound possesses anti-yeast and mild anti-bacterial activity (*51*).

Phytoalternarins A, B, and C are produced by *A. kikuchiana* Tanaka. Phytoalternarin A is a colorless solid; B is a yellow fluorescent liquid, and C is a colorless solid, melting at 235°C (*5*). All three give positive ninhydrin, Lieberman, and Xanthoproteic tests, but negative Fehling and Biuret reactions (*52*).

Synthetic Methods

Alternariol was first synthesized by coupling 2-bromo-4,6-dimethoxybenzoic acid with 3,5-dihydroxytoluene in the presence of basic copper sulfate. The resulting material was methylated giving a compound identical to alternariol trimethyl ether (*18*). A more elegant synthesis of alternariol has recently been described (*19*). The dibenzyl ether of methyl orsellinate was condensed with dilithioacetylactone to give a triketone derivative. The triketone was carboxylated with lithium di-isopropylamide and esterified with diazomethane. Removal of the benzyl protective groups caused spontaneous cyclization to a chroman derivative. Treatment of the chroman with sodium acetate gave alternariol in 52% yield (Figure 3). Alternariol presumably is formed by an aldol condensation between positions two and seven, followed by dehydration and lactonization. Since alternariol can be selectively methylated to alternariol methyl ether, this constitutes a synthesis of the methyl ether as well (*20*). By use of the appropriate benzoic acid analogs this method could also provide synthetic routes to altenusin, dehydroaltenusin, and altertenuol.

Tenuazonic acid is synthesized by condensing L-isoleucine with diketene. The product is methylated with diazomethane and cyclized by refluxing with the sodium methoxide in benzene. The compound is purified by recrystallization of its copper (*37*) or its N,N'-dibenzylethylenediamine salt (*34*).

Altenin has been prepared by the condensation of ethyl glyoxalate with 3-acetoxy-acetylacetone in the presence of potassium amide (*3*). The synthetic material was identical to the naturally occurring compound in phytopathologic activity as well as spectroscopy.

The only anthraquinone metabolite that has been synthesized is macrosporin monomethyl ether (*54*). The method involved condensing α-resorcylic acid with 3-methoxy-4-methylbenzoic acid by heating with

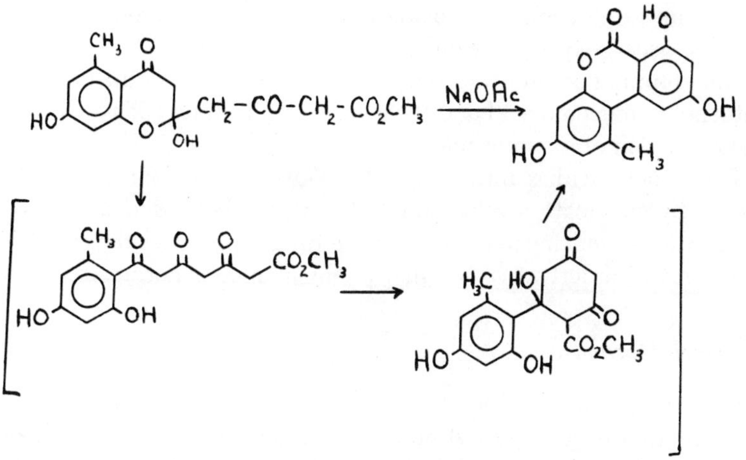

Figure 3.   Biogenetic type synthesis of alternariol

concentrated sulfuric acid and boric anhydride. Methylation of this material gave macrosporin monomethyl ether. Although two isomers were possible, only that one corresponding to naturally-occurring macrosporin was isolated.

Biosynthetic Pathways

The biosynthesis of alternariol has been discussed in relation to the polyketide hypothesis (56). This theory maintains that a long poly-β carbonyl chain is formed by head-to-tail condensations of acetate with malonyl-CoA units. The resultant chain may then cyclize by aldol or Claissen-type reactions and lead to the observed products. The theory involves only slight modification of that believed to be responsible for fatty-acid synthesis.

The enzyme complex responsible for alternariol synthesis has been purified by gel filtration on Sephadex G-25 (16). The enzyme utilizes acetyl-CoA and malonyl-CoA as substrate but is inhibited by excessive concentrations of either reagent. Optimum velocity was observed with a ratio of malonyl pantotheine to acetyl-CoA of 6:1 which is the ratio of malonate to acetate found in alternariol. The optimum activity was observed at pH 7.8 at 28°C (17). It was also demonstrated that the addition of S-adenosylmethionine to the reaction mixture caused the formation of alternariol methyl ether.

The degradation of alternariol methyl ether could account for most of the other dibenzo-pyrone metabolites (Figure 4). Altenusin would be the result of hydroxylation followed by reductive opening of the lactone ring. Dehydroaltenusin and altenuene could arise from altenusin by oxidation and reduction. The oxidation of the carbon–methyl group followed by decarboxylation would lead to altertenuol. Oxidation of the catechol grouping of altenusin—in a manner analogous to the degradation of catechol to muconic acid and then to muconolactone (56)—would lead to the formation of altenuic acid.

Tenuazonic acid is formed by the N-acetoacetylation of iso-leucine followed by enzymatic cyclization (57). It has been demonstrated that adding valine or leucine to cultures of the fungus produces the corresponding tetramic acid derivative but that phenylalanine is not utilized (58).

Analytical Methods

Few analytical methods have been reported for the *Alternaria* metabolites. Alternariol, the methyl ether, and altenuene have been analyzed by gas chromatography as silyl ethers (59). The silyl ethers are chromatographed on 3% OV-17 at 100°–250°C at 8°/min. Under these condi-

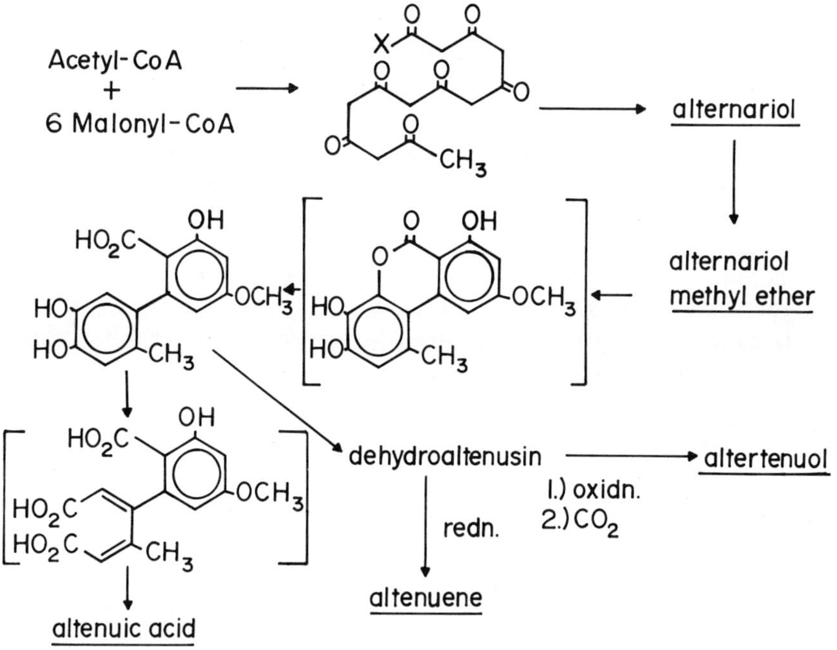

Figure 4.   Possible biosynthetic pathway for the dibenzo-pyrone metabolites of the Alternaria

tions altenuene has a retention time of 23 min, alternariol 27 min, and the methyl ether, 29 min. This method has also been used for several commonly occurring fungal metabolites such as stearic acid, palmitic acid, succinic acid, erythritol, and mannitol. It is also useful for some metabolites of other fungi, e.g., kojic acid, penicillic acid, and patulin (60). Thin layer chromatography has been used recently to detect alternariol and the methyl ether in grain samples (61). The method was of value in distinguishing between alternariol, zearelenone, and aflatoxin in infected grains. Tenuazonic acid has been analyzed by a spectrophotometric method (62) and a gas chromatographic method (63).

Toxicity

Crude *Alternaria* extracts are lethal to mice (ip injection) at 300 mg/kg (50). Similar levels of toxicosis occur in rats with oral dosage. The major mammalian toxin is believed to be tenuazonic acid (64). Several investigators demonstrated the toxicity of tenuazonic acid to mice (38, 65), rats, dogs, monkeys and guinea pigs (65).

Sodium tenuazonate is highly inhibitory to the human adenocarcinoma (HAd1) in the egg host system at 0.1 mg/egg and toxic to the embryo at 0.48 mg/egg (*34*). The D-allo and D-isomers as well as structural analogs of tenuazonic acid, substituted in the carbon-five position, were much less active against tumors. Analogs substituted on nitrogen showed an increased antibacterial activity but a reduced antitumor activity. Against *Bacillus megaterium,* analogs substituted at carbon-five were about as active as the parent compound. Against *B. megaterium,* L- and D-sodium tenuazonate were equally active (*38*).

Sodium tenuazonate and isotenuazonate were equally effective against enteroviruses (ECHO-9, Coxsackie B), respiratory viruses [parainfluenza-3, (HA-1), Salisbury HGP], vaccinia, herpes simplex HF, and 'B' virus at 100–500 μg/ml. Sodium tenuazonate was effective against poliovirus MEF1, whereas sodium isotenuazonate was not. Neither was active in tissue culture against polyoma virus or in mice against Asian influenza, rabies, or Friend leukemia (*66*).

Tenuazonic acid inhibits the incorporation of amino acids into protein *in vivo* in Sprague-Dawley rats and *in vitro* in Ehrlich Ascites tumor cells. It is believed that tenuazonic acid interferes with the release of newly-formed protein from the ribosomes thus preventing the ribosomes from accepting amino acids from transfer RNA (*67*). Tenuazonic acid is also known to block peptide bond formation in protein synthesis of human tonsil and pig-liver ribosomes (*68*).

Tenuazonic acid has a protective effect on *in vivo* cell death of intestinal crypt epithelial cells after exposure to 1-β D-arabinofuranosylcytosine, nitrogen mustard, or x-irradiation. At 30–75 mg/kg in male rats tenuazonic acid inhibits leucine incorporation into protein and thymidine incorporation into DNA but not uridine incorporation into RNA. The protective effect was attributed to the inhibition of protein synthesis (*69*).

Several other metabolites have been examined for cytotoxicity (*50, 70*) and teratogenicity (*50*). Alternariol and the methyl ether exhibited a synergistic effect against bacteria and as teratogens. Altenuene, altenuisol, and the altertoxins were all active against HeLa cells, with ID_{50} values from 0.5–28 μg/ml (*50*).

The toxicity of the remaining *Alternaria* metabolites has not been studied extensively. No data exist for altertenuol, altenusin, dehydroaltenusin, altenuic acid, or the anthraquinone pigments. Brassiciolin A has low antibacterial activity but fair antiyeast and antifungal properties. This and other metabolites of *A. brassicicola* need further study since strains of this type were the most consistently active against bacteria, molds, and yeast (*14*). Even though α,β-dehydrocurvularin has not been investigated for antibiotic or phytotoxic activity, it is similar in structure to zearelenone, a *Fusarium* metabolite which has strong estrogenic activity, and may be of interest in studies of that type.

Phytotoxicity

Several *Alternaria* metabolites have been associated with phytotoxicity (5). Tentoxin is responsible for seedling chlorosis of cotton and citrus fruits. The purified compound interferes with chlorophyll formation in many higher plant species. Most dicotyledons are sensitive with the exception of tomato and the Cruciferae (71). The compound does not affect the alga *Euglena gracilis*, bacteria, the yeast *Saccharomyces cerevisiae*, or filamentous fungi at concentrations that cause 100% chlorosis of cucumber cotyledons.

Altenin is capable of causing black spots on susceptible Japanese pear at 2×10^{-5} mg/ml. The active moiety is believed to be the enediolcarbonyl grouping (3).

Zinniol is responsible for leaf spot and seedling blight of zinnia, sunflower, and marigold. Plants with severe infection often wilt and die. At 500 ppm zinniol inhibits the germination of zinnia, tomato, lettuce, watermelon, and carrot seeds. At 1000 ppm it causes complete withering of cut seedlings of watermelon, squash, spinach, beet, tomato, oat, corn, pea, and bean. The compound is mildly inhibitory to Actinomycetes at 485 μg/disc (42).

Alternaric acid was isolated from cultures of *A. solani,* the fungus responsible for early blight of tomatoes and potatoes, an economically significant plant disease in the United States (44, 72). At 5–10 μg/ml it causes wilting and death to seedlings of radish, cabbage, mustard, and carrot.   At 2–20 μg/ml it causes necrotic lesions in tomato and potato shoots. It also possesses some antifungal activity, inhibiting the germination of *Absidia, Myrothecium,* and *Stachybotrys* at 0.1–1.0 μg/ml. At 200 μg/ml it inhibits the rate of germination of *Botrytis, Fusarium,* and *Penicillium* (5).

Alternariol methyl ether has also been shown to cause chlorosis in tobacco leaves (73). When solutions of the material are injected into tobacco leaves, chlorotic zones, proportional in size to concentration, were formed within 48 hr. The level of activity was between 10–25 μg/ml. It was also observed that the methyl ether was produced by growing *A. alternata* on tobacco substrate. The compound was rapidly metabolized and was nondetectable 72 hr after injection into living tissue. This is supported by the fact that other workers failed to find alternariol or the methyl ether in extracts of naturally moldy tobacco (74).

Phytoalternarins A, B, and C have been isolated by chromatography on alumina columns. Phytoalternarin A has the same host specificity as the fungus itself. A correlation is observed between tissue age and optimum temperature for symptom development between the fungus and pure toxin. Phytoalternarins B and C are toxic to susceptible varieties of Japanese pear (5).

Summary

The importance of the *Alternaria* toxins as environmental hazards has not yet been firmly established. Human populations would not be expected to receive acutely toxic doses in highly-developed nations. However in underdeveloped areas there is a greater possibility of human exposure to infected food crops. More important is the possibility of effects arising from continued low-level exposure to the metabolites. The limited fetotoxicity data implies some combined activity for alternariol and the methyl ether, but the majority of the metabolites have not been tested. The authors feel that continued research is necessary to evaluate the potential hazards of the *Alternaria* toxins particularly at the chronic level of exposure.

Literature Cited

1. Christensen, C. M., *Cereal Chem.* (1951) **28**, 408.
2. Christensen, C. M., *et al.*, Cancer Res. (1968) **28**, 2293.
3. Sugiyama, N., *et al.*, *Bull. Chem. Soc., Jap.* (1966) **39**, 2470.
4. Lucas, G. B., "Diseases of Tobacco," p. 228, Scarecrow, New York, 1959.
5. Templeton, G. E., in "Microbial Toxins," Vol. VII, (S. Kadis et al., Eds.), pp. 169–192, Academic, New York, 1972.
6. Lucas, G. B., *Tob. Sci.* (1971) **15**, 37.
7. Joffe, A. Z., *Bull. Res. Counc. Isr., Sect D.* (1960) **9**, 101.
8. Doupnik, B. Jr., Sobers, E. K., *Appl. Microbiol.* (1968) **16**, 1596.
9. Slifkin, M. K., Spalding, J., *Toxicol. Appl. Pharmacol.* (1970) **17**, 375.
10. Forgacs, J., *et al.*, *Am. J. Vet. Res.* (1958) **19**, 744.
11. Forgacs, J., *et al.*, *Avian Dis.* (1962) **6**, 363.
12. Hamilton, P. B., *et al.*, *Appl. Microbiol.* (1969) **18**, 570.
13. Sobers, E. K., Doupnik, B., Jr., *Appl. Microbiol.* (1972) **23**, 313.
14. Lindenfelser, L. A., Ciegler, A., *Dev. Ind. Microbiol.* (1969) **10**, 271.
15. Thomas, R., *Biochem. J.* (1961) **78**, 748.
16. Gatenbeck, S., Hermodsson, S., *Acta. Chem. Scand.* (1965) **19**, 65.
17. Sjoland, S., Gatenbeck, S., *Acta. Chem. Scand.* (1966) **20**, 1053.
18. Raistrick, H., *et al.*, *Biochem. J.* (1953) **55**, 421.
19. Hay, J. V., Harris, T. M., *J. Chem. Soc., Chem. Comm.* (1972) 953.
20. Thomas, R., *Biochem. J.* (1961) **80**, 234.
21. Pero, R. W., *et al.*, *Tetrahedron Lett.* (1973) **12**, 945.
22. Pridham, J. B., Ed., "Methods in Polyphenol Chemistry," p. 120, Macmillan, New York, 1964.
23. Pero, R. W., *et al.*, *Biochem. Biophys. Acta.* (1971) **230**, 170.
24. McPhail, A. T., *et al.*, *J. Chem. Soc., Chem. Comm.* (1973) 682.
25. Coombe, R. G., *et al.*, *Aust. J. Chem.* (1970) **23**, 2343.
26. Rogers, D., *et al.*, *J. Chem. Soc., Chem. Comm.* (1971) 393.
27. Rosett, T., *et al.*, *Biochem. J.* (1957) **67**, 390.
28. Williams, D. J., Thomas, R., *Tetrahedron Lett.* (1973) **9**, 639.
29. Stoessl, A., *J. Chem. Soc., Chem. Comm.* (1967) 307.
30. Stoessl, A., *Can. J. Chem.* (1969) **47**, 767.
31. Suemitsu, R., *et al.*, *Bull. Agric. Chem. Soc. Jap.* (1959) **23**, 547.
32. Kinoshita, T., *et al.*, *Ann. Phytopathol. Soc. Jap.* (1972) **38**, 397.
33. Iwasaki, S., *et al.*, *Tetrahedron Lett.* (1972) **1**, 13.

34. Kaczka, T., *et al.*, *Biochem. Biophys. Res. Comm.* (1964) **14**, 54.
35. Stickings, C. E., *Biochem. J.* (1959) **72**, 332.
36. Umetsu, Y., *et al.*, *Agric. Biol. Chem.* (1973) **37**, 451.
37. Harris, S. A., *et al.*, *J. Med. Chem.* (1965) **8**, 478.
38. Gitterman, C. O., *J. Med. Chem.* (1965) **8**, 483.
39. Meyers, W. L., *et al.*, *Tetrahedron Lett.* (1971) **25**, 2357.
40. Koncewicz, M., *et al.*, *Biochem. Biophys, Res. Comm.* (1973) **53**, 653.
41. Meyer, W. L., *et al.*, *Biochem. Biophys. Res. Comm.* (1974) **56**, 234.
42. White, G. A., Starrat, A. N., *Can. J. Bot.* (1967) **45**, 2087.
43. Starrat, A. N., *Can. J. Chem.* (1968) **46**, 767.
44. Brian, P. W., *et al.*, *J. Gen. Microbiol.* (1951) **5**, 619.
45. Grove, J. F., *J. Chem. Soc.* (1952) 4056.
46. Bartels-Keith, J. R., Grove, J. F., *Proc. Chem. Soc.* (1959) 398.
47. Starrat, A. N., White, G. A., *Phytochemistry* (1968) **7**, 1883.
48. Munro, H. D., *et al.*, *J. Chem. Soc.*, (*C*) (1967) 947.
49. Slifkin, M. K., *et al.*, *Mycopathol. Mycol. Appl.* (1973) **50**, 241.
50. Pero, R. W., *et al.*, *Environ. Health Perspectives* (June 1973) 87.
51. Ciegler, A., Lindenfelser, L. A., *Sep. Exp.* (1969) **25**, 719.
52. Hiroe, I., Aoe, S., *J. Fac. Agric.*, *Tottori Univ.* (1954) **2**, 1.
53. Shimizu, M., Ohta, G., *J. Pharm. Soc. Jap.* (1951) **71**, 879.
54. Suemitsu, R., *et al.*, *Agric. Biol. Chem.* (1961) **25**, 100.
55. Light, R. J., *J. Agric. Food Chem.* (1970) **18**, 260.
56. Sistrom, W. R., Stanier, R. Y., *J. Biol. Chem.* (1954) **210**, 821.
57. Gatenbeck, S., *Acta. Chem. Scand.* (1973) **27**, 1825.
58. Gatenbeck, S., Sierankiewicz, J., *Antimicrob. Agents Chemother.* (1973) **3**, 308.
59. Pero, R. W., *et al.*, *Anal. Biochem.* (1971) **43**, 80.
60. Pero, R. W., Harvan, D. J., *J. Chromatogr.* (1973) **80**, 255.
61. Seitz, L. M., *et al.*, *J. Agric. Food Chem.* (1975) **23**, 1.
62. Mikami, Y., *et al.*, *Agric. Biol. Chem.* (1971) **35**, 611.
63. Harvan, D., Pero, R., *J. Chromatogr.* (1974) **101**, 222.
64. Meronuck, R. A., *et al.*, *Appl. Microbiol.* (1972) **23**, 613.
65. Smith, E. R., *et al.*, *Cancer Chemother. Rep.* (1968) **52**, 579.
66. Miller, F. A., *et al.*, *Nature* (1963) **200**, 1338.
67. Shigeura, H. T., Gordon, C. N., *Biochemistry* (1962) **2**, 1132.
68. Carrasco, L., Vasquez, D., *Biochem. Biophys. Acta.* (1973) **319**, 209.
69. Lieberman, M. W., *et al.*, *Cancer Res.* (1970) **30**, 942.
70. Spalding, J. W., *et al.*, *J. Cell Biol.* (1970) **47**, 199a.
71. Templeton, G. E., *et al.*, *Proc. Mycotoxin Res. Seminar* (1967), p. 27, U.S. Dept. Agric., Wash., D.C.
72. Pound, G. S., Stahmann, M. A., *Phytopathology* (1951) **41**, 1104.
73. Pero, R. W., Main, C. E., *Phytopatholgy* (1970) **60**, 1570.
74. Lucas, G. B., *et al.*, *J. Agric. Food Chem.* (1971) **19**, 1275.

RECEIVED November 8, 1974.

16

Phytoalexins, Plants, and Human Health

J. KUĆ

Department of Plant Pathology, University of Kentucky, Lexington, Ky. 40506

W. CURRIER

Purdue University, Lafayette, Ind. 47907

Plants accumulate many different compounds as a result of infection or stress. Some (the phytoalexins) are toxic to microorganisms and rapidly accumulate in resistant plants following infection. Others accumulate in susceptible host–parasite interactions and may be precursors or degradation products of phytoalexins or unrelated to them. Phytoalexin accumulation can be caused by: living organisms, products of living organisms, chemical toxicants, ethylene, pesticides, and temperature stress. Plant breeders developing new resistant varieties may select for plants which accumulate phytoalexins. The presence of phytoalexins and related compounds in foods obtained from new varieties, stressed plants, plants treated with pesticides and infected plants is a potential hazard to human health.

People naturally are most aware of human diseases. However the world's population depends as much on the control of the diseases of plants and animals that comprise our living environment as it does on the control of human disease. Starvation is the world's number one killer, and its control requires a healthy agriculture and living environment. Early man recognized that if he survived some diseases, he subsequently became immune to them. Eventually the concept of immunization was accepted and, together with antibiotics, has been responsible for the control of many of man's most deadly diseases in some parts of the world. Starvation has not been controlled, and any hope of control depends on the control of plant diseases. Yet little support has been given to elucidate the nature of disease resistance in plants relative to the support for work with human disease.

The basic mechanism for resistance in man is twofold. First, there are physical and chemical barriers to keep infectious agents out of the body. Second, there are response mechanisms which inhibit infectious agents and eliminate those that have penetrated. These basic mechanisms also explain disease resistance in plants. This paper considers one aspect of the complex mechanisms for disease resistance in plants; the presence or production of compounds in response to infection. Since these compounds can occur in common foodstuffs or products derived from such foodstuffs and since some have demonstrated toxicity to animals, their implications to human health will also be considered.

A phenomenon similar to induced immunity in animals was reported with the potato by Muller and Borger (*1*). They found that tubers developed localized resistance to a pathogenic race of *Phytophthora infestans* if they were first inoculated with a race of the fungus to which they were resistant. This observation lead to the "Phytoalexin Theory." The basic concept of this theory is that chemical compounds, phytoalexins, are produced by plant cells as a result of metabolic interaction between host and infectious agent. Generally pathogens are either not sensitive to the phytoalexins or not able to cause their accumulation to toxic levels soon enough after penetration. Plants in the families Leguminosae and Solanaceae and their interactions with fungi have been studied most often. In general, phytoalexins from members within a family appear structurally related, though the phytoalexins produced by an individual species may not be.

Pisatin

Pisatin accumulates in the pods of the garden pea *Pisum sativum* L. inoculated with fungi. It is a weak antibiotic with a broad biological spectrum. Fungi pathogenic to pea are generally insensitive to the amounts of pisatin accumulating after infection, whereas nonpathogens of pea are generally sensitive. Pisatin accumulation is stimulated by many fungi, metabolic inhibitors, spore-free germination fluids, ethylene, ultraviolet radiation, DNA intercalating compounds, and many microbial metabolites including well known antibiotics. Pisatin is degraded by several pathogens of pea, and the ability to detoxicate pisatin may determine pathogenicity. Since pisatin is not a stable end product in plant tissues, degradation by the plant itself is also a consideration.

Phaseollin

Phaseollin is the major phytoalexin in diffusates from seed cavities of green bean pods *Phaseolus vulgaris* inoculated with a nonpathogen of bean *M. fructicola*. Recently several compounds structurally related to phaseollin have also been isolated from diffusates or tissues inoculated with fungi, bacteria, and viruses: phaseollidin (*2*); phaseollidin, phaseol-

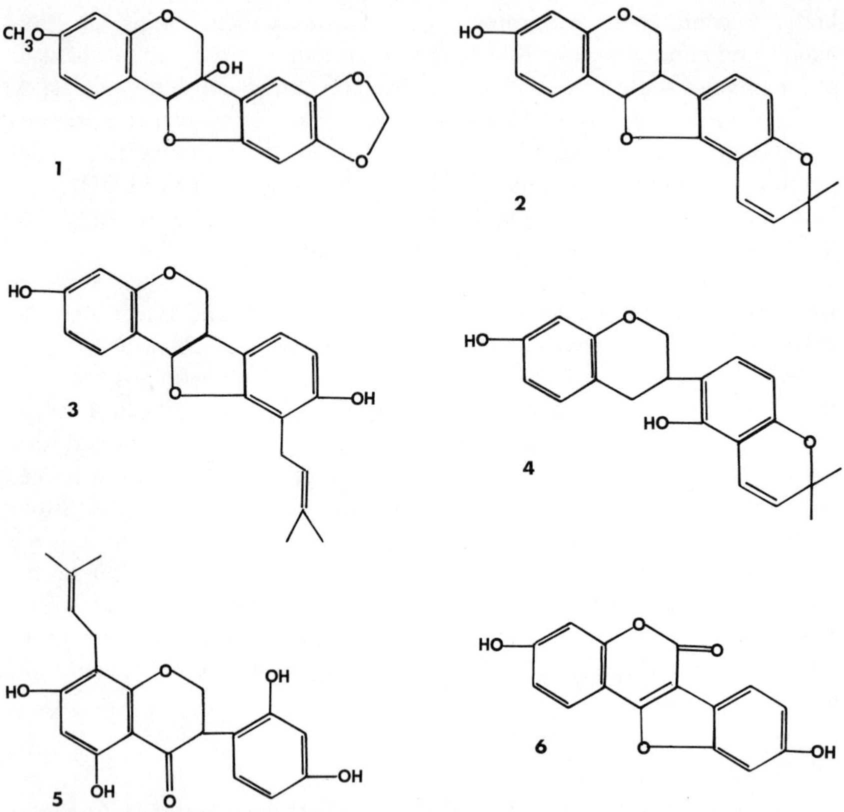

Figure 1. Phytoalexins in pea and green bean. Pea: (1) pisatin. Green bean: (2) phaseollin, (3) phaseollidin, (4) phaseollinisoflavan, (5) kievitone, (6) coumesterol.

linisoflavan, and kievitone (3); kievitone (4); coumesterol (5). In addition several degradation products of phaseollin have been reported in infected tissue, culture filtrates of fungi, and diffusates from infected tissue (6, 7, 8). Accumulation of phaseollin and phaseollin-like compounds appears associated with a mechanism for varietal resistance to *Colletotrichum lindemuthianum* as well as resistance to nonpathogens. The time of accumulation and its magnitude, rather than the ability to accumulate the phytoalexin, distinguish susceptibility from resistance (9), and the phaseollin concentration in infected resistant hypocotyls appears sufficient to inhibit growth of the fungus (10). Bean hypocotyls inoculated with an incompatible (nonpathogenic) race or heat-attenuated compatible (pathogenic) race of *C. lindemuthianum* are protected from disease when subsequently inoculated with a compatible race (11, 12, 13, 14), and protection is expressed at a distance from the sight of inoculation with an incompatible race. Protection is induced in varieties of bean

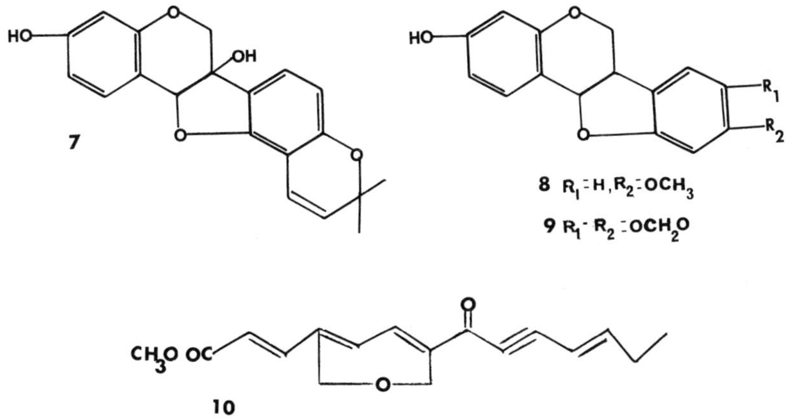

Figure 2. Phytoalexins in soybean, alfalfa, red clover, and broad bean. Soybean, (7) Glyceollin; Alfalfa, (8) Medicarpan; Red Clover, (8) Medicarpan (9) maackiain; Broad Bean, (10) Wyerone.

susceptible to all races of *C. lindemuthianum* by *Colletotrichum* sp. nonpathogenic on green bean (*15*). Skipp and Deverall (*16*) demonstrated that culture filtrates of compatible and incompatible races caused protected tissue to produce an inhibitor of spore germination, and Berard, Kuć and Williams (*17, 18*) reported the presence of a nonfungitoxic substance in cell-free diffusates from incompatible, but not compatible, interactions which caused protection. Phaseollin accumulation is also caused by low concentrations of heavy metal ions, metabolic inhibitors, and antibiotic inhibitors of nucleic acid and protein synthesis.

Glyceollin

Several fungitoxic compounds accumulate in open soybean pods and hypocotyls inoculated with nonpathogens of soybeans. One of these (*19, 20*) originally identified as 6 α-hydroxyphaseollin and subsequently characterized as glyceollin (*21*), was isolated from soybean hypocotyls inoculated with *Phytophthora sojae.* The compound is closely related to pisatin and phaseollin, and it accumulates 10–100 times faster in hypocotyls challenged with an incompatible as compared with a compatible race of the fungus. In incompatible and compatible reactions the concentration of glyceollin is 100–400 and 1–4 times the ED_{50} concentration for inhibiting mycelial growth of the fungus. As with other phytoalexins, resistance and susceptiblity apparently depend on the speed and magnitude of accumulation. Protection is induced against pathogens by varietal non-

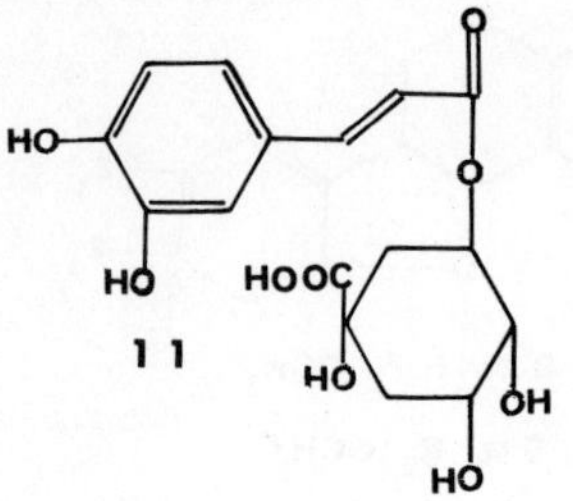

11

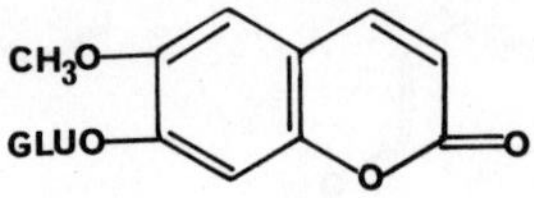

12

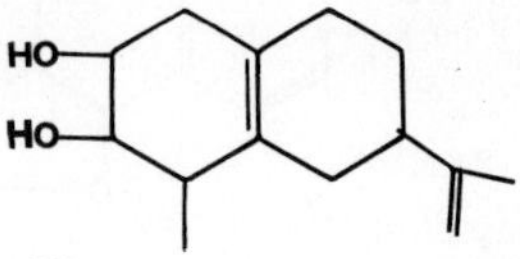

13

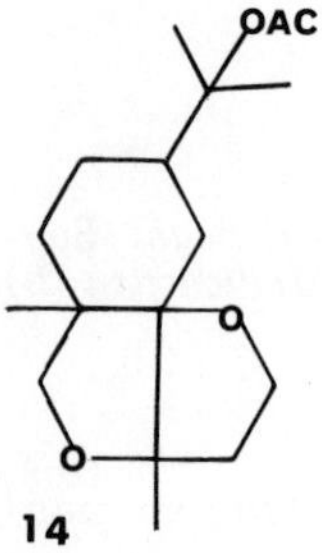

14

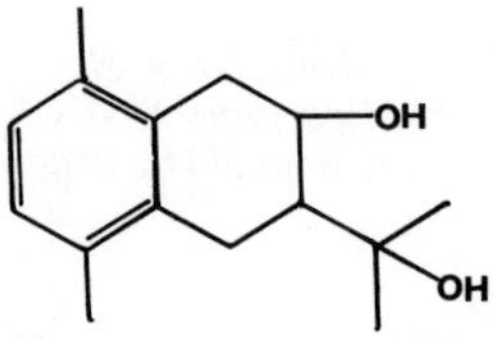

15

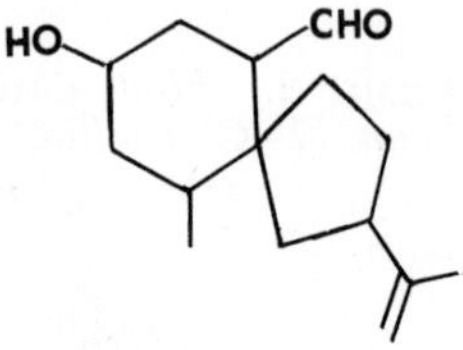

16

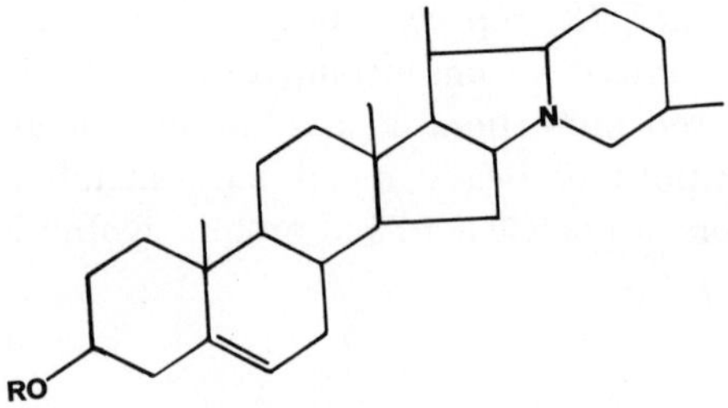

17 R:GLU,RHA,RHA
18 R:GAL,GLU,RHA

*Figure 3. Phytoalexins in potato: (**11**) chlorogenic acid, (**12**) scopolin, (**13**) rishitin, (**14**) phytuberin, (**15**) rishitinol, (**16**) lubimin, (**17**) α-chaconine, (**18**) α-solanine.*

pathogenic races of pathogens or nonpathogens. Several fungicides, uv radiation, and tobacco necrosis virus also induce accumulation of glyceollin (*22, 23, 24*). Glyceollin, daidzein, coumesterol, and sojagol may accumulate in infected hypocotyls because of a general activation of isoflavonoid biosynthesis with metabolites directed to the biosynthesis of pterocarpans.

Coumesterol, Medicarpin, Maackiain, and Wyerone

Coumesterol and many other flavonoid aglycones and glycosides accumulate in infected alfalfa, and the concentration of coumesterol is directly related to the degree of infection (*25*). Medicarpin has been isolated from alfalfa leaves inoculated with spores of the corn pathogen *Helminthosporium turcicum* (*26*), and the pathogen *Stemphylium botryosum*, but not *H. turcicum*, degrades medicarpin to noninhibitory compounds. *Colletotrichum phomoides*, a nonpathogen, and *S. loti*, a weak pathogen of alfalfa, also degrade medicarpin, but the degradation products are inhibitory to these fungi. Two phytoalexins, medicarpin and maackiain, were isolated from red clover foliage infected with *H. turcicum* (*27*); wyerone and wyerone acid were found in broad bean (*28*).

Phenolic Acids, Rishitin, and Steroid Glycoalkaloids

Chlorogenic and caffeic acids, scopolin, α-chaconine, and α-solanine are fungitoxic compounds found in potato peel. They accumulate in mechanically injured or infected tubers. Rishitin, rishitinol, phytuberin, and lubimin accumulate in infected tubers, and after treatment with some chemicals; they do not accumulate after mechanical injury. Quinones of chlorogenic and caffeic acid have been suggested to be phytoalexins, and they also form polymers which may limit microbial development. Reactive quinones are toxic to plant cells as well as infectious agents, and their production may explain the necrosis often associated with hypersensitive resistance. Polymerization may represent a detoxication mechanism to prevent extensive injury to the plant. Recently Clarke (*29*) reported that scopolin accumulates in potato tissue in response to infection by viruses, fungi, and an actinomycete. The greatest accumulation occurs in tissue infected by virulent isolates of pathogens, including *P. infestans*. Little or none accumulates in response to wounding, avirulent isolates, or nonpathogens.

Another group of phytoalexins accumulating in potato after infection are isoprenoid derivatives including the bicyclic norsesquiterpene alcohol rishitin (*30*). Rishitin is first detected when the growth of *P. infestans* is inhibited in resistant cultivars; it accumulates rapidly to levels many times that necessary to completely prevent it. Little accumulates after infection in susceptible cultivars. Browning and restricted cell death induced by many chemicals and physiological stimuli do not cause rishitin accumulation, but it and other isoprenoid derivatives accumulate in response to inoculation with nonpathogens of potato. Cell-free sonicates of *P. infestans* cause rishitin to accumulate in susceptible and resistant cultivars of potato. A consistent response of tubers to infection in resistant cultivars includes rapid necrosis and the accumulation of rishitin (*31*), phytuberin, a recently characterized aliphatic, unsaturated, sesquiterpene acetate ($C_{17}H_{26}O_4$) (32), rishitinol (33), lubimin (34), and several spirovetiva derivatives (35). The potential for resistance apparently exists in completely susceptible cultivars, but this potential is not expressed. A race (compatible) of P. infestans on a susceptible cultivar suppresses both necrosis and the accumulation of rishitin and phytuberin in tubers subsequently inoculated with a race unable to attack (incompatible). The supression of the response to the incompatible race, or inoculation with the compatible race alone, is accompanied by the accumulation of nonfungitoxic terpenoids which are not detected in incompatible reactions (36). A compatible interaction also suppresses the hypersensitive host-response to cell-free sonicates of the fungus.

At least two steroid glycoalkaloids, α-solanine and α-chaconine, may also be associated with resistance as part of a general wound response. They occur in tubers and foliage and appear localized around sites of injury in tubers. The steroid glycoalkaloids are largely restricted to the peel of whole tubers, and they are the major antifungal compounds in potato peel. The accumulation of α-solanine and α-chaconine at the surface of cut tissue slices is markedly suppressed by inoculation with P. infestans. The suppression is most marked after inoculation with incompatible races of the fungus (37, 38).

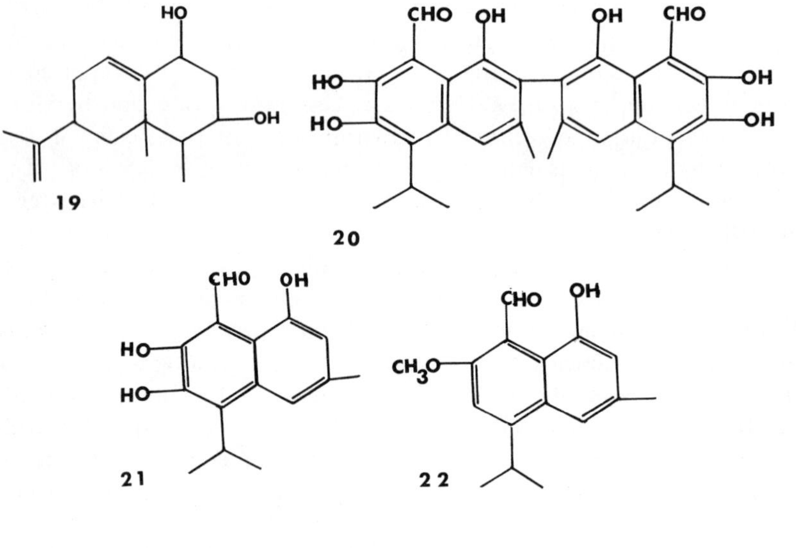

Figure 4.   Phytoalexins in pepper and cotton. Pepper: (19) capsidiol. Cotton: (20) gossypol, (21) hemigossypol, (22) vergosin.

Capsidiol

The sesquiterpene phytoalexin capsidiol was isolated from the fruit of sweet pepper *Capsicum frutescens* L. inoculated with several fungi (*39, 40, 41*). Capsidiol accumulates rapidly in some interactions, but in others it is rapidly oxidized to capsenone.

Gossypol

Gossypol is one of many ether-soluble phenols accumulating in boll cavities or xylem vessels of excised stems of *Gossypium hirsutum* or *Gossypium barbadense* 24–72 hr after inoculation with conidia of the pathogen *Verticillium albo-atrum*. The rate of accumulation of gossypol and gossypol-like compounds in stem sections and intact plants is directly related to host resistance and inversely related to virulence of the pathogen.

Heat-killed conidia or conidia attenuated by heat in stem sections cause gossypol accumulation and increase resistance. Avirulent strains of the fungus also protect against damage from subsequent inoculation with virulent strains. Like the many phytoalexins discussed in preceding sections, gossypol synthesis is activated by low concentrations of many toxic chemicals and by wounding and chilling. Vergosin and hemigossypol may be the major antifungal phenols accumulating in cotton in response to infection (*42*). The chemical structure of vergosin is still in doubt. Zaki, Keen, and Erwin (*43*) reported that a protein–lipopolysaccharide complex isolated from culture filtrates of *V. albo-atrum* elicites accumulation of gossypol derivatives in cotton. Though susceptibility to disease appears directly related to sensitivity to the complex, Keen, Long, and Erwin (*44*) found the complex elicited *ca.* four times the accumulation of gossypol derivatives in a susceptible as compared to a resistant variety.

Ipomeamarone, Phenolic Acids, and Coumarins

Infection, injury, or treatment with chemicals all lead to the accumulation of chlorogenic acid, isochlorogenic acid, caffeic acid, scopoletin, esculetin, umbelliferone, and ipomeamarone in sweet potato root. The peel of sweet potato also contains all of the above.

Ipomeamarone, ipomeanine, ipomeanic acid, and numerous other furanoterpenes accumulate more rapidly in several varieties resistant to black rot (caused by *Ceratocystis fimbriata*) as compared to susceptible varieties. Ipomeamarone markedly inhibits growth of the fungus *in vitro* at concentrations found in infected tissue.

The development of prune and coffee isolates of *C. fimbriata* is severely restricted in sweet potato roots; however the accumulation of

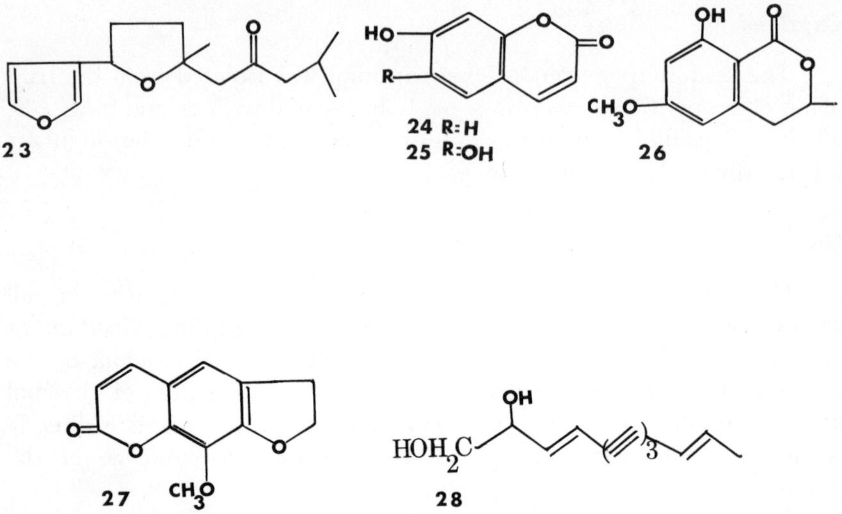

Figure 5. *Phytoalexins in sweet potato, carrot, parsnip, and safflower. Sweet potato: (23) ipomeamarone, (24) umbelliferone, (25) esculetin. Carrot: (26) 6-methoxymellein. Parsnip: (27) xanthotoxin. Safflower: (28) safynol.*

furanoterpenes is less than in tissue infected by a pathogenic isolate. Thus it appears that furanoterpene accumulation may not be the sole or primary determinant of disease resistance.

6-Methoxymellein and Xanthotoxin

Chlorogenic acid and 6-methoxymellein reach fungitoxic levels around infection sites within 24 hr after inoculation with several fungi nonpathogenic to carrot. The accumulation of 6-methoxymellein has been reported with seven isolates of *C. fimbriata* as well as with five varieties of carrot. Accumulation of 6-methoxymellein can also be induced by chemicals, cold treatment, and ethylene (45, 46). The compound is responsible for the condition of bitter carrot, a physiological disorder of carrots resulting from storage at suboptimal temperatures. Recently xanthotoxin has been demonstrated to accumulate in parsnip root inoculated with fungi, and it may act as a phytoalexin (47).

Polyacetylenes

The polyacetylene safynol has been identified in healthy and wounded hypocotyls of safflower and rapidly accumulates to fungitoxic levels in resistant tissue after infection. It appears, as with other phytoalexins studied, that a series of polyacetylenic compounds may accumulate (48).

Summary

This paper is not intended to present an exhaustive literature review. Several reviews are available (*49–60*), and these consider in depth the earlier work with pisatin, phaseollin, ipomeamarone, 6-methoxymellein, and gossypols. Only the more recent publications are cited in this paper. Several general observations appear valid. The phytoalexins are not produced as a specific response to infection. They may occur in trace quantities in apparently healthy plants, and they accumulate in tissues treated with some microbial metabolites, antibiotics, low concentrations of metabolic inhibitors, ultraviolet radiation, pesticides, or after mechanical injury or temperature stress. They may be part of a general tissue repair mechanism which may have a role in resistance. Inoculation with some bacteria, viruses, and fungi causes phytoalexins to accumulate, though evidence implicating phytoalexins in resistance to bacterial or virus diseases is meager. In most host–parasite interactions several phytoalexins accumulate. Some are structurally related, and some are not. Phytoalexin accumulation after infection is not restricted to a resistant or immune plant, and a specific phytoalexin is not produced for each infectious agent. Specificity of phytoalexin accumulation appears to reside in both the time and magnitude of accumulation.

The most powerful weapon in our battle against plant disease is the development of new disease resistant varieties. Though the application of chemicals to control disease is extremely important with some crops, it would be impossible to feed the world's population if disease control depended solely on the use of existing chemicals. The large increase in production costs, scarcity of supply, and the problem that residues would cause to all animal and plant life make dependence on chemical control impractical.

Disease resistant plants however do not provide a solution without its share of problems. New strains of pathogens develop which can attack resistant plants, and there are many diseases of a single crop. Against which disease does the breeder develop resistant plants? Can new strains of old pathogens be predicted? In addition, high yield and quality must also be incorporated into crops together with disease resistance. Finally a food crop must be nutritious and safe for animal or human consumption. It may be comforting, but unwise, to think that a resistant cultivar is identical to a susceptible cultivar except for a single factor which controls resistance, and this factor does not affect the safety of the crop for animal consumption. Although today's foods have stood the test of time, is last year's potato the same as a newly developed resistant variety? What factors have been incorporated along with the genetic information for resistance when crosses are made with inedible species? We have detected two steroid glycoalkaloids, α- and β-solamarine, in injured potato tubers of the variety Kennebec which is resistant to certain races of *P. infestans* (*61*). These compounds are not detected in either of the two parents from which this variety was developed.

Phaseollin, glyceollin, phytoalexins of green bean, soybean, and medicarpan (a phytoalexin of alfalfa and red clover) cause lysis of bovine erythrocytes at $\leq$ 0.35 m*M*. Phaseollin also lysis human erythrocytes (*62, 63*). Glyceollin and phaseollin can be isolated from infected pods. The steroid glycoalkaloids of potato have a long history of toxicity to animals (*64, 65, 66, 67*). Usually 20 mg/100 g of potato is considered toxic (*65*), though as little as 3 mg/kg body weight has been reported toxic to man (*67*). Under certain conditions of stress the levels in tubers can exceed this concentration (*37, 38*). Recently a variety of potato, Lenape, was released and subsequently withdrawn because of its extremely high levels of steroid glycoalkaloids even when growing under normal conditions (*68*). Ipomeamarone derivatives, 4-ipomeanol, 1-ipomeanol, ipomeanine, and 1,4-ipomeadiol, which are all part of the phytoalexin complex of furanoterpenoids in sweet potato, produce pulmonary toxicity in animals (*69*). These toxicants can accumulate to high levels in minimally blemished potatoes infected with any of a broad spectrum of fungi, and they are not destroyed by cooking (*69*). Two phytotoxic psoralens, 4, 5', 8'-trimethyl psoralen and 8-methoxypsoralen (xanthotoxin), were isolated and characterized from celery heads and stalks infected with pink rot caused by *Sclerotinia sclerotiorum* (*70, 71*). The later psoralen has also been reported as a phytoalexin in parsnip root (*47*). The two psoralens in infected celery appear responsible for the blistering cutaneous disorder common with celery workers. The compounds are not detected in healthy celery. Coumesterol and other isoflavonoid derivatives are phytoalexins in several legumes, and many have oestrogenic, insecticidal, piscicidal, and antifungal activity (*72, 73, 74, 75*). Gossypol and gossypol derivatives, phytoalexins of cotton, also have a long medical history of toxic effects (*76*).

The development of new varieties does introduce new chemical factors, some of which may be phytoalexins. It seems imperative that these new varieties should be screened before being released for animal consumption. Efforts to regulate genetic manipulation of food crops have been initiated by the Food and Drug Administration (*77*). These efforts should be expanded to include studies of toxic phytoalexins produced under conditions of infection and stress. The fact that compounds occur naturally does not speak for their safety.

Literature Cited

1. Muller, K., Borger, H., *Arb. Biol. Reichsanst. Land Forstwirtsch, Berlin-Dahlem* (1940) **23**, 189.

2. Perrin, D., Whittle, C., *Tetrahedron Lett.* (1972) **17**, 1673.
3. Burden, R., Bailey, J., Dawson, G., *Tetrahedron Lett.* (1972) **41**, 4175.
4. Smith, D., Van Etten, H., Serum, J., Jones, T., Bateman, D., Williams, T., Coffen, D., *Physiol. Plant Pathol.* (1973) **3**, 293.
5. Rathmell, W., Bendall, D., *Physiol. Plant Pathol.* (1971) **1**, 351.
6. Cruickshank, I., Biggs, D., Perrin, D., Whittle, C., *Physiol. Plant Pathol.* (1974) **4**, 261.
7. Heath, M., Higgins, V., *Physiol. Plant Pathol.* (1973) **3**, 107.
8. van den Heuvel, J., Van Etten, H., *Physiol. Plant Pathol.* (1973) **3**, 107.
9. Rahe, J., Kuć, J., Chuang, C., Williams, E., *Neth. J. Plant Pathol.* (1969) **75**, 58.
10. Skipp, R., Deverall, B., *Physiol. Plant Pathol.* (1972) **2**, 357.
11. Rahe, J., Kuć, J., Chuang, C., Williams, E., *Phytopathology* (1969) **59**, 1641.
12. Rahe, J., *Phytopathology* (1973) **63**, 572.
13. Rahe, J., Kuć, J., *Phytopathology* (1970) **60**, 1006.
14. Elliston, J., Kuć, J., Williams, E., *Phytopathology* (1971) **61**, 1110.
15. Elliston, J., Williams, E., *Phytopathology* (1972) **62**, 756.
16. Skipp, R., Deverall, B., *Physiol. Plant Pathol.* (1973) **3**, 299.
17. Berard, D., Kuć, J., Williams, E., *Physiol. Plant Pathol.* (1972) **2**, 123.
18. Berard, D., Kuć, J., Williams, E., *Physiol. Plant Pathol.* (1973) **3**, 51.
19. Sims, J., Keen, N., Honward, V., *Phytochemistry* (1972) **11**, 827.
20. Keen, N., *Physiol. Plant Pathol.* (1971) **1**, 265.
21. Burdin, R., Bailey, J., *Phytochemistry* (1975) **14**, 1389.
22. Bridge, M., Klarman, W., *Phytopathology* (1973) **63**, 606.
23. Klarman, W., Hammerschlag, F., *Phytopathology* (1972) **62**, 719.
24. Reilly, J., Klarman, W., *Phytopathology* (1972) **62**, 1113.
25. Sherwood, R., Olah, A., Oleson, W., Jones, E., *Phytopathology* (1970) **60**, 684.
26. Smith, D., McInnes, A., Higgins, V., Millar, R., *Physiol. Plant Pathol.* (1971) **1**, 41.
27. Higgins, V., Smith, D., *Phytopathology* (1972) **62**, 235.
28. Letcher, R., Widdowson, B., Deverall, B., Mansfield, J., *Phytochemistry* (1970) **9**, 249.
29. Clarke, D., *Physiol. Plant Pathol.* (1973) **3**, 347.
30. Katsui, N., Murai, A., Takasugi, M., Imaizumi, K., Masamune, T., Tomiyama, K., *Chem. Comm.* (1968) 43.
31. Varns, J., Kuć, J., Williams, E., *Phytopathology* (1971) **61**, 174.
32. Hughes, D., Coxon, D., *Chem. Comm.* (1974) 822.
33. Katsui, N., Matsunaga, A., Imaizumi, K., Masamune, T., Tomiyama, K., *Tetrahedron Lett.* (1971) **2**, 83.
34. Stoessl, A., Stothers, J., Ward, E., *Chem. Comm.* (1974) 709.
35. Coxon, D., Price, K., Howard, E., Osman, S., Kolan, E., Zaccharius, M., *Tettrahedron Lett.* (1974) **34**, 2921.
36. Subramanian, S., Varns, J., Kuć, J., *Proc. Indiana Acad. Sci.* (1970) **80**, 367.
37. Shih, M., Kuć, J., Williams, E., *Phytopathology* (1973) **63**, 821.
38. Shih, M., Kuć, J., *Phytopathology* (1973) **63**, 826.
39. Stoessl, A., Unwin, C., Ward, E., *Phytopathol. Z.* (1972) **74**, 141.
40. Gordon, M., Stoessl, A., Stothers, J., *Can. J. Chem.* (1973) **51**, 748.
41. Stoessl, A., Unwin, C., Ward, E., *Phytopathology* (1973) **63**, 1225.
42. Zaki, A., Keen, N., Erwin, D., *Phytopathology* (1972) **62**, 1402.
43. Zaki, A., Keen, N., Erwin, D., Sims, J., *Phytopathology* (1972) **62**, 1398.
44. Keen, N., Long, M., Erwin, D., *Physiol. Plant Pathol.* (1972) **2**, 317.
45. Jaworski, J., Kuć, J., Williams, E., *Phytopathology* (1973) **63**, 408.
46. Jaworski, J., Kuć, J. *Plant Physiol.* (1974) **53**, 331.
47. Johnson, C., Brannon, D., Kuć J., *Phytochemistry* (1973) **12**, 2961.

48. Allen, E., Thomas, C., *Phytopathology* (1971) **61**, 1107.
49. Kuć, J., *Ann. Rev. Microbiol.* (1966) **20**, 337.
50. Kuć, J., in "The Dynamic Role of Molecular Constituents in Plant–Parasite Interaction," C. Mirocha, I. Uritani, Eds., p. 183, Bruce, St. Paul, Minn., 1967.
51. Kuć, J., *World Rev. Pest Control* (1968) **7**, 42.
52. Kuć, J., *Ann. Rev. Phytopathol.* (1972) **10**, 207.
53. Kuć, Jr., in "Microbial Toxins," Vol. VIII, S. Ajl, G. Weinbaum, S. Kadis, Eds., p. 211, Academic Press, New York, 1972.
54. Kuć, J. *Teratology* (1973) **8**, 333.
55. Cruickshank, I., *Ann. Rev. Phytopathol.* (1963) **1**, 351.
56. Cruickshank, I., Perrin, D., in "Biochemistry of Phenolic Compounds," J. Harborne, Ed., p. 511, Academic Press, New York, 1965.
57. Cruickshank, I., Biggs, D., Perrin, D. J., *Indian Bot. Soc.* (1971) **50A**, 1.
58. Ingham, J., *Bot. Rev.* (1972) **38**, 343.
59. Kosuge, T., *Ann. Rev. Phytopathol* (1969) **7**, 195.
60. Stoessl, A., *Rec. Advan. Phytochem.* (1970) **3**, 143.
61. Shih, M., Kuć, J., *Phytochemistry* (1974) **13**, 997.
62. Van Etten, H., *Phytopathology* (1972) **6,2** 795.
63. Van Etten, H., Bateman, D., *Phytopathology* (1971) **61**, 1363.
64. Oslage, H., *Kartoffelbau* (1956) **7**, 204.
65. Sapeika, N., "Food Pharmacology," N. Kugelmass, Ed., pp. 67, 72, Thomas, Springfield, 1969.
66. Nishie, K., Gumbmann, M., Keyl, A., *Toxic. Appl. Pharmacol.* (1971) **19**, 81.
67. Swinyard, C., Chaube, S., *Teratology* (1973) **8**, 349.
68. Zitnak, A., Johnston, G., *Amer. Potato J.* (1970) **47**, 256.
69. Boyd, M., Burka, L., Harris, T., Wilson, B., *Biochim. Biophys. Acta* (1973) **337**, 184.
70. Scheel, L., Perone, V., Larkin, R., Kupel, R., *Biochemistry* (1963) **2**, 1127.
71. Perone, V., Scheel, L., Meitus, R., *J. Invest. Dermatol.* (1964) **42**, 267.
72. Bickoff, E., Loper, G., Hanson, C., Graham, J., Witt, S., Spencer, R., *Crop Sci.* (1967) **7**, 259.
73. Geissman, T. in "The Chemistry of Flavonoid Compounds," T. Geissman Ed., p. 1, Macmillan, New York, 1962.
74. Beck, A., *Aust. J. Agric. Res.* (1964) **15**, 223.
75. Loper, G., Hanson, C., Graham, J., *Crop Sci.* (1967) **7**, 189.
76. Adams, R., Geissman, T., Edwards, J., *Chem. Rev.* (1960) **60**, 555.
77. Miller, J., *Science* (1974) **185**, 240.

RECEIVED November 8, 1974. Work supported in part by a grant from the Herman Frasch Foundation and Cooperative State Research Service, USDA, Research Agreement 316–15–51.

Stress Metabolites of White Potatoes

GARNETT E. WOOD

Division of Chemistry and Physics, Bureau of Foods, Food and Drug
Administration, U.S. Department of Health, Education, and Welfare,
Washington, D.C. 20204

*Many compounds are produced in white potatoes as a result
of physiological stress imposed on the tissues. Stress conditions in a potato may result from exposure to light, injury,
certain microorganisms, and extreme temperatures. The imposed stress may alter normal metabolic pathways in the
potato resulting in the synthesis of abnormal amounts of a
particular compound or may cause different metabolic pathways to be utilized thus giving rise to new or unusual compounds. The stress phenomenon results in the production of
certain compounds including chlorogenic acid, scopolin, solanine, and chaconine in levels greater than that found in
the normal tissue and in the production of other compounds
like rishitin, phytuberin, lubimin, alpha-solamarine, and
beta-solamarine which are not found in nonstressed tissue.
The chemistry of these metabolites is reviewed, and the
potential toxicological significance of the presence of these
compounds in potatoes is discussed.*

White potatoes (*Solanum tuberosum*) are widely used in many parts
of the world as a staple food for man. Potatoes are susceptible to
attack by various microorganisms and insects while in the field and during
storage; they may also be subjected to mechanical damage during the
harvesting operation. The imposition of any of these conditions on healthy
potatoes will upset some normal physiological sequences thereby causing
"stress" on the metabolic system. Stress can also be induced by certain
chemical toxicants as well as by variations in temperature and environmental factors. Stressed potatoes may be found to contain increased
amounts of certain compounds that are normal constituents of the tissue
or certain compounds that are not normally found in the tissue. In the
latter case the pathways for the synthesis of these compounds must exist

in the tissue, yet they may not be activated or utilized unless the usual metabolic pathways become altered or damaged as a result of stress conditions. In plants stress metabolites are synthesized by modifying either the shikimic acid, acetate–malonate, or acetate–mevalonate pathways.

Unusual compounds produced by plants in response to various exogenous stimuli are generally referred to as phytoalexins. This term was introduced by Müller and Börger (1) to define a chemical compound produced only when the living cells of the host are invaded by a parasite and undergo necrobiosis. That definition was later modified by Müller (2) as a result of further studies and was restated as "antibiotics which are produced as a result of the interaction of two metabolic systems, host and parasite, and which inhibit the growth of microorganisms pathogenic to plants." A detailed description of the properties of phytoalexins and their role in host–parasite interactions was presented in reviews by Cruickshank (3) and Cruickshank and Perrin (4). A more recent review on phytoalexins was written by Kuć (5) based on the concept that "the term phytoalexins should serve as an umbrella under which chemical compounds contributing to disease resistance can be classified whether they are formed in response to injury, physiological stimuli, and the presence of infectious agents or are the products of such agents." A similar definition was used by Kira'ly (6) who defined phytoalexins as substances produced by plants after infection and adverse treatments and responsible for resistance to infecting agents.

Prior to 1972 interest in compounds produced in plants as a result of stress conditions was centered around the development of an understanding of the biochemical basis of disease resistance in plants. Excellent reviews on phytoalexins and compounds accumulating in plants after infection have been presented by Kuć (5, 7). Currently, particular emphasis is on stress metabolites that accumulate in the tubers of white potatoes because of a report by Renwick (8) which implied that certain potatoes contained a specific but unidentified compound that caused birth defects in humans. The compound (compounds) was believed to be produced as a result of exposure of the potato to stress conditions, particularly exposure to the mold *Phytophthora infestans*, the causative agent of late blight. This hypothesis was supported by epidemiological data that showed correlations between incidence of birth defects, potato blight, and potato consumption by geographic region, year, and income group. Experimental evidence supporting the presence of a teratogenic agent in blighted potatoes was later presented by Poswillo et al. (9). This evidence was based on observations made when cotton-eared marmosets were fed a diet which included sprouted, unpeeled, irradiated, boiled, freeze-dried blighted potatoes. Four of eleven fetuses from six females that had consumed the diet for a period of time showed abnormal cranial defects; no defects were observed in fetuses from females in a control group that did not consume potatoes in their diet. In further experiments in which pregnant marmosets were given a mixture of potatoes that were blighted and otherwise damaged no gross abnormalities were observed, but behaviorial defects were noted (*10*). Since then, other investigators have cited data, epidemiological and experimental, which show inconsistencies in the relationship between the consumption of blighted potatoes and birth defects (*11, 12, 13, 14, 15*).

The purpose of this paper is to reveal those compounds that are considered stress metabolites in white potatoes and to review their chemistry and information that is known about their toxicity. A report concerning metabolites accumulating in potato tubers following infection and stress recently appeared in the literature (*16*).

Normal Constituents Whose Concentrations Increase Because of Stress

The structure and chemical composition of the potato tuber was reviewed by Schwimmer and Burr (*17*). The chemical composition of the potato differs with the variety, age, condition of growth, and even individual differences, but these variables fall within well-defined limits (*18*).

Glycoalkaloids. Although the potato contains many types of compounds, some of which have intrinsic toxic properties, only solanine or the glycoalkaloids are hazardous to man (*19*). The alkaloids that are normally found in the white potato are derivatives of the steroid base solanidine (Figure 1). This base (aglycone) contains an alcohol hydroxyl group, a reducible double bond and a tertiary nitrogen that does not bear a methyl group and has four C-methyl groups and the composition $C_{27}H_{43}ON$ (*20*). The alkaloids in potatoes are referred to as glycoalkaloids because they

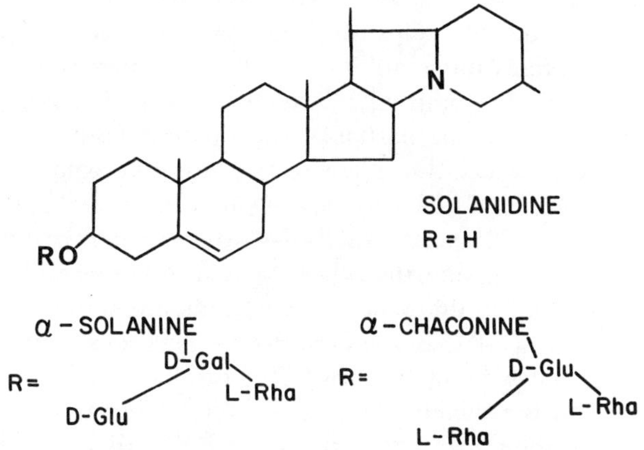

SOLANIDINE
R = H

RO

α – SOLANINE

R =

D⁻Gal
L⁻Rha
D-Glu

α – CHACONINE

R =

D⁻Glu
L⁻Rha
L⁻Rha

Figure 1.   Major glycoalkaloids in white potatoes

exist as glycosides or acetals resulting from a combination of a steroid base with various sugars. The two major glycoalkaloids in potatoes are α-solanine and α-chaconine; both contain the solanidine base but differ in their carbohydrate components. Solanine contains one mole of glucose, one mole of galactose, and one mole of rhamnose; chaconine contains one mole of glucose and two moles of rhamnose. α-Solanine and α-chaconine account for 95% of the total glycoalkaloids in potatoes (21). Other glycoalkaloids found in smaller amounts include β- and γ-solanine and β- and γ-chaconine (22); these are products resulting from the partial hydrolysis of α-solanine and α-chaconine. The presence of glycosidases in potato sprouts that hydrolyze α-solanine and α-chaconine was demonstrated by Guseva and Paseshnichenko (21). Most studies have been conducted on α-solanine and α-chaconine because they are usually the major components of the potato alkaloids. In many reports the term solanine is used to refer to a mixture of the two compounds since they are not easily separable. These compounds have been reported to exist in a ratio of one solanine to two chaconine in several varieties of potatoes (23, 24). Some reports in the literature contain data on total glycoalkaloids without differentiating between solanine and chaconine.

The amount of total glycoalkaloids in normal healthy potatoes can be affected by such factors as location, conditions of growth, variety, and storage conditions. In a detailed study by Wolf and Duggar (25) involving 32 varieties of potatoes grown in Wisconsin the total glycoalkaloid content in healthy potatoes ranged from 1.8–13 mg% with 75% of the varieties between 3.2 and 9.4 mg%. In a more recent study by Sinden and Webb (26) five commercial varieties of potatoes grown at 39 locations throughout the United States were analyzed for total glycoalkaloids content. The average glycoalkaloid content of the five varieties tested in 1970 was 7.2 mg/100 g. In 1971 the average content for three commercial varieties was 9.0 mg/100 g for all locations. Excessive (20 mg/100 g) glycoalkaloid contents for samples of the five varieties from certain locations were attributed to unusual environmental conditions or postharvest handling procedures at the particular location. The solanine content of potatoes has been observed to increase as a result of exposure to light of various intensities (27, 28, 29) and various temperatures (30). In studies by Salunkhe et al. (30) potato slices were divided into two groups: one was stored in the dark, and the other exposed to fluorescent light. Each group was subjected to different storage temperatures ranging from 0°– 24°C. After 48 hr at 24°C in the dark the solanine level had increased to seven times as much as in the original control samples; after 48 hr as 24°C in the light the solanine level was three to four times greater than that observed in the dark. The authors concluded that this phenomenon may be a form of physiological defense mechanism in tubers or slices when exposed to a stress such as high light intensity that might occur in grocery stores or wounding as in the case of slices or strips prepared for chips or french fries. In an earlier study by Kuć (*31*) it was observed that the levels of solanine and chaconine increase significantly in potato slices that were stored in the dark at room temperature for three days.

Solanidine, the aglycone of solanine and chaconine, has been noted to accumulate in certain varieties of potatoes. Zitnak (*32*) found that under conditions of intense solar radiation alternated with exposure to near freezing temperatures, which frequently occur during the potato harvest in northern areas, solanidine is rapidly produced in excess of amounts that could be bound as solanine.

The level of solanine and chaconine in potatoes is known to increase as a result of wounding (*33*). Locci and Kuć (*34*) noted an increase in these alkaloids in aged noninoculated sliced tissue. They concluded that the alkaloids accumulated in response to physiological stress which was induced by mechanical injury. It has been demonstrated that alkaloids are largely restricted to the peel of whole potatoes, but injury caused by slicing results in increased synthesis and accumulation in peeled potatoes (*24*). Other investigators have also observed an accumulation of glyco-alkaloids at the surface of cut tissue (*35, 36, 37*). Shih et al. (*37*) noted however that the accumulation is suppressed significantly if the cut tissue is inoculated with *Phytophthora infestans*. This suggests that the bio-synthetic pathway for glycoalkaloid production can be further altered as a result of additional stress imposed by infection with microorganisms.

Many cases of human poisoning have been attributed to the consumption of potatoes (*38*). In some of the reported cases, analyses of the suspected potatoes for total glycoalkaloids were made, and it was found that all of the potatoes involved had an abnormally high solanine content. A glycoalkaloid content of 20 mg/100 g of potato tissue is considered toxic for humans (*39*). In experiments with humans it was found that an oral dose of 200 mg of solanine can cause drowsiness and labored breathing; higher doses caused vomiting and diarrhea (*40*). An extensive pharma-cological study of solanine was carried out by Nishie et al. (*41*). Solanine was found to be toxic to chick embryos, mice, rats, and rabbits when ad-ministered parenterally. The LD_{50} values in chick embryos (yolk sac injection) and in mice and rabbits (ip) were 18.8, 42, and 20 mg/kg, respectively. Oral administration of 1 g/kg produced no toxic effects in mice. Solanidine, the aglycone, was less toxic than solanine; it was non-toxic to mice at 500 mg/kg IP. These investigators concluded from their findings that the relatively rare occurrence of solanine poisoning from potatoes and the low oral toxicity of solanine for laboratory animals may be explained on the basis of poor absorption from the gastrointestinal tract, rapid urinary and fecal excretion of metabolites, and gastrointestinal

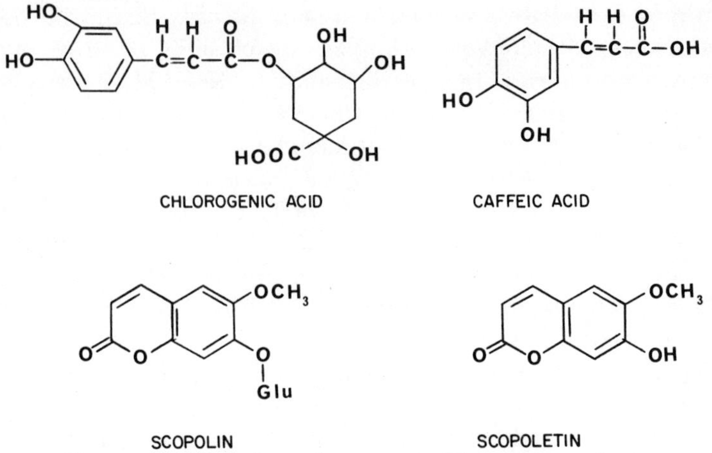

CHLOROGENIC ACID   CAFFEIC ACID

SCOPOLIN   SCOPOLETIN

Figure 2.   Phenols and coumarin-like compounds in
white potatoes

hydrolysis of solanine to the less toxic solanidine. No information is available on the toxicity and pharamcological properties of α-chaconine, the second major glycoalkaloid of the potato.

Phenolic Compounds. Chlorogenic and caffeic acids are present in all parts of the potato. The levels of caffeic acid (*42*) and chlorogenic (*43*) have been observed to increase in potatoes after slicing (Figure 2). Chlorogenic acid is the principal phenol that accumulates in cut tissue. Caffeic acid can be formed by the hydrolysis of chlorogenic acid; certain fungi are capable of facilitating this hydrolysis and metabolizing the hydrolysis product (*44*). Zucker (*45*) found that brief exposure of potato disks to light of low intensity doubled the synthesis of chlorogenic acid in the dark; continued exposure of disks to light of high intensity for up to 40 hr resulted in higher levels of the compound. In other studies (*46*) it was found that the production of the enzyme phenylalanine deaminase in potato disks was greatly stimulated by white light, and its induction was directly proportional to the production of chlorogenic acid; the enzyme was not present in fresh tissue. One can therefore conclude that the light imposes stress on the potato and that it serves as an inducer of phenolic synthesis. Phenylalanine deaminase is considered the key enzyme in the biosynthetic pathway of chlorogenic acid synthesis.

Although injury to the potato usually results in an increase in chlorogenic and caffeic acids, injury also can cause rapid oxidation of these acids (*5*). Oxidation products of these acids are toxic to many microorganisms. In one study (*47*) chlorogenic acid in the culture medium stimulated the growth of *Phytophthora infestans,* although it also undergoes transformation (by oxidation) to quinic and caffeic acids. Quinic acid had a stimulating effect on the growth of the organism, but caffeic acid was toxic and therefore inhibited growth. Chlorogenic and caffeic acids are believed associated with the disease resistance of potatoes. The lethal ip dose of chlorogenic acid in mice was found to be 3.5 g/kg; 4–5 g/kg oral or SC gave no toxic manifestations (48). Toxicity data from other animal species should be obtained before one can safely say that the production of increased amounts of chlorogenic and caffeic acid does not pose a threat to human health.

Scopolin and Scopoletin. Scopolin and scopoletin are coumarin-type compounds that are normally present in potatoes. Scopolin accumulates to a greater extent than other coumarin-type compounds in tissue that has been infected with fungi, bacteria, or viruses (49). Mechanical wounding of tissue slices alone did not induce the accumulation of scopolin. The content of caffeic acid and scopoletin in tubers is reported to change in response to various physiological states. Korableva et al. (50) found that the content of these compounds is highest in the period when the tubers are in profound dormancy (Sept.–Oct.). During the emergence from dormancy (Dec.–Jan.) the content of these substances decreases. The increased amounts of these compounds was attributed not only to direct synthesis but also to the hydrolysis of glucosides since beta-glucosidase activity is highest in tubers in a state of profound dormancy.

Unusual Compounds Produced in Response to Stress

The compounds included in this category are not normally found in healthy potatoes; they are produced or synthesized when the potato is subjected to physiological stress (Figure 3). The stress conditions that result in production of these compounds include aging of sliced potatoes and inoculation or treatment of potatoes with certain microorganisms or cell-free extracts of certain fungi. The latter stress conditions have been reported elsewhere (51).

Alkaloids. The presence of two new glycoalkaloids in the leaves and aged slices of Kennebec potatoes was recently reported by Shih and Kuć (52). These glycoalkaloids, identified as alpha- and beta-solamarine, contain the spirosolane, tomatidenol (tomatid-5-en-3β-ol), as the aglycone instead of solanidine which is found in solanine and chaconine. The presence of the spirosolane aglycone in potatoes was reported by Schreiber in 1957 when a small amount was isolated from the hydrolysate of a crude solanine preparation (53). Tomatidenol is the major aglycone in alkaloids of *Solanum dulcamara* (woody nightshade or bittersweet), a toxic plant belonging to the potato family. Alpha- and beta-solamarine were not found in tuber peel or freshly sliced tubers of Kennebec or in 20 other cultivars; they were only found in the leaves of Kennebec tubers and accumulated at the cut surface of aged Kennebec tuber slices in amounts equal to that of solanine and chaconine. Although the solamarines con-

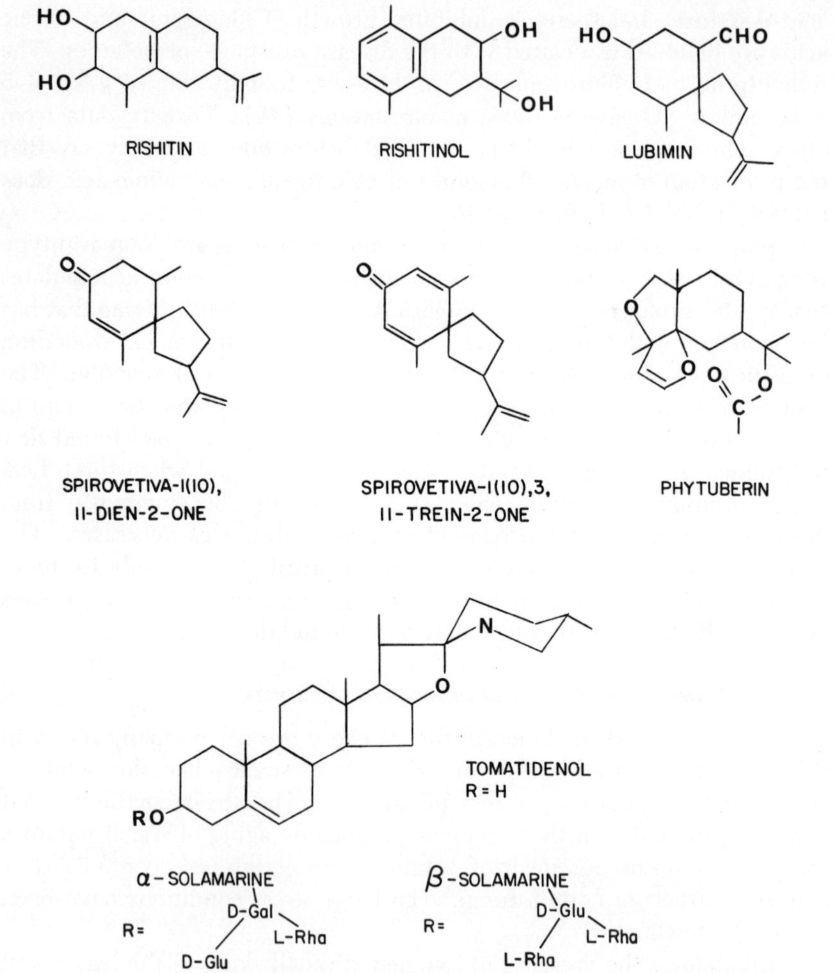

Figure 3. *Compounds not present in healthy white potatoes but which are produced in response to stress*

tain the spirosolane aglycone, they are structurally related to the solanidine alkaloids in that the trisaccharide moiety of alpha-solamarine is identical to that of alpha-solanine, and the trisaccharide moiety of beta-solamarine is identical to that of alpha-chaconine. Shih and Kuć (52) suggest that the spirosolane aglycone may have been inherited by the Kennebec variety as a result of cross-breeding with wild plant species when efforts were made to produce new varieties of potatoes resistant to late blight. Since the Kennebec variety of potatoes is very popular and widely consumed in certain areas of the United States, the production of these new alkaloids at the surface of aged slices of potatoes is of great concern from the standpoint of human health.

Terpenes. Terpenoid compounds that accumulate in potatoes as a result of stress include rishitin, rishitinol, phytuberin, lubimin, two new vetispirane derivatives, and others not yet identified. These compounds are produced in response to stress conditions created by the inoculation of potato tubers with numerous nonpathogens of potatoes and with *Phytophthora infestans* or by treatment with cell-free sonicates of *P. infestans* (*16*). These compounds accumulate at levels that are fungitoxic around the site of infection and are thought to be a part of the mechanism of disease resistance of the potato. The greatest accumulation of these compounds seems to be in potato varieties that are resistant to *P. infestans*.

Rishitin ($C_{14}H_{22}O_2$) was originally isolated from the Rishiri variety of potatoes by Tomiyama et al. (*54*) and was determined to be a bicyclic norsesquiterpene alcohol (*55*). Rishitin was not found in intact healthy potatoes, but trace amounts were found in sliced noninoculated tissue. Rishitin accumulated to significant levels in sliced tubers inoculated with certain fungi. In other studies (*56*) traces of rishitin were found in sliced noninoculated aged tissue; also rishitin and another terpene, phytuberin ($C_{17}H_{26}O_4$), were found to accumulate in 11 cultivars that were inoculated with *P. infestans* (*57*). Rishitin is active biologically as an antifungal agent (*58*). The hydroxyl group on carbon 3 in the molecule is believed to be indispensable for its antifungal activity.

Phytuberin was isolated by Varns et al. (*57*) and described as an aliphatic, unsaturated, sesquiterpene acetate. The structure of phytuberin was recently determined by Hughes and Coxon (*59*). The accumulation of rishitin and phytuberin in tissue slices is usually preceded by necrosis. In later studies by Varns et al. (*60*) it was found that the induction of necrosis in tissue by physical or chemical means does not cause the accumulation of the terpenes in the absence of the fungus or fungal products. Recently, Deahl (*61*) reported that tubers which do not show significant accumulation of terpenoid compounds on infection with *P. infestans* did accumulate significant quantities of rishitin, phytuberin, and unidentified terpenoids when allowed to wound-heal for 72 hr prior to inoculation.

The presence of rishitinol ($C_{15}H_{22}O_2$), a sesquiterpenoid alcohol, in potatoes infected with *P. infestans* was reported in 1971 (*62*). The structure and configuration of the molecule were deduced from spectral and chemical data and confirmed by synthesis (*63*). No other information on this compound has been reported.

Lubimin ($C_{15}H_{24}O_2$) is a sesquiterpenoid hydroxyaldehyde first isolated from the Soviet Lyubimets variety of potatoes infected with *P. infestans* (*64*). Its structure was derived from ir, NMR, and mass spectra of the isolate, its deuterated and monoacetyl derivatives, and its 2,4-dinitrophenylhydrazone (*65*). A revised structure for lubimin was recently reported (66). Lubimin has greater biological activity as an anti-fungal agent than rishitin (67).

Two new vetispirane derivatives, Spirovetiva-1(10),11-dien-2-one and Spirovetiva-1(10),3,11-trien-2-one, were recently isolated simultaneously and independently by research groups in the United States and England from potatoes infected with *P. infestans* (68).

Toxicological Studies

To obtain information on the toxicity of compounds that accumulated in potatoes subjected to stress by infection and by slicing and aging, a preliminary study was conducted in our laboratory (69). The potatoes (Kennebec variety) were separated into two main groups: one group (A) was inoculated with *Phytophthora infestans* (wild type—provided by courtesy of Gary A. McIntye, Dept. of Plant Pathology, University of Maine), and the second group (B) was used to produce alkaloids by allowing slices to age in lined petri dishes stored in the dark for 96 hr. The potatoes in group A were surface sterilized, sliced, and placed in large sterile flasks. The flasks were inoculated with *P. infestans* suspended in phosphate buffer. Noninoculated control slices were treated with only phosphate buffer. The flasks were incubated at 16°C for six days. Terpenoid compounds were extracted from one portion of the incubated slices with methanol by using the procedure described by Varns et al. (57). Glycoalkaloids were extracted from a second portion of the incubated slices and from the aged slices with chloroform–acetic acid–methanol (50:5:45) using the procedure described by Shih et al. (37). Similar extracts were prepared from the noninoculated slices treated with phosphate buffer and from freshly sliced healthy potatoes. All extracts were examined by thin-layer chromatography. The methanolic extract from the infected tissue contained rishitin, phytuberin, and unidentified compounds that were not observed in the control tissue extract. The glycoalkaloid extract from nonaged tissue contained two compounds with R_f values corresponding to solanine and chaconine; the extract from the infected tissue contained additional compounds not observed in control extracts; and the extract from the aged tissue also contained additional compounds two of which had R_f values corresponding to alpha- and beta-solamarine (70). The crude extracts along with adequate control samples were evaporated to dryness, suspended in ethanol and injected into non-incubated and four day-incubated, fertile chick eggs via yolk sac route, at 400 μg/egg for the terpene-containing extracts and up to 80 μg/egg for glycoalkaloid containing extracts. The nonincubated eggs were used to detect any neural tube defects which should show up during the first 24–48 hr of incubation. No toxic or teratogenic effects were observed in embryos injected with the methanolic extract which contained the terpenes from the infected potatoes. In contrast, moderate toxicity and scattered abnormalities were observed in embryos that were injected with glycoalkaloids from uninoculated, infected, and aged tissue. The most severe abnormalities were in the embryos injected with glycoalkaloids from the aged tissue. The abnormalities included crossed beaks, deformed eye cavities, and malformed wings; no spinal or brain defects were noted. There was no apparent specific abnormality associated with any fraction.

Swinyard and Chaube (*15*) conducted studies to determine if blighted potatoes (potatoes infected with *P. infestans*), solanine, and total glycoalkaloids extracted from potato blossoms were teratogenic for experimental animals. No teratogenic effects were observed in pregnant rats given a known quantity of homogenized blighted potatoes by gavage on days 7–16 of gestation. Solanine and total glycoalkaloids (suspended in carboxymethylcellulose) were relatively nontoxic to maternal and fetal rats at ip doses of 5 and 10 mg/kg/day when given on days 5–12 of gestation, but a high incidence (44%) of relatively minor abnormalities were observed. By comparision on a mg/kg/day basis the total glycoalkaloid sample was about seven times more toxic to fetuses at 10 mg/kg/day than was solanine. This suggests that the total glycoalkaloid sample contained other material more toxic than solanine. Daily ip injections of 5 mg/kg of solanine in pregnant rabbits on days 0–8 of gestation produced abortions and resorptions but no teratogenesis. Yolk sac injections of 5–20 mg/kg of solanine in embryonated chick eggs produced 63–90% mortality without significant teratogenesis. The mortality was high in both the experimental and control groups. A single ip injection of 40 mg/kg of total glycoalkaloid extract and two injections of 20 mg/kg of solanine killed adult rhesus monkeys in 48 hr.

Ruddick et al. (*71*) fed rats a diet containing freeze-dried blighted potatoes (75 g/kg/day) during days 1–22 of gestation and found no teratogenic effects. Oral administration of α-solanine, α-chaconine, and scopoletin given on days 6–15 of gestation also failed to elicit teratogenic effects in rats.

Gull et al. (*72*) reported that the growth rate of rats was suppressed when they were fed a diet containing 200 mg of solanine per 100 g of food. The LD_{50} for ip injection of solanine was 7.5 mg/100 g of body weight and 59 mg/100 g when the compound was administered by stomach tube. Russian investigators (*73*) found that pregnant rats given 25–50 mg/kg of solanine–HCl with their food gave birth to litters with survival rates below that of controls. Administration of the compound before or after pregnancy did not affect rats born during subsequent pregnancies.

Mun et al. (*74*) reported on the teratogenic effects in chick embryos of solanine and glycoalkaloids from potatoes infected with *Phytophthora*

infestans. Solanine or total glycoalkaloid extracts from the infected potatoes that were injected into 0–26 hr incubated chick eggs at 130–260 μg/
egg (yolk sac injection) resulted in 22–27% mortality and 16–22% abnormal embryos. At the solanine level of 15 μg/egg, 25% of the embryos
were abnormal, but there was no mortality. Some abnormalities and
deaths were also observed in embryos injected with control solutions. The
most conspicious defect noted was the absence of the tail or trunk below
the wing bud; this defect was not observed in embryos injected with
control solutions.

Toxicological studies on solanine were mentioned earlier; however
the toxicity of the new glycoalkaloids, alpha- and beta-solamarine, have
not been investigated. Beta-solamarine is reported to show tumor-inhibi-
tory activity against sarcoma 180 in mice (75). Alpha- and beta-solamarine are structurally related to cyclopamine, a steroid alkaloid isolated
from *Veratrum californicum* that produces teratogenic effects in sheep
(76). The terminal portion of cyclopamine consists of a fused furano-
piperidine ring; the terminal portion of the solamarine molecule consists
of a furan moiety fused to the steroidal portion of the molecule rather
than to the piperidine ring. According to Keeler (77) the fused furano-
piperidine arrangement is the essential structural feature necessary for
teratogenicity among the Veratrum alkaloids. He postulated that potato
alkaloids that possess a terminal furan and a piperidine ring could possibly
be teratogens according to the structural and configurational similarity to
the known Veratrum teratogens (78). In view of this it is tempting to
suggest that the abnormalities observed in our studies in chick embryos
with extracts from aged tissue were attributed to the presence of alpha-
and beta-solamarine in the extracts; solanine and chaconine do not contain a furan ring. The above finding suggests that the glycoalkaloids of
stressed and nonstressed white potatoes should be thoroughly investigated
toxicologically. Toxicological data from chronic studies using pure solanine and chaconine are needed. The toxicity of the new stress metabolites
alpha- and beta-solamarine, should be investigated in several animal
species. Most of the terpenoid stress metabolites are toxic to various fungi,
but no data are available on their toxicity for other animal species. Several research groups have already initiated studies on many of the known
stress metabolites. The results from these studies may be delayed because
of problems involved in obtaining a sufficient amount of the pure compounds for toxicological studies in experimental animals. The use of the
chick embryo as a rapid bioassay system may prove very advantageous in
obtaining preliminary information on the toxicity of these compounds.

Biosynthetic Studies

The chemistry of the Solanum alkaloids was reviewed by Schreiber

(*22*). From a biogenetic viewpoint steroid alkaloids are considered pseu-doalkaloids in that they are derivatives of generally occurring nitrogen-free compounds. Nitrogen is introduced into the structure of steroid alkaloids at some stage during their biosynthesis from nitrogen-free deriva-tives. Studies on the biosynthesis of the sterol cholesterol were reviewed by Bloch (*79*). The sequences involved in the biosynthesis of the steroids and terpenoids proceeded via the acetate–mevalonic acid pathway, and squalene, a polyisoprenoid hydrocarbon, was a key intermediate. Since solanidine, the aglycone moiety of the alkaloids in potatoes, possesses a carbon skeleton related to cholesterol, it has been assumed that both have common precursors. In studies on the biosynthesis of alkaloids in potato seedlings, Guseva et al. (*80*) observed a significant incorporation of acetate-2-^{14}C and DL-mevalonic acid-2-^{14}C into the alkaloids and solanidine, thus suggesting that these compounds are intermediates in the pathway. Tschesche and Hulpke (*81*) found that radioactive cholesterol applied to leaf surfaces of potato plants was metabolized to solanidine, indicating that cholesterol can be a precursor. The conversion of the sterols lanos-terol and cycloartenol to solanidine and tomatine has recently been re-ported (*82*). In more recent studies using labelled compounds Jadhav et al. (*83*) found that β-hydroxy-β-methylglutaric acid (HMG), leucine, alanine, and glucose were incorporated into the glycoalkaloids of potato sprouts; the percent of incorporation was less for these precursors than for mevalonic acid. They also observed that certain chemicals effectively re-duced alkaloid synthesis in the sprouts.

Stress metabolites in plants are synthesized by altering either the shikimic acid, acetate-malonate, or acetate-mevalonate pathways or by joint participation of all three pathways (*84*). Experimental evidence sug-gests that the biosynthesis of glycoalkaloids and terpenoid compounds in stressed potatoes involves the use of the same pathway. Ozeretskovskaya et al. (*36*) observed a decrease in the glycoalkaloid level in damaged potato tissue infected with *P. infestans* and concluded that the fungus could decompose the alkaloids. They also found that in wounded tissue mevalonate was used to synthesize glycoalkaloids, but in necrotic tissue (resulting from fungal infection) glycoalkaloids were not formed, and all mevalonate was used to synthesize lubimin and rishitin. Shih et al. (*37*) found that the accumulation of glycoalkaloids in potato slices was sup-pressed when the cut surface was inoculated with *P. infestans;* this sup-pression was associated with the accumulation of high levels of rishitin. In further studies (*85*) using ^{14}C-labelled acetate and mevalonate they found that the accumulation of the glycoalkaloids and rishitin in potato tubers after cutting or cutting and inoculation with *P. infestans* appeared to arise from de novo synthesis via the acetate–mevalonate pathway. The branch point in the synthetic pathway which leads to rishitin or the glycoalkaloids appears to be after mevalonate. Phytuberin, which is usually produced along with rishitin when resistant varieties of potatoes are infected with *P. infestans,* is believed to be synthesized by a pathway different from rishitin. In studies (86) using 2-chloroethylphosphonic acid, which exhibits growth-regulating properties on certain plants, it was found that the chemical stimulated phytuberin synthesis in potato slices inoculated with *P. infestans* but had the opposite effect on rishitin accumulation in the same tissue. Further studies are needed to elucidate the biosynthetic pathway involved in the synthesis of other stress metabolites.

Future Research

Abnormal concentrations of various constituents in potatoes and the production of new or unusual compounds in this widely used plant food under various conditions of stress have stimulated much research and concern for the effects of these compounds on human health. The results of studies that have been conducted in experimental animals indicate that the glycoalkaloids are not only toxic but may be teratogenic in certain animals. Although solanine is toxic for humans, detailed studies are needed on the other glycoalklaloids, terpenes, phenols, and other compounds that accumulate in response to various stress conditions. It is possible that some of the products resulting from the degradation of these compounds may also be toxic.

There is a need for a continual evaluation of new varieties of potatoes for their acceptability and safety for humans. In 1970 the Lenape variety of potatoes was withdrawn from commercial use because of its high glycoalkaloid content (87). In future evaluations all known stress metabolites should be included in the screening process. Plant breeders should be informed and aware of all non-nutritive compounds that have been identified in normal, healthy potatoes and conditions under which additional compounds may be produced as a result of stress. They should also have a knowledge of the types of compounds present in nonedible varieties of solanaceous plants, so that in the breeding program, the possible introduction of deleterious compounds to edible varieties can be avoided.

Literature Cited

1. Müller, K., Börger, H., "Experimentelle Untersuchungen uber die Phytophthora-Resistenz der Kartoffel," *Arb. Biol. Reichsanst. Land. Forstwirt., Berlin-Dahlem* (1940) **23**, 189-231.
2. Müller, K., "Einige Einfache Versuchenzum Nachweis von Phytoalexinen," *Phytopathol. Z.* (1956) **27**, 237–54.
3. Cruickshank, I. A. M., Phytoalexins, *Ann. Rev. Phytopathol.* (1963) **1**, 351–374.
4. Cruickshank, I. A. M., Perrin, D. R., "Pathological Function of Phenolic Compounds in Plants," in "Biochemistry of Phenolic Compounds," J. B. Harborns, Ed., pp. 511–544, Academic, London, New York, 1964.
5. Kuć, J., "Phytoalexins," *Ann. Rev. Phytopathol.* (1972) **10**, 207–232.
6. Kira'ly, Z., Barna, B., Ersek, T., "Hypersensitivity as a Consequence, Not

the Cause, of Plant Resistance to Infection," *Nature* (1972) **239**, 456–458.

7. Kuć, J., "Compounds Accumulating in Plants After Infection," in "Microbial Toxins," Vol. VIII, S. J. Ajl, G. Weinbaum, S. Kadis, Eds., pp. 211–247, Academic Press, New York, 1971.

8. Renwick, J. H., "Hypothesis:Anencephaly and Spina Bifida Are Usually Preventable by Avoidance of a Specific but Unidentified Substance Present in Certain Potato Tubers," *Brit. J. Prev. Soc. Med.* (1972) **26**, 67–88.

9. Poswillo, D. E., Sopher, D., Mitchell, S., "Experimental Induction of Foetal Malformation with 'Blighted' Potato: A Preliminary Report," *Nature* (1972) **239**, 462–464.

10. Poswillo, D. E., Sopher, D., Mitchell, S. J., Coxon, D. T., Curtis, R. F., Price, K. R., "Investigations into the Teratogenic Potential of Imperfect Potatoes," *Teratology* (1973) **8**, 339–348.

11. Knox, E. G., "Anencephalus and Dietary Intakes," *Brit. J. Prev. Soc. Med.* (1972) **26**, 219–223.

12. Chaube, S., Swinyard, C. A., Daines, R. H., "Failure to Induce Malformations in Fetal Rats by Feeding Blighted Potatoes to Their Mothers," *Lance* (1973) **1**, 329–330.

13. Lorber, J., Stewart, C. R., Ward, A. M., "Alpha-Fetoprotein in Antenatal Diagnosis of Anencephaly and Spin Bifida," *Lancet* (1973) **1**, 1187.

14. Emanuel, I., Sever, L. E., "Questions Concerning the Possible Association of Potatoes and Neural-Tube Defects, and an Alternative Hypothesis Relating to Maternal Growth and Development," *Teratology* **8**, 325–332.

15. Swinyard, C. A., Chaube, S., "Are Potatoes Teratogenic for Experimental Animals?" *Teratology* (1973) **8**, 349–358.

16. Kuć, J., "Metabolites Accumulating in Potato Tubers Following Infection and Stress," *Teratology* (1973) **8**, 333–338.

17. Schwimmer, S., Burr, H., "Structure and Chemical Composition of the Potato Tuber," in "Potato Processing," W. F. Talburt, O. Smith, Eds., pp. 12–43, Avi, Westport, Conn., 1959.

18. Lampitt, L. H., Goldenberg, N., "The Composition of the Potato," *Chem. Ind.* (1940) **18**, 748–761.

19. Coon, J. M., "Naturally Occurring Toxicants in Foods," *Food Technol.* (1969) **23**, 1041–1045.

20. Bentley, K. W., "The Alkaloids," Part II, pp. 98–141, Interscience, New York, 1965.

21. Guseva, A. R., Paseshnichenko, V. A., "Enzymic Degradation of Potato Glycoalkaloids," *Biochemistry (USSR)* (1957) **22**, 792–799.

22. Schreiber, J., "Steroid Alkaloids: The Solanum Group," in "The Alkaloids Chemistry and Physiology," Vol. 10, R. H. F. Manske, Ed., pp. 1–192, Academic, New York, 1968.

23. Paseshnichenko, V. A., "Content of Solanine and Chaconine in the Potato During the Vegetation Period," *Biochemistry (USSR)* (1957) **22**, 929–931.

24. Allen, E. H., Kuć, J., "α-Solanine and α-Chaconine as Fungitoxic Compounds in Extracts of Irish Potato Tubers," *Phytopathology* (1968) **58**, 776–781.

25. Wolf, M. J., Duggar, B. M., "Estimation and Physiological Role of Solanine in the Potato," *J. Agric. Res.* (1946) **73**, 1–32.

26. Sinden, S. L., Webb, R. E., "Effect of Environment on Glycoalkaloid Content of Six Potato Varieties at 39 Locations," Technical Bulletin No. 1472, Agric. Res. Ser., U.S.D.A., Washington, D.C., 1974.

27. Conner, N. W., "The Effect of Light on Solanine Synthesis in the Potato Tubers," *Plant Physiol.* (1937) **12**, 79.

28. Gull, D. D., Isenberg, F. M., "Chlorophyll and Solanine Content and Distribution in Four Varieties of Potato Tubers," *Proc. Amer. Soc. Hortic.*

Sci. (1960) **75**, 545–556.
29. Patil, B. C., Salunkhe, D. K., Singh, B., "Metabolism of Solanine and Chlorophyll in Potato Tubers as Affected by Light and Specific Chemicals," *J. Food Sci.* (1971) **36**, 474–476.
30. Salunkhe, D. K., Wu, M. T., Jadhav, S. J., "Effects of Light and Temperature on the formation of Solanine in Potato Slices," *J. Food Sci.* (1972) **37**, 969–970.
31. Kuć, J., "Phenolic Compounds and Disease Resistance in Plants," in "Phenolics in Normal and Diseased Fruits and Vegetables," V. Runeckles, Ed., pp. 63–81, Imperial Tobacco Co., Montreal, 1964.
32. Zitnak, A., "The Occurrence and Distribution of Free Alkaloid Solanidine in Netted Gem Potatoes," *Can. J. Biochem. Physiol.* (1961) **39**, 1257–1265.
33. McKee, R., "Host Parasite Relationships in the Dry-Rot Disease of Potatoes," *Ann. Appl. Biol.* (1955) **43**, 147–148.
34. Locci, R., Kuć, J., "Steroid Alkaloids as Compounds Produced by Potato Tubers Under Stress," *Phytopathology* (1967) **57**, 1272–73.
35. Ishizaka, N., Tomiyama, K., "Effect of Wounding or Infection by *Phytophthora infestans* on the Contents of Terpenoids in Potato Tubers," *Plant Cell Physiol.* (1972) **13**, 1053–1063.
36. Ozeretskovskaya, O. L., Davylova, M. A., Vasyukova, N. I., Metlitskii, L. V., "Glycoalkaloids in Sound and Injured Potato Tubers," *Dokl. Akad. Nauk SSR* (1971) **196(6)**, 1470–1473.
37. Shih, M., Kuć, J., Williams, E. B., "Suppression of Steroid Glycoalkaloid Accumulation as Related to Rishitin Accumulation in Potato Tubers," *Phytopathology* (1973) **63**, 821–826.
38. Willimott, S. G., "An Investigation of Solanine Poisoning," *Analyst* (1933) **58**, 431–438.
39. Wilson, G. S., "A Small Outbreak of Solanine Poisoning," *Mon. Bull. Med. Res. Council* (1959) **18(12)**, 207–210.
40. Rühl, R., "Beitrag zur Pathologie und Toxikologie des Solanins," *Arch. Pharm.* (1961) **284**, 67–74.
41. Nishie, K., Gumbmann, M. R., Keyl, A. C., "Pharmacology of Solanine," *Toxicol. Appl. Pharmacol.* (1971) **19**, 81–92.
42. Kuć, J., Henze, R. E., Ullstrup, A. J., Quackenbush, F. W., "Chlorogenic and Caffeic Acids as Fungistatic Agents Produced by Potatoes in Response to Inoculation with *Helminthosporium carbonum*," *J. Amer. Chem. Soc.* (1956) **78**, 3123–3125.
43. Sakuma, T., Tomiyama, K., "The Role of Phenolic Compounds in the Resistance of Potato Tuber Tissue to Infection by *P. infestans*," *Ann. Phytopathol. Soc., Jap.* (1967) **33**, 48–58.
44. Lee, S., Le Tourneau, D., "Chlorogenic Acid Content and Verticillium Wilt Resistance of Potatoes," *Phytopathology* (1958) **48**, 268–274.
45. Zucker, M., "Influence of Light on Synthesis of Protein and of Chlorogenic Acid in Potato Tuber Tissue," *Plant Physiol.* (1963) **38(5)**, 575–580.
46. Zucker, M., "Induction of Phenylalanine Deaminase by Light and Its Relation to Chlorogenic Acid Synthesis in Potato Tuber Tissue," *Plant Physiol.* (1965) **40(5)**, 779–784.
47. Sokolova, V. E., "Toxicity of Chlorogenic Acid and Its Derivatives Caffeic and Quinic Acids for *Phytophthora infestans* Fungus," *Izv. Akad. Nauk SSR, Ser. Biol.* (1963) **28(5)**, 707–718.
48. Chassevent, F., "Physiological and Pharmacological Action of Chlorogenic Acid," *Ann. Nutr. Aliment.* (1969) **23(1)**, 1R–14R.
49. Clarke, D. D., "The Accumulation of Scopolin in Potato Tuber Tissue After Infection by *Phytophthora infestans* and Its Role in Pathogenesis," *Phytochemistry* (1969) **8**, 7.
50. Korableva, N. P., Morozova, E. V., Metlitskii, L. V., "Participation of

Phenolic Growth Inhibitors in the Regulation of the Dormancy of Potato Tubers and Their Resistance to *Phytophthora infestans*," *Dokl. Akad. Nauk SSR* (1973) **212(4)**, 1000–1002.

51. Kuć, J., Currier, W., "Compounds Accumulating in Plants After Infection," Abstracts, 168th National Meeting of the American Chemical Society, Atlantic City, N. J., Sept. 1974, Division of Agricultural and Food Chemistry, 102.

52. Shih, M., Kuć, J., "α- and β-Solamarine in Kennebec *Solanum Tuberosum* Leaves and Aged Tuber Slices," *Phytochemistry* (1974) **13**, 997–1000.

53. Schreiber, K., "Solanum Alkaloids, V. Isolation of Δ^5-Tomatidin-3β-ol and Yamogenin from Potatoes," *Angew. Chem.* (1957) **69**, 483.

54. Tomiyama, K., Sakuma, T., Ishizaka, N., Sato, N., Katsui, N., Takasugi, M., Masamune, T., "A New Antifungal Substance Isolated from Resistant Potato Tuber Tissue Infected by Pathogens," *Phytopathology* (1968) **58**, 115–116.

55. Katsui, N., Murai, A., Takasugi, M., Imaizumi, K., Masamune, T., "The Structure of Rishitin, a New Antifungal Compound from Diseased Potato Tubers," *Chem. Commun. (Sect. D)* (1968) 43–44.

56. Varns, J., "Biochemical Response and Its Control in the Irish Potato Tuber (*Solanum tuberosum*)—*Phytophthora infestans* Interaction," Ph.D. Thesis, Purdue University, Lafayette, Ind., 1970.

57. Varns, J., Kuć, J., Williams, E. B., "Terpenoid Accumulation as a Biochemical Response of the Potato Tuber to *Phytophthora infestans*," *Phytopathology* (1971) **61**, 174–177.

58. Ishizaka, N., Tomiyama, K., Katsui, N., Murai, A., Masamune, T., "Biological Activities of Rishitin, an Antifungal Compound Isolated from Diseased Potato Tubers, and Its Derivatives," *Plant Cell Physiol.* (1969) **10**, 183–192.

59. Hughes, D. L., Coxon, D. T., "Phytuberin; Revised Structure From the X-Ray Crystal Analysis of Dihydrophytuberin," *J. Chem. Soc., D.* (1974) 822–823.

60. Varns, J., Currier, W., Kuć, J., "Specificity of Rishitin and Phytuberin Accumulation by Potato," *Phytopathology* (1971) **61**, 968–971.

61. Deahl, K. L., "The Effect of Wound-Healing on Phytoalexin Production and Invasion by *Phytophthora infestans* in Potato Tuber Tissues," Abstracts of Meeting. Annual Meeting of American Phytopathology Society, 1974.

62. Katsui, N., Matsunaga, A., Imizumi, K., Masamune, T., "The Structure and Synthesis of Rishitinol, a New Sesquiterpene Alcohol from Diseased Potato Tubers," *Tetrahedron Lett.* (1971) No. 2, 83–86.

63. Katsui, N., Matsunaga, A., Imaizumi, K., Masamune, T., "The Structure and Synthesis of Rishitinol. Sesquiterpene Alcohol from Diseased Potato Tubers," *Bull. Chem. Soc., Jap.* (1973) **45**, 2871–2877.

64. Metlitskii, L. V., Ozeretskovskaya, O. L., Chalova, L. I., Vasyukova, N. I., Davydova, M. A., "Lubimin, a Potato Phytoalexin," *Mikol. Fitopatol.* (1971) **5(3)**, 263–271.

65. Metlitskii, L. V., Ozeretskovskaya, O. L., Vul'fson, N. S., Chalova, L. I., "Chemical Nature of Lubimin, a New Phytoalexin of Potatoes," *Dokl. Akad. Nauk SSR* (1971) **200(6)**, 1470–1472.

66. Stoessl, A., Stothers, J. B., Ward, E. W. B., "Lubimin: A Phytoalexin of Several Solanaceae. Structure Revision and Biogenetic Relationships," *J. Chem. Soc., D.* (1974) 709–710.

67. Metlitskii, L. V., Ozeretskovskaya, O. L., Vul'fson, N. S., Chalova, L. I., "Effects of Lubimin on Potato Resistance to *Phytophthora infestans* and Its Chemical Identification," *Mikol. Fitopatol.* (1971) **5(5)**, 439–443.

68. Coxon, D. T., Price, K. R., Howard, B., Osman, S. F., Kalan, E. B., Zacharius, R. M., "Two New Vetispirane Derivatives; Stress Metabolites from

Potato *(Solanum tuberosum)* Tubers," *Tetrahedron Lett.* (1974) **34**, 2921–2924.

69. Wood, G. E., Mislivec, P. B., Verrett, M. J., "Characterization of Abnormal Plant Metabolites," unpublished data, 1973.
70. Boll, P. M., "Alkaloidal Glycosides from *Solanum dulcamara*. II. Three New Alkaloidal Glycosides and a Reassessment of Soladulcamaridine," *Acta Chem. Scand.* (1962) **16**, 1819–1830.
71. Ruddick, J. A., Harwig, J., Scott, P. M., "Nonteratogenicity in Rats of Blighted Potatoes and Compounds Contained in Them," *Teratology* (1974) **9**, 165–168.
72. Gull, S. D., Isenberg, F. M., Bryan, H. H., "Alkaloid Toxicology of *Solanum tuberosum*," *Hortic. Sci.* (1970) **5**, 316.
73. Sklyarevskii, L. Y., Tereshkor, G. F., "Effect of Solanine on Pregnancy in Rats and Survival of Their Offspring," *Tr. Vses. Nauch-Issled. Inst. Lek. Rast.* (1971) **14**, 97–102; *Chem. Abstr.* (1973) **79**, 496082.
74. Mun, A. M., Barden, E. S., Wilson, J. M., Hogan, J. M., "Teratogenic Effects of Solanine and Glycoalkaloids from Potatoes Infected with Late Blight," *Teratology* (1974) **9** (3), A–30.
75. Kupchan, S. M., Barboutis, S. J., Knox, J. R., LauCam, C. A., "Beta-Solamarine: Tumor Inhibitor Isolated from *Solanum dulcamara*," *Science* (1965) **150**, 1827–28.
76. Keeler, R. F., "Teratogenic Compounds of *Veratrum californicum* (Durand), VI. The Structure of Cyclopamine," *Phytochemistry* (1969) **8**, 223–225.
77. Keeler, R. F., "Teratogenic Compounds in *Veratrum californicum* (Durand), IX. Structure-activity Relation," *Teratology* (1970) **3**, 169–174.
78. Keeler, R. F., "Comparison of the Teratogenicity in Rats of Certain Potato-Type Alkaloids and the Veratrum Teratogen Cyclopamine," *Lancet* (1973) **1**, 1187–1188.
79. Bloch, K., "The Biological Synthesis of Cholesterol," *Science* (1965) **150**, 19–28.
80. Guseva, A. R., Paseshnichenko, V. A., Borikhina, M. G., "Synthesis of Radioactive Mevalonic Acid and Its Use in the Study of the Biosynthesis of Steroid Glycoalkaloids from *Solanum*," *Biochemistry (USSR)* (1961) **26**, 631–635.
81. Tschesche, R., Hulpke, H., "Biosynthesis of Steroid Derivatives in Plants, VIII. Biogenesis of Solanidine from Cholesterol," *Z. Naturforsch.* (1967) **22b**, 791.
82. Ripperger, H., Moritz, W., Schreiber, K., "Biosynthesis of Solanum Alkaloids from Cycloartenol or Lanosterol," *Phytochemistry* (1971) **10**, 2699–2704.
83. Jadhav, S. J., Salunkhe, D. K., Wyse, R. E., Dolvi, R. R., "Solanum Alkaloids: Biosynthesis and Inhibition by Chemicals," *J. Food Sci.* (1973) **38**, 453–455.
84. Kuć, J., "Resistance of Plants to Infectious Agents," *Annu. Rev. Microbiol.* (1966) **20**, 337–70.
85. Shih, M., Kuć, J., "Incorporation of ^{14}C from Acetate and Mevalonate into Rishitin and Steroid Glycoalkaloids by Potato Tuber Slices Inoculated with *Phytophthora infestans*," *Phytopathology* (1973) **63**, 826–829.
86. Shih, M., "The Accumulation of Isoprenoids and Phenols and Its Control as Related to the Interaction of Potato (*Solanum Tuberosum* L.) with *Phytophthora infestans*," Ph.D. Thesis, Purdue University, Lafayette, Ind., 1972.
87. U.S. Department of Agriculture, Press Release 423-70, Washington, D.C., Feb. 11, 1970, New potato variety withdrawn.

RECEIVED November 8, 1974.

Toxic Furanosesquiterpenoids from Mold-Damaged Sweet Potatoes (*Ipomoea batatas*)

LEO T. BURKA and BENJAMIN J. WILSON

Center in Environmental Toxicology, Vanderbilt University, Nashville, Tenn. 37232

Sweet potatoes (Ipomoea batatas) *when infected with fungus or under certain other stress conditions produce several 3-substituted furans; some of these have now been isolated and identified. Of these the hepatotoxic sesquiterpene ipomeamarone is perhaps the best known and has been investigated for many years. As a result of outbreaks of pulmonary disease in cattle which consumed mold-damaged sweet potatoes, recent investigations have concentrated on the causative agents of this disease which has been described as atypical interstitial pneumonia. In addition to ipomeamarone and other hepatotoxins, a series of 1-(3-furyl)-1,4-dioxygenated pentanes has been isolated from sweet potatoes infected with* Fusarium solani. *These compounds, especially 1-(3-furyl)-4-hydroxy-1-pentanone (4-ipomeanol), show marked pulmonary toxicity in laboratory animals. It seems likely that these compounds are also the toxic factors in the bovine disease. The isolation, identification, synthesis, and toxicity of several of these furans are discussed.*

In response to stress conditions the sweet potato produces several metabolites which normally are absent or present in only minute amounts. These stress metabolites are formed under a variety of conditions including fungus infection, treatment with heavy metal salts and other compounds (*1*), and mechanical injury from slicing (*2*) or weevil infestation (*3*). The known stress metabolites fall into two general classes: hydroxycinnamic acid derivatives (including coumarins) and furanosesquiterpenes. Although several of the cinnamic acid derivatives seem important to the defense mechanism of the plant (*4*), the emphasis of this review focuses on the furan metabolites since some of these are apparently causative agents in the enzootics of livestock poisoning that result from ingestion of mold-damaged sweet potatoes (5, 6). The furans thus far identified fall into two categories: those containing a normal unrearranged sesquiterpene skeleton, and those containing less than fifteen carbon atoms but retaining the sesquiterpene skeleton. The latter compounds are probably the result of metabolic degradation of the sesquiterpenes.

Among the stress metabolites produced by the sweet potato impomeamarone (1) is perhaps the best known. The compound was first isolated by Hiura (7), and early structural studies were performed by

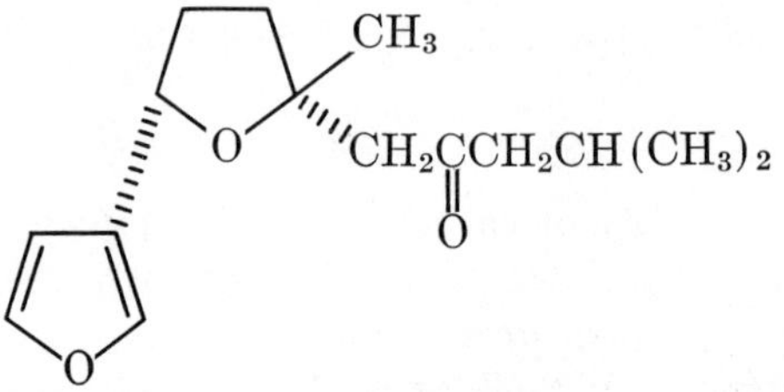

several Japanese groups (8, 9, 10). Final structure determination was accomplished by Kubota and co-workers (11).

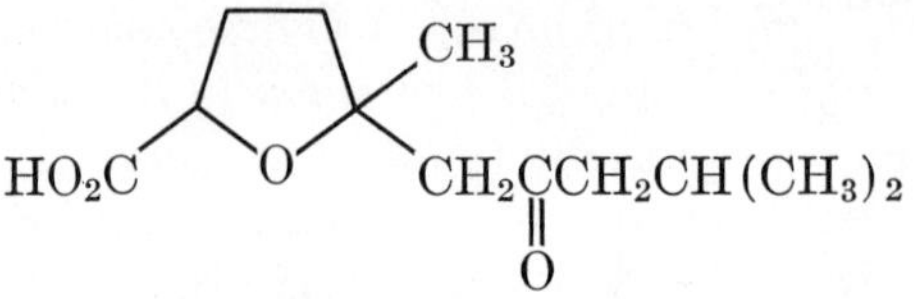

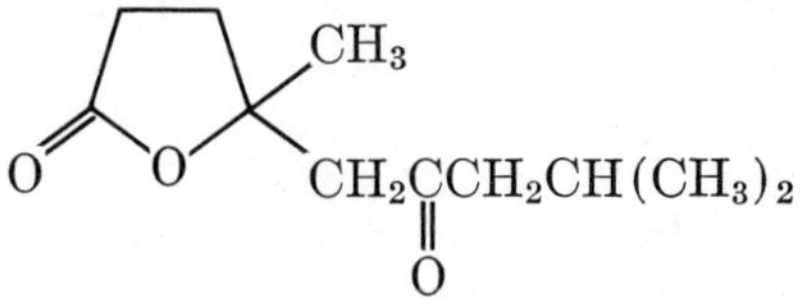

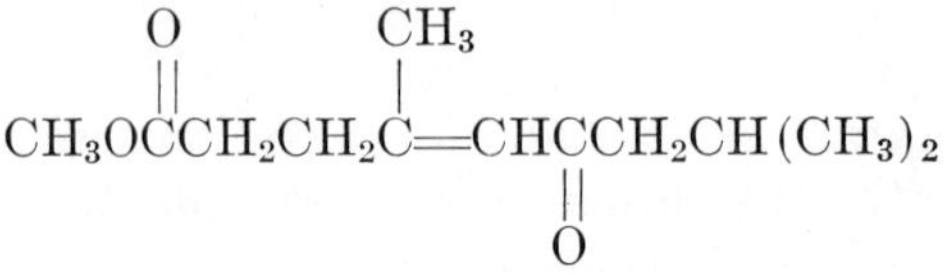

Structural determination was based primarily on identification of the products of oxidative degradation. Ozonolysis of 1 gave two products: ipomeanic acid (2) and ipomic lactone (3) (11). The latter was converted to methyl anhydroipomate (4) by saponification, dehydration, and reesterfication. The semicarbazone of 4 was ozonized; methyl levulinate and the bissemicarbazone of isobutylglyoxal were isolated. Barbier-Wieland decomposition allowed the conversion of **2** to **3**. Compound **3** was subsequently synthesized. Alder-Rickert degradation of **1** gave furan-3,4-

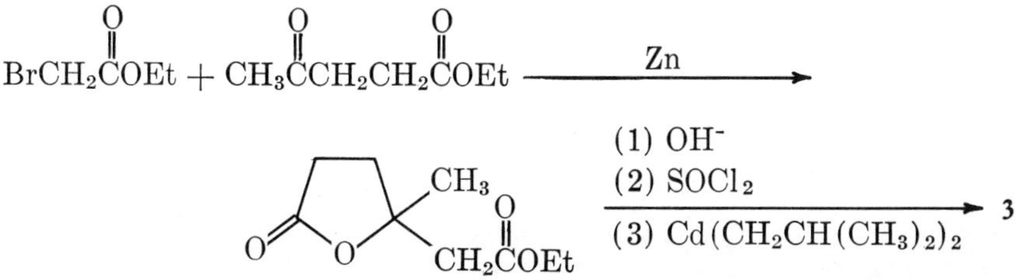

$$BrCH_2\overset{O}{\overset{\|}{C}}OEt + CH_3\overset{O}{\overset{\|}{C}}CH_2CH_2\overset{O}{\overset{\|}{C}}OEt \xrightarrow{\quad Zn \quad}$$

$$\xrightarrow[\qquad]{\begin{array}{l}(1)\ OH^-\\(2)\ SOCl_2\\(3)\ Cd(CH_2CH(CH_3)_2)_2\end{array}} \mathbf{3}$$

dicarboxylic acid indicating that the furan ring in Structure **1** must be β-substituted. This information, coupled with identification of the ozonolysis products established Structure **1** as ipomeamarone except for the stereochemistry about the tetrahydrofuran ring.

Contempory with Kubota's work, groups from Australia were investigating ngaione, a toxic principle of the Ngaio bush (*Myoporum laetum*) and related plants, which was first described by McDowall (*12, 13, 14*). The similarity between ngaione and ipomeamarone was noted (*15*), and after some initial confusion (*16*) they were established as enantiomorphs (*11, 17*). Thus the unusual situation exists in which a major phytoalexin of the sweet potato is the enantiomer of a normal constituent of several species of *Myoporum* and *Eremorphila*.

A synthesis of racemic ipomeamarone was described by Kubota (*11, 17*). The last step in this reaction sequence, treatment of the acid chloride **6** with diisobutyl cadmium, gave the tricyclic ketone **7** as the major product and a minor product (**8**) which was similar to **1** but dif-

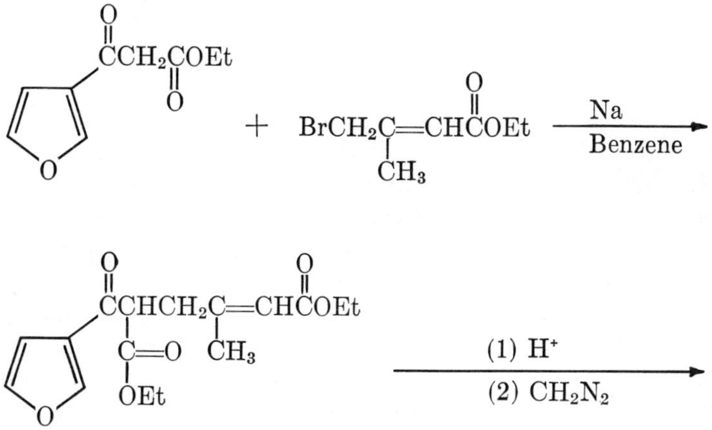

$$+ \quad BrCH_2\overset{CH_3}{\underset{|}{C}}=CH\overset{O}{\overset{\|}{C}}OEt \xrightarrow[\text{Benzene}]{Na}$$

$$\xrightarrow[\qquad]{\begin{array}{l}(1)\ H^+\\(2)\ CH_2N_2\end{array}}$$

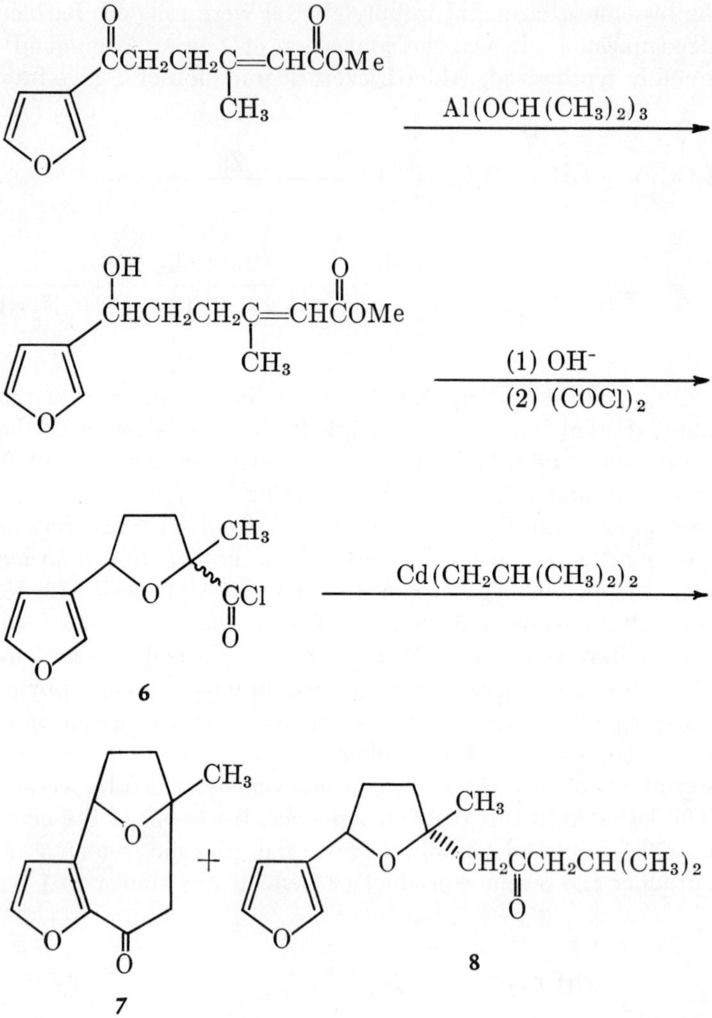

$\overset{O}{\overset{||}{C}}CH_2CH_2\overset{CH_3}{\overset{|}{C}}{=}CH\overset{O}{\overset{||}{C}}OMe$

$Al(OCH(CH_3)_2)_3 \longrightarrow$

$\overset{OH}{\overset{|}{C}}HCH_2CH_2\overset{CH_3}{\overset{|}{C}}{=}CH\overset{O}{\overset{||}{C}}OMe$

(1) OH^-
(2) $(COCl)_2$ $\longrightarrow$

CH_3
$\overset{|}{C}Cl$
$\overset{||}{O}$

6

$Cd(CH_2CH(CH_3)_2)_2 \longrightarrow$

CH_3

7

$+$

CH_3
$CH_2\overset{O}{\overset{||}{C}}CH_2CH(CH_3)_2$

8

ferent in spectral characteristics. It was argued that since most of the cis acid chloride cyclized to give **7**, **8** must have a trans configuration about the tetrahydrofuran ring. Ipomeamarone, it is postulated, must be the corresponding cis compound. Compound **8**, so-called epingaione, has been isolated from *Myoporum* sp (*18*).

To complete the synthesis of **1** Kubota relied on a reaction from the early work on ngaione, *i.e.*, treatment with potassium acetate in acetic anhydride to give the ring-opened acetate **9** (*12, 13, 14*). The hydrolysis of **9** had been reported to give racemic **1**, implying that cyclization occurred to give the cis configuration at the tetrahydrofuran ring (*16*).

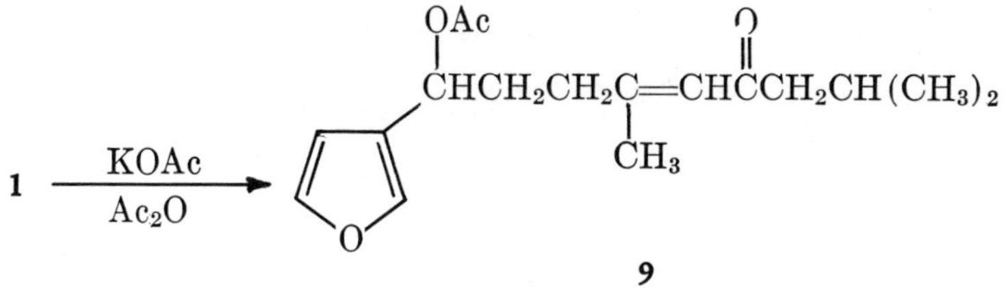

$$1 \xrightarrow[\text{Ac}_2\text{O}]{\text{KOAc}}$$

Structure **9**: furan ring with side chain
$$\overset{\text{OAc}}{\overset{|}{\text{CHCH}_2\text{CH}_2\text{C}}}=\text{CH}\overset{\text{O}}{\overset{\|}{\text{C}}}\text{CH}_2\text{CH(CH}_3)_2$$
with CH_3 substituent

9

Thus when synthetic **8** was treated with potassium acetate and acetic anhydride, then saponified, the cyclized material was identical to that obtained by treating natural **1** in the same way (*11, 17*).

As a result of the need for a source of **1** to further investigate the toxicity of ipomeamarone, Burka et al. described a second synthesis of **1** (*19*). It was found that **9** could be synthesized in good yield from 1-ipomeanyl acetate (**10**) (vide infra) and the phosphonate Wittig

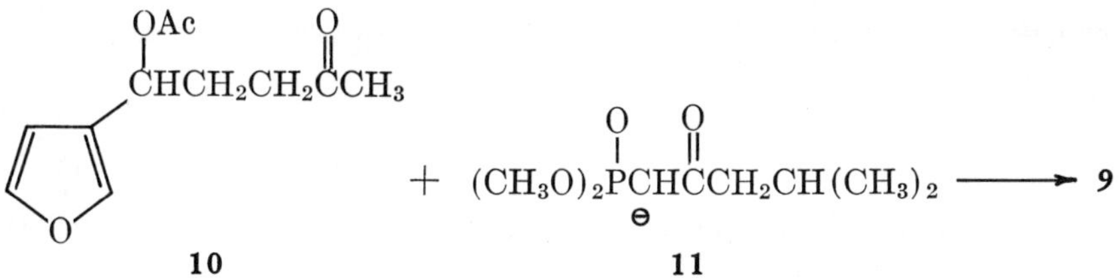

Structure **10**: furan ring with side chain
$$\overset{\text{OAc}}{\overset{|}{\text{CHCH}_2\text{CH}_2}}\overset{\text{O}}{\overset{\|}{\text{C}}}\text{CH}_3$$

10

$$+ \quad (\text{CH}_3\text{O})_2\overset{\text{O}}{\overset{|}{\underset{\ominus}{\text{P}}}}\text{CH}\overset{\text{O}}{\overset{\|}{\text{C}}}\text{CH}_2\text{CH(CH}_3)_2 \longrightarrow \textbf{9}$$

11

reagent **11**. Hydrolysis of **9** resulted in formation of 1:1 mixture of epimers **1** and **8** which could be separated by high pressure liquid chromatography. The saponification was further investigated by scanning repeatedly the NMR spectrum of a solution of **9** in methanolic sodium hydroxide. It was determined that **1** and **8** were formed at about the same rate and that their relative concentrations did not change with equilibration. Apparently the ring closure is not stereospecific.

Two sesquiterpenes, which are similar structurally to **1** have been isolated from mold-damaged sweet potatoes. The first of these, ipomeamaronol (**12**) was simultaneously isolated and identified by Yang et al. (*20*) and by Kato *et al.* (*21, 22*). The structure elucidation was determined mainly from spectral data. Oguni *et al.* recently reported the isolation of dehydroipomeamarone (**13**) from *C. fimbriata* infected sweet potatoes (*23, 24, 15*). Compound **13** had previously been isolated from *Anthenasia* sp by Bohlmann and Rao (*26*) and from *Myoporum* sp by Hamilton et al. (*18*). No synthesis of **12** or **13** has been reported.

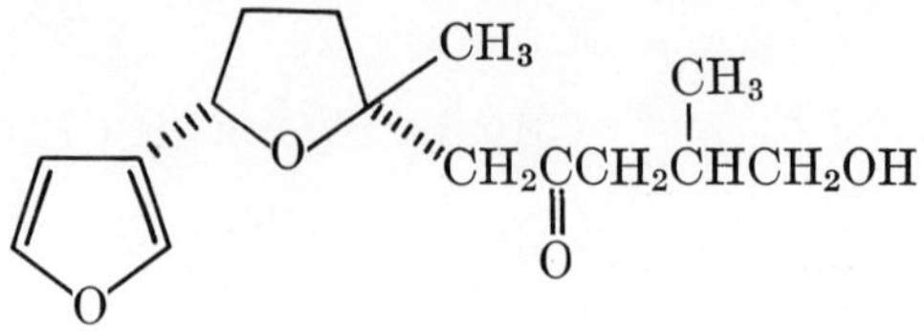

12

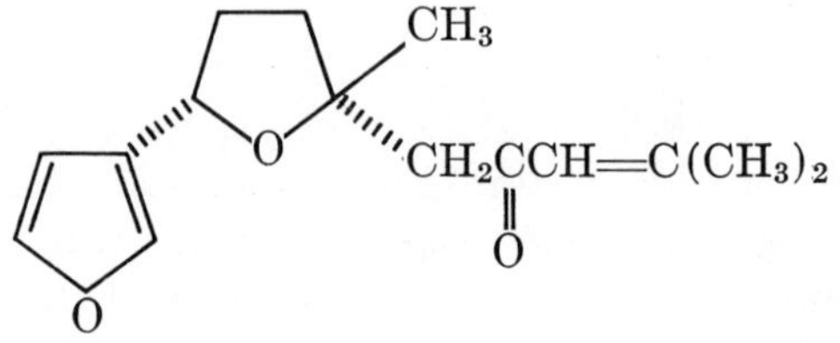

13

An additional sesquiterpene, 7-hydroxymyoporone (14), has been isolated which does not contain the tetrahydrofuran ring found in 1, 12, and 13 (27). Compound 14 was identified by spectral means and by oxidative degradation to the acid 15 which in turn was synthesized.

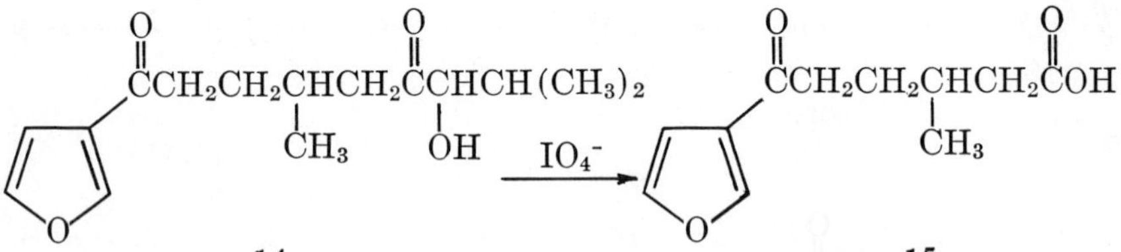

14

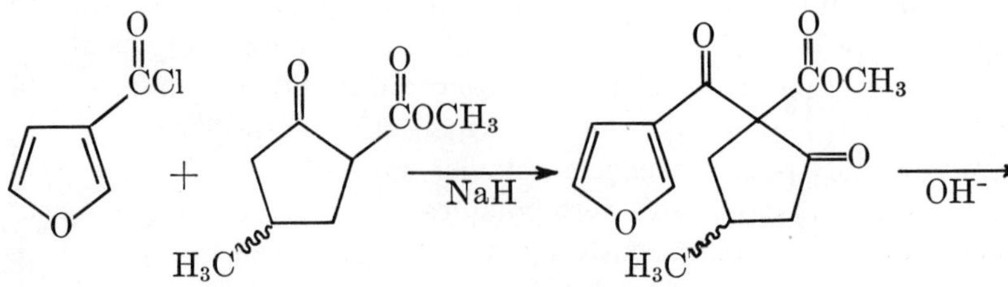

15

Ogawa and Hirose reported the presence of dendrolasin (16) and the ketone 17 in fusel oil resulting from fermentation of sweet potatoes (28), but Akazawa could not establish the presence of 16 and 17 in *C. fimbriata* infected sweet potatoes (29).

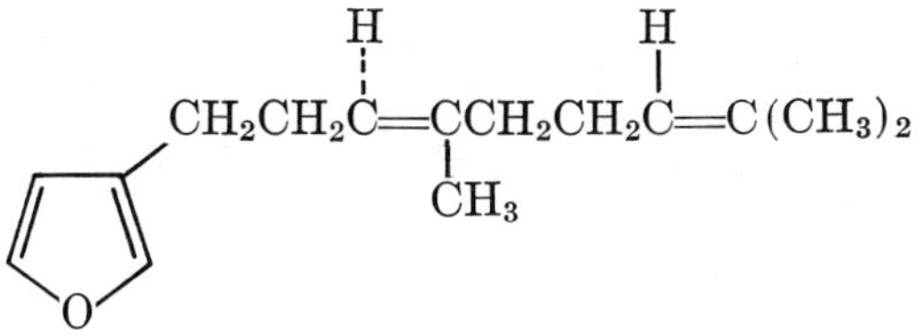

$$CH_2CH_2\overset{\overset{\displaystyle H}{|}}{C}\!\!=\!\!\underset{\underset{\displaystyle CH_3}{|}}{C}CH_2CH_2\overset{\overset{\displaystyle H}{|}}{C}\!\!=\!\!C(CH_3)_2$$

16

$$CH_2CH_2CH_2\underset{\underset{\displaystyle CH_3}{|}}{C}HCH_2\overset{\overset{\displaystyle O}{\|}}{C}CH_2CH(CH_3)_2$$

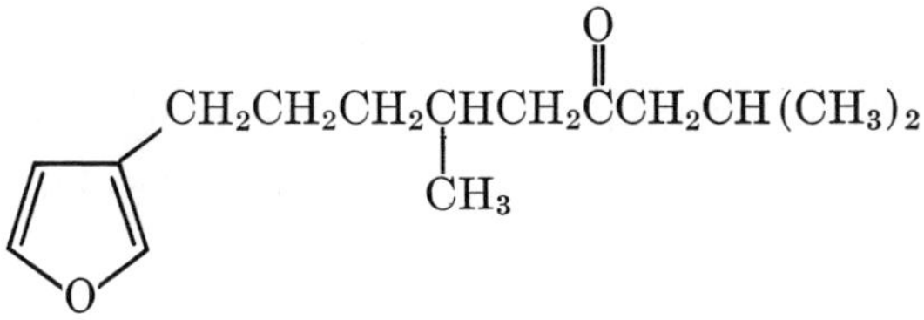

17

Seawright and Mattocks found that ngaione (the enantiomer of **1**), epingaione, and ipomeamarone (**1**) are all hepatotoxic; LD_{50} values for the compounds center about 200 mg/kg (*30*). Seawright and O'Donahoo made a detailed study of the pathology of ngaione toxicity in the mouse liver (*31*). Involvement of organs other than the liver was not mentioned. The toxicities of compounds **12, 13,** and **14** have not been studied in detail, but apparently the compounds are hepatotoxic and are about as potent as **1** (*18, 20, 27*).

Several compounds that have been isolated from mold-damaged sweet potatoes contain fewer than fifteen carbons and seem to be formed as a result of sesquiterpene catabolism. Two of these are 3-furoic acid (**18**) and batatic acid(**19**) (*11*). The structure of **19** was confirmed by

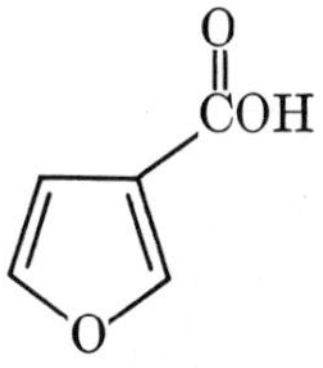

$$\overset{\overset{\displaystyle O}{\|}}{C}OH$$

18

$$\overset{\overset{\displaystyle O}{\|}}{C}CH_2CH_2\underset{\underset{\displaystyle CH_3}{|}}{C}H\overset{\overset{\displaystyle O}{\|}}{C}OH$$

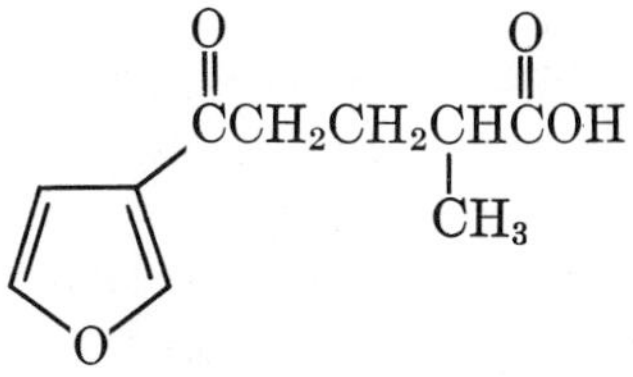

19

Kubota from isolating α-methylglutaric acid after ozonolysis and from synthesis of **19** (*11*).

Of greater interest is a series of compounds containing nine carbon atoms which have been researched by Wilson and co-workers for several years. When this research began, ipomeamarone was the only sweet potato phytoalexin whose toxicity had been studied. The primary target organ in cattle poisoned by mold-damaged sweet potatoes was the lung (*5, 6*). This observation suggested that the hepatotoxic ipomeamarone might not be the causative agent. Realization of this inconsistency prompted a search by Wilson for a so-called lung edema factor in sweet potatoes infected with *Fusarium solani*. As a result of this search a compound causing lung edema in mice was isolated by using a combination of column chromatography and gas chromatography. The structure of the compound, 4-ipomeanol (**20**), was established by spectral means (*32, 33*). Subsequently two similar lung edemagenic compounds, 1-ipomeanol (**21**)

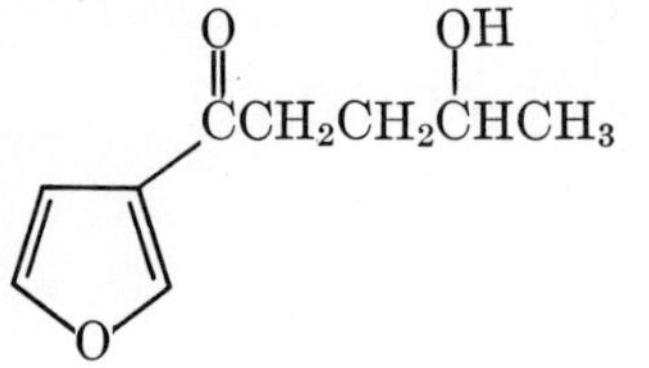

and 1,4-ipomeadiol (**22**), were isolated and identified in the same manner (*34*). A fourth compound in this series, ipomeanine (**23**), had been isolated from *C. fimbriata* infected sweet potatoes by Kubota, but its toxicity apparently had not been investigated (*11*).

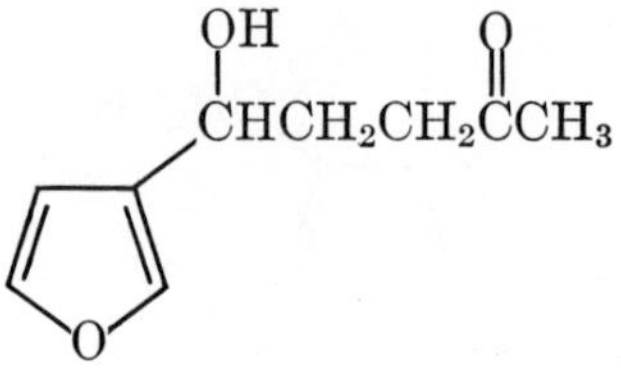

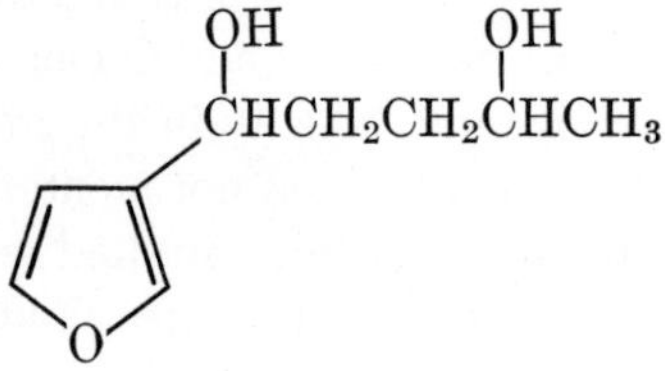

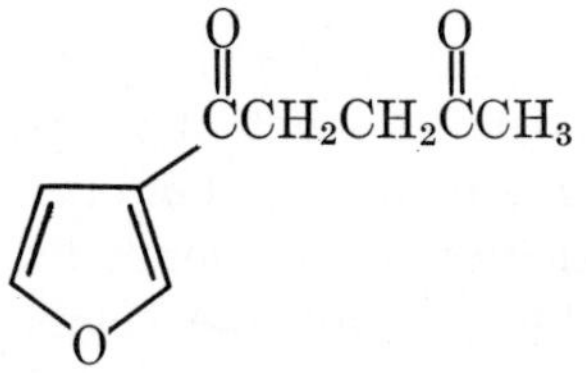

To establish unequivocally the structure of compounds **20–22** and to provide material for further testing, each was synthesized as shown below (*34*). Ipomeanine had previously been synthesized by Kubota, and that synthesis is included in the scheme. The syntheses are straightforward and provide a good source for these interesting compounds.

Compounds **20–23** all demonstrated an acute pulmonary toxicity in rodents which was indistinguishable from the acute response produced by administering crude extract from *F. solani* infected sweet potatoes. The LD_{50} of the synthetic edemagens ranges from: 25 mg/kg for **23** to 67 mg/kg for **22**—IP, male mice (*34*). It should be noted that these compounds are considerably more toxic than ipomeamarone.

The lung edemagens demonstrate a specific toxic action on the lungs. Mice which died within 24 hr of toxication did not show (by light microscopy) significant pathology in organs other than the lungs. In mice surviving the initial pulmonary attack renal necrosis was often observed several days after administration of **21** and **22** (*34*).

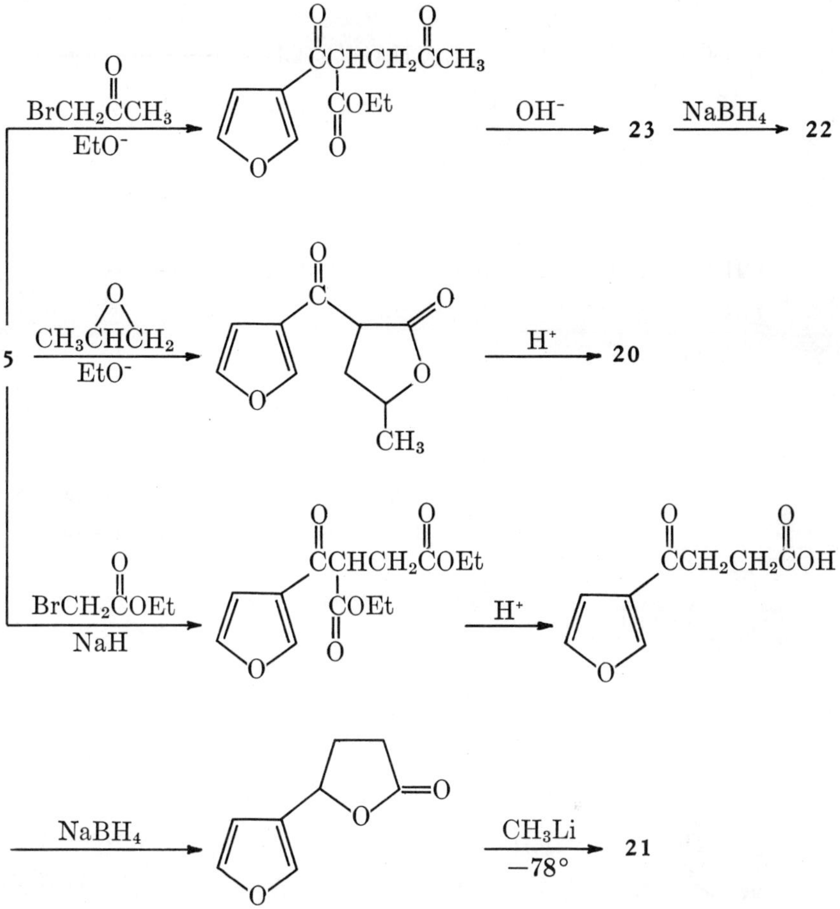

Boyd et al. investigated the distribution of radiolabelled **20** in the rat. Radioactivity is rapidly accumulated in the lungs, liver, and kidneys and remains in these organs long after most of the radioactivity has been eliminated from the rest of the body (*35*). It has been postulated that the pulmonary toxicity is associated with the covalent binding of **20** or a metabolite of **20** to macromolecules in the lungs (*36*).

The elaboration of furanoid metabolites in mold-damaged sweet potatoes has, not unexpectedly, inspired considerable interest in their biogenesis. Nearly all the information on the biosynthesis of furanoterpenoids in the sweet potato has been derived from Japanese work and relates primarily to ipomeamarone. These studies have been confined to sweet potato stimulation with the black-rot organism *C. fimbriata*. The nature of the stimulus which modifies sweet potato metabolism is not clear but appears to have a somewhat specific etiologic basis since only certain

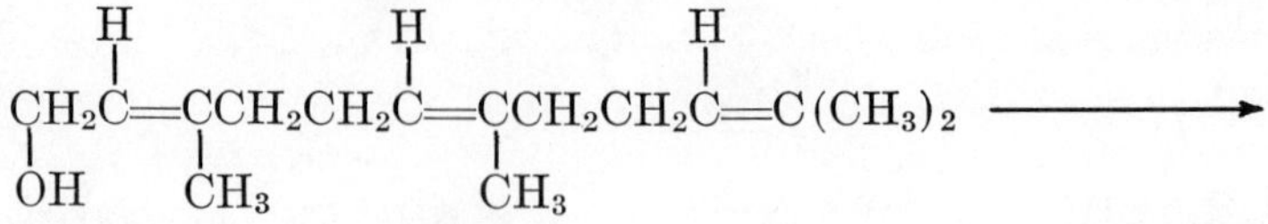

$$\underset{\underset{OH}{|}}{CH_2}\overset{\overset{H}{|}}{C}{=}\underset{\underset{CH_3}{|}}{C}CH_2CH_2\overset{\overset{H}{|}}{C}{=}\underset{\underset{CH_3}{|}}{C}CH_2CH_2\overset{\overset{H}{|}}{C}{=}C(CH_3)_2 \longrightarrow$$

24

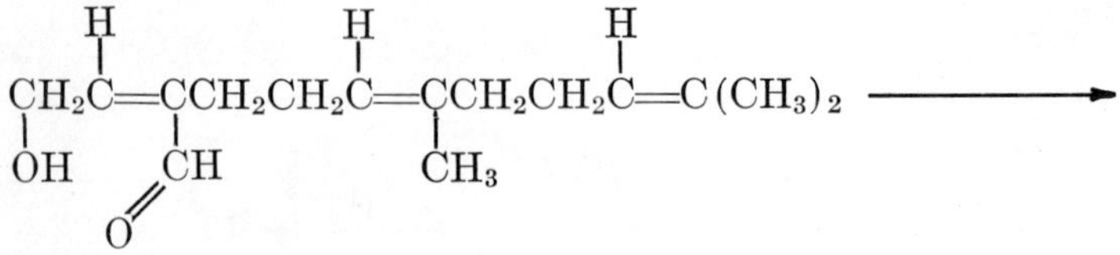

$$CH_2\overset{\overset{H}{|}}{C}{=}\underset{\underset{\overset{||}{O}}{CH}}{C}CH_2CH_2\overset{\overset{H}{|}}{C}{=}\underset{\underset{CH_3}{|}}{C}CH_2CH_2\overset{\overset{H}{|}}{C}{=}C(CH_3)_2 \longrightarrow$$
OH

25

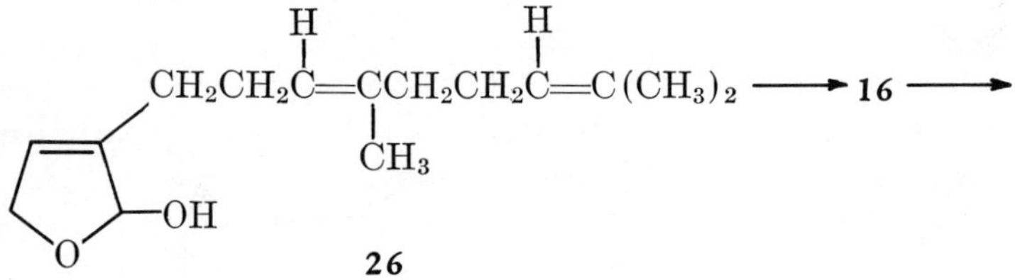

$$CH_2CH_2\overset{\overset{H}{|}}{C}{=}\underset{\underset{CH_3}{|}}{C}CH_2CH_2\overset{\overset{H}{|}}{C}{=}C(CH_3)_2 \longrightarrow 16 \longrightarrow$$
—OH

26

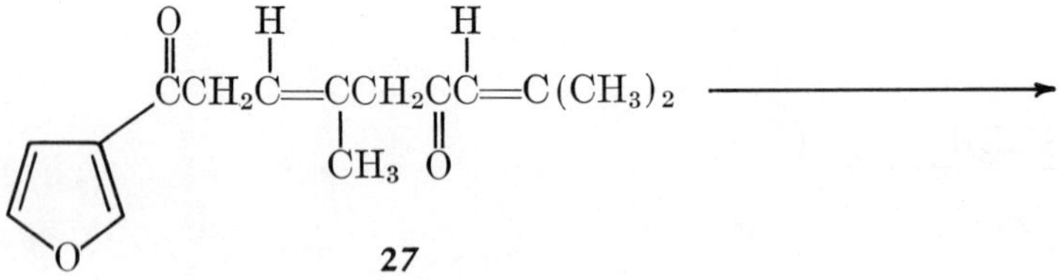

$$\overset{\overset{O}{||}}{C}CH_2\overset{\overset{H}{|}}{C}{=}\underset{\underset{CH_3}{|}}{C}CH_2C\overset{\overset{H}{|}}{C}{=}C(CH_3)_2 \longrightarrow$$

27

$$\overset{\overset{OH}{|}}{CH}CH_2CH_2\overset{}{C}{=}\underset{\underset{CH_3}{|}}{C}HC\overset{\overset{H}{|}}{C}{=}C(CH_3)_2 \longrightarrow 13 \longrightarrow 1$$

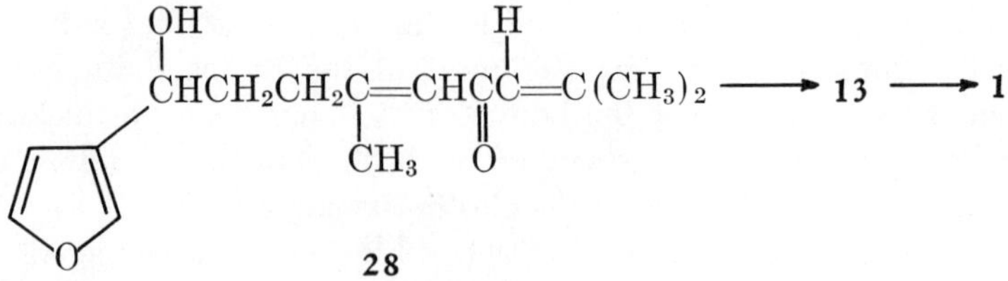

28

fungi are capable of inducing these toxic metabolites. In fact, some strains of *C. fimbriata* isolated from sources other than sweet potato stimulate furanosesquiterpene production minimally or not at all (*37, 38*).

The incorporation of acetate (*29, 38, 39, 40, 41*), mevalonate (*29, 40, 42*), pyruvate (*41*), citrate (*41*), ethanol (*43*), leucine (*44*), and farnesol (*45, 46*) into ipomeamarone has been demonstrated. Little experimental information is available concerning the steps in the biosynthetic pathway beyond farnesol. In their studies on furanosesquiterpenes from the Ngaio tree and related plants Sutherland and Park suggested that furanosesquiterpenes from those sources could result from oxidation of allylic carbons in farnesol followed by cyclization (47). By applying this idea to biosynthesis in the sweet potato a pathway can be postulated. Farnesol (24) could be oxidized to oxofarnesol (25) which could cyclize to hemiacetal 26 and undergo 1,4-dehydration to form dendrolasin (16). Further modifications of 16 could account for formation of the remaining furanosesquiterpenes—*e.g.*, allylic oxidation to give 27 followed by reduction of one of the keto groups and rearrangement of a double bond to give 28 which could cyclize Michael-fashion to give 13. The conversion of 13 to 1 by *C. fimbriata* infected sweet potatoes has been demonstrated by Oguni and Uritani (23, 25). Variations in this scheme would allow for formation of the other observed products. Since 16 has not been found in *C. fimbriata* infected sweet potatoes, it may be that oxidation at other sites precedes furan ring formation leading to 27 or some similar precursor without the intermediacy of 16.

The biosynthetic origin of the furans which comprise the lung edema factor is not yet clear. It is possible that the compounds are formed from metabolism of the C-15 compounds by the sweet potato, by the fungus, or both. For instance one can imagine hydrolysis of the tetrahydrofuran ring in ipomeamarone to form the β-hydroxyketone 29 which after a retroaldol reaction would give 1-ipomeanol. Further oxidation or reduction of 21 would lead to the other lung edemagens. We recently isolated a compound similar to 29, 4-hydroxymyporone (30), in which oxidation of the carbon adjacent to the furan ring has taken place (48). It seems likely that this compound is a key intermediate in the biosynthesis of the lung toxins.

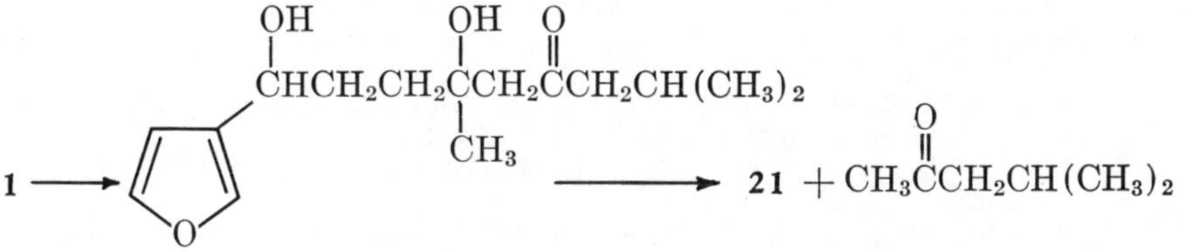

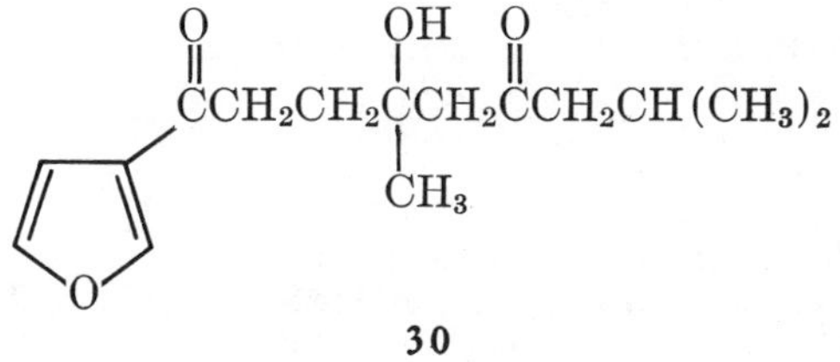

30

Extensive research remains to be done on the sweet potato stress metabolites. Livestock poisoning generally occurs after acute exposure to the toxins; the chronic effects of these compounds have not been investigated. Study of the effects of chronic exposure seems important especially with respect to human health. Reliable analytical techniques are available only for ipomeamarone. It is imperative that suitable analytical procedures for the lung edemagens be developed if the implication to health is to be elucidated.

The pharmacological aspects of the toxicity of the lung edemagens also provide an area for further research. There are few known lung toxins, especially those exhibiting the specificity for the lungs shown by 20 and 23. The reason for this specificity or the mode of action of the toxins has not yet been established.

The biosynthesis of the stress metabolites is also incompletely understood. Further investigation is needed not only to understand the intermediate steps from acetate to ipomeamarone and the lung toxins but also to determine the triggering mechanism for sesquiterpene metabolism in the sweet potato.

Acknowledgement

The authors wish to thank T. M. Harris and M. R. Boyd for helpful discussions.

Literature Cited

1. Uritani, I., Uritani, M., Yamada, H., *Phytopathology* (1960) **50**, 30.
2. Akazawa, T. Wada, K., *Plant Physiol.* (1961) **36**, 139.
3. Akazawa, T., Uritani, I., Kubota, H., *Arch. Biochem. Biophys.* (1960) **88**, 150.
4. Uritani, I., Akazawa, T., "Plant Pathology," Vol. I (J. G. Horsfall, A. E. Dimond, Eds.), 349 ff, Academic, New York, 1959.
5. Peckham, J. C., Mitchell, F. E., Jones, O. A., Doupnik, B. Jr., *J. Am. Vet. Med. Assoc.* (1972) **160**, 169.
6. Wilson, B. J., Yang, D. T. C., Boyd, M. R., *Nature* (1970) **227**, 521.
7. Hiura, M., *Rept. Gifu Agr. Coll.* (1943), **50**, 1.
8. Takeuchi, T., *Sci. Insect Control* (1946), **12**, 26; *Chem. Abstr.* (1949) **43**, 8453.
9. Ohno, T., Toyao, M., *Bull. Chem. Soc. Jap.* (1952) **25**, 414.
10. Watanabe, H., Nishiyama, S., *J. Agric. Chem. Soc.* (1952) **26**, 200; *Chem. Abstr.* (1953) **47**, 2361.
11. Kubota, T., *Tetrahedron* (1958) **4**, 68.
12. McDowall, F. H., *J. Chem. Soc.* (1925) **127**, 2200; McDowall, F. H., *ibid.* (1927) 731; McDowall, F. H., *ibid.* (1928) 1324.
13. Brandt, D. W., Ross, D. J., *J. Chem. Soc.* (1949) 2778.
14. Birch, A. J., Massy-Westropp, R., Wright, S. E., *Aust. J. Chem.* (1953) **6**, 385.
15. Ohno, T., *Bull. Chem. Soc. Jap.* (1952) **25**, 222.
16. Birch, A. J., Massy-Westropp, R., Wright, S. E., Kubota, T., Matsuura, T., Sutherland, M. D., *Chem. Ind.* (1954) 902.

17. Kubota, T., Matsuura, T., *J. Chem. Soc.* (1958) 3667.
18. Hamilton, W. D., Park, R. J., Perry, G. J., Sutherland, M. D., *Aust. J. Chem.* (1973) **26**, 375.
19. Burka, L. T., Harris, T. M., Wilson, B. J., *J. Org. Chem.* (1974) **39**, 2212.
20. Yang, D. T. C., Wilson, B. J., Harris, T. M., *Phytochemistry* (1970) **10**, 1653.
21. Kato, N., Imaseki, H., Nakashima, N., Uritani, I., *Tetrahedron Lett.* (1971) 843.
22. Kato, N., Imaseki, H., Nakashima, N., Uritani, I., *Plant Cell Physiol.* (1973) **14**, 597.
23. Oguni, I., Uritani, I., *Agric. Biol. Chem.* (1973) **37**, 2443.
24. Oguni, I., Uritani, I., *Phytochemistry* (1974) **13**, 521.
25. Oguni, I., Uritani, I., *Plant Physiol.* (1974) **53**, 649.
26. Bohlmann, F., Rao, N., *Tetrahedron Lett.* (1972) 1039.
27. Burka, L. T., Bowen, R. M., Harris, T. M., Wilson, B. J., *J. Org. Chem.* (1974) **39**, 3241.
28. Ogawa, S., Hirose, Y., *J. Chem. Soc. Jap.* (1962) **83**, 747; *Chem. Abstr.* (1963) **59**, 1565.
29. Akazawa, T., *Arch. Biochem. Biophys.* (1964) **105**, 512.
30. Seawright, A. A., Mattocks, A. R., *Experientia* (1973) **29**, 1197.
31. Seawright, A. A., O'Donahoo, R., *J. Pathol.* (1972) **106**, 251.
32. Boyd, M. R., Wilson, B. J., *J. Agric. Food Chem.* (1972) **20**, 428.
33. Wilson, B. J., Boyd, M. R., Harris, T. M., Yang, D. T. C., *Nature* (1971) **231**, 52.
34. Boyd, M. R., Burka, L. T., Harris, T. M., Wilson, B. J., *Biochim. Biophys. Acta* (1974) **337**, 184.
35. Boyd, M. R., Burka, L. T., Wilson, B. J., Sastry, B. V. R., "Abstracts of Papers," 13th Annual Meeting, Society of Toxicology, Washington, D.C., 1974.
36. Boyd, M. R., Burka, L. T., Neal, R. A., Wilson, B. J., Holsher, M. M., *Fed. Proc.* (1974) 33, Abstract No. 175.
37. Weber, D. J., Stahmann, M. A., *Science* (1964) **146**, 929.
38. Hyodo, H., Uritani, I., Akai, S., *Phytopathology* (1968) **58**, 1032.
39. Akazawa, T., Uritani, I., *Agric. Biol. Chem.* (1962) **26**, 131; *Biol. Abstr.* (1962) **39**, 7792.
40. Akazawa, T., Uritani, I., Akazawa Y., *Arch. Biochem. Biophys.* (1962) **99**, 52.
41. Oba, K., Shibuta, H., Uritani, I., *Plant Cell Physiol.* (1970) **11**, 507.
42. Oshima, K., Uritani, I., *Agric. Biol. Chem.* (1968) **32**, 1146.
43. Oguni, I., Uritani, I., *Agric. Biol. Chem.* (1971) **35**, 357.
44. Oshima-Oba, K., Sugiura, I., Uritani, I., *Agric. Biol. Chem.* (1969) **33**, 586.
45. Oguni, I., Uritani, I., *Agric. Biol. Chem.* (1970) **34**, 156.
46. Oguni, I., Uritani, I., *Plant Cell Physiol.* (1971) **12**, 507.
47. Sutherland, M. D., Park, R. J., "Terpenoids in Plants" (J. B. Pridham, Ed.), pp. 154–157, Academic, New York, 1967.
48. Burka, L. T., Kuhnert, L., Wilson, B. J., Harris, T. M., *Tetrahedron Lett.* (1974) 4017.

RECEIVED November 18, 1974. This work was supported by the USPHS through Training Grant 5 TO1 ES00112-07 and by the Center in Toxicology Grant ES00267.

INDEX

INDEX

The text of this book is set in 10 point Caledonia with two points of leading. The chapter numerals are set in 30 point Garamond; the chapter titles are set in 18 point Garamond Bold.

The book is printed offset on Text White Opaque, 50-pound. The cover is Joanna Book Binding blue linen.

Jacket design by Linda McKnight.
Editing and production by Joan Comstock.

The book was composed by the Service Composition Co., Baltimore, Md., printed and bound by The Maple Press Co., York, Pa.